ACSM's Worksite Health Handbook

Second Edition

A Guide to Building Healthy and Productive Companies

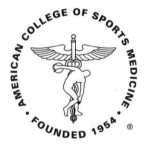

Nicolaas P. Pronk, PhD, FACSM

Editor

Vice President for Health Management, HealthPartners
Health Science Officer, Journeywell
Senior Research Investigator, HealthPartners Research Foundation
Minneapolis, MN

Endorsed by the International Association for
Worksite Health Promotion, an affiliate society of the
American College of Sports Medicine

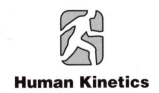

Human Kinetics

Library of Congress Cataloging-in-Publication Data

ACSM's worksite health handbook : a guide to building healthy and
productive companies / American College of Sports Medicine ; Nicolaas
P. Pronk, editor. -- 2nd ed.
     p. / cm.
  Rev. ed. of: ACSM's worksite health promotion manual / American
College of Sports Medicine ; [Carolyn Cox, editor]. c2003.
  Includes bibliographical references and index.
  ISBN-13: 978-0-7360-7434-6 (hard cover)
  ISBN-10: 0-7360-7434-1 (hard cover)
  1. Employee health promotion--Handbooks, manuals, etc. I. Pronk,
Nicolaas P. II. American College of Sports Medicine. III. ACSM's
worksite health promotion manual. IV. Title: Worksite health handbook.
  [DNLM: 1. Health Promotion--organization & administration. 2.
Occupational Health. 3. Workplace. WA 400 A187 2009]
  RC969.H43A825 2009
  658.3'82--dc22

2008045915

ISBN-10: 0-7360-7434-1 (print)   ISBN-10: 0-7360-8579-3 (Adobe PDF)
ISBN-13: 978-0-7360-7434-6 (print) ISBN-13: 978-0-7360-8579-3 (Adobe PDF)

This book is a revised edition of *ACSM's Worksite Health Promotion Manual,* published in 2003 by Human Kinetics, Inc.

The Web addresses cited in this text were current as of September 2008, unless otherwise noted.

Acquisitions Editor: Michael S. Bahrke, PhD; **Managing Editor:** Melissa J. Zavala; **Copyeditor:** Jocelyn Engman; **Proofreader:** Sarah Wiseman; **Indexer:** Nancy Ball; **Permission Manager:** Dalene Reeder; **Graphic Designer:** Joe Buck; **Graphic Artist:** Yvonne Griffith; **Cover Designer:** Keith Blomberg; **Photographer (cover):** © Human Kinetics; **Photo Asset Manager:** Laura Fitch; **Photo Production Manager:** Jason Allen; **Art Manager:** Kelly Hendren; **Associate Art Manager:** Alan L. Wilborn; **Illustrator:** Alan L. Wilborn; **Printer:** Thomson-Shore, Inc.

Printed in the United States of America   10 9 8 7 6 5 4 3 2 1

Human Kinetics
Web site: www.HumanKinetics.com

United States: Human Kinetics
P.O. Box 5076
Champaign, IL 61825-5076
800-747-4457
e-mail: humank@hkusa.com

Canada: Human Kinetics
475 Devonshire Road Unit 100
Windsor, ON N8Y 2L5
800-465-7301 (in Canada only)
e-mail: info@hkcanada.com

Europe: Human Kinetics
107 Bradford Road
Stanningley
Leeds LS28 6AT, United Kingdom
+44 (0) 113 255 5665
e-mail: hk@hkeurope.com

Australia: Human Kinetics
57A Price Avenue
Lower Mitcham, South Australia 5062
08 8372 0999
e-mail: info@hkaustralia.com

New Zealand: Human Kinetics
Division of Sports Distributors NZ Ltd.
P.O. Box 300 226 Albany
North Shore City
Auckland
0064 9 448 1207
e-mail: info@humankinetics.co.nz

Contents

Part I Setting the Context   1

Chapter 1 Population Health Management at the Worksite 2

Nicolaas P. Pronk, PhD, FACSM

Chapter 2 Employee Health Promotion: A Historical Perspective 10

R. William Whitmer, MBA

Chapter 3 Workplace-Based Health and Wellness Services 21

Raymond J. Fabius, MD, CPE, FACPE, and Sharon Glave Frazee, PhD

Chapter 4 State of the Worksite Health Promotion Industry: The 2004 National Worksite Health Promotion Survey 31

Laura A. Linnan, ScD, CHES

Chapter 5   Health Promotion Programming in Small, Medium, and Large Businesses **41**

Heather M. Bowen, MS, RD, LD; Todd D. Smith, MS, CSP, ARM; Mark G. Wilson, HSD; and David M. Dejoy, PhD

Chapter 6   Employee Health Promotion: A Legal Perspective **49**

Alison Cline Earles, Esq., and LuAnn Heinen, MPP

Chapter 7   Health Care Policy and Health Promotion **58**

John M. Clymer, AB; Garry M. Lindsay, MPH, CHES; Jennifer M. Childress, MS, CHES; and George J. Pfeiffer, MSE, FAWHP

Chapter 8   The Case for Change: From Segregated to Integrated Employee Health Management **66**

Ann L. Yaktine, PhD, and Mike D. Parkinson, MD, MPH, FACPM

Chapter 17 Organizational Assessment for Health

Thomas Golaszewski, EdD

Chapter 18 Assessment Tools for Employee Productivity 160

Nicolaas P. Pronk, PhD, FACSM

Chapter 19 Calculating the Economic Return of Health and Productivity Management Programs. 165

Seth Serxner, PhD, MPH, and Daniel B. Gold, PhD

Chapter 20 Using Claims Analysis to Support Intervention Planning, Design, and Measurement 175

David H. Chenoweth, PhD, and Jeff A. Hochberg, MS

Part IV Program Design and Implementation   182

Chapter 21 Organizing Intelligence to Achieve Increased Consumer Engagement, Behavior Change, and Health Improvement . . .183

Stephanie Pronk, MEd

Chapter 31 Programs Designed to Improve Employee Health Through Changes in the Built Environment 269

Mireille N.M. van Poppel, PhD, and Luuk H. Engbers, PhD, PT

Chapter 32 The Design, Implementation, and Evaluation of Medical Self-Care Programs 277

Don R. Powell, PhD, and Jeanette D. Karwan, RD

Chapter 33 Disease Management for Employed Populations 286

Dennis E. Richling, MD

Chapter 34 From the Basics to Comprehensive Programming 296

Mary M. Kruse, MS, ATC

Part V Case Studies   308

Chapter 38   Introducing Environmental Interventions at the Dow Chemical Company to Reduce Overweight and Obesity Among Workers 336

Ron Z. Goetzel, PhD; Jennie D. Bowen, MPH; Ronald J. Ozminkowski, PhD; Cheryl A. Kassed, PhD, MSPH; Enid Chung Roemer, PhD; Maryam J. Tabrizi, MS, CHES; Meghan E. Short, BA; Shaohung Wang, PhD; Xiaofei Pei, PhD; Heather M. Bowen, MS, RD, LD; David M. Dejoy, PhD; Mark G. Wilson, HSD; Kristin M. Baker, MPH; Karen J. Tully, BS; John M. White, PhD; Gary M. Billotti, MS; and Catherine M. Baase, MD

Foreword

This book could not be more timely. It summarizes evidence and provides solutions to three major concerns of employers: out of control health care cost increases; the impact of obesity and unhealthy lifestyles on workplace costs and productivity; and the need for a strong, healthy workforce to fuel our economic engine to maintain our standard of living and quality of life, which are seriously threatened.

Historically, employers have focused primarily on meeting customer needs, growing revenues, and controlling costs to be profitable if they are businesses or to have an operating margin if they are non-profits or even government agencies. U.S. employers are most worried, usually number 1 or 2 in annual surveys, about the high costs of medical claims and prescription drugs for employees, dependents, and retirees. Starting in the 1980s and continuing through 2003, employer-initiated efforts to control costs included an array of "managed care" tools, care systems, and other resources. Strategies included utilization management, pharmacy benefit managers, care management, Preferred Provider Organizations (PPOs), Health Maintenance Organizations (HMOs), Point of Services (POS) plans, higher cost sharing, and many other cost-control tactics. Where new methods were developed and implemented well, employers saw modest, relative gains that may be defined as controlling medical spending compared to the average nationwide or by region, albeit that there were almost always health care cost increases that were considerably higher than all other indicators of growth, even for the best managed plans. Employers learned that managing or eliminating health risks, moderating illness, and preventing injuries are the only sure ways to reduce costs.

Since the 1980s, the United States has also seen a substantial increase in the number of employees or associates and dependents who are seriously overweight or obese and suffer from related debilitating illnesses, such as diabetes. These employees also are less productive, sick more often, and stay out of work longer. In addition to excess weight, other health-related risk factors, such as smoking, physical inactivity, or alcohol misuse, also exert their toll on employee work performance, excess medical care resource use, and poor personal health. Consider that, as a nation, our future is literally in the hands of the people in the workforce now who are under 55 years of age. We already know that Gen-Xers, Millennials, adolescents, and children are overall considerably less healthy than their older counterparts when those groups were in a similar life stage. Hence, we now face challenges never faced before.

This book also is aimed at companies outside the United States, and while other countries have vastly different health systems, especially in terms of financing, they all have productivity challenges. Whether headquartered in the United States or not, more and more companies are truly global. Often their greatest challenge is productivity related—affected by both environmental and personal health hazards. Consider that the variability in worker safety protections remains large among countries and despite the abundance of evidence on the detrimental health impacts of tobacco use, workers in many countries are still allowed to smoke at the worksite.

Although knowing how very important it is for employers to use their leverage and resources to help improve the health and productivity of their workforces and their dependents, there has been a surprisingly modest amount of resources applied to research on what works and identification of best practices, especially considering the billions of dollars at stake. This is especially problematic as evidence of effectiveness and a positive return on investment are often essential for employers to persuade the C-Suite to invest in programs that can be relatively expensive and may require internal resources that managers may be loathe to redeploy away from revenue-producing operations. In corporations, there is always pressure to keep headcount to a minimum, especially overhead staff. In what is a sea change of perspectives and strategies, employers now understand that they have to tackle these problems head-on. They understand that all of the plan design and cost sharing tools will barely make a dent in controlling costs if the underlying population is ill or suffering from injuries because of their poor lifestyle-related health habits: smoking, no seat belt or helmet use, excessive weight gain, use of nutritionally barren foods, sedentary lifestyles, consumption of too much alcohol, and use of addictive drugs. The beauty of this book is that it has the right mix of research, evidence, and practical solutions—exactly what is needed yet has been missing heretofore.

Employers now fully understand in a way rarely grasped before that the good health and high productivity of their employees are competitive advantages and key assets. Whatever their otherwise more noble reasons for investing in employee or associate health, investing wisely and strategically in their employees' health is a business imperative, not just nice or the right thing to do.

It is certainly true that some employers may have higher turnover so the value of their investments may be more difficult to achieve as compared to other employers with longer tenured employees. Yet, even high turnover sectors usually have a significant portion of their workers or associates stay a long time so service-based benefits can help balance the costs with the pay-off to the company. In addition, there are particular health behaviors such as smoking, where the pay-off for quitting is immediate both for the individual and for their family members.

The combination of these three major forces—high and constantly increasing costs, more and more "demand" for services due to obesity, and the constant challenge of worker productivity—makes this book essential reading for all employers, medical directors, health plan administrators, occupational health practitioners, public health practitioners, and anyone working with employers and employees to improve the health of workers and their dependents. In addition, those educating future practitioners, students, and researchers will both enjoy and learn from this comprehensive book.

As this book illustrates so well, programmatic solutions can succeed when there are the following elements: a comprehensive strategy led by and supported at the highest level of the organization, consistent with the corporate culture; strong incentives; benefits aligned with the strategy; a mission-critical focus on improving and protecting the health and productivity of all workers; and programs that reach dependents. With *ACSM's Worksite Health Handbook, Second Edition*, edited by the authoritative and widely admired Nicolaas Pronk, PhD, every reader will have an excellent foundation for a practical, successful strategy to improve workforce health, just in time to affect our threatened future.

Helen Darling, President and CEO
National Business Group on Health
Washington, DC

Contributors

Edward W. Aberger, PhD
Clinical Assistant Professor, Community Health, Brown University Medical School, Providence, RI and Senior Vice President, Abacus Health Solutions, Cranston, RI

David K. Ahern, PhD
Senior Scientist, The Abacus Group, Cranston, RI and National Program Director, Health e-Technologies Initiative, Brigham Women's Hospital, Boston, MA

Calvin U. Allen, MBA, CHIE
Senior Vice President, Corporate Strategic Planning and Human Resources, HealthPartners, Bloomington, MN

Benjamin C. Amick III, PhD
Scientific Director, The Institute for Work and Health, Toronto, Ontario and Professor, Department of Health Promotion and Behavioral Science, The University of Texas School of Public Health, Health Science Center at Houston, Texas

David R. Anderson, PhD
Vice President, Program Strategy & Development, StayWell Health Management, St. Paul, MN

Catherine M. Baase, MD
Global Director, Health Services, The Dow Chemical Company, Midland, MI

Kristin M. Baker, MPH
Research Analyst, Health and Productivity Research, Department of Health Promotion & Behavior, College of Public Health, University of Georgia, Thomson Healthcare, Athens, GA

Gary M. Billotti, MS
Health and Human Performance Leader, The Dow Chemical Company, Midland, MI

Heather M. Bowen, MS, RD, LD
Project Coordinator, The Workplace Health Group, Department of Health Promotion and Behavior, University of Georgia, Athens, GA

Jennie D. Bowen, MPH
Research Analyst, Health and Productivity Research, Thomson Healthcare, Washington, DC

Lauren Buckel, BA
Research Associate, Abacus Management Techologies, LLC, Cranston, RI

Thomas J. Chapel, MA, MBA
Senior Health Scientist, Office of Workforce and Career Development, Centers for Disease Control and Prevention, Atlanta, GA

David H. Chenoweth, PhD
President, Chenoweth & Associates, Inc. & Professor, Department of Health Education and Promotion, East Carolina University, New Bern, NC

Yosuke Chikamoto, PhD
Director of Research, Health Fitness Corporation, Bloomington, MN

Jennifer M. Childress, MS, CHES
Senior Fellow and Program Officer, Partnership for Prevention, Washington, DC

John M. Clymer, AB
President, Partnership for Prevention, Washington, DC

Jessica Colling, BSC, MSC
Head of Health Promotion Program Development, vielife, Ltd., London, UK

K. Andrew Crighton MD, CPE
Vice President and Chief Medical Officer, Prudential Financial, Inc, Newark, NJ

Kathleen K. Cross, RN, CANP
Health Services Manager, BAE Systems, Minneapolis, MN

David M. DeJoy, PhD
Professor, Health Promotion and Behavior and Director, The Workplace Health Group, University of Georgia, Athens, GA

Alison Cline Earles, Esq.
Chief Executive Officer, ACE Ideas, LLC, Atlanta, GA

Luuk H. Engbers, PhD, PT
TNO Quality of Life, Leiden and Body@Work, Research Center Physical Activity, Work and Health, TNO-VUmc, VU University Medical Center, Leiden, The Netherlands

Raymond J. Fabius, MD, CPE, FACPE
President and Chief Medical Officer, CHD Meridian Healthcare, Chadds Ford, PA

Jonathan E. Fielding, MD, MPH, MBA
Director and Health Officer, Los Angeles Department of Health Services, University of

California–Los Angeles School of Public Health, University of California–Los Angeles School of Medicine, Los Angeles, California

Michael J. Follick, PhD
President and Chief Executive Officer, Abacus Health Solutions, Cranston, RI and Clinical Professor, Community Health, Brown University Medical School, Providence, RI

Edward M. Framer, PhD
Director, Health and Behavioral Sciences, Research, Development and Outcomes, Health Fitness Corporation, Plano, TX

Jason M. Gallagher, MBA
Director of Health Informatics, HealthPartners, Inc., Bloomington, MN

David Gimeno, PhD
Senior Research Fellow, International Institute for Society and Health, Department of Epidemiology and Public Health, University College–London, London, England, United Kingdom

Karen Glanz, PhD, MPH
Director, Emory Prevention Research Center, Behavioral Sciences & Health Education, Emory University, Rollins School of Public Health, Atlanta, GA

Sharon Glave Frazee, PhD
Vice President, Health Informatics, CHD Meridian Healthcare, Nashville, TN

Ron Z. Goetzel, PhD
Research Professor and Director, Institute for Health and Productivity Studies, Department of Health Policy and Management, Rollins School of Public Health, Emory University, and Vice President, Consulting and Applied Research, Health and Productivity Research, Thomson Healthcare, Washington, DC

Thomas Golaszewski, EdD
Professor, Department of Health Science, SUNY at Brockport, Brockport, NY

Daniel B. Gold, PhD
Principal, Mercer Health and Benefits, Minneapolis, MN

Matt Griffith, MPH
ORISE Research Fellow, The Community Guide, US Centers for Disease Control and Prevention, Atlanta, GA

Jessica Grossmeier, MPH
Director, Research, StayWell Health Management, St. Paul, MN

LuAnn Heinen, MPP
Director, Institute on the Costs and Health Effects of Obesity, National Business Group on Health, Washington, DC

Jeff A. Hochberg, MS
President, The Outcomes Group, Inc., Palm Harbor, FL and Fellow, Association for Worksite Health Promotion

David P. Hopkins, MD, MPH
Epidemiologist, Guide to Community Preventive Services, Division of Health Communication and Marketing, Centers for Disease Control and Prevention, Atlanta, Georgia

Jeanette D. Karwan, RD
Director, Product Development, American Institute for Preventive Medicine, Farmington Hills, MI

Cheryl A. Kassed, PhD, MSPH
Health and Productivity Research, Thomson Healthcare, Washington, DC

Nicole R. Keith, PhD
Assistant Professor, Department of Exercise Science, Indiana University–Purdue University, Indianapolis, IN

Mary M. Kruse, MS, ATC
Director, HealthSource, Park Nicollet, Minneapolis, MN

Jason E. Lang, MPH, MS
Team Lead, Workplace Health Programs, National Center for Chronic Disease Prevention and Health Promotion, Centers for Disease Control and Prevention, Atlanta, GA

Kimberly D. Leeks, PhD, MPH
Research Public Health Analyst, Health, Social Science and Economic Research, Research Triangle Institute International, Atlanta, GA

Joseph A. Leutzinger, PhD
Principal, Health Improvement Solutions, Omaha, NE

Garry M. Lindsay, MPH, CHES
Managing Senior Fellow and Senior Program Officer, Partnership for Prevention, Washington, DC

Laura A. Linnan, ScD, CHES
Associate Professor, Department of Health Behavior and Health Education, University of North Carolina Chapel Hill School of Public Health, Chapel Hill, NC

Timothy J. McDonald, PA, MSHA
Director, Health Management Consulting, Employer Solutions, Ingenix, Eden Prairie, MN

Peter Mills, MD
Chief Medical Officer, vielife, Ltd., and Physician, Department of Respiratory Medicine, Whittington Hospital, London, UK

Shirley Musich, PhD
Senior Researcher, Employer Solutions, Ingenix, Eden Prairie, MN

Daniel Newton, PhD
Director of Total Health Management, Resolution Health, Inc., Columbia, MD

Steven P. Noeldner, PhD
Principal, Health and Productivity Management, Mercer Health and Benefits, Newport Beach, CA

Ronald J. Ozminkowski, PhD
Consulting Economist, Ann Arbor, MI

LaVaughn Palma-Davis, MA
Senior Director, University Health & Well Being Initiatives, University of Michigan, Ann Arbor, MI

Michael D. Parkinson, MD, MPH, FACPM
President, American College of Preventive Medicine, Washington, DC

Xiaofei Pei, PhD
Economist, Health and Productivity Research, Thomson Healthcare, Washington, DC

George J. Pfeiffer, MSE, FAWHP
President/Founder, The WorkCare Group, Inc., Charlottesville, VA

Don R. Powell, PhD
President and CEO, American Institute for Preventive Medicine, Farmington Hills, MI

Nicolaas P. Pronk, PhD, FACSM
Vice President, Health Management; Health Science Officer, JourneyWell; Senior Research Investigator, HealthPartners Research Foundation

Stephanie Pronk, MEd
Vice President, Employer and Health Management Consulting, Ingenix, Inc., Minneapolis, MN

Lisa Quintiliani, PhD
Research Fellow, Center for Community Based Research, Dana-Farber Cancer Institute and Research Fellow, Society, Human Development and Health, Harvard University, Boston, MA

Dennis E. Richling, MD
Vice President, Clinical Strategy, Matria Healthcare, Inc., Rosemont, IL

Delia B. Roberts, PhD, FACSM
Instructor, School of University Arts and Sciences, Selkirk College, Castlegar, BC

Enid Chung Roemer, PhD
Senior Research Associate, Institute for Health and Productivity Studies, Department of Health Policy and Management, Rollins School of Public Health, Emory University, Washington, DC

Margaret Sabin, MHSA
CEO, Sutter Health Partners and Vice President, New Product Development, Sutter Health Partners, Sacramento, CA

Howard Schubiner, MD
Mind-Body Center of Providence, Southfield, MI and Clinical Professor, Internal Medicine, Wayne State University, Detroit, MI

Seth Serxner, PhD, MPH
Principal, Health and Productivity Management, Mercer Human Resource Consulting, Los Angeles, CA

Meghan E. Short, BA
Research Analyst, Health and Productivity Research, Thomson Healthcare, Washington, DC

Todd D. Smith, MS, CSP, ARM
Doctoral student, The Workplace Health Group, Department of Health Promotion and Behavior, University of Georgia, Athens, GA

Neal S. Sofian, MSPH
Director of Behavioral Interventions, Resolution Health, Inc. Seattle, WA

Robin E. Soler, PhD
Coordinating Scientist, The Guide to Community Preventive Services, Centers for Disease Control and Prevention, Atlanta, GA

Glorian Sorensen, PhD, MPH
Director, Center for Community-Based Research, Dana-Farber Cancer Institute and Professor, Society, Human Development and Health, Harvard School of Public Health, Boston, MA

Maryam J. Tabrizi, MS, CHES
Senior Research Analyst, Health and Productivity Research, Thomson Healthcare, Washington, DC

N. Marcus Thygeson, MD
Vice President & Medical Director, Consumer Health Solutions, HealthPartners, Inc., Bloomington, MN

A. Janet Tomiyama, MA
Graduate student, Department of Psychology, UCLA College of Letters and Sciences, Los Angeles, CA

Karen J. Tully, BS
Global Health Promotion Leader, The Dow Chemical Company, Midland, MI

Mireille N. M. van Poppel, PhD
Associate Professor, Department of Public and Occupational Health, VU University Medical Center, EMGO-Institute, Amsterdam and Body@Work, Research Center Physical Activity, Work and Health, TNO-VUmc, VU University Medical Center, Leiden, The Netherlands

Jeffrey J. VanWormer, MS
Director, Heart of New Ulm Project, Minneapolis Heart Institute Foundation, Minneapolis, MN

Shaohung Wang, PhD
Senior Statistician, Health and Productivity Research, Thomson Healthcare, Cambridge, MA

John M. White, PhD
Texas Region Health Services Leader, The Dow Chemical Company, Freeport, TX

R. William Whitmer, MBA
President and CEO, Health Enhancement Research Organization (HERO), Birmingham, AL

Mark G. Wilson, HSD
Associate Professor, The Workplace Health Group, Department of Health Promotion and Behavior, University of Georgia, Athens, GA

Ann L. Yaktine, PhD
Senior Program Officer, Institute of Medicine, The National Academies, Washington, DC

Antronette K. (Toni) Yancey, MD, MPH
Professor, Department of Health Services, Center to Eliminate Health Disparities, and Division of Cancer Prevention and Control Research, UCLA School of Public Health, Los Angeles, CA

Preface

In recent years, recognition of the influence of worker health status on excess health care expenditures and health-related productivity losses has become increasingly apparent. An ever-increasing body of knowledge supports the contention that healthy workers have less need for medical care, use those resources less frequently, and have higher occupational performance (i.e., productivity) than their less healthy counterparts. Whereas the research community expeditiously publishes reports on these issues, new developments in the worksite health field and industry as a whole outpace the research and find the practitioner in need of support to address strategic, tactical, and operational challenges. Therefore, the quality and effectiveness of our health promotion efforts in the worksite setting are at least partially dependent on our understanding of research-based evidence that tells us what works. However, the research knowledge should be complemented with practice-based learnings of quality program design, efficient implementation processes, and optimal context so that our solutions and applications are at once affordable, scalable, and sustainable.

The need for a book that connects worksite health research and practice has become evident. *ACSM's Worksite Health Handbook, Second Edition,* is a completely revised and updated text following the first edition published in 2003. It is a comprehensive and contemporary resource on worksite health, which is broadly defined as an integrated set of initiatives designed to promote and protect the health of those associated with the worksite setting—individually as well as collectively. This resource also provides appropriate context in which worksite health initiatives reside, such as the historical development of the field, the legal and regulatory aspects, the changing nature of the organization of work, the role of health insurance benefits, the workplace culture, and the importance of health policy. This book makes available to practitioners, administrators, academicians, and students the raw materials needed to design and implement successful programs. It represents a collaborative effort of more than 80 of the finest scientists, practitioners, and thought leaders in the field who hail from Canada, Europe, and the United States.

ACSM's Worksite Health Handbook, Second Edition, has 38 chapters organized into five parts. Part I provides a synthesis of important contextual issues, including the worksite-based intervention opportunities for population health, the history of the field, the current state of the industry, the legal perspectives, the role of health policy, and the need for change in order to improve health in the worksite setting. Part II shifts the focus to the role of evidence of effectiveness in employer-sponsored health programs. This section includes an overview of the role of evidence in making decisions about resource allocations, the processes to generate evidence-informed intervention solutions, the systematic reviews and best practices of what works in the worksite setting, the effect of the organization of work on health, and the relationship between health and productivity. Part III emphasizes assessment, measurement, and evaluation. Chapters in this section present information related to an integrated evaluation model; an in-depth look at health and productivity assessment tools for individuals, populations, and companies; an estimation of economic returns of health improvement programs; and a discussion of the appropriate use of claims-based analysis and planning. Part IV contains an in-depth discussion of the various aspects of program design and implementation. From considering the basics of behavior change theory to new and innovative approaches of using data to engage employees in programs, various aspects of technology use, social networks, and programmatic design features that connect health to business aspects, this section outlines the key features of best-practice programs. This section also addresses diversity, health literacy, the built environment, medical self-care, disease management, healthy workplace culture, incentives, communications, and the effectiveness of integration. It concludes by pulling all these issues together into a chapter that walks the practitioner through the process of implementing a program in order to present all the pieces as a cohesive whole. Finally, Part V is dedicated to four in-depth case studies that serve as examples of successful applications. The first case study presents an innovative method to apply principles of sport science to occupational performance of tree planters in the Pacific Northwest.

The second case study illustrates the potential of an employer–health plan partnership focused on improving health and managing cost trends in a midsize employer. The next case study reports on the efforts of a large multinational company from the United Kingdom to affect health and productivity outcomes using a pilot study method. Finally, the last case study describes the process followed by a large multinational company to introduce environmental interventions aimed at addressing excess weight among employees using a formal research approach.

This book was not designed to be an exhaustive academic reference text, and undoubtedly the reader will notice that the chapters are relatively concise and appropriately, not extensively referenced. This reflects the objective to focus on access to important concepts that are supported by both research and practice-based learnings with an eye toward serving the practitioners' needs. Each chapter concludes with a brief set of chapter review questions to assist the reader in identifying key concepts and issues. The format of the book allows for cover-to-cover reading or for use as a reference or resource text. The use of the information and ideas proposed across all chapters is intended to support the introduction and continued use of effective interventions that generate improvements in worker health and business performance.

Acknowledgments

The publication of a book of this kind reflects the collaborative efforts of many. It started out with the interest to create a second edition of the *ACSM's Worksite Health Promotion Manual* as expressed by the members of the Publications Committee of the American College of Sports Medicine (ASCM). The rapid and dramatic evolution of the field of worksite health promotion over the past 5 to 10 years warranted for the second edition to be an entirely updated version—and this work was supported by many who deserve credit for their efforts.

First and foremost, I am deeply grateful to the chapter contributors of this book, without whom there would be no final product. Without exception, they all dedicated selflessly their time, energy, and expertise to this project. They all submitted high-quality manuscripts and were positive on editorial changes when those applied. As a result, they made the editing work for the final manuscript an enjoyable process. In addition, we had a remarkable review team that conducted a rigorous review of the material and ensured feedback for the final manuscript. The resulting text was strengthened because of it. The review team consisted of Greg Heath, PhD (Review Team Editor); Shawna Mercer, PhD; Leigh Ramsey, PhD; Yvonne Ingram-Rankin; and Reed Engel (Review Team Coordinator).

Paul Couzelis, PhD, Reed Engel, Lauve Metcalf, and Heather Turner have been stellar colleagues in managing the ACSM Interest Group on Worksite Health Promotion and laying the foundations for the International Association for Worksite Health Promotion (IAWHP), the ACSM affiliate society endorsing this book. They deserve a lot of credit for their support and guidance throughout the process of planning this new edition.

A deeply felt thank you goes out to Jeanette Tschida, who served as project manager on this effort. Jeanette's expertise, process management skills, and amazing attention to detail made the entire process of coordinating administrative tasks, deadlines, and timelines with more than 80 contributors and reviewers a seemingly simple one. The staff at Human Kinetics was always there to support the successful completion of this endeavor—special thanks to Mike Bahrke, Maureen Eckstein, and Melissa Zavala.

Although great care went into the assurance of quality and prevention of any errors and inconsistencies, I take full responsibility for any errors or omissions that may remain in the book. I truly appreciate the efforts of all.

Part

I

Setting the Context

When implementing health promotion programs at the worksite, the environment in which such programs are implemented has much to do with how well they are received, how much health they generate, and how well they support business performance. This context may be considered an important factor in program effectiveness. Part I is all about the context in which worksite health is implemented.

There are eight chapters in Part I. The first chapter introduces the overall framework for the book. Chapter 2 presents the history of the still relatively young but emerging worksite health promotion field with emphasis on the last three decades. Chapter 3 describes the integration of a broad array of health services in workplace-based clinics. Chapter 4 presents the results of the major national health promotion surveys and as a result, paints a picture of the current state of the industry. Chapter 5 discussed the importance and context of the size of a business. Chapter 6 presents legal issues that every employer, vendor, and health plan that provides worksite health promotion services need to consider. Chapter 7 introduces the role and importance that health policy plays in health promotion initiatives. Finally, Chapter 8 gives a succinct review of the major reasons why a new approach to generating health is needed. All chapters in Part I are intended to introduce important considerations that will aid you in placing other chapters of the book in the proper context.

Population Health Management at the Worksite

Nicolaas P. Pronk, PhD, FACSM

There is a relatively new term in search of an accepted definition (14). *Population health* is the aggregate level of health among the individuals who make up the group. Whereas population health refers to a state, population health management refers to a process. It infers an active, dynamic, and integrated process designed to improve the health outcomes for both the individual and the group. Applied to a population associated with a place of employment, population health management is intended to improve health outcomes of employees—one at a time—in order to lower company expenses in the areas of health care, productivity, worker replacement, disability management, and absenteeism, among others. In this book, the population of primary interest is the group of active employees, although secondary populations may include spouses, dependents, early retirees, and others associated with the company. The importance of improving the health of each individual cannot be overstated, but it is recognized that all individuals aggregate into the larger group and thus become the population of interest. For the purpose of this book, population health management is defined as *the strategic and operational processes used to generate the health outcomes of a defined group of individuals collectively associated with a company's health improvement efforts.*

It is the purpose of this chapter to provide a brief historical context related to population health at the workplace, to discuss the population health management concept, to outline a population health model that may be applied to the workplace and that will serve as a guide for the remainder of this book, and to introduce best-practice employee health management elements and concepts that may prove important for continued improvement in the field.

A Look at the Past

The role of health has long been recognized as an important feature in securing a safe and prosperous existence. Healthy, strong, and well-trained warriors were vital to protecting the interests of the community and the country as long ago as we can remember. Certainly these ideas are substantiated by early writings from ancient Greece, where military training was connected to functioning in society, being a productive citizen, and the general importance of education. Athenians considered moral training an important part of overall education, and through physical education youngsters developed self-discipline, courage, humility, determination, and good sporting behavior. In addition, in pursuit of their ideal to unite the "man of action" with the "man of wisdom," Athenians participated in arduous exercises to become all-around citizens with physical, mental, and spiritual well-being and vigor (5). Aristotle (384-322 BC), a Greek philosopher and student of Plato, departed from his teacher's support for a Spartan-type system of military training and recommended healthy diets and plenty of exercise that would not be so severe as to hinder growth among children and strength and health among all. In his *Aristotelis De Moribus ad Nicomachum,* Aristotle states (1) ". . . that it is the nature of such things to be destroyed by defect and excess, as we see in the case of strength and health (for to gain light on things imperceptible we must use the evidence of sensible things); both excessive and defective exercise destroys the strength, and similarly drink or food which is above or below a certain amount destroys the health, while that which is proportionate both produces and increases and preserves it."

This view of exercise and nutrition in appropriate balance seems particularly salient in today's society, where overweight is the norm and physically active lifestyles are the exception.

The Roman poet Juvenal, who lived in the late first and early second century, ascribed to the same principles put forth by Aristotle; his now centuries-old dictum to pray for a sound mind in a sound body *(mens sana in corpore sano)* rings more true today than ever before. Experimental studies continue to support the role of physical activity in the delay of neurocognitive decline (18).

Fast-forward to more modern times—in 1700, Bernardino Ramazzini, widely considered the father of industrial medicine, published his first book on occupational diseases, *De Morbis Artificum Diatriba (The Diseases of Workmen)*. This publication became the foundation for the development of the occupational medicine discipline and may well represent the first recognition of the worksite as an important setting for population health interventions. Not long thereafter, in 1761, the Italian Austrian physician Giovanni Antonio Scopoli published his book *De Hydroargyro Idriensi Tentamina* (11) on the symptoms of mercury poisoning among miners. Dr. Scopoli may well be the first known company medical director.

Leap to post–World War II times, when one of the earliest recorded mentions of the term *health promotion* arrives on the scene. In 1946, Henry E. Sigerist, the renowned medical historian and social visionary, defined the four tasks of medicine as (1) the promotion of health, (2) the prevention of illness, (3) the restoration of the sick, and (4) rehabilitation (25). Sigerist had also noted that medical care should be a system of health institutions and medical personnel available to all, responsible for the people's health, and ready and able to advise and help the people in the maintenance of health and in its restoration when prevention has broken down (24). In this sense, he well may have been speaking of population health management as we think of it today, since he also included health education, proper working and living conditions, appropriate means for rest and recreation, and research and training as components of such a program.

A significant marker was reached in the development of occupational health and health and safety at the worksite when U.S. President Richard M. Nixon signed the Occupational Safety and Health Act on December 29, 1970. As a result of this act, both the National Institute for Occupational Safety and Health (NIOSH) and the Occupational Safety and Health Administration (OSHA) were created. NIOSH was established to help assure safe and healthful working conditions by providing research, information, education, and training in the field of occupational safety and health. As part of its services, NIOSH provides national and world leadership to prevent work-related illness, injury, disability, and death by gathering information, conducting scientific research, and translating the knowledge gained into products and services.

The field of health promotion has been greatly influenced by international initiatives such as the Ottawa Charter for Health Promotion, which was developed and adopted at an international health promotion conference sponsored by the World Health Organization (WHO), Health Canada (formerly known as Health and Welfare Canada), and the Canadian Public Health Association and held October 17 through October 20, 1986, in Ottawa, Ontario, Canada. The creation of supportive environments, including work environments, is called out and placed into the broader context of society.

In addition, the establishment of the European Network for Workplace Health Promotion (ENWHP) in 1996 recognized the increasingly important role worksites play in protecting and promoting the health and safety of the population. ENWHP was established in response to the European Union's interest in health promotion and has successfully brought together an international collaborative that produces standardized criteria for quality programs, reports on best-practice models, and disseminates learnings through national and international forums.

The American Association of Fitness Directors in Business and Industry (AAFDBI; later named the Association for Fitness in Business, or AFB, and eventually the Association for Worksite Health Promotion, or AWHP) was an organization founded in 1974 to advance worksite health promotion around the world. AWHP was particularly active in supporting the needs of practitioners and led the way in many aspects of the development and evolution of the industry. In early 2000, AWHP closed its doors. Despite less visibility, continuation of service to the field was provided by the Interest Group on Worksite Health Promotion under the American College of Sports Medicine (ACSM). In late 2008, The ACSM

Interest Group on Worksite Health Promotion morphed into the International Association for Worksite Health Promotion (IAWHP), an ACSM affiliate society. IAWHP's mission is to advance the global community of worksite health promotion practitioners through high-quality information, services, educational activities, personal and professional development, and networking opportunities.

Chapter 2 in this book is dedicated to a more detailed overview of the evolution of worksite health promotion and employee health management over the course of the past three decades. It is often true that the emergence of an innovation occurs when the circumstances allow it to do so. This fast-paced journey through time has provided a partial overview of the circumstances that, as a whole, shaped and molded the context through which a focused effort on health promotion at the worksite has emerged.

Managing the Health of Defined Populations

Managing the health of populations is not a new endeavor. In some form or another, the roots of this interest go back a long way in time. Yet today, perhaps more so than at any other time in history, the interest in population health is of global significance. The world is shrinking due to advancements in almost any field imaginable. Innovative, and sometimes disruptive, technologies of all sorts affect the nature of work, and humans are struggling to keep up (20). This struggle, in turn, has a profound effect on the life of individuals—at work, at home, in the community—and this effect aggregates across populations. In many instances, these phenomena negatively influence the health status of various populations, including but not limited to those associated with the worksite—workers, early retirees, dependents. Lack of physical activity, weight-related concerns, depression and mental health issues, diabetes and chronic conditions, just to name a few health concerns, are increasingly associated with employer- and employee-related struggles around health care costs and productivity. Examples of companies that struggle with these issues include General Motors, a company that announced its health care spending exceeded its steel bill (13), and Starbucks, a corporation announcing its health care costs have now surpassed its spending on coffee (10). Although these companies have publicly expressed their situations, many others

share their pain even though they may not make the headlines. Fortunately, population health management may well be one of the most important strategies to not only manage the ever-increasing trend of health care but also ensure that health care remains not only a viable but also an *affordable* option for employers. For the United States, at least, generating health, not treatment, is central to the issue of health care affordability.

While it is true that health care spending is a major culprit to U.S. employers, productivity concerns may drive the need for change in other parts of the world where the employer is not responsible for employee health care coverage. Regardless of whether it is driven by health care costs, productivity, absence management, attracting and retaining quality employees, improving employee morale, improving workplace safety, or some other goal, the need for better health among individual workers and worker populations has become a clear objective.

Across the population, a relatively small group of people is responsible for the majority of the health care expenses. Typically, this distribution follows the Pareto principle—20% of the people incur 80% of the costs. This distribution is depicted in figure 1.1 and, in the absence of thoughtful multiyear analyses, tends to lead to the conclusion that there is a dire need to intervene with those who incur high costs (22). However, once the same population is being considered across multiple years, it becomes clear that more than 50% of the high-cost cases in year two were actually low-cost cases in year one (8). Such analyses make a convincing case that in order to address health care costs for the population of covered lives, a total population health management strategy is needed, not merely a focus on high-cost subpopulations—this proposition is supported by several scientific findings (14,15). Keeping healthy workers healthy allows for a population health management strategy to positively affect medical care cost trends and reduce health-related productivity losses. In short, healthy workers are central to a healthy company.

The Population Health Management Framework

A population health management approach recognizes that health improvement needs to occur at the individual level, aggregates up to the population level, and is supported at the environmental level. The use of an integrative

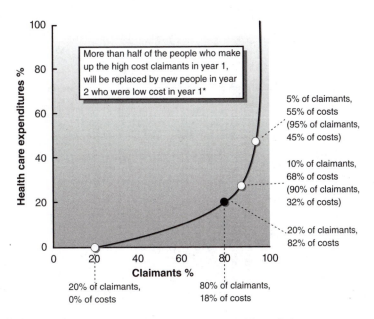

Figure 1.1 — chart content:

More than half of the people who make up the high cost claimants in year 1, will be replaced by new people in year 2 who were low cost in year 1*

5% of claimants, 55% of costs (95% of claimants, 45% of costs)

10% of claimants, 68% of costs (90% of claimants, 32% of costs)

20% of claimants, 82% of costs

20% of claimants, 0% of costs

80% of claimants, 18% of costs

Health care expenditures %

Claimants %

Figure 1.1 The typical distribution of U.S. health care spending in a commercial population.

and robust framework may provide grounding for the individual components of a total population health management approach. Such a framework is depicted in figure 1.2. The overall goal is to achieve optimal health and productivity levels for the defined population. The population of interest needs to be defined clearly upfront and may, for example, be all company employees, all employees and dependents, all benefits eligibles, and so on. The framework walks through components such as assessments, approaches to stratification or segmentation, and strategies that support improvement of population health. The various components are supported by examples of action steps on the right-hand side of the figure. These examples are programs, services, and functions that need to be integrated at the level of the worksite through effective data and communication strategies. It is recognized that this goal may only be achieved over time; the arrows inside the population segmentation step represent this time dimension by indicating subpopulation movement from higher risk to lower risk and prevention of movement into higher risk for those at a given risk level in the framework.

As part of the framework, definitions of levels of disease prevention are indicated. Specifically, four levels of prevention are outlined, namely, primordial, primary, secondary, and tertiary prevention. Disease prevention not only includes activities intended to prevent disease in the first place but also includes those intended to detect disease early or to mitigate its progress or reduce its consequences once established. A brief description of the four levels of disease prevention is outlined in table 1.1.

What Works?

Effective means of improving population health should follow strategies and tactics that have a high likelihood of being worth the investment. That means that if there is evidence available that shows a particular health improvement intervention causes health to improve for a population and, ideally, lowers overall costs for that population as well, we should prioritize such a solution high on the list of programs that are worthy of investment. Such an approach may be referred to as *evidence-based health* and should be supported by literature in the form of systematic reviews, cost-benefit or cost-effectiveness studies, or business case studies with appropriate context to infer an acceptable degree of causality. Chapters 7, 9, 10, 30, and 32 and the case studies presented in chapters 35 through 38 all support this contention.

While the research support continues to improve, there is a general lack of well-designed studies in the area of employee health management that allow for strong recommendations to be generated that may guide the investment decisions of employers. However, it should be

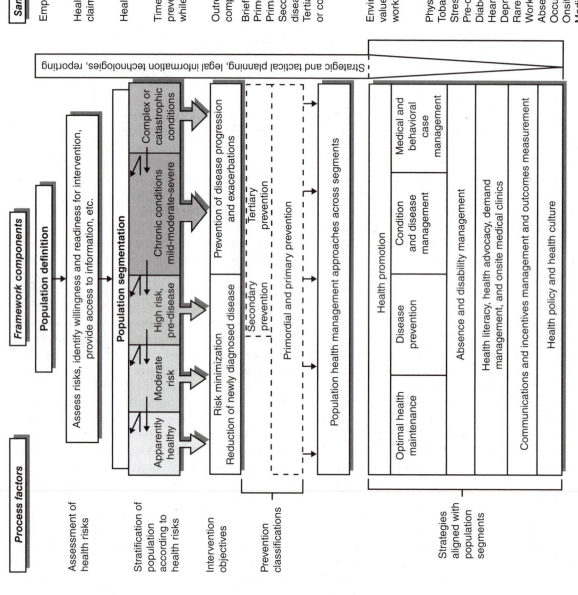

Figure 1.2 The population health management framework.

Process factors

Assessment of health risks

Stratification of population according to health risks

Intervention objectives

Prevention classifications

Strategies aligned with population segments

Framework components

Population definition

Assess risks, identify willingness and readiness for intervention, provide access to information, etc.

Population segmentation

Apparently healthy | Moderate risk | High risk, pre-disease | Chronic conditions mild-moderate-severe | Complex or catastrophic conditions

Risk minimization
Reduction of newly diagnosed disease

Prevention of disease progression and exacerbations

Secondary prevention

Tertiary prevention

Primordial and primary prevention

Population health management approaches across segments

Health promotion

Optimal health maintenance | Disease prevention | Condition and disease management | Medical and behavioral case management

Absence and disability management

Health literacy, health advocacy, demand management, and onsite medical clinics

Communications and incentives management and outcomes measurement

Health policy and health culture

Sample characteristics, factors, or definitions

Employees, dependents, early retirees

Health assessment, biometric screenings, claims analysis, readiness to change

Health data analytics, predictive modeling

Time dimension; over time, the objective is to prevent progression to the right of the framework while shifting the population to the left

Outreach, engagement, participation, completion, behavior change

Brief definitions of prevention classifications:
Primordial: Prevention of risk factors in the population
Primary: Prevention of new disease (incidence)
Secondary: Prevention of increases in disease prevalence
Tertiary: Prevention of disease progress or complications

Environmental and cultural initiatives, organizational values, benefits design, organization of work, workplace safety, workplace health policies

Physical activity
Tobacco cessation
Stress management
Pre-diabetes risk reduction
Diabetes management
Heart disease management
Depression management and EAP
Rare and chronic condition management
Worker's compensation and return-to-work
Absence management
Occupational health and safety
Onsite clinic
Medical self-care
Health advocacy
Health policy

Table 1.1 Prevention Classifications and Definitions

Level of disease prevention	Brief description
Primordial	Primordial prevention addresses the underlying conditions that may lead individuals or populations to become exposed to causative factors for disease—it is intended to prevent the occurrence of risk factors in the population. The goal is to address social and environmental conditions that create health-damaging exposures and susceptibilities among the population. Primordial prevention strategies may apply to subgroups (of particular interest due to exposure to specific conditions) or to the total population.
Primary	Primary prevention intends to limit the incidence of disease by controlling causes and risk factors. It may apply to the total population with the aim of reducing average (overall) population risk, to particular subgroups of interest, or to individuals at high risk for a particular condition.
Secondary	Secondary prevention is intended to cure patients and reduce the more serious consequences of disease through early diagnosis and treatment. It is directed at the point in time between onset of disease and diagnosis and aims to reduce the prevalence of disease. The target populations for secondary prevention are population subgroups at elevated risk and established patients.
Tertiary	Tertiary prevention is intended to reduce, mitigate, or limit the progress or exacerbations of diagnosed disease and is an important aspect of therapeutic and rehabilitative medicine. Its target population is established patients.

recognized that often the research considered for inclusion in such reviews is limited to standards relatively inappropriate for the worksite setting; in other words, randomized controlled trials are the gold standard for generating recommendations. In the worksite setting, mainly due to business-specific rationale, it is often difficult, if not impossible, to randomize the population to treatment and control conditions. More acceptable designs may be the quasi-experimental designs and in-depth case studies, the gold standard for business practice, as exemplified by Jim Collins' analysis of a small number of business case studies in his book *Good to Great* (4). Evidence of effectiveness may be generated based on a different evidence scale than is typically used in medical or behavioral research.

Chapter 12 presents an overview of benchmarking and best practices and introduces methods that help identify characteristics of programs that are considered successful. Using this approach, we can identify what kinds of program components are essential elements to be considered in a total population health management program at the worksite. Regardless of how many elements may be identified, key principles to be addressed in such a list include organizational culture and leadership, program design, program implementation and resources, and program evaluation.

By studying several benchmarking and best-practice projects that have been conducted over the past several years, it is possible to generate a list of characteristics strongly associated with best practices (3,6,7,17,23). Whereas it is difficult to ascribe relative importance to this list, some characteristics appear more frequently on the list of key ingredients than others do—which does not necessarily mean they are more important (it could be that they were easier to implement than other, more critical ones). As a result, the list outlined in table 1.2 is an aggregate view of characteristics that have been identified in companies that have documented program outcomes consistent with best practices. Applying them to any given company should be based on the unique situation and specific goals. Other characteristics that may be considered critical for success were identified as part of an in-depth effort by the Institute of Medicine's Committee to Assess Worksite Preventive Health Program Needs for NASA to delineate recommendations for future worksite-based health promotion and protection programs (12). In addition to listing valuable characteristics, table 1.2 also indicates which chapter in this book addresses the characteristics.

These best-practice characteristics also allow programs to be comprehensive in scope and not merely focus on particular risk factors (e.g., high blood pressure or tobacco use). In addition, they allow programs to happen without time limits and thus avoid short-term effects without long-term success. Participation can be increased to include the large majority of employees and even dependents as opposed to only the salaried personnel or those already interested (and in better general health). Finally, these characteristics open the door to effective integration of health promotion and disease prevention programs into

Table 1.2 Employee Health Management Best-Practice Characteristics

	Characteristic	Chapter numbers
Leadership and strategy	Organizational commitment (including management support)	4, 8, 12, 23, 34
	Shared program ownership (leadership inclusive of all staff levels)	26, 34
	Identified wellness champion	12, 34
	Program connected to business objectives	12, 24, 26
	Supportive policy, physical, and cultural environment	7, 26, 31
Operations	Clearly defined plan of operations	34
	Effective communications	28, 29, 34
	Scalable, sustainable, and accessible programs	3, 5, 11, 29, 34
	Scalable and effective assessment, screening, and triage	10, 16
	Effective interventions	9-12, 19, 22, 30, 31
	Meaningful participation incentives	6-8, 28
Evaluation	Program measurement and evaluation	10, 12, 14-20
Integration and data practices	Integration of program components at the point of implementation	6, 8, 21, 30
	Integration across multiple organizational functions and departments	
	Integrated data systems	
	Efficient and effective data practices	
	Relentless focus on safeguarding personal health information privacy and confidentiality	

traditional health protection programs under the mission of occupational health and safety (19,21). In fact, NIOSH has also generated a list of essential elements of effective workplace programs and policies for improving worker health and well-being. This list is organized around organizational culture and leadership, program design, program implementation and resources, and program evaluation and provides a comprehensive view of what it takes to address these essential elements of successful programs (see www.cdc.gov/niosh/worklife for more information).

A Glimpse of the Future

The population health management field is rapidly changing. Globally, it is an emerging field with the multinational companies leading the way (2). Health assessment is the most frequently implemented program component, with technology-driven tools such as Web portals, online programs, and personal health records being the fastest growing program components. Corporate culture is increasingly recognized as an important determinant of successful population health management. As a result, the intersection of individual behavior, corporate culture, environmental support, and enabling technologies appears to be a sweet spot for attention, as it brings together key elements for successful solutions.

As employer-sponsored health management programs continue to grow, programmatic solutions will become increasingly sophisticated. It is likely there will be growing demand for comprehensive programs patterned after the list of characteristics outlined in the previous section (and in table 1.2) to be implemented at the worksite. In the current literature, programs that drive a positive return on investment (ROI) tend to be multilevel, multicomponent, and comprehensive programs. These programs are also the ones seeking integration into occupational health and safety in an effort to enhance their effect on health maintenance, injury prevention, and productivity (12).

The need for increased confidence that programs will succeed and justify their investment for the company will be substantiated through a measurement process that will drive the need for accreditation. Objective measurement will warrant standardization in the industry, and the need for independent audits and certification of providers will be provided by trusted accreditation organizations. As a result, the field will improve its service quality, its general performance, and its overall outcomes.

Finally, innovations in the use of technologies and tailored messaging will start to address the issues of engagement and participation in programs. Chapter 21 presents a discussion on what is possible today, although major advancements in this area are anticipated in the short-term future. Since the objective is to improve health, it stands to reason that the voluntary nature of participation remains central to program design. Participation incentives need to be cleverly designed so as to ensure that ultimately the choice to participate remains with the individual—after all, it is not possible to force people into health.

Conclusion

This chapter has provided some background on historical events that collectively led up to the formation of employer-sponsored programs designed to improve the health and productivity of defined populations, introduced key principles and program elements that are associated with the most successful programs today, and introduced some thoughts on where the industry is heading over the course of the coming decades. Details necessary to provide deeper insight into any of these issues are provided in the various chapters of this book. Those details may be grounded by

the framework outlined in figure 3.1, which was created as context for this book and is presented to support and guide an internal or group dialogue of any given element, intervention, or principle presented anywhere in this book. Where does a particular issue or topic fit? How does it relate to other key principles or design elements? Where does measurement come into play? Any of such questions may be considered or addressed in the context of this framework. The work generates health and productivity as proximal outcomes, and cost effects represent distal outcomes since monetary investment returns cannot be generated without health improvement or reductions in health-related productivity losses. This is an observation consistent with various views on population health (16) and consistent with the time needed for interventions to bring about their intended effects.

Chapter Review Questions

1. Define population health and population health management.

2. Explain the Pareto principle application.

3. Does the Pareto principle to health care costs apply each successive year when considering the population of a given company?

4. Who introduced the dictum *mens sana in corpore sano* and what does it mean?

5. Name and discuss at least 10 best-practice characteristics of successful programs.

2

Employee Health Promotion
A Historical Perspective

R. William Whitmer, MBA

In trying to identify the person who invented wellness and was the first advocate for the concept, one could go back to Galen, who was second only to Hippocrates as the founder of modern medicine. Sometime around 185 AD, Galen wrote, "Both in importance and in time, health precedes disease. Therefore, *we ought to consider first how health may be preserved,* and then how one may best cure disease" (38; italics added). Within more current times, the person most often given the credit as being the founder of wellness is Halbert L. Dunn, MD, PhD, who was responsible for establishing a national vital statistics system for the United States. The Halbert L. Dunn Award is one of the most prestigious annual awards presented in the field of biostatistics. In the late 1950s, at a church in Washington, DC, Dunn facilitated a regular series of lectures on the values of a healthy lifestyle. In 1961, he published a book entitled *High Level Wellness* (16). The book was never a big seller, but it did find its way into the hands of the early wellness pioneers who expanded on some of his concepts to move wellness to its first level of national awareness. What was Dunn up against? As late as 1960, magazine and radio commercials proclaimed, "More doctors smoke Camels than any other cigarette" (15, p. 24).

It is generally agreed that attempts to provide and monitor the delivery of programs and services to help employees learn about and become proactive in taking better care of their health started about 30 years ago. I have been involved in this effort from the beginning. In 1976, I founded and became CEO of Wellness South, a full-service worksite wellness provider and consultant firm; I maintained this position until 1996. From 1996 until the present, I have served as the president and CEO of the Health Enhancement Research Organization (HERO). Over those 30 y, I have had the pleasure of knowing and, in many cases, working closely with many of the corporate and provider employee health management thought leaders. In the preparation of this brief historical chronicle, a number of these colleagues were contacted and invited to provide information, experiences, and opinions about their involvement and perception of employee health promotion. Their input is greatly appreciated. In this process, there is no doubt that events and accomplishments thought to be significant by some are not recognized or discussed. This limitation is driven by the space available and is in no way intended to overlook important historical events or contributions.

The following analysis of the history of efforts to improve the health of employees via work-based initiatives is divided into three segments and identified by terminology that was popular during those times. The segments are Worksite Wellness—1975 to 1985, Employee Health Promotion—1986 to 1995, and Employee Health Management—1996 to the Present.

Worksite Wellness— 1975 to 1985

The early days of worksite wellness required a large helping of passion and deep determination to become involved. There was little published research, little behavioral change know-how, and minimal interest in employee health. Health care cost was not a significant factor. According to A. Foster Higgins, a health care consulting firm, in 1980 the total health care cost was $246 billion U.S., which was 9.1% of the gross national product.

Health care cost for a family of four averaged $920.00 U.S. per year (11). It was not uncommon for employers to state that an employee's health was a personal thing and should not be of interest to the company. The only health risk appraisal (HRA) was a crude two-page questionnaire available through the Centers for Disease Control and Prevention (CDC). Then, in 1976, the U.S. Congress created the Office of Disease Prevention and Health Promotion (ODPHP). Efforts began to create and operate a national worksite wellness professional association. Although not plentiful, worksite wellness research was starting to be conducted and published. Those who first molded worksite wellness into a viable business were often solo operators who had the perseverance to fight through the obstacles. To a certain extent, the first decade of worksite wellness can be accurately described as the time of trial and error.

Two of the very early pioneers of the wellness movement were John (Jack) Travis, MD, MPH, and Don Ardell, PhD. Both of these trendsetters are still going strong and continue to be prolific innovators. In 1972, Travis obtained the copyright for the illness–wellness continuum, which is a sliding scale between two endpoints: premature death on one end and high-level wellness on the other end (34,35,40). According to Travis, every person is always moving in one direction or the other, toward either premature death or high-level wellness. In explaining the continuum, he wrote, "A 'well' being is not necessarily a strong, brave, successful, young, or even illness-free person. You can pursue wellness even if you are physically disabled, aged, scared in the face of challenge, in pain, imperfect. Sounds familiar? The direction in which you are headed is what's important."(34, p. 15)

From the start Travis was a prolific writer, having written and published a number of wellness-oriented books, the first of which was completed in 1974 (34). In 1976, he opened what he believes to be the first wellness center in the world, which was in Mill Valley, California. In 1991, he switched his focus to infant wellness and became the founder of the Alliance for Transforming the Lives of Children, which centers on how upbringing and environmental factors affect the wellness of infants and young children. He currently lives in Victoria, Australia.

Don Ardell's interest in wellness started in the early 1970s, when he was executive director of the United States' largest health planning agency, which was located in San Francisco, California.

This effort centered on the medical system, especially medical facilities, services, and personnel. According to Ardell, "We did not recognize at that time, that the way to promote well being and save costs was to inform, motivate, convince, inspire, guide, and otherwise support people to take better care of themselves without relying on the medical system" (32). To illustrate this concern, his doctoral dissertation was *High Level Wellness: An Alternative to Doctors, Drugs, and Disease,* which was later published by Rodale Publishing (4). Ardell has published 12 books, the first of which was published in 1977. When summing up 30 y of experience, Ardell suggests "Wellness is positive. The focus is not hazards and risks, but rather on satisfaction and pleasure. It is comprehensive, not just about fitness, nutrition and managing stress but also entails critical thinking, humor and play, emotional intelligence and the quest for added meaning and purpose in life. It is based on science and reason, not New Age wishful thinking and reliance or even inclusion of 'alternative' or other therapies, modalities, or healing systems. It is also a mindset or philosophy founded on personal responsibility and accountability." (5) Ardell's current interests center on helping senior citizens achieve high-level wellness.

In 1976, the U.S. Congress created the ODPHP. In 1997, Michael McGinnis, MD, who was Deputy Assistant Secretary for Health at the Department of Health, Education, and Welfare (later named the Department of Health and Human Services), became director of the ODPHP. McGinnis also served as the chairman of Secretary Joseph A. Califano's Task Force on Disease Prevention and Health Promotion. This effort resulted in the creation of a series of prevention activities for a number of government public health service agencies, such as the first *Healthy People* report. McGinnis also was chairman of the National Coordinating Committee on Worksite Health Promotion from 1979 to 1987; this committee was designed to raise the awareness of worksite wellness. The ODPHP remains active, as illustrated by the release of *Healthy People 2000, Healthy People 2010,* and *Dietary Guidelines for America—2005,* among other initiatives that apply to the worksite setting.

In the mid-1970s, William (Bill) Kizer, who was a chairman of an insurance company, developed interest in creating a well workplace. It did not take long for him to realize that credible resources from which to secure information and expertise did not exist. To this end, in the early 1980s he formed the Wellness Councils of America (WELCOA). Kizer's vision was to "establish a national resource that could be easily accessed by large corporations, health care agencies, government organizations, small businesses, and institutes of higher learning" (37). To make this vision a reality, he engaged individuals from the corporate world and various health promotion provider organizations. The vision that Kizer developed 25 y ago for WELCOA is live and well today.

One of the first peer-reviewed and published worksite wellness studies appeared in 1986 in the *Journal of the American Medical Association (JAMA;* 7). The study, which took place from 1979 to 1983, involved more than 11,000 Johnson & Johnson employees in 18 states. Those participating in intervention programs were compared with those not involved in intervention programs from a health care cost perspective. Over the years of the study, savings of about $1 million U.S. were reported. This was the first complete financial analysis of a comprehensive worksite wellness program to be published. The other interesting point about this study is that it was published in a top-tier medical journal, a feat which has not often been duplicated. This study was the genesis of the Johnson & Johnson Live for Life program.

In the mid-1970s, the CEO of Control Data Corporation, William Norris, speculated that health care costs would become a major social and economic issue in the future. At the time, Control Data, a pioneer in mainframe computing, was a *Fortune* 200 company with more than 50,000 employees in the United States. Using his foresight, Norris led an effort to create a portfolio of health care services, one of which was employee wellness. Part of this strategy was for Control Data to acquire the Life Extension Institute (LEI), a company that conducted executive physical examinations and had developed a fully computerized health risk assessment instrument to support its wellness efforts. LEI registered the trademark StayWell Health Management for its wellness products. In 1987, Control Data joined Milliman and Robertson in publishing a significant study, "Health Risks and Behavior: The Impact on Medical Costs," (9) which was another of the early large-scale studies to link employee health risks directly to employer medical costs. During this time, Control Data failed to anticipate the importance of microcomputer technology and continued to center on mainframe computer operations. This caused the company to go back to its core business. As a result, the StayWell Health Management segment of the business was spun off (D.R. Anderson; personal correspondence, March, 2008).

During the latter part of the first decade of worksite wellness, an attempt was made to provide networking and education opportunities for the discipline. To this end, the AAFDBI was organized and launched. After several years, the name was changed to the AFB. As worksite wellness developed, it involved much more than fitness activities. In order to expand its reach and recognize and accommodate the multifaceted nature of worksite wellness, AFB morphed into the AWHP. At its peak, AWHP had more than 2,500 members and operated at the national and regional levels. The 20th annual AWHP conference, which took place in 1994, had a registration of more than 1,000 individuals. AWHP ceased to exist as a stand-alone volunteer organization in 2000, but continued service was provided through the adoption of the worksite health promotion agenda by the ACSM Interest Group on Worksite Health Promotion.

Although not plentiful, the publication of worksite wellness research projects continued to increase. In 1985, DuPont reported on the effect of a comprehensive worksite wellness program on the reduction of disability days. The study groups were 29,315 employees who participated in the worksite wellness programs and 14,573 employees who were nonparticipants. Over 2 y, the participating employees had 11,726 fewer disability days. This study was one of the first to demonstrate the effect of a comprehensive worksite wellness program on absenteeism (6).

Employee Health Promotion—1986 to 1995

This decade was a very interesting time for employee health promotion. During the first 5 y, the discipline started to become a little better organized. While it could not be concluded that employee health promotion had become sophisticated, it was starting to move in that direction. From 1988 to 1991, health care costs went ballistic, and employers started to become concerned about them. The U.S. National Institutes of Health (NIH) and an employer funded a major $3 million U.S. research project. The first national health promotion scientific journal was launched, along with a national conference. The latter part of the decade was dominated by a federal government attempt to take control of the health care system. In response to this effort, the employee health promotion discipline consolidated efforts to assure that if there was socialized medicine, it would include employer financial incentives for qualified employee health *promotion programs. The quality and quantity of research started to increase during this decade. A study was published that defined the actual causes of death. Something called* stage of change *was starting to be discussed. The second decade of employee health promotion was characterized by enhanced organization and the start of multiple events that brought together a variety of people with interest in the discipline.*

In 1984, Michael O'Donnell, PhD, wrote the business plan for what became the *American Journal of Health Promotion (AJHP)* while working as the health promotion director at San Jose Hospital. According to O'Donnell, the rationale for creating the business plan was, "My reference book, *Health Promotion in the Workplace,* had just been published. Scrambling through the literature to find concepts and data for that book made me realize that the field needed a reference journal and a more rigorous scientific foundation in order to progress to the next level" (M.P. O'Donnell; personal correspondence; January, 2008). The first issue was mailed in June 1986. The second quarterly issue was 2 mo late, and it took 2 y to get on a publishing schedule of every 4 mo. Publication was increased to six issues per year in 1989 as the volume of submissions grew. "Editorial goals of the *AJHP* were to narrow the gap between science and practice and provide a format for discussion among the many diverse fields involved in health promotion," O'Donnell said (M.P. O'Donnell; personal correspondence; January, 2008). In 1989, the *AJHP* launched the Art and Science of Health Promotion (ASHP) conference. The creation and availability of the *AJHP* and the ASHP conference have had a significant effect on all facets of health promotion.

The NIH and the City of Birmingham, Alabama, funded a $3 million U.S. employee health management research project, which took place from 1985 to 1990 (19). The 4,000 city employees served as the study subjects. This was the largest investment ever made in employee health management research in the United States up to that point in time. One of the significant elements of this research project was the all-employee annual health assessment. Over the 5 y of the study, 97.5% of the covered employees participated each year. This was accomplished by making the employee health promotion program an integral part of the health care plan, which was a pioneering effort at the time. The health care plan document outlined that participation in a confidential, no-cost health assessment was a prerequisite for health care coverage. Over the 5 y of the study and compared

to other Alabama employers, the cost savings for the City of Birmingham was $7,146,878 U.S. (1990 dollars).

From 1985 to 1990, the University of Michigan Health Management Research Center conducted a research study for Steelcase (39). The study found that employees who went from high to low risk decreased health care costs from $1,155 to $537 U.S. annually and that those who moved from low to high risk had costs that increased from $1,155 to $1,677 U.S. annually. High risk was defined as three or more risks, while low risk was two or fewer risks. The risks evaluated were blood pressure, smoking, fitness, cholesterol, relative body weight, medications, alcohol consumption, and seat belt use. Continued focus on long-term analysis using the University of Michigan employee database has resulted in a body of employee health promotion research that shaped the direction of the field and continues to do so today.

In 1993, William Foege, MD, former director of the CDC, and Michael McGinnis, MD, published a review entitled "Actual Causes of Death in the United States." The report, which was published in *JAMA,* pointed out that in 1990, tobacco use caused 400,000 deaths, diet and activities patterns caused 300,000 deaths, alcohol use caused 100,000 deaths, microbial agents caused 90,000 deaths, toxic agents caused 60,000 deaths, firearms caused 35,000 deaths, sexual behavior caused 30,000 deaths, motor vehicles caused 25,000 deaths, and illicit drug use caused 20,000 deaths (24). This added up to 1,060,000 (49.3%) of the total 2,150,000 deaths for 1990. Later, the CDC collaborated with McGinnis and Foege to replicate their work and create "Actual Causes of Death in the United States—2000," which was published in *JAMA* in 2004 (25).

During the middle of this decade there was an increase in publications on financial effect, methodology, and ROI. Over a 10 y time frame, Kenneth Pelletier, PhD, published an ongoing review and analysis of cost effectiveness (29). Steve Aldana, PhD, published literature reviews on financial effect and methodology (1,2). Michael O'Donnell, PhD, reported on methodological quality (27). Larry Chapman published on cost effectiveness (13), and Ron Goetzel, PhD, evaluated the ROI (18). These and similar publications added significantly to the field.

To set the stage for the middle decade of employee health promotion, it is important to understand what happened relative to health care cost increases. Figure 2.1 shows the results of a survey from Mercer and Foster Higgins that

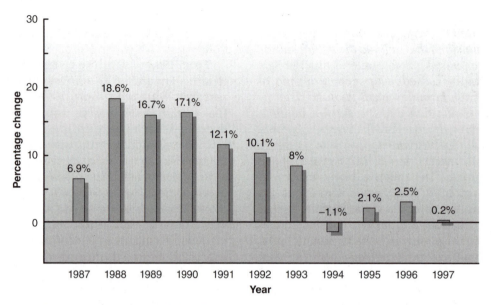

Figure 2.1 Annual change in average total health benefit cost for active and retired employees.
Graph reprinted by permission from Mercer LLC.

included data from nearly 4,000 employers on the total health care costs for active and retired employees (33).

The years from 1988 to 1997 produced some of the most volatile changes in health care cost ever recorded. In 1988, health care costs increased 18.6%. This was followed by an increase of 16.7% in 1989, 17.1% in 1990, 12.1% in 1991, 10.1% in 1992, and 8% in 1993. Then abruptly everything reversed. In 1994, there was a 1.1% decrease followed by increases of 2.1% in 1995, 2.5% in 1996, and 0.2 % in 1997. The ultimate question is: What caused the precipitous rise and fall in health care cost increases?

To address this question, it is important to consider what was happening to the health care system, what transpired in politics, and what was happening in employee health promotion during these 10 y. From 1988 to 1991 there were few checks and balances on health care costs, which resulted in extraordinary increases. The employer purchasing coalitions were not yet operational and health maintenance organizations (HMOs) were just beginning to step forward in large scale. In late 1991, the presidential primaries started with most candidates addressing health care costs and socialized medicine. From 1988 to 1992, the health care provider system built significant financial reserves. An attempt at health care reform failed in 1994. This caused the HMO industry to move forward aggressively with the message that it would control health care costs, and it did from 1994 to 1997. This was accomplished by reducing costs through the use of financial reserves. When the reserves were exhausted, costs began to increase again in 1998.

In September of 1993, President Clinton spoke to the joint houses of the U.S. Congress and presented a plan for the federal and state governments to assume control of the health care system. Due to the enormous size of this effort, five congressional committees were assigned the responsibility of discussing, debating, and creating legislation for governmental takeover. The two committees in the U.S. Senate were Labor and Human Resources and Finance, and the three committees in the U.S. House of Representatives were Education and Labor, Energy and Commerce, and Ways and Means. The Clinton proposal was only one of a number of bills that were debated. Some the others were the Kennedy plan, the Managed Competition Act, the Chafee plan, the House-GOP plan, and the MediSave Plan. To suggest that confusion reigned supreme in the U.S. Congress at this time would not be an overstatement.

One of the key features of nearly all the proposed and debated bills was that health care costs would be capitated, which means that there would be a flat fee per person or family. The concept of capitation or of *community rating,* as it was called, concerned those with interest in employee health promotion, because with fixed health care costs, employers could not realize a reduction in cost increases based on a healthier workforce. To address this situation, in early 1994 a group of individuals representing the AWHP, American Corporate Health, the *AJHP,* the ACSM, the American Association of Occupational Health Nurses (AAOHN), Johnson & Johnson, Human Kinetics, the Health Project, Fitness Systems, Group Health Cooperative, Union Pacific Railroad, the University of North Texas, WELCOA, and Wellness South created the Worksite Health Promotion Alliance (WHPA), which was a 501(c)(5) political lobbying corporation.

WHPA took no position on health care reform. If health care reform became law, the mission was for the legislation to contain language that would give financial incentives to employers who provided qualified worksite health promotion programs. Influencing something as complex as congressional legislation is no simple task. For this reason, WHPA hired a prominent Washington, DC, legal firm specializing in health care to help make the mission become a reality. This effort was supplemented by hundreds of hours of lobbying by individuals who represented the WHPA members. The result was that four of the five U.S. House and Senate committees used language that would provide the desired financial incentives for employers. At the beginning of the health care reform debate, the majority of the U.S. adult population favored health care reform. As the process moved into the summer of 1994 and more and more details became available, the public turned against the concept. The tipping point for the demise of health care reform was an austere black and white television message that played across the country, saying, "If you like the compassion of the Internal Revenue Service, the efficiency of the U.S. Postal Service, and the cost effectiveness of the Defense Department, you are going to love government controlled health care." All health care reform efforts came to a halt in October of 1994. Paying attention today to this experience is important, because the interest in health care reform could again become part of the political scene.

In 1993, a research study reported on the financial effects of the health promotion program at Union Pacific Railroad (22). The Union Pacific program started in 1987 with a single fitness facility at the corporate headquarters in Omaha, Nebraska, and later expanded operations to 59 sites, which were called *System Health Facilitators (SHFs).* The SHFs were used by more than 20,000 of the company's 28,000 employees. To investigate cost effects, one of the Union Pacific provid-

ers, Johnson & Johnson Health Management, conducted an analysis using its lifestyles claims analysis (LCA). According to Ron Goetzel, PhD, a researcher at Johnson & Johnson, "We figured out what percentage of total health plan costs are associated with poor health habits, which gives us the best opportunities for cost saving." (R. Goetzel, personal communication, December 2007) This research effort was somewhat unorthodox in that the Union Pacific health care rates were determined through negotiations among management, unions, and health care providers for the entire railroad industry. For this reason Union Pacific data were compared with the industry-wide data. The results were that stress was associated with 35% of costs, driving safety with 21%, tobacco use with 16%, obesity with 15%, hypertension with 10%, and no exercise with 10%. The Union Pacific program has advanced to become one of the most highly recognized and successful programs.

One of the early attempts at employee health promotion incentives or disincentives was at A.E. Miller, a wholly owned subsidiary of ConAgra Foods, a diversified food products company located in Omaha, Nebraska (26). There were 1,280 employees and 3,200 covered lives. In 1987, health care cost increases were 25%, growing from $1.6 to $2 million U.S. In 1988, three incentives, or disincentives, depending on one's point of view, were launched: (1) Employees and spouses who did not attend prenatal seminars were not reimbursed for the cost of delivery or the baby's care in the hospital. To qualify for benefits, the mother-to-be was required to visit a physician in the first trimester. (2) The company became smoke free. Smokers paid $66 U.S. toward their premiums versus $30 U.S. for nonsmokers. Smoking cessation programs were provided at no cost. (3) The company did not cover any medical costs associated with an automobile accident if the driver was under the influence of drugs or alcohol or was not using a seat belt. Health care cost increases went from a high 25% in 1988 to a 0% increase in 1992 and a 7% increase in 1993.

In 1992, Dr. Roger Porter, assistant to President George H.W. Bush, asked Carson Beadle and Daniel Wright if there was a way to save health care costs by keeping people healthy. In response, the Health Project, a private–public organization formed to bring about critical attitudinal and behavioral changes in the American health care system and dedicated to the furtherance of better health and lower medical costs by reduction in the need and demand for medical services, announced in 1994 the first C. Everett Koop National Health Awards. The award recipients were Aetna; the Dow Chemical Company; L.L. Bean; the Quaker Oats Company; Steelcase; and Union Pacific Railroad. Over the years, some of the other organizations to receive the award were Johnson & Johnson, Pitney Bowes, Motorola, DaimlerChrysler (now Chrysler), Glaxo Welcome (now GlaxoSmithKline), Fairview Health Services, Marriott, USAA, Pepsi Bottling Group, and We Energies. In determining the organizations to receive the award, there are three considerations: (1) The program must share the Health Project's goal of reducing the need and demand for medical services, (2) the program must be directed at the *Healthy People 2000* or *Healthy People 2010* health promotion targets, and (3) the program must include cost reduction as a major program element. C. Everett Koop, MD, a former U.S. Surgeon General, was the initial chairman of the Health Project and is now honorary chairman. Carson Beadle was the first president and currently serves as the chairman. James Fries, MD, is the current president. For 15 y, the C. Everett Koop National Health Award has been, and will continue to be, a guiding light for employee health management excellence. Other important recognition programs are the American College of Occupation and Environmental Medicine (ACOEM) Corporate Health Achievement Award, American Psychological Association (APA) Psychologically Healthy Workplace Award, Institute for Health and Productivity Management (IHPM) Corporate Health and Productivity Management Award, National Business Group on Health (NBGH) Best Employers for Healthy Lifestyle awards, and WELCOA Well Workplace Award.

James Prochaska, PhD, created the transtheoretical model of health behavior change (30). The concept proposes that health behavior change moves through six defined changes: precontemplation, contemplation, preparation, action, maintenance, and termination. This model proved to be a major step forward in addressing the predictability of health behavior change. The use of this approach advanced to the point that in 1997 the *AJHP* published a special issue on the Transtheoretical Model and the Stages of Change (30). Use and basic research suggested that for at-risk populations, 40% are in precontemplation, 40% are in contemplation, and 20% are in preparation to change. The stage of change construct was an important development since it brought a systematic method to behavioral change, and as a result it has become widely used, including its application via the Internet.

Employee Health Management— 1996 to the Present

The third decade of employee health management was one of ongoing development, sophistication, and success. The discipline developed to the point that mergers and acquisitions started to occur early in the decade and accelerated during the latter part. In 1997, one of the first national conferences on health and productivity took place, which reflected the growing interest and activity devoted to the topic. As the interest in health and productivity increased, attention turned to the creation of self-administered instruments to measure the effect of different diseases on productivity. The Internet increasingly became a part of employee health management as effective programming for health screening, education, and behavioral change became available. The quality and quantity of research increased. Employers for the first time began to recognize that health care costs would continue to escalate annually and that prevention and a healthier workforce were not only desired but required. Because of this, in 2002 employer interest in employee-dependent health management started to increase. Over time, this interest developed into unprecedented acceptance and activation of comprehensive programs. As of 2007, this growth pattern continues. The last 10 y of employee health management can be described best as the beginning of the age of maturity.

In 1996, HERO, a coalition of large employers and selected providers, became operational. Initial activities centered on the creation of a large-scale research database that defined the effects of 10 modifiable health risks on individual health care costs (18). The initial project was a joint effort by StayWell Health Management, the Medstat Group (now Thompson Medstat), and HERO. The risks evaluated were body weight, blood glucose level, cholesterol, depression, excessive alcohol use, exercise habits, nutritional habits, stress level, former smoker, current smoker, and nutrition. The initiative analyzed 5 y of cost data for about 46,000 employees. The most costly risks, in descending order, were found to be depression, excess stress, and elevated blood glucose; body weight, tobacco use, and hypertension; lack of exercise, high cholesterol, and excess alcohol consumption. This research project was peer reviewed and published in the fall of 1998. Several other research projects were generated by the HERO database, one of which was a group-level assessment of health care costs, which was published in 2000 (3). In 2003, the HERO Think Tank was created. It assumed the responsibility to create and disseminate national employee health management (EHM) policy, strategy, leadership, and infrastructure.

Health and productivity came to the forefront around 1997. Researchers at Harvard Medical School, in collaboration with researchers at Kaiser Permanente (Denver), the Group Health Center for Health Studies, the HealthPartners Research Foundation (HPRF), American Airlines, and the WHO (21), started a process to create a validated, self-administered instrument that employees complete and that measures the effect of 10 medical conditions on work performance. These conditions were cancer, irritable bowel syndrome, migraine, neurasthenia (fatigue), sleep problems, allergy, arthritis, depression, generalized anxiety disorder, and panic attacks. The psychometricians designing the instrument made contact with several employers who were collecting definitive health and work performance data. One of these was an airline that was monitoring its reservationists for the number of reservation calls received, the number of reservations made, the dollar volume of tickets sold, the time involved, and other outcomes. Another was a telephone company that was monitoring employee activities relative to the number of equipment units installed, the number of callbacks, the number of complaints, and other measures of work performance. Over time, employees at these companies completed the health and work performance questionnaire so that work performance standards could be compared and validated. The instrument that evolved from these efforts is known as the Health and Productivity Questionnaire (HPQ; see www.hpq.org). This instrument was used in 2000 in the WHO World Mental Health (WMH) Survey Initiative (see www.hcp.med.harvard.edu/wmh/ for more information) to evaluate 120,000 individuals in 25 countries (36). At least six other health and work performance instruments are currently available.

In 1997, the Institute for Health and Productivity Management (IHPM) became operational. Its purpose was "to make employee health an investment in corporate success, through enhanced work productivity. IHPM grew out of work done earlier under the 'Two Pens' Project on Healthcare Value, carried out jointly by the National Business Coalition on Health and the National Association of Managed Health Care Physicians." (20)

IHPM provides information on health and productivity through the Measuring Employee Productivity: A Guide to Self-Assessment Tools series (23). In addition, IHPM facilitates regular conferences in the United States and a number of foreign countries. The Integrated Benefits Institute (IBI) is another leader in the field of health and productivity and other areas related to health. IBI research explores how health, disability, and absence benefits can be designed and provided in order to maximize their effect. IBI has a substantial track record of facilitating national meetings that center on health, productivity, and absence. In regard to health and productivity, IBI offers the Health and Productivity Intelligence Suite (see www.ibiweb.org/ and conduct site search).

In 1999, Hewitt Associates published a study comparing the Fortune 100 Best Companies to Work For with 100 employers who were not on this list (14). Two outcomes were evaluated, which were the number of applications for employment received in a year and the turnover for the same year. Of the 100 Best Companies, 42% had on-site fitness centers compared with 26% of the companies who were not on the list, 52% provided stress management compared with 37% of the companies not on the list, and 63% offered on-site immunizations compared with 45% of the companies not on the list. During the 1 y spent on the evaluation, the 100 Best Companies employers received 18,040 applications for employment while the other companies received 11,380 applications. Turnover at the 100 Best Companies was 13% compared with 26% in the other companies.

One of the very early employee health management providers was Fitness Systems, which was acquired, renamed Health Fitness Corporation (HFC), and turned into a publicly traded company. In 2003, HFC acquired the Johnson & Johnson Health & Fitness Services Division, which had been providing fitness and health service programs for employees in the United States, Canada, and Latin America since 1986. The merger of HFC and the Johnson & Johnson division created what was at the time one of the larger employee health management companies to provide both traditional employee health management programming and services and fitness center management. It also was the beginning of other significant acquisitions and mergers. CorSolutions was acquired by Matria Healthcare. Harris HealthTrends was acquired by Axia Health Management, which in turn was acquired by Healthways. CHD Meridian Healthcare acquired ProFitness Health Solutions.

In 1999, HealthPartners published a study in *JAMA* that involved 5,689 adults enrolled in the HealthPartners health care plans (31). A research data set was created that included information from a behavioral questionnaire and 18 mo of health care costs. The analysis involved smoking, obesity (body mass index, or BMI), and physical activity. When current smokers were compared with nonsmokers, costs were 18% more for current smokers. When never smokers were compared with former smokers, former smokers' costs were 25.8% more. For every day of exercise performed per week, costs decreased from the median by 4.7%. For every increase in BMI increment, costs increased from the median by 1.9%. Research design permitted each of these factors to be evaluated as independent variables.

In 2003, employee health management providers started reporting that the employer interest in programs and services was on the rise. Employers who had moderately sized programs were expanding and those with no programs were becoming involved. Initially it was not known if the increasing interest was a momentary blip on the radar screen or the beginning of something more substantial. Now that the situation has been monitored for several years, there is reason to believe that a paradigm shift may be taking place. This shift is reflected in the growing sophistication, acceptance, and success of employee health management programming and services.

A logical question is what caused this somewhat abrupt upturn in employee health management. The answer is a number of things. Increasing numbers of employers began feeling that employees and dependents should take greater responsibility for their health and well-being and that the provision of employee health management programs and services is a way to make this happen. There has been a growing interest in health and work performance issues. On an increasing basis, a comprehensive and quality employee health management program is being recognized as a major employee benefit. These and related issues are all part of the employee health management growth equation. However, the most significant driving force has been the relentless increase in health care costs.

In 2005, the cost of health care was $2.0 trillion U.S., which is an amount that the human mind has difficulty to comprehend (12). One way to bring the cost of health care into sharper focus is to compare it with the U.S. federal budget for the same year. In 2005, the federal budget was $2.5 trillion U.S. (28). So, how big is the cost of health care? It is about 80% of what is expended to pay for the operation of the entire U.S. government domestically and around the world. This kind of information is helping employers and others to understand the incomprehensible cost of health care. Corporations are also devoting more attention to long-term health care cost projections. According to federal forecasts, the cost of health care in the United States in 2015 will be about $11,700 U.S. per person (not to be confused with per employee). At this point, health care costs will be $4 trillion U.S. annually, or double the cost in 2005 (8). Given these and similar forecasts, employers are accepting the fact that health care cost increases are not going to moderate and that substantial investment in human capital is required to change employee and dependent lifestyles and reduce the occurrence of preventable disease.

An illustration of the concern that top-level corporate executives have for health care cost is evident in one of the surveys conducted by the Business Roundtable (10). The Business Roundtable is a national coalition of about 160 corporate CEOs, mostly from Fortune 200 companies. In 2003 the CEOs were asked, "What cost is your greatest concern?" Of the 160 CEOs, 81%, or 140, responded as follows: 43% said health care costs, 20% said litigation, 19% said energy, 12% said materials, 3% said labor, and 3% said pensions. There is little doubt that the concern about health care costs has invaded the executive suite and is a dominant factor in the growing interest in employee health management.

Former and Current Providers

Providers of employee health management programs have played a critical role in the development of this industry. Along with researchers, academicians, educators, policy makers and shapers, human resource managers, medical and benefits directors, business leaders, and other stakeholders, providers have been central in shaping the field of employee health management. They have been thought leaders and innovators as well as dedicated and persistent advocators. Unfortunately, an in-depth review of all providers that have played a role in shaping the industry is beyond the scope of this chapter. However, it is appropriate to address activities and contributions providers have performed or made as a group and a brief overview of significant activities conducted by providers or health-related organizations has been outlined in table 2.1.

During the first decade of worksite wellness, provider companies were made up of a small number of individuals who were innovators with a high passion for worksite wellness. The basic programs included a self-administered HRA

Table 2.1 Significant Events or Activities: 1975-2007

Year	Organization	Event or activity
1970-1975	Centers for Disease Control and Prevention (CDC)	Developed HRA for use among CDC employees
1974	Association for Worksite Health Promotion (AWHP)	Began as the American Association of Fitness Directors in Business and Industry and in 1983 changed its name to the Association for Fitness in Business; in 1993, changed its name to the Association for Worksite Health Promotion to reflect the evolution of the industry into a broader and more comprehensive approach to employee health promotion
1976	*Healthwise*	Introduced the first edition of the *Healthwise Handbook* (42)
1972-1977	John Travis, MD	Copyrighted the illness-wellness continuum (1972) and published the Wellness *Workbook for Health Professionals* (1977) (40)
1976	U.S. Congress	Created the Office of Disease Prevention and Health Promotion
1985-1990	University of Alabama at Birmingham and Wellness South	Implemented a $3 million U.S. worksite health promotions trial (funded by the NIH) for employees of the City of Birmingham, Alabama
1986	Johnson & Johnson	Published comprehensive worksite health promotion financial analysis in *JAMA*
1986	*American Journal of Health Promotion (AJHP)*	Debuted as the first scientific publication devoted to health promotion
1987	Milliman and Robertson and Control Data Corporation	Published the study titled "Health Risk and Behaviors: The Impact on Medical Cost" (41)
1991	University of Michigan, Health Management Research Center	Reported on health care costs when health risks were reduced or increased
1997	James Prochaska, PhD	Created the stages of change, which brought a systematic method to behavioral change
1998	Health Enhancement Research Organization (HERO)	Created the largest database to define the effects of risks or costs
1999	HealthPartners Research Foundation (HPRF)	Defined the effects of smoking, obesity, and inactivity on medical care costs and published the report in *JAMA*

with confidential participant reports that were provided to the employees. Usually, the HRA was accompanied by biometric evaluations that determined weight and height, blood glucose, cholesterol levels, and blood pressure. Often the employer was provided with an aggregate report minus any employee identification. For those found to be at risk, there were follow-up group and, on occasion, individual behavioral change programs. The programs most often centered on smoking, nutrition, weight management, exercise, and stress management. Often, the HRA was repeated on an annual basis. The incentive for employee participation was usually a baseball cap, running shirt, or coffee cup. Disease management as it is known today did not exist. Health benefits consultants had not yet figured out their role and health care plans, and providers usually did not want to know about prevention and worksite wellness. The providers were often multitaskers. The individual who did the market-

ing sometimes worked at the medical screens and often was a behavior change expert. Many provider companies operated for a year or two and then disappeared because of a lack of cash flow. However, a small number of program providers that became operational in the first decade or shortly thereafter remain in business today. Some of these are Fitness Systems (which was acquired and became Health Fitness Corporation), MediFit Corporate Services, StayWell Health Management, Summex Health Management (acquired by WebMD Health Services), American Institute for Preventive Medicine, CorSolutions (acquired by Matria Healthcare), Harris HealthTrends (acquired by Healthways), Wellsource, and ProFitness Health Solutions (acquired by CHD Meridian Healthcare). The first-decade providers are recognized for their vision and for the foundation they provided on which others would build.

During the second decade of employee health promotion, the provider network expanded. The health benefits consulting firms became active in providing various kinds of advice and analytical information. The size of provider companies expanded substantially. Instead of having a dozen employees, companies now had hundreds. Some companies started placing full-time employees at large corporations to deliver programs on-site. The number of providers that designed and managed on-site fitness centers increased. Telephonic nurse consultants were starting to be part of the provider package. By the end of this decade, nearly all major providers had started making program services available on the Internet. In the second decade, health and benefits consulting firms increasingly became involved not as program providers but as sources of valuable information. Companies such as Hewitt Associates, Mercer, PricewaterhouseCoopers, Towers Perrin, and others conducted annual, large-scale employer surveys that provided important information on employee health management patterns of use, outcomes, projections for future growth, and other parameters. At the same time consulting firms such as SHPS, Ingenix, Thompson Medstat, and Health Data Management Solutions provided program cost-effectiveness and other analytical consulting services. The second-decade providers are recognized for the development of the discipline.

The third decade of employee health management has been a time of amazement. Some provider companies have thousands of employees. During the latter part of this decade, employer acceptance of employee health management expanded significantly. Today, it is not unusual for multiple providers to work together to deliver comprehensive programs and services for a single large employer. Health and productivity services have started to become commonplace. The defining of outcomes has improved. Total integration is no longer a dream, but a reality. The use of incentives has become a science. Increasingly, providers have become an integral part of the corporate environment as employers strive to control heath care cost increases, enhance work performance, and elevate employee well-being. Involvement of health care providers and plans in the delivery of employee health management programs has become more common during the decade, though several providers such as SwedishAmerican Health System, HealthPartners, Kaiser Permanente, and the Mayo Clinic had been involved much earlier. More recently, Intermountain Healthcare, Sutter Health Partners, AtlantiCare, and a number of Blue Cross Blue Shield plans (Rhode Island, Massachusetts, North Carolina, Tennessee, and Arizona) have become involved. Several other

key provider organizations of this decade are IncentOne, OptumHealth, and Quest Diagnostics. The third-decade providers are recognized for being ready and successful in responding to sharp increases in employer and employee acceptance of employee health management.

Conclusion

Following this look back over the first 30 y of what we now call *employee health management,* it can be surmised that the future is bright and filled with high potential. However, this is no time to relax. With employee health management at new levels of acceptance and success, the prime question is: What is required to sustain and enhance the growth? The answer is twofold. First, efforts must continue to elevate the levels of innovation and effectiveness. In addition, the documentation of outcomes must continue to improve. Second, the employee health management discipline must interact on a regular schedule with top-level corporate executives to create dialogue and remain informed on what kind of information and data are required in order to keep the investment in human capital a top priority. This must occur on a discipline-wide basis so that the information, requirements, and expectations are shared with all providers and other stakeholder organizations. These activities are not optional, because between 2006 and 2016 health care costs will double (8). This provides an unprecedented opportunity for employee health management to step forward and establish prevention as the method of choice to enhance the health and well-being of employees and covered dependents and thereby control cost increases and maximize work performance.

Chapter Review Questions

1. From 1988 to 1997, health care costs went from 5 y high double-digit increases to 4 y of nearly no increases. What factors were responsible for these cost shifts?

2. During the health care reform debate that took place from 1993 to 1994, what transpired to cause employer financial incentives to be part of the legislation being debated in the U.S. Senate and House of Representatives?

3. What caused the increased interest in employee health management that began in 2004?

4. What is required to assure that the growth in the interest in employee health management that began in 2004 will be sustained and enhanced?

3

Workplace-Based Health and Wellness Services

Raymond J. Fabius, MD, CPE, FACPE, and Sharon Glave Frazee, PhD

That men in general should work better when they are ill fed than when they are well fed, when they are disheartened than when they are in good spirits, when they are frequently sick than when they are generally in good health, seems not very probable. Years of dearth, it is to be observed, are generally among the common people years of sickness and mortality which cannot fail to diminish the produce of their industry.

–Adam Smith, *Wealth of Nations,* 1776 (47)

To gain efficiencies, corporations, particularly large employers, have built or at least organized significant campuses to manage and house large populations of workers. The workplace is where working adults spend many of their waking hours. Having concentrations of employees in one location offers employers a chance to provide effective health-related programs to keep their well workers healthy and to assist their less-well employees in managing medical issues in order to remain productive. As it becomes increasingly clear that a healthy workforce is a competitive advantage, employers have been investing in health. That investment has even included building large, full-service primary care centers with integrated pharmacies and dental and optical centers to serve not just employees but also dependents, contracted vendor staff, and retirees. Workplace health and wellness encompasses a broad array of services and programs that are focused within a workplace setting and are designed to improve the lives of employees, increase worker productivity, and create value for the business community. This chapter explores some of the options available in the realm of workplace-based health and wellness services.

Business leaders today are increasingly recognizing the need to invest in the health of their employees for more than altruistic reasons—investment in health is critical to the bottom line of the company (12). In the United States, employers have sponsored health insurance for their employees since the 1940s (6). By 1950, more than 90% of the American workforce was covered by employer-sponsored health benefits. Even though the percentage of employees with employer-sponsored health insurance has dropped to 61% today (31), the annual increases of direct health care costs paid by employers continue to rise even before the costs of absenteeism, presenteeism, and other factors that make up the full cost of poor health are taken into account. According to a recent Mercer survey, the 2007 health benefits costs to U.S. employers rose at twice the rate of inflation, with an average cost of $7,983 U.S. per employee (31). If the health and productivity of employees are not improved, health costs will continue to erode business profitability.

Businesses see workplace health as one way to wrestle some control out of the health care system. They also recognize the lost-time savings that can be realized since employees can take care of health care needs quickly on-site rather than taking a half or even an entire day off to see a health care provider in the community. Evidence is gathering to suggest that when access to care is easier and faster, employees and patients take better care of their health, obtain preventive care and screenings, make better lifestyle choices, and do the things that will lower health care costs for the employer as well as improve their productivity in the long run. Business leaders cannot change the aging workforce demographic or significantly influence what community health care providers charge, but they can create an atmosphere of good stewardship for personal health among their employees.

The benefits of workplace health and wellness services for employees are many and include acces to services employees might otherwise not have or be willing to seek out, services designed to maximize their employee benefits plan, and services provided in a convenient location with out-of-pocket costs that are typically lower than those of similar services in the community. Both convenience and lower cost encourage increased use of preventive services, more timely use of services for acute conditions, and even use of services that might not be readily available in the community, such as health coaching.

It is easy to see how improving the health and productivity of employees can benefit both the employer and the employee, and recent debate posits that improved health might even be good for communities. Healthy employees help create fiscally healthy and more productive companies that can then pay employees more without raising prices for goods and services. Better paid employees support a healthier local economy that can then invest more into the health, education, and overall enrichment of the community. An article published in *Science* in 2000 started an interesting debate over the direction of the relationship between health and income (5). Traditionally, it was thought that health was the result of wealth, but the *Science* article poses that wealth is actually the result of health due in large part to increased labor productivity. While the *Science* article was proposing this relationship for nations, it seems reasonable to apply it to smaller units of analysis as well, such as communities, businesses, or even individuals. The idea that healthy workers are more productive is not a new idea—on the contrary, it was proposed by Adam Smith in the *Wealth of Nations,* first published in 1776, making this emerging field of health and productivity at least 225 y in the making.

Workplace health in the broadest sense acknowledges that many factors within the workplace greatly influence health and productivity. Workplaces are an optimal setting in which to deliver health promotion and health care and can also be a key determinant of health itself. The policies and practices of a workplace create a culture that can drive and sustain health in the employees who work there. With such a wide definition, workplace health can encompass an almost unlimited number of programs or activities. These typically range from traditional occupational health services focused on managing risk to medical management activities such as case management to population management programs such as on-site primary care with integrated pharmacies. Workplace health is no longer just treating workplace injuries and providing annual flu shots—workplace health can now truly aspire to be the home of medical care for employees and their dependents. An example of such a home is the Toyota Family Health Center in San Antonio, Texas. In November 2006, the Toyota Motor Corporation spent $9 million U.S. to open this center with its vast array of services (8). Today as never before business leaders are recognizing that workplace health care can contain medical costs, improve productivity and morale, promote wellness, retain staff, and assist corporations in achieving status as an employer of choice. In other words, workplace health is good business.

Brief History of Workplace Health Centers

Workplace health centers are hardly a new phenomenon. As early as 1860, railroads and mining companies began to employ company doctors. While these doctors typically did not operate actual health centers at the workplace, they were employed to provide health care to employees, typically using their home or private office as the infirmary. During the 19th century, the role of the company physician was primarily limited to the treatment of occupational injuries, with little attention paid to occupational diseases (34). The first American industries to employ company doctors— railroads, mining companies, lumber companies, iron works, steel mills, and other heavy manufacturing companies—had several things in common, including dangerous work conditions, high accident rates, and often remote locations with little access to health care outside the company (39). Railroad work conditions were particularly dangerous. In 1900 there were more than 1 million railroad workers in the United States. According to the Interstate Commerce Commission, 1 of every 28 employees was injured and 1 of every 399 was killed on the job in the year ending June 30, 1900 (26). Other industries did not have it much better. A survey of workplace fatalities occurring in Allegheny County, Pennsylvania (41), from July 1906 to June

1907, found that during this 1 y, 526 workers died in work accidents, 195 of which were steelworkers (9). The National Safety Council estimates that in 1912, work-related injuries resulted in between 18,000 and 21,000 deaths across the United States; in 1913 the Bureau of Labor Statistics documented approximately 23,000 industrial deaths among a workforce of 38 million, a rate of 61 deaths per 100,000 workers (9). Mining was a dangerous occupation. In fact, the first recorded company physician of modern times, J. A. Scopoli (1723-1788), was assigned to the mercury mines in what is now Slovenia because of the large number of accidents occurring there (20). In 1900 there were 448,541 coal miners in the United States and 1,489 workplace fatalities, or 331 deaths per 100,000 workers (43). Miners were challenged not only with frequent accidents and injuries but also with occupational diseases such as mercury poisoning and occupational lung cancer (20). The combination of frequent accidents and geographic isolation from preexisting medical systems made creating company-owned health clinics necessary for both the employees and their families (38). Thus, in many places, industrial medicine became the community's medicine as well, a precursor to today's full-service primary care and pharmacy health centers offered by some large employers (33).

Industrial medicine evolved alongside the general health care field. Company physicians began to conduct periodic as well as preemployment health examinations of employees and became more involved in the health supervision of workers in general. This change occurred around the same time the state workers' compensation laws were enacted (around 1911) and was partially fueled by the rise in popularity of Frederick Taylor's theories of scientific management. The focus of workplace health care slowly began to shift from injury response to preventive medicine and medical engineering (38).

Workplace health was greatly influenced by Kaiser Steel during World War II when the corporation and its foundation formed a group practice called *Kaiser Permanente*. Using hospitals located on company property near the shipyards, Kaiser operated a full-service medical program to treat employees and their dependents. Kaiser was arguably one of the first large companies to make health care part of its organizational philosophy (14). Many other companies hired doctors and developed variations of the Kaiser model of company medicine; these include New York Bell's primary care clinics for employees and their family members and the in-house wellness programs operated by Tenneco and Uniroyal (14).

During the 1950s to 1970s, industrial hygiene and safety often reported to the company doctor, but by the late 1970s these disciplines had been largely removed from the company doctor's supervision. In this new model, environmental affairs, safety, and industrial hygiene reported directly to plant managers or vice presidents, whereas the medical department was demoted to reporting to human resources, making it much more difficult for occupational physicians to influence plant activities. With the medical department in this weakened position, members of management sometimes wondered if they were getting their money's worth, and many joined the outsourcing bandwagon of the late 1980s and 1990s.

Even with the weakening of traditional occupational medicine, interest in promoting health continued, particularly as the cost of health care skyrocketed and started cutting into company profits. Major companies, including Johnson & Johnson and AT&T, started to make major investments in health promotion for their employees during the 1980s. Economic analysis of these activities indicated that they were not only cost effective but also a good ROI (22). This encouraged other corporations to make investments in health promotion.

Today, workplace health is stronger than ever, with some of the largest and most innovative companies opening workplace health centers, installing workplace fitness facilities, promoting wellness and healthy lifestyles through healthy food options in cafeterias and vending machines, providing disease management programs for employees and family members with chronic diseases, providing health coaching to encourage positive health changes, and creating many other types of services. Some of these services are described in the sections to follow.

From Occupational Health to Population Health

When a company makes a commitment to offer medical services at the workplace, it is making a significant investment in time, effort, and money. Physical facilities have to be designed, medical equipment must be purchased, clinicians must be hired, and an organizational philosophy must be developed to determine which services will be provided to employees, contracted workers, retirees, and dependents. Occupational health is often the starting point for companies as they strive to manage risk and meet regulatory guidelines. Occupational health services include those performed both before and during employment, such as preplacement evaluations and periodic monitoring of employees. Types of occupational health services include medical surveillance exams, treatment of occupational injuries and illnesses, ergonomics, emergency response, OSHA reporting, workers' compensation, and employee assistance programs (EAP) behavioral health. Medical surveillance is the periodic assessment of individual workers in terms of occupational history, medical history, and symptoms or signs related to hazardous substances or conditions at the workplace. Surveillance may include biological screening such as blood or urine testing performed either as a routine or as part of a special investigation related to exposure to hazardous conditions or substances (46). Additionally, occupational health usually includes the treatment and rehabilitation of occupational injuries and illnesses, which is among the most direct ways that occupational health services improve the productivity of a workforce—with appropriate and timely care for injuries and illnesses that occur on the job, employees may return to work quickly. Since approximately two-thirds of workers' compensation costs are wage replacement for lost time, reducing the time an employee is away from the job can have a huge effect on costs.

As the research in the area of health and productivity advances, business leaders are recognizing the need to do more than focus on occupational health. This has led to investments and the migration to other forms of workplace health, including primary care, pharmacy, case management and medical management, wellness, and

fitness (16). The migration from risk management to case management to population management is illustrated in figure 3.1.

Workplace-based health and wellness services can be broadly categorized into risk management, medical management, and population management, although some types of services may fall into more than one category. Figure 3.1 illustrates the most commonly purchased benefits and services offered at the workplace but is by no means exhaustive. While risk management is the traditional starting point of workplace health, it encompasses only about 25% of the total cost of health care to the employer. The far greater portion of employer-paid health care costs can be affected by the right-hand side of the spectrum of services, as is shown in figure 3.1.

Services that focus on the individual employee, such as medical management, are often the next step in the migration from occupational to population health. Medical and case management can help supervise the treatment of both occupational and nonoccupational illness and injury, help manage costs and improve outcomes for the employee by reducing duplication of services, help ensure that quality health care providers are selected, and help employees navigate the often confusing medical system so they can return to full health and functionality as soon as possible. This benefits the employee, the employer, and the coworkers as well as the family members of the employee.

Population health recognizes that while case and medical management focus on the needs of

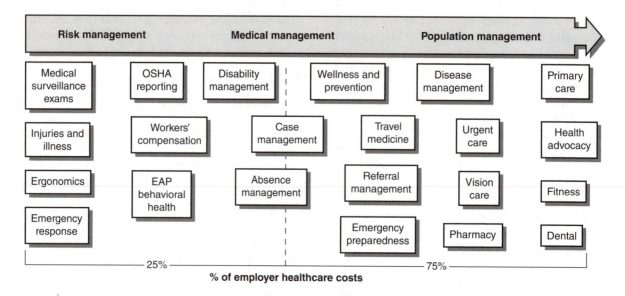

Figure 3.1 The migration from risk management to population management.

a particular employee, the largest gains are made by focusing on mitigating the direct and indirect costs of poor health and lifestyle choices for the entire employee population. This can include clinical services such as workplace primary care that allow employees and often employee family members increased access to medical services, regular follow-up for employees with disease, and evidence-based screening for chronic conditions. Such services reduce absenteeism, as employees can access medical care in usually less than half an hour. Wellness and other health promotion services improve the health of the employee community by encouraging healthy lifestyle choices; providing access to fitness facilities, coaching, and guidance on how to make and maintain healthy changes; and acting as health advocates for the employees.

In the past, employee health services tended to focus on individuals more than populations, on treatment rather than prevention, and on disease status more than health status. This traditional focus often led to segregated health management systems and missed some of the largest gains possible from employee health programs. Employers are now beginning to recognize that meeting the challenge of managing their entire community of covered lives means keeping the well population healthy and helping the population with health issues make health improvements. Integration, including the integration of health and wellness, disease management, on-site fitness centers, and health advocacy, is often the key to success in this endeavor. Dental and vision services are also being added to provide convenient, one-stop access for employees and to reduce lost work time. Workplace pharmacies integrated with workplace primary care centers build the foundation of a clinical team that can prevent, diagnose, treat, and ensure compliance to therapeutic regimes in ways that are significantly improved when compared with nonintegrated community services (18).

How Worksite Health Promotion Fits In

The recent focus on preventive health has spurred the demand for worksite health promotion. As employers face an aging workforce and rising health care costs, they are trying to shift health care spending toward prevention with the hope that treatment costs will decrease as more employees and their families engage in healthier lifestyles. Worksite health promotion addresses the source by focusing upstream on improving employee lifestyles to make employees healthier. Early worksite wellness and health promotion programs typically focused on programs thought to have substantial ROI, such as safety instruction, smoking cessation, stress management, nutrition, and weight control (17). The scope of worksite health promotion has widened to encompass a variety of programs that closely integrate with and support the benefits plan structures and business goals set up by employers (24).

The increased demand for worksite health promotion is seen in the rise in the number of employers offering on-site clinics and fitness centers as well as those offering an assortment of health promotion programs. A survey conducted by Watson Wyatt in 2007 found that 23% of the 573 large employers questioned had an on-site clinic and that an additional 6% planned on opening an on-site clinic in 2008 (44). The same survey found that 72% of these employers were offering HRAs, 42% had weight reduction programs, and 28% offered reduced health insurance premiums for participation in health management programs.

Health promotion programs have many benefits. They can lead to improvements in lifestyle habits that reduce the likelihood that health problems will arise over time. Just as regular maintenance of an automobile can prevent large and expensive problems later on, addressing health risk factors is less expensive and more effective than simply addressing medical problems after they occur. If health promotion programs are well integrated into the overall health and productivity management system of the organization, they can spur additional savings by complementing the goals of other programs and can create an environment of wellness that supports and maintains health (23). In addition, these programs can save employers vast amounts of lost productivity due to absenteeism and presenteeism. It is well documented that unhealthy employee behaviors or health risks contribute greatly to employer costs such as salary paid to absent employees, medical expenses, workers' compensation awards, distress to other employees caused during absence, cost of temporary replacement, and administrative costs (10). While medical services are dedicated to the treatment of illness, health promotion and workplace fitness centers can touch all of the covered lives of an employer population. Moreover, these efforts can go a long way toward keeping the healthy employees well. This is at least equally important to caring for the ill since the well workers are the ones doing the majority of the work and studies show that a comprehensive health and productivity effort can result in health risk reductions for the community as a whole (15).

The advantage of providing health promotion and fitness centers at the workplace is the same as the advantages of providing illness and other preventive services. Making exercise easy and available reduces the hurdle people refer to when considering participation. Changing the environment where people spend the majority of their waking hours can contribute greatly to healthy lifestyles. Promoting healthy food options in the cafeterias, banning smoking on campus, and building inviting fitness facilities can go a long way toward building a culture of health. Supporting these efforts with trusted clinicians such as doctors, pharmacists, health educators, and sport physiologists dedicated to the care of the lives covered by the employer can make a large difference in employee health.

Workplace Health as a Point of Integration

Integration of workplace health programs is becoming more important than ever. The Institute of Medicine (IOM; 25) suggests that the key to success for workplace health is integration of programs. An integrated health approach brings together health promotion, medical benefits, short- and long-term disability, workers' compensation, disease management, case management programs, primary care, pharmacy, and other health programs into a single process that emphasizes improving outcomes, measurement and benchmarking, coordination of services, and creating synergy between programs and services (22). Nearly every recent publication on workplace health recommends integration, and there is encouraging evidence that employers are moving to an integrated model in order to reap the full value of health and wellness programs and thus increase the value of their human capital. This is evidenced by the number of recent national conferences such as the NIOSH WorkLife Initiative, the joint Disease Management Association of America (DMAA) and National Association of Manufacturers (NAM) meetings that focus on the need for integration.

Workplace health clinics are at the intersection between work and health. Given that the worksite is where most American adults spend a substantial portion of their time, it is an appropriate setting in which to promote and protect health. Work plays a dominant role in the lives of adults, and the social and environmental aspects of the workplace and the people within it can profoundly influence health. Studies have found that accessible, comprehensive, and well-integrated primary care is associated with better outcomes and lower costs (37). American adults with an accessible source of primary care are more likely to receive preventive care and less likely to encounter coordination problems, and they experience fewer disparities in health care when compared with those lacking accessible primary care (2). Perhaps at no time in history has this need been greater, as the shortage of primary care physicians reduces access to this important source of health care. Given this evidence, creating workplace primary care centers as the medical home for employees and their dependents and providing ready access to a medical home and then using these primary care centers as the hub for integration can promote health through preventive services, coordinated care, and programs that reduce the long-term costs associated with disease and disability. This is illustrated in figure 3.2.

The silo approach to managing health costs has proven to be inefficient. Decreases in one area often lead inadvertently to increases in other areas when a business tries to purchase and implement employee health and productivity programs in piecemeal fashion. For example, increased drug co-payments may result in lower pharmacy costs for the business but at the cost of lower drug compliance and subsequent higher hospital costs. In addition, failure to integrate makes it nearly impossible to obtain a full understanding of the true cost of health to the business or the effect of health promotion programs on the population since the data are often disparate and difficult to bring together (30).

There is also growing evidence that integrating all health and wellness programs at the workplace with an on-site health center drives results and improves the overall value of employer-sponsored health and productivity programming (18, 19). Strong evidence that coordinating health and productivity services through trusted clinicians at the workplace and that aligning caregivers— be they physicians, nurses, pharmacists, fitness specialists, physical therapists, or health coaches to name a few—into a single, integrated model will bring the business closer to realizing the ultimate value of population health management. Clinicians who treat patients at workplace health centers have better knowledge of the work environment—of its stressors and hazards as well

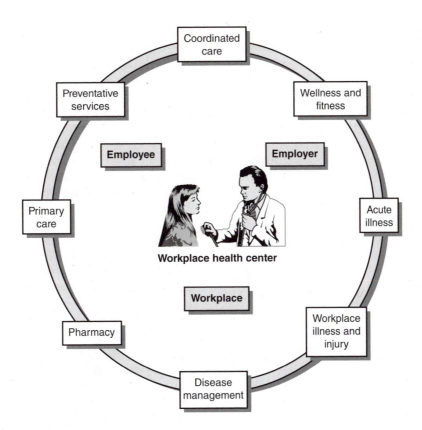

Figure 3.2 Workplace health centers as the hub for integration.

as its benefits. Recent research on the integration of health services at the workplace has shown that participation rates in disease management programs are 3 to 5 times higher than industry norms (19). Research on integrating workplace primary care with workplace pharmacies has shown dramatic improvements in appropriate prescribing of antibiotics, provision of evidence-based care for patients, and cost savings for employers (18).

Workplace physicians, nurses, therapists, and pharmacists are challenged to incorporate wellness and health promotion into their delivery of health care services. Historically this may not have been done at all, may have been remotely provided to workers by health plans, or may have been delivered independently by various wellness vendor organizations. However, just as doctors write prescriptions to be filled at a pharmacy or make referrals to a medical specialist, they should also direct patients to health educators and personal exercise trainers for individualized wellness programs and services. Because trusted clinicians at the workplace are perhaps the greatest driver of successful lifestyle behavior change, making referrals for fitness and wellness in a less coordinated fashion makes little sense. Workplace health

centers also provide dedicated clinicians who, unlike those who practice in the community, need to be aware of only one benefits plan, one referral network, and one formulary. This integration yields dramatically better benefits administration in network referrals and formulary compliance. Additionally, when clinicians are unencumbered by dealing with dozens of health plans, they can spend more time with their patients and thus reduce the need for specialty referral and improve patient satisfaction (32). This in return increases treatment compliance and medication adherence (36).

The Value of Workplace Health

Until the late 1990s worksite wellness and fitness centers were seen as just a nice thing to do for employees, but today the decision to provide these services has truly become a business decision, benefiting the company with lower medical costs, greater productivity, and less absenteeism. The cost of doing nothing keeps rising. Even the most conservative studies have found that health risks account for at least 25% to 30% of excess medical costs (45), although other studies find this to be as high as 43% (28). If a company is self-insured, one heart attack can easily cost in excess of $100,000 U.S. If the company can prevent 10 or 20 heart attacks, the savings can run into the millions. An integrated service model covering the entire employee health continuum is the best strategy to help companies maximize these savings.

Today, an ever-increasing number of employers are trying to help employees become healthier and more physically active. By doing so, employers experience the benefits of

- lower health care costs,
- increased employee productivity,
- reduced absenteeism,
- less employee turnover, and
- improved ability to attract and retain high-performance employees.

In fact, according to a 2007 survey by Hewitt Associates, The Road Ahead: Emerging Health Trends (48), 63% of the employers surveyed indicated that they will become much more involved in the health of their employees in the future as they try to manage health- and productivity-related costs.

Potential cost savings when providing primary care at the workplace can be produced via multiple channels, including reduced direct medical costs, better referral management (high-performance network for workers' compensation and primary care), more appropriate use of generics, and reduced use of hospital and outpatient services as well as emergency room services. Add to this the reduction in health risks and the increase in productivity that are garnered from wellness programs and the value of workplace health becomes extremely high.

The quality of care also adds to the value of workplace health. Workplace health, particularly on-site primary care, allows greater control over the management of care. Instead of attempting to manage a network of providers through a third-party administrator workplace, employers can use health centers to capture the vast majority of a workforce community within a single practice. If the employer is interested in having its employees cared for using electronic medical records (EMRs), it can encourage the throngs of doctors who treat its employees to do so or it can build an on-site facility for care, create benefits advantages to use the facility, and install an EMR system from the beginning. Additionally, such primary care centers can manage and direct specialty referrals, funneling them to a high-performance

network of physicians and hospitals with proven evidence-based protocols and results. Workplace clinicians typically have more time to spend with patients and can provide primary care education during teachable moments. They are also more able to fully address all of the patient's questions. Efficiencies in care and service can be created by applying the industry-touted Toyota Production System (TPS) and Six Sigma used to reduce variations in service and outcomes. Scorecards and dashboards, much like those used for other business practices, can be applied to the health delivery for employees, allowing business executives and operations staff to track progress over time and to identify anomalies quickly.

In the last decade, epidemiological research has shown the cost-effectiveness of interventions that manage and prevent conditions that affect employee health and productivity (35). Kessler's seminal work on the influence of undertreated physical and mental health conditions on work performance clearly shows that the effects of these conditions are substantial (27). His work is backed by other research that clearly shows the association between poor health and low work productivity (7). The ability of health promotion programs to affect employee health has been the subject of many published research manuscripts and reviews (11). Reviews of the effectiveness of many interventions have shown promising results. Of particular recent interest are programs that focus on keeping the well population healthy by supporting maintenance of healthy behaviors. For instance, Edington found that reducing health risk factors, including stress, reduced medical costs and that for each healthy employee kept healthy, future health care costs were reduced by $350 U.S. per year (15). This strategy is estimated to have the greatest effect on influencing the health of a workplace population and exemplifies the core of worksite health promotion—prevention and detection.

Improving employee productivity is an important component of workplace health programs. Productivity improvements can be seen in saved work time (access convenience—acute care visits take 30 min rather than half a day), reduced absenteeism (earlier treatment, better compliance), reduced disability and workers' compensation claims (ergonomics, early intervention, employer of choice), and reduced presenteeism (higher performance at work).

A literature review by Aldana found that the majority of published studies support the hypothesis that worksite health promotion programs lower absenteeism (1). When workplace health and wellness services achieve best practices through integration, as much as a 25% reduction in the overall employee cost of health, turnover, absenteeism, disability, and workers' compensation programs has been shown (21). In fact, one study of a comprehensive workplace health program implemented at DuPont, a company with 110,000 employees at more than 100 locations, produced an average hourly employee absenteeism reduction of 12.5%, with some high- participation worksites showing absenteeism rates as much as 46.5% lower than baseline rates (3). Even when only workplace primary care is available, the reductions in absenteeism are considerable, as shown in a study by Stempien and colleagues that found that employees who used a workplace health clinic averaged 3.3.d less absenteeism than those who used community care only (39).

Disability days can also be affected by workplace health programs. A pre- and postcontrol group study on a blue-collar workforce found that after the implementation of a comprehensive workplace health program, disability days dropped by 10.5% after 1 y compared with a 1.5% increase at nonprogram locations (4). Reducing the number of disability days not only reduces absenteeism but also reduces the costs associated with medical treatment during disability leave, the replacement costs for the employee who is disabled, and the exponential effect on coworkers' productivity that is wrought when a key team member is absent.

The value of workplace health, however, has many factors, including the success of the integration of the health and wellness programs, the breadth and depth of the programs, and the workplace culture toward health and productivity. Towers Perrin, a leading human resources consulting firm, found that high-performing companies have health costs that are about $1,500 U.S. less per employee when compared with costs of low performers and can offer health benefits to employees at an employee out-of-pocket cost that on average is 23% less than the out-of-pocket costs of employees at low-performing companies (40). The difference between high-performing and low-performing companies had more to do with a culture of wellness, the provision of health and productivity programs, rigorous attention to measurement and transparency, and high levels of employee engagement than cost cutting, reducing benefits, and passing more of the health care costs to the employee. This culture of wellness can be achieved through integrated workplace health programs with management support and a commitment to the long-term health of the employees.

The health of the workforce affects all of us, and making the effort to implement health and wellness programs is a worthy goal on many levels. While health care for the workforce is primarily funded by employers, the government is trying to encourage wellness programs through goals and tax incentives. The U.S. Department of Health and Human Services has established a goal of having 75% of all firms provide comprehensive wellness programs by 2010 (42). To provide incentives to businesses to implement comprehensive wellness programs for their employees, legislation has been introduced to provide a tax credit of up to 50% of the costs of employee wellness programs for employers who provide comprehensive wellness programs to their employees. If passed, the bipartisan Healthy Workforce Act of 2007 (S. 1753 IS; 29), introduced in July 2007 by Senators Tom Harkin (D-IA) and Gordon Smith (R-OR), will provide these credits for 10 y to employers whose programs meet at least 3 of 4 provisions including health awareness programs, behavioral change programs, an employee engagement committee, and an environment to encourage employee participation that includes offering incentives such as lower health insurance premiums. Perhaps though, the greatest proof of the value of workplace health and wellness programs is found outside the United States. In countries where the majority of health costs are borne by the state, such as Canada and the United Kingdom, workplace health and productivity programs are being embraced by businesses that find value in reducing job stress, absenteeism, presenteeism, and disability and realize that a healthy workforce is a productive workforce (13).

What Does the Future Offer?

The future of workplace health will include exciting advances in data integration and cost-effectiveness analysis. Connecting within the confines of the Health Insurance Portability and Accountability Act (HIPAA) regulations, data resources to patient care can have extraordinary influence on the health of a population. When large employer purchasers can tie the costs of health care, disability, and workers' compensation claims with productivity losses from absenteeism and presenteeism, their ability to promote and purchase effective programs will be enlightened. Additionally, these health-related productivity calculations will take into account secondary effects such as employee turnover and coworker effects as well as the influence that family illness and other personal issues can have on reduced performance of the index worker. The most sophisticated systems will be able to value four key drivers for large employer purchasers: workplace safety, quality of care, health care cost efficiencies, and employer of choice status.

Any and all efforts to improve the health of the workforce can come alive through integrated workplace efforts. The future will demonstrate near-perfect participation rates in wellness and disease management programs as companies develop a culture of health. To accomplish this employers will utilize communications, marketing, sales, facilities, environmental health and safety, and new product development as well as medical and benefits departments. It will require a village to build a culture of health. Those companies that demonstrate best practices receive support for these efforts from the CEO down. Coordinating a healthy work environment with strategic value-based benefits designs and comprehensive worksite medical services will demonstrate the most significant returns on the investment. Some companies will develop their own health plan, leveraging trusted clinicians working on-site to navigate employees to a directly contracted high-performance specialty network to improve the quality and the value of medical dollars spent. Providing these services will engender strong ties to employees, reduce turnover, and attract the best talent. As the reporting and analysis of the effects health can have on productivity mature, we will see more investment into human capital. Great companies will seek out people with the knowledge base necessary to do the job as well as the motivation to perform with excellence. Future human resource organizations will then be charged with keeping this group emotionally, spiritually, and physically well. Great companies in the future will pursue workforces with the skill and

the will to perform at high levels and will invest in keeping this valuable workforce from becoming ill. This will translate into significant productivity gains that yield community prosperity. Workplace health centers will be in the forefront of this effort. Accessible, available, and dedicated doctors, pharmacists, nurses, therapists, and sport physiologists will collaborate on-site to deliver a quantum improvement in health care delivery. And this care will provide industry-leading and innovative employers with a competitive edge.

Conclusion

As proposed by Adam Smith in the Wealth of Nations as early as 1776, healthy workers tend to be more productive workers, and this benefits the company as well as the employee. Workplace health centers have the ability to provide a set of services that positively impact the health of the employees and provide a point of integration for occupational health services and health promotion programs. As a result, workplace health centers represent an important component in a company's population health strategy. The results of implementing an integrated workplace health center program have shown significant improvements in absenteeism rates, overall productivity, worker's compensation claims, staff turnover, disability days, and health care costs.

Chapter Review Questions

1. Name seven or more components of occupational health services.
2. Identify eight or more health- or care-related programs that may be integrated through the use of a workplace health center.
3. Describe two examples of projects or studies that successfully associate health-related improvements with health-related expenses.

State of the Worksite Health Promotion Industry

The 2004 National Worksite Health Promotion Survey

Laura A. Linnan, ScD, CHES

Beginning in 1980, health professionals reached consensus on efforts that should be implemented to improve the public's health. National health objectives were developed and monitored over a 10 y time frame. *Healthy People 2010* is the current set of national objectives and includes two overall goals: (1) to improve the health and quality of life of the U.S. population and (2) to eliminate health disparities (15). In the service of those two goals, more than 400 specific, measurable objectives were established (the complete list of objectives can be found at http://healthypeople.gov). An important *Healthy People 2010* objective (number 7-5) directly targeted to worksites is to increase—to at least 75%—the proportion of worksites that offer a comprehensive employee health promotion program (15). National, state, and local health departments, private businesses, health agencies, managed care organizations, governmental agencies, and other employers are encouraged to integrate *Healthy People 2010* objectives into their strategic planning efforts.

Monitoring progress toward achieving this worksite-related objective has occurred as part of a series of national worksite health promotion surveys of employers. Specifically, nationally representative samples of employers completed phone surveys in 1985, 1992, 1999, and, most recently, 2004. The purpose of this chapter is to briefly review previous national monitoring efforts and to share selected results from the 2004 National Worksite Health Promotion Survey (NWHPS). In addition to monitoring national progress, employers may use these results as benchmarks for

achieving worksite-specific plans and establishing standards for success.

Monitoring Worksite Health Promotion Objectives— National Surveys (1985, 1992, 1999)

The first U.S. national worksite survey was conducted in 1985 with 1,358 completed interviews and a response rate of 83% (5). The exclusion criteria of the survey involved employers with less than 50 employees, public worksites, and governmental agencies. The instrument included questions about the responding employer, the employee demographics, and the presence or absence of nine different types of health promotion activities. Overall, 65.5% of responding worksites reported offering at least one type of health promotion activity, and larger worksites were more likely than smaller worksites to offer health promotion activities. Respondents from the western United States (73.4%) were somewhat more likely to offer health promotion activities than were worksites from other geographic regions. When all activities were considered, worksites were most likely to report (5) offering smoking cessation (35.6 %), which was followed by health risk assessments (29.5%), back problem prevention and care (28.5%), stress management (26.6%), exercise and fitness (22.1 %), and accident prevention (19.8%).

In 1992, the second national worksite survey was conducted to assess employer policies, practices, services and facilities, information, and activities related to employee health promotion. A total of 1,507 private U.S. worksites were included, representing 74% of eligible worksites (13). Again, worksites were categorized by industry, worksite size, and U.S. region. Similarly to the 1985 survey, employers with less than 50 employees, public worksites, and governmental agencies were excluded. Results indicated that 81% of responding worksites reported offering at least one health promotion activity, compared with 66% in 1985. Specifically, increases in the number of worksites reporting programs or activities addressing physical fitness and exercise, nutrition, weight control, stress management, back care, and blood pressure and cholesterol reduction were realized. An overall increase in preventive services (physical exams, cancer screening, blood sugar tests, blood pressure screening, or cholesterol tests) was also observed. In addition, the percentage of worksites with formal policies prohibiting or severely restricting smoking at the workplace more than doubled, increasing from 27% to 59%. As in 1985, larger worksites (750 or more employees) were more likely than smaller worksites to offer any type of health promotion activities. Some differences by industry type were identified (e.g., service and transportation industries were more likely to offer health risk appraisals and screenings), but no regional differences were observed.

In 1999, the NWHPS was conducted, garnering 1,544 completed worksite interviews among sites with 50 or more employees (14). The response rate was 60%, and the sample was stratified by size but not by industry type. Overall, 90% of worksites reported offering at least one health promotion activity for their employees, a number that was up from 81% in 1992. Across all worksites, physical activity programs (36%), substance abuse programs (28%), and stress management programs (26%) were offered most frequently. The screening programs most commonly offered were blood pressure (29%) and blood cholesterol (22%); cancer screenings (9%) were conducted far less often. As in previous surveys, larger worksites reported offering more health promotion programs and more screening or preventive services, and they were more likely to offer policies that support employee health. Additional questions on this survey queried respondents about the value of employee health and the business implications of poor health. For example, health care costs were identified most commonly by respondents as a serious threat to their ability to promote or maintain employee health and well-being (14).

In summary, these first three national surveys attempted to monitor progress toward achieving key national objectives for worksite health promotion. A first observation is that encouraging gains in the number and type of health promotion programs or activities have been reported by employers over time. Although this finding is promising, it is important to note that the definition of what qualifies as offering a health promotion program has evolved over time. Specifically, in 1985, an employer who reported offering any type of health promotion activity, program, or service was counted the same as an employer who offered a comprehensive, multilevel intervention. While subsequent surveys added measures to discern the number of activities offered, phone survey methods are not well-suited to assess the quality of the programming offered. Moreover, it is possible that some worksite respondents overreported health promotion activities to give a socially desirable response to the interviewer. Finally, these surveys have not provided insights into program effectiveness. While there have been positive trends since 1985, more details about the type and potential effects of these programs are warranted.

A second important observation from the previous survey results is that smaller worksites are significantly less likely than larger worksites to offer health promotion programs, preventive services, and supportive health policies. This trend is clear given that all three previous surveys have stratified by the same categories of employee size. Additionally, in most cases there is a clear dose–response relationship between worksite size and health promotion programming such that the smaller the worksite, the less likely it is to offer any type of programming, policy support, or preventive service. While differences by industry type changed over the survey years, differences by worksite size persisted. The remainder of this chapter focuses on the most recent national worksite health promotion survey and offers selected results to help clarify whether observations from previous surveys held true in 2004.

2004 National Worksite Health Promotion Survey

The 2004 national survey was developed, pilot tested, implemented, and analyzed by a national work group including worksite health promotion experts from the CDC, National Center for Health Statistics, Office of Disease Prevention and Health Promotion, Partnership for Prevention, Watson Wyatt Worldwide, and University of North Carolina at Chapel Hill. Support for the survey was provided by the U.S. Department of Health and Human Services, and the Robert Wood Johnson Foundation provided initial funding to Partnership for Prevention for staff support.

The aim of the work group was to develop a survey that would monitor progress toward the worksite-related *Healthy People 2010* objectives and allow for, when possible, meaningful comparisons between the 2004 survey and the previous survey results. In addition, working group members desired to address the fact that previous surveys had included private employers but not government employers or worksites with less than 50 employees. Thus, efforts were made to include these worksites in the sample drawn for 2004. However, only the results from nongovernment worksites and employers with at least 50 employees are reported here to facilitate comparisons with previous surveys.

Survey Sample and Key Measures

A cross-sectional, nationally representative sample of U.S. worksites was drawn from the Dun & Bradstreet database (3) of all private and public employers in the continental United States. The survey used a disproportionate stratified sampling design with 35 strata defined by two categories: (1) worksite size by number of employees (less than 50, 50-99, 100-249, 250-749, and 750 or more) and (2) industry type based on the U.S. Standard Industrial Classification (SIC) system (agriculture, mining, and construction; finance, insurance, and real estate; transportation, communications, and utilities; business and professional services; manufacturing; wholesale and retail trade; and public administration and government). Importantly, as in similar surveys, respondents were asked to answer questions for a specific worksite rather than for the company to which the worksite belonged.

The survey asked about selected health promotion programming, screening services, health-supportive environmental supports and policies, and several items addressing program supports, incentives, and benefits or challenges to offering worksite health promotion programs. In addition, the 2004 survey attempted to address the issue of whether an employer offered a comprehensive health promotion program as defined by *Healthy People 2010*. Such a program includes five key components: (1) health education (e.g.,

skill development and lifestyle behavior change along with information dissemination and awareness building), (2) supportive physical and social environments (e.g., an organization's implementation of policies and structures that promote health), (3) integration of the worksite program into the organization's structure (e.g., budget, dedicated staff, facilities), (4) linkage to related programs (e.g., safety, EAPs, and programs to help employees balance work and family), and (5) worksite screening programs (linked to medical care to ensure follow-up and appropriate treatment). If the respondent answered *yes* to all five elements, the program was designated as comprehensive.

Data Collection Procedures and Analysis Plan

Although initially the plan was to develop a Web-based version of the 2004 survey, response rates to initial testing of the instrument proved very low, and the work group returned to the phone survey format. The 20 min survey was conducted with the person at each worksite who was identified as being directly responsible for health promotion and wellness or who had an in-depth knowledge of these types of programs at the worksite. Once the data were collected and the initial cleaning was performed, analyses were carried out with the Surveyfreq and Surveylogistic procedures in SAS/STAT, version 9.1 of the SAS System (12). These procedures use a Taylor expansion approximation to calculate standard errors and corresponding 95% confidence intervals for stratified weighted data (1). Weights were computed as the inverse of selection probabilities and were adjusted for nonresponse. The Rao-Scott χ^2 statistic was used to assess differences by size and industry type (11), with a p-value of .05 or less indicating statistically significant results. The Surveylogistic procedure and Wald χ^2 statistic were used to fit logistic regression models comparing groups with and without a comprehensive health promotion program (7).

Results

The results of the 2004 NWHPS are presented in several sections. These include an overview of general characteristics of programs, health promotion activities and disease management programs, environmental activities, and comprehensive programs.

General Characteristics of Responding Worksites and Their Programs

Overall, 1,553 surveys were completed, which is a 59.7% response rate. After government employers and worksites with fewer than 50 employees were set aside, 730 respondents remained, including those with an employee size of 50 to 99 (n = 179), 100 to 249 (n = 229), 250 to 749 (n = 211), and more than 750 (n = 111). Industry categories by SIC included manufacturing (n = 198), finance (n = 85), wholesale and retail (n = 117), transportation (n = 73), agriculture (n = 86), and business and professional (n = 171).

Approximately 61% of the 2004 survey respondents held the title of director or manager, and the majority (52.7%) were from either the human resources or the benefits department. Most respondents identified themselves as being for-profit private organizations (63.4%), with fewer identifying themselves as for-profit, public (25.4%), and nonprofit (11.3%) organizations. The majority of worksites (64.6%) employed at least one full-time or part-time staff person directly responsible for health promotion and worksite wellness. Regarding history of offering worksite health promotion programs, among those with a program, the majority (60.8%) indicated that their program was in place for 5 y or less, while 30.5% of respondents indicated that their program was in place for 10 or more y and 8.7% had programs in place for 6 to 9 y. Nearly 70% of respondents believed that the worksite health promotion program was supportive of the organization's business strategy, but slightly less than 50% of respondents reported using data to guide the direction of the program. While 67.5% described their health promotion program as integrated into the health care strategy of the organization, only 30.2% of worksites had a 3 to 5 y plan in place for worksite health promotion.

Employers were also asked about funding for worksite health promotion programs. Health plans were the primary funder of most programs, and these were followed by the employer and shared funding (between the employee and the organization). For example, the majority of worksites that responded (68.1%) reported that the organization's health plan funded disease management programs. Additionally, 25.9% of worksites reported offering incentives to employees with the aim of increasing participation in worksite health programs; the decision to offer incentives did not differ by worksite size or industry type. Worksites reported similar barriers and challenges to the success of health promotion programs, regardless of industry type or worksite size. Lack of employee interest (63.5%) and lack of staff resources (50.1%) were cited as the most common barriers, followed by lack of management support and funding and low employee participation.

Health Promotion Classes and Activities, Screenings, and Disease Management Programs

Table 4.1 summarizes programs, activities, disease management programs, and preventive screenings offered overall and by worksite size. Across all programs and activities, 45.0% of respondents reported offering back injury prevention programs, and 44.7% offered EAPs. The next most prevalent programs offered were stress management (24.9%), nutrition (22.7%), health care consumerism (21.6%), and weight management (21.4%). Although industry type did not affect the offerings, there were statistically significant differences by worksite size in the prevalence of all programs offered, except for health care consumerism.

Among all respondents, the most prevalent screening program offered was high blood pressure (36.4%); it was followed by alcohol and drug abuse (35.9%), blood cholesterol (29.4%), diabetes (27.4%), and cancer (21.8%). Larger worksites were statistically more likely than smaller worksites to offer all screening programs. For example, 84.9% of worksites with 750 or more employees versus 27.1% of employers with 50 to 99 employees offered blood pressure screening.

For disease management programs, the most frequently offered program for all responding worksites was cardiovascular disease (CVD; 26.1%), followed by diabetes (25%), hypertension (22.8%), cancer (22.5%), and depression (20.5%). There were no statistical differences by worksite size among employers offering CVD or diabetes programs, but larger worksites were statistically more likely to offer all other disease management programs.

Selected Environmental Programs or Policies

Among all responding worksites, environmental supports for physical activity included access to on-site fitness facilities (14.9%), access to on-site shower facilities (27.6%), and signage to encourage stair use (6.2%). While 24% of worksites reported having access to an on-site cafeteria, the majority

Table 4.1 Selected Health Promotion Programs, Classes, and Screenings by Size of Workforce

Programs, classes, or activities	All worksites (n = 730) %, (95% CI)	50-99 employees (n = 179) %, (95% CI)	100-249 employees (n = 229) %, (95% CI)	250-749 employees (n = 211) %, (95% CI)	750+ employees (n = 111) %, (95% CI)
EAPs	44.7 (39.28, 50.13)	32.4 (23.49, 41.28)	48.07 (39.03, 57.12)	63.3 (52.40, 74.24)	84.2 (69.70, 98.62)
Smoking cessation	18.6 (14.51, 22.46)	8.8 (3.51, 14.12)	19.4 (12.66, 26.08)	32.0 (21.92, 42.17)	68.1 (53.13, 83.14)
Physical activity	19.6 (15.54, 23.67)	9.0 (3.67, 14.30)	23.6 (16.11, 31.11)	28.5 (19.50, 37.42)	66.1 (49.15, 83.10)
Cholesterol reduction	19.9 (15.55, 24.14)	16.4 (9.02, 23.87)	17.5 (11.41, 23.55)	29.3 (19.78, 38.86)	42.1 (23.80, 60.45)
Nutrition	22.7 (18.16, 27.24)	11.0 (4.61, 17.34)	30.4 (21.92, 38.85)	34.0 (23.50, 44.45)	43.0 (24.71, 61.35)
Stress management	24.9 (20.10, 29.86)	17.6 (9.92, 25.19)	27.7 (19.44, 35.92)	32.3 (22.20, 42.49)	54.3 (35.18, 73.39)
Weight management	21.4 (16.94, 25.93)	11.3 (5.11, 17.40)	24.8 (16.79, 32.86)	34.1 (23.81, 44.43)	56.1 (37.14, 75.14)
Back injury prevention	45.0 (39.28, 50.65)	37.2 (27.70, 46.67)	46.1 (37.08, 55.11)	55.7 (44.88, 66.56)	81.5 (71.80, 91.17)
Health care consumerism ns	21.6 (16.76, 26.48)	16.5 (8.64, 24.34)	27.0 (18.59, 35.35)	22.7 (14.69, 30.69)	27.6 (13.20, 42.02)
HIV/AIDS ns	14.6 (10.53, 18.70)	11.3 (4.55, 18.12)	14.2 (7.54, 20.92)	24.9 (15.51, 34.38)	16.8 (6.97, 26.72)
Screenings or counseling services					
Cancer screening	21.8 (17.45, 26.09)	14.3 (7.82, 20.74)	22.1 (14.90, 29.27)	29.4 (20.06, 38.67)	70.2 (55.57, 84.85)
Diabetes screening	27.4 (22.47, 32.25)	19.0 (11.50, 26.56)	27.7 (19.67, 35.68)	39.9 (29.39, 50.32)	70.2 (54.99, 85.46)
Blood pressure screening	36.4 (30.98, 41.74)	27.1 (18.22, 35.92)	35.8 (27.15, 44.35)	51.5 (40.41, 62.69)	84.9 (73.16, 96.63)
Blood cholesterol screening	29.4 (24.50, 34.39)	21.8 (13.77, 29.91)	26.8 (19.13, 34.49)	43.5 (32.94, 54.20)	80.5 (68.00, 93.01)
Alcohol or drug abuse support	35.9 (30.76, 41.09)	28.6 (20.14, 37.03)	37.3 (28.96, 45.65)	45.0 (34.20, 55.78)	70.7 (54.39, 86.94)
Disease management programs					
Diabetes	25.0 (20.10, 29.83)	21.8 (13.45, 30.08)	22.4 (15.40, 29.39)	33.6 (23.67, 43.53)	48.2 (28.63, 67.73)
Asthma ns	19.1 (14.84, 23.39)	15.8 (8.64, 22.95)	20.8 (13.97, 27.65)	18.7 (12.08, 25.37)	39.4 (19.10, 59.66)
Cancer ns	22.5 (17.66, 27.28)	17.5 (9.61, 25.44)	25.8 (17.78, 33.74)	27.9 (18.39, 37.38)	28.3 (14.62, 41.88)
Depression ns	20.5 (16.11, 24.87)	15.5 (8.44, 22.64)	24.3 (16.88, 31.69)	25.6 (16.92, 34.36)	23.2 (11.51, 34.95)
Hypertension ns	22.9 (18.10, 27.60)	20.1 (11.87, 28.31)	23.3 (15.94, 30.72)	28.1 (19.44, 36.77)	29.6 (13.94, 45.26)
Back pain ns	20.1 (15.59, 24.57)	16.1 (8.71, 23.42)	22.3 (14.86, 29.72)	23.4 (14.75, 31.95)	32.3 (15.71, 48.96)
CVD	26.1 (21.14, 31.10)	20.1 (12.73, 29.22)	27.8 (20.04, 35.59)	30.3 (20.51, 40.04)	50.9 (31.34, 70.36)
Chronic obstructive pulmonary disease ns	15.6 (11.62, 19.61)	13.3 (6.59, 19.98)	14.3 (8.55, 20.05)	21.7 (13.07, 30.25)	29.3 (9.53, 49.06)
Obesity	16.4 (12.22, 20.53)	11.9 (5.12, 18.61)	16.8 (10.00, 23.56)	29.1 (19.27, 38.92)	16.6 (7.70, 25.56)
High-risk pregnancy	18.6 (14.22, 22.94)	14.8 (7.39, 22.14)	18.8 (12.35, 25.21)	22.7 (14.43, 31.05)	41.4 (21.23, 61.49)

ns = statistically not significantly different; CI = confidence interval.

(79.6%) had vending machines with food and beverages available for employees. Moreover, 37.4% of worksites reported labeling healthy food choices, and 5.6% of worksites offered promotions for choosing healthy foods. Nearly all worksites had policies prohibiting alcohol use (91.1%) and drug use (93.4%), while 85.8% had policies prohibiting firearms. The majority of responding worksites had restrictive smoking policies; 56.5% restricted smoking to outside areas and 39.9% prohibited smoking on the property. Statistically significant differences by worksite size were observed for the majority of environmental programs and policies (table 4.2).

Table 4.2 Selected Environmental and Policy Characteristics by Worksite Size

	All worksites (n = 730) %, (95% CI)	50-99 employees %, (95% CI)	100-249 employees %, (95% CI)	250-749 employees %, (95% CI)	750+ employees %, (95% CI)
Physical environment					
On-site fitness center	14.6 (9.97, 19.14)	9.8 (2.20, 17.30)	13.17 (5.63, 20.71)	17.5 (9.46, 25.50)	49.6 (29.98, 69.24)
On-site shower facilities	27.6 (22.87, 32.36)	20.9 (13.59, 28.15)	29.7 (21.43, 37.99)	32.4 (23.28, 41.50)	63.8 (45.54, 82.11)
Signage to promote stair use	6.2 (3.57, 8.85)	2.1 (0.12, 4.01)	11.7 (5.14, 18.32)	4.2 (1.57, 6.74)	11.4 (3.45, 19.24)
Fitness or walking trails	13.5 (9.66, 17.28)	7.7 (2.17, 13.13)	13.9 (7.22, 20.64)	22.1 (12.62, 31.59)	40.5 (21.83, 59.16)
Cafeteria	24.0 (19.39, 28.65)	12.9 (5.92, 19.97)	24.5 (17.02, 31.95)	41.9 (30.75, 52.98)	74.1 (59.13, 88.71)
Labeling of healthy food choices	37.4 (26.32, 48.56)	34.6 (6.50, 62.75)	28.8 (11.39, 46.26)	32.4 (16.50, 48.37)	73.1 (53.64, 92.63)
Special promotions	5.6 (3.07, 8.09)	3.9 (0.00, 8.03)	5.4 (1.37, 9.42)	7.4 (3.62, 11.12)	18.6 (4.46, 32.71)
Vending with healthy food and beverage choices	79.6 (74.5, 84.7)	70.8 (61.47, 80.17)	82.1 (74.16, 90.01)	95.9 (92.67, 99.21)	95.4 (91.12, 99.61)
Policies					
Fitness breaks provided	12.4 (8.59, 16.21)	11.0 (4.59, 17.48)	13.0 (7.02, 18.95)	13.5 (6.08, 20.97)	17.6 (4, 21, 31.37)
Catering policy	6.1 (0.00, 11.49)	6.3 (0.85, 11.79)	5.7 (1.37, 9.93)	4.7 (0.00, 10.35)	12.4 (1.69, 23.09)
Smoking completely prohibited on property	39.9 (34.12, 45.65)	34.2 (24.66, 43.73)	45.6 (36.52, 54.61)	40.8 (29.98, 51.60)	48.5 (28.91, 68.26)
Smoking restricted to designated areas inside	34.7 (27.81, 41.48)	32.0 (21.01, 43.03)	36.4 (25.25, 47.46)	39.3 (25.88, 52.73)	36.3 (18.94, 53.56)
Smoking restricted to outside	56.5 (49.24, 63.77)	50.8, (38.90, 62.67)	56.5 (44.59, 68.35)	70.3 (59.31, 81.30)	77.4 (64.17, 90.61)
Alcohol policy	91.1 (87.46, 94.75)	86.3 (79.55, 92.96)	93.2 (87.67, 98.75)	98.5 (97.02, 100.00)	99.2 (98.18, 100.00)
Drug policy	93.4 (90.30, 96.54)	91.8 (86.37, 97.36)	94.4 (89.46, 99.30)	94.2 (88.36, 100.00)	99.2 (98.18, 100.00)
Occupant protection	45.0 (39.18, 50.98)	49.0 (39.22, 59.00)	38.9 (29.83, 48.00)	45.6 (34.40, 56.72)	53.2 (35.54, 71.03)
Firearms prohibited	85.8 (81.75, 90.01)	83.0 (75.66, 90.43)	87.5 (81.09, 93.97)	87.4 (79.72, 95.05)	96.3 (92.11, 100.00)

CI = confidence interval.

Comprehensive Worksite Health Promotion Programs

When all worksites were considered, 6.9% offered all five key elements of a comprehensive worksite health promotion program (table 4.3); statistically significant differences were observed by worksite size. For example, 24.1% of worksites with 750 or more employees offered a comprehensive program, compared with 4.6% of worksites with 50 to 99 employees, 6.0% of worksites with 100 to 249 employees, and 11.3% of worksites with 250 to 749 employees. Here, industry type revealed differences, as manufacturing and business and

professional services sectors were significantly more likely than all other industry types to offer comprehensive programs. Among the five key elements, linkages to related programs such as EAPs and programs to help employees balance work and family (41.3%) were most commonly reported, followed by a supportive social and physical environment (29.9%), integration of programs into the organizational structure (28.6%), health education programming (26.2%), and worksite screening programs with appropriate follow-up and treatment (23.5%).

Worksites with fewer employees were less likely to offer a comprehensive program and were

Table 4.3   Five Key Elements of a Comprehensive Health Promotion Program by Worksite Size

	All worksites ($n = 730$)	50-99 employees ($n = 179$)	100-249 employees ($n = 229$)	250-749 employees ($n = 211$)	750+ employees ($n = 111$)	p-value
All elements	6.9 (3.87, 10.02)	4.6 (0.00, 9.36)	6.0 (1.72, 10.33)	11.3 (3.80, 18.76)	24.1 (4.03, 44.21)	.03
Health education	26.2 (21.54, 30.84)	17.8 (10.37, 25.32)	26.2 (18.80, 33.67)	38.1 (27.61, 48.49)	70.3 (54.22, 86.40)	.0001
Supportive social and physical environment	29.9 (24.67, 35.03)	24.0 (15.28, 32.73)	32.5 (24.40, 40.68)	33.5 (23.43, 43.63)	53.7 (34.70, 72.80)	.04
Integration	28.6 (23.37, 33.74)	20.6 (12.24, 29.05)	33.3 (24.85, 41.75)	30.9 (20.62, 41.17)	61.4 (43.20, 79.54)	.0015
Linkage with EAPs	41.3 (35.87, 46.71)	29.6 (20.68, 38.43)	43.7 (34.66, 52.70)	59.3 (47.87, 70.82)	80.5 (65.61, 95.36)	<.001
Worksite screening	23.5 (18.68, 28.27)	15.8 (8.07, 23.49)	25.3 (17.58, 33.05)	30.5 (20.99, 39.96)	62.4 (44.10, 80.76)	<.001

also less likely to offer any one of the five key elements. For example, while 80.5% of worksites with 750 or more employees offered linkages to EAPs, only 29.6% of those with 50 to 99 employees, 43.7% of those with 100 to 299 employees, and 59.3% of those with 250 to 749 employees offered linkages (table 4.3). Logistic regression analyses revealed that after controlling for worksite size, years of experience with a wellness program, and industry type, a worksite with a dedicated staff person was more than 10 times more likely than a worksite without a dedicated staff person to have a comprehensive worksite wellness program (8).

Discussion

A worksite-related *Healthy People 2010* objective aims to increase, to at least 75%, the percentage of employers that offer a comprehensive worksite health promotion program (15). Previous national worksite health promotion surveys (1985, 1992, 1999) and the recent 2004 survey have monitored the extent to which a nationally representative sample of worksites is progressing toward this objective. Results from the 2004 survey indicated that only 6.9% of worksites offered all five key elements included in the definition of a comprehensive program. There were statistically significant differences among worksites by size such that 24.1% of worksites with 750 or more employees offered a comprehensive program, compared with only 4.6% of worksites with 50 to 99 employees. When considering the extent to which worksites offered at least one or more of the five key elements, 9.7% of all worksite respondents answered *yes* to offering health education programming, a supportive worksite environment, and worksite screening programs (three key elements), and 16.7% of respondents reported *yes* to offering at

least health education programming and a supportive worksite environment (two key elements). However, even with these more inclusive ways of describing the extent to which worksites are offering health promotion programs, the 2004 survey found that, compared to earlier surveys, fewer worksites offered health promotion programs, and significant differences continued to persist by worksite size (e.g., smaller worksites were less likely to offer these elements). Thus, it remains clear that much improvement is needed to achieve the national objective of at least 75% of worksites offering a comprehensive worksite health promotion program.

A second important observation from the 2004 NWHPS results is that worksites with 750 or more employees typically offered more health promotion programs, screening programs, disease management programs, environmental supports, and health-supportive policies than smaller worksites offered. This trend has persisted over the past three decades, and it is imperative to understand why these patterns exist so that small businesses can begin to share in the many benefits of employee health promotion programs. Several plausible reasons are offered here. First, smaller worksites are resource constrained (direct costs) and are less likely to have experienced staff or resources to dedicate to worksite health promotion programs (indirect costs). Most small worksites must attend to the survival of the business; time, effort, and resources (people and money) are dedicated to keeping the business viable rather than to starting new initiatives. Thus, the direct and indirect costs of offering worksite wellness programs may be too big a barrier for small businesses to overcome. On a related note, small businesses may face competing demands for time and resource allocations to meet production or service goals, to operate efficiently, and to grow the business. As human capital needs and resources are constantly being juggled, employee health promotion may be low on the list of priorities for small-business owners.

A second reason why this problem has persisted is that fewer small businesses offer health insurance for their employees. For example, while 98% of businesses with 200 or more employees offer health benefits, only 59% of firms with less than 200 workers offer health benefits to employees (2). This lack of health insurance severely limits access to health and medical care for employees, so that employees of small businesses are at high risk if any type of medical problem or accident occurs. Because health insurers are the leading source of funding for most behavior change, preventive screening, and disease management programs, it is not surprising that employers that do not offer health insurance are less likely to have these programs available.

Wilson (16) conducted a nationally representative survey of small businesses and learned that employers with 50 to 99 employees differed from those with less than 50 employees in nearly all categories. For example, employers in the 50 to 99 category were more likely to offer employee health insurance, had more formalized health-related policies and practices, and offered more health promotion programming. These employers were also more likely to have dedicated staff for health promotion, occupational health and safety, and EAPs (16). The 2004 NWHPS results point out the importance of having a dedicated staff person because doing so increases the likelihood that comprehensive worksite health promotion programs can be implemented. Small businesses are less likely to have dedicated staff or health insurance.

One final reason why small businesses are less likely to offer worksite health promotion programs is linked to the small-business culture and the leadership tendencies of the owners. Eakin (4) conducted an important study in which she interviewed 53 small-business owners to investigate the role of manager beliefs and attitudes in framing the meaning and experience of work in small-business environments. Her results revealed that the prevailing way of managing health and safety issues is to leave it up to the workers, as is exemplified when owners say they do not want to meddle in the private lives of employees.

Comparing the 2004 NWHPS results with those of previous years is challenging due to differences in the wording and phrasing of a number of questions. However, it is important to note that, over time, health promotion programming has remained relatively stable among worksites with more than 750 employees, while a noticeable decline in programming appears to have occurred in worksites with fewer than 750 employees. While it is possible that a real drop-off has occurred among smaller worksites in that 5 y time frame, measurement error may account for some of the difference. While results were reported from a nationally representative sample in each survey, the surveys were all cross-sectional—therefore, direct comparisons from year to year are subject to differences based on different samples, changes in the larger social context, or chance. Moreover, despite efforts to ask comparable questions, even small changes in the way that questions were worded or asked may have influenced responses.

It is worth noting, however, that the 2004 and 1999 surveys asked identical questions regarding perceived barriers to offering worksite health promotion programs (14). In 2004, 63.5% of worksites reported that lack of employee interest was a barrier to offering health promotion programs, compared with only 49.6% of worksites in 1999 ($p = .003$). Thus, responding worksites in 2004 reported an increase in perceived barriers to offering worksite health promotion programs. Logically, an increase in perceived (or actual) barriers may be associated with a decline in health promotion programs offered.

Finally, in the 2004 survey results, almost no differences by industry type were observed when health promotion programs, activities, classes, screenings, disease management programs, physical environment, and policies were considered. Thus, while it may be important to tailor worksite wellness programs to a particular work environment, assisting smaller worksites within a given industry sector seems as important as targeting a particular industry type.

Implications for Practice

Much work is needed if we are to achieve the *Healthy People 2010* objective of at least 75% of employers offering a comprehensive worksite health promotion program. An important recommendation is that employers identify and then allocate at least a portion of staff time to worksite wellness. Having a dedicated staff person significantly increases the likelihood of having a comprehensive program, making this an important recommendation for worksites of all sizes.

Dedicated facilities and budgets are also likely to be helpful, but dedicated staff is paramount.

Increasing the likelihood that health promotion is integrated into the organizational structure is needed as well. EAPs offer a wide range of mental health programs and services that improve the mental and emotional health of employees. Since stress and depression are among the leading health care costs in most work environments (9), finding ways to link and cross-promote EAPs as part of health promotion is a win–win situation. Moreover, integrating safety and health-related programs is another approach that can tie into ongoing initiatives, creating economies of scale in resource-constrained environments.

Creating a health-supportive work environment is likely to be a cost-efficient way to offer wellness programming. Policy changes (e.g., healthy food and catering policies) may be relatively inexpensive to implement, and some policies (e.g., restrictive smoking policies or total smoking bans) may stimulate cost savings to employers by reducing facility cleaning costs or fire insurance premiums. Changes in the physical environment (e.g., installing showers, developing walking trails, or offering a salad bar) may have higher initial costs but may produce added benefits in improved employee morale and health in the future. Moreover, both policies and environmental supports are relatively permanent changes for the work environment. For example, the majority of worksites in the 2004 NWHPS, regardless of size, reported having food or beverage vending machines. An employer that advocates for healthy food or beverage options to be added to the current list of offerings may be able to improve access to healthy food options at work at no additional cost.

Partnerships with insurance providers, local health agencies and hospitals, health departments, and unions may lead to an increase in the offering of disease management programs, screening programs, and other health promotion services. For example, local universities or community colleges may have student nurses who need to practice conducting blood pressure screenings and might be willing to offer such screenings for an employer group. Partnerships, especially for small businesses, can help fill gaps in programs and services at a relatively low cost to the employer. Evaluating the success of these programs and building the business case for offering worksite health promotion programs— particularly for small businesses—should be an ongoing priority. Taken together, these strategies offer suggestions for increasing the likelihood that worksites of all sizes can meet each of the five key elements of a comprehensive worksite health promotion program.

Implications for Research

The 2004 NWHPS results reveal several important areas for future research. First, it is essential that monitoring of employer-based worksite health promotion continue on a regular basis. Thus, at least every 5 y, a national survey that allows for comparisons of trends should be sponsored. It would also be useful to ensure that questions related to safety, the five elements of comprehensive programs, and employee participation in programs are included. Second, it would be extremely beneficial to monitor employee participation in worksite health promotion efforts. Such participation was studied using National Health Interview Survey data reporting on access to and participation in worksite health promotion programs by employed people in the general population (6). This information can assist in monitoring the *Healthy People 2010* objective to increase to at least 75% employee participation in worksite health promotion programs (15). Third, research that helps clarify how safety and health programs are best integrated would be helpful. NIOSH has funded several Centers for Excellence that are working to address this issue (9). Finally, in addition to monitoring employers, it would be useful to do qualitative research involving in-depth interviews or case studies of worksites that have experienced great success (or extreme challenges) in carrying out a worksite health promotion program.

Conclusion

Regular monitoring of the worksite health promotion activity across the United States provides data sources for benchmarking purposes and can serve as an important surveillance and planning source for national health objectives such as *Healthy People 2010*. The 2004 NWHPS shows that only 6.9% of responding worksites offer comprehensive worksite health promotion programs. Significant differences in the number of comprehensive programs as well as the number of activities offered within such programs exist across companies of different size—smaller employers lag significantly behind larger employers. Increasing the number, quality, and types of worksite health promotion programs represents an important goal for the corporate setting in order to address health care cost trends and remains an important public health goal.

Chapter Review Questions

1. Describe the five key elements of a comprehensive worksite health promotion program as defined by *Healthy People 2010*.

2. Explain three reasons why small worksites are less likely to offer worksite health promotion programs for their employees.

3. List at least three strategies employers might use to increase the likelihood that their worksites offer all five elements of a comprehensive worksite health promotion program.

4. State two implications of the NWHPS results for improving practice.

5. State two research implications of the NWHPS results.

5

Health Promotion Programming in Small, Medium, and Large Businesses

Heather M. Bowen, MS, RD, LD; Todd D. Smith, MS, CSP, ARM; Mark G. Wilson, HSD; and David M. Dejoy, PhD

During the past two decades, health promotion activities and services have become increasingly common in American workplaces. This growth has been documented through a series of national worksite health promotion surveys beginning in 1985. In the 1985 survey, about 66% of private companies with 50 or more employees indicated that they offered at least one health promotion activity to their employees; this number increased to 81% in 1992 and 90% in 1999. The national surveys show quite clearly that the prevalence of health promotion activities varies considerably between large employers and small employers, with large employers (i.e., those with 750 or more employees) typically offering the most programs and activities to their employees (1,6,25).

With this background provided by the national surveys as the starting point, this chapter compares and contrasts program design features and health promotion offerings among small, medium, and large employers and presents recommendations for improving program quality, availability, and access, making special reference to smaller organizations. From our perspective, small-business employees are a huge and underserved market in terms of worksite health promotion. According to the U.S. Bureau of Labor Statistics, in 2004 more than 40% of the American private sector workforce worked for businesses of 50 or fewer employees (23). More than 70% worked for businesses with fewer than 250 employees. We begin this chapter by discussing some of the distinguishing characteristics of small employers.

Characteristics of Small Versus Large Employers

There are no hard-and-fast rules about how many employees constitute a small, medium, or large business. Even the U.S. Small Business Administration (SBA) uses different definitions for its many programs and services. In some instances, employers with 500 or fewer employees are considered small businesses, while in other instances the defining number may be 250 or 100 employees. The SBA definitions also vary from industry to industry in terms of the numerical values used to identify qualifying small businesses (26). In some instances, annual revenues are factored into the classification process. To add to the confusion, the definitions pertinent to small business that are used by other governmental agencies sometimes refer to *business establishments* and at other times to *business firms*. According to the U.S. Office of Management and Budget (21), "an establishment is an economic unit, generally at a single physical location, where business is conducted or where services or industrial operations are performed." An establishment may be a branch plant or a warehouse facility of a larger company rather than an independent entity. In contrast, a firm is a separate and independent operation; it may or may not consist of multiple establishments.

Small and large businesses possess other distinguishing characteristics that present both challenges and opportunities for health promotion programming. For example, employment in small businesses is not distributed uniformly across industries. Industries such as construction, wholesale trade, and retail trade have large proportions of their total workforce in small businesses. Employees working in the manufacturing, transportation, and public utilities sectors, on the other hand, are more likely to work for large employers (32). Small businesses are also more likely to be located in rural areas and to be of more recent origin (27,28). The mix of employees is also different in small businesses. Small businesses have fewer employees in management, administrative support, and sales and a larger proportion of employees directly involved in production or service delivery.

Small firms tend to employ more workers who are under age 25 or over age 65. There are also some differences in workforce diversity among small and large businesses. Overall, Whites and Hispanics are somewhat more likely to work in smaller firms, while Asians, Blacks, and women are somewhat less likely to work in these firms. With the notable exception of medical and certain other professional practice firms, small businesses tend to have more employees with a high school education or less (12). In addition, many low-wage earners work for small businesses, and a higher proportion of small-business employers are likely to be receiving some form of public assistance. Small businesses also have more part-time workers, and these workers are less likely to have access to employer-provided health insurance and other benefits. Fewer small businesses are offering health benefits due to increasing costs, and those who do offer health insurance are increasing employee contributions, changing insurance companies, and changing to policies with higher deductibles (17). Unfortunately the smallest businesses that do not provide health benefits also tend to have lower wages, a younger workforce, more part-time workers, and more women and minority employees who are unlikely to have the resources to purchase individual health plans on their own (7).

Availability of Health Promotion Activities and Services

Current knowledge about the availability of health initiatives in American workplaces comes almost exclusively from national surveys conducted in 1985, 1992, 1999, and 2004. These surveys assessed the prevalence of health promotion activities rather than health promotion programs,

simply asking employers whether they had offered employees any information or activities during the previous 12 mo. Nevertheless, these surveys do provide a useful gauge of the range of topics addressed by employers of different sizes. From these surveys, we know that larger businesses, defined as having 750 or more employees, are more likely to offer health promotion programs, classes, and activities as well as screenings and disease management programs (1,14,25). The percent of worksites offering at least one health promotion activity increases with the size of the worksites. In 2004, the most commonly reported programs, classes, and activities were EAPs, back injury prevention, and stress management (14). Despite the increasing incidence of chronic health problems related to poor diet and lack of physical activity, there are large differences in the availability of lifestyle programs. For example, less than 10% of businesses with 50 to 99 employees reported providing physical activity programs, classes, or activities, whereas approximately 50% of businesses with 750 or more employees reported providing such programs.

One gap in these surveys is that none of them reported data for businesses with fewer than 50 employees. Wilson and colleagues (33) analyzed data for businesses with as few as 15 employees. Using a set of health promotion questions contained in the CDC national Business Responds to AIDS survey, they found that worksites with 15 to 99 employees offered significantly fewer programs than businesses with 100 or more employees offered. The smaller worksites were also less likely to offer nutrition and weight management programs, blood pressure and cholesterol screening, and health risk appraisals (HRAs). The Wilson and colleagues study (33) also assessed programs instead of activities. Programs were defined as "formal, planned sessions that address any health-related issue and that are offered on a regular basis" (p. 360). McMahan and associates (15) sampled 1,846 small businesses in California and divided the businesses into three size categories: 2 to 14 employees, 15 to 99 employees, and 100 to 500 employees. Business size was a strong predictor of programming, with smaller companies offering fewer health promotion activities. Furthermore, the activities offered by smaller employers tended to emphasize safety-related topics (15). This focus on safety-related topics among small businesses has been noted by other researchers (2,33).

Another limitation of the U.S. national surveys is that they only sampled employers from the private sector. Governmental workers at the local, state, and federal levels are a considerable portion of the labor market, making up about 16% of the total American workforce (23). Grosch and colleagues (11) analyzed data from the 1994 National Health Interview Survey (NHIS) and included as respondents those employed in either the private or the public sector. Although these researchers did not provide results in terms of employer size, they found that employees of the federal government enjoyed the highest availability of most types of health promotion services, while private-sector employees had the least access to such services. State and local employees fell in between these groups.

Because the Grosch and colleagues study (11) analyzed data collected from individual employees, they were able to examine availability as a function of demographics (see table 5.1). Availability did not vary as a function of gender, but the very youngest category of workers (aged 18-24) reported less availability than did older workers. Availability was somewhat lower for Blacks than it was for other ethnic groups, but these differences were not large. On the other hand, availability increased consistently with increasing level of education.

Access to Health Promotion Activities and Services

While employees cannot access programs that do not exist, the mere existence of activities and services is no guarantee that all employees have equal access to them. In today's work world, any number of factors at both the individual and the organizational level may facilitate or hinder access. Data directly pertinent to program access are quite limited, and we often rely on program participation data to draw conclusions about access. In the previously mentioned Grosch and colleagues study (11), the authors reported that about 82% of respondents indicated that at least one health program activity or service was available at their workplace during the preceding 12 mo. Close to 50% of respondents reported having used an activity or a service during this same time. As shown in table 5.1, reported participation levels did not vary appreciably by either gender or educational level. Differences were somewhat more apparent for age and ethnicity. Perhaps most interesting is that while Blacks have slightly

Table 5.1 Health Promotion Program Availability and Participation by Gender, Age, Race, and Education

	% Available	% Participated
Gender		
Male	39.9	40.6
Female	39.4	39.7
Age (y)		
18-24	26.4	35.5
25-39	39.7	41.6
40-54	43.7	40.7
55+	38.6	35.2
Race		
Black	39.9	44.7
White	42.9	39.7
Other	42.1	38.3
Education		
0-11 y	24.6	39.8
High school degree	34.5	41.9
Some college	41.9	42.2
College or more	48.8	37.4

Data from J.W. Grosch, T. Alterman, M.R. Peterson, and L. Murphy, 1998, "Worksite health promotion programs in the US: Factors associated with availability and participation, *American Journal of Health Promotion* 13(1):36-45.

fewer programs available to them, they tend to participate at higher levels. Program availability increased steadily with level of education, though participation remained relatively constant—that is, better-educated workers did not participate more than did workers with less education.

Although larger businesses may offer a wider array of health promotion activities and services, their participation levels are not necessarily higher. In fact, a California small-business survey (15) found that smaller companies enjoyed higher participation levels in six different programming areas: weight management, violence prevention, immunization, mental health, ergonomics, and first aid training. Quite clearly, employers can enhance access through the adoption of supportive policies and work rules, the investment of financial and organizational resources, the provision of supportive environmental features, and the use of various incentives to encourage employees to participate in health promotion programming. Larger employers are more likely to have separate departments and dedicated staff for programming (33), but there does not seem to be wide variation in the use of financial and other incentives among companies of differing sizes (14). For example, in the 2004 survey, about 23% of the small employers (with 50-99 employees) used incentives to promote participation, compared with about 29% of the largest employers (with 750 or more employees). On the other hand, larger worksites are more likely to offer an environment supportive of physical activity and healthy eating, with features such as shower facilities, fitness centers, walking trails, and cafeterias. The larger worksites are also more likely to have policies to support good health practices. For example, 34% of businesses with 50 to 99 employees completely banned smoking on their premises, compared with 49% of businesses with 750 or more employees.

Quality of Health Promotion Activities and Services

Unfortunately, we have very little direct evidence that speaks to the quality of health promotion programming being offered in organizations of varying sizes. With respect to health promotion programming in general, there are no established or consensus standards pertaining to quality.

We sometimes use employee participation rates to gauge quality or to show program value, but the fact remains that effectiveness—not participation—is the core element of quality. In simplest terms, we can define effectiveness by asking the following: Does the program, activity, or service do what it is supposed to do for employees? Good evaluation data are crucial to determining effectiveness and thus quality. The published research literature mostly contains studies conducted on very large and well-known companies, and in general, we do know that comprehensive programs and multi-component programs are more effective than less-comprehensive efforts (5,13,20).

As noted earlier in this chapter, large employers typically offer more health promotion activities and services to their employees, but this alone does not qualify as comprehensive programming. According to *Healthy People 2010* (24), a comprehensive program should contain five elements: (1) health education programs, (2) supportive social and physical environments, (3) integration of health promotion into the organization's structure, (4) linkages to related programs such as EAPs, and (5) worksite screening programs with medical follow-up as needed. On the 2004 worksite survey, employers were asked whether each of these elements was part of their health promotion efforts. Combining worksites of all sizes showed that only about 7% included all five elements, and the percentage of worksites offering each element almost doubles

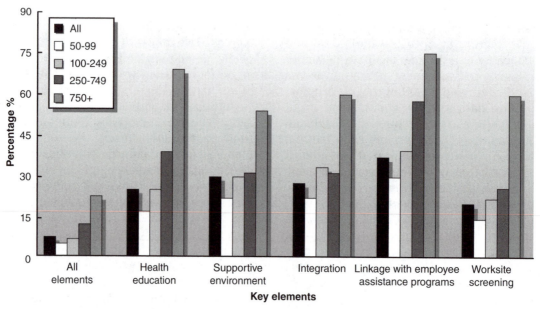

Figure 5.1 Percentage of U.S. worksites providing the key elements of a comprehensive worksite health promotion program.
Data from L. Linnan et al. 2008, "Results of the 2004 national worksite health promotion survey," *American Journal of Public Health* 98:1503-1509 (14).

from the smallest worksites to the largest worksites (see figure 5.1). Of the largest companies (750 or more employees), slightly less than 1 in 4 (24%) met the *Healthy People 2010* definition of comprehensive programming. Comprehensive efforts were most likely to be available in the manufacturing and business and professional services sectors and least likely to be available in the wholesale and retail, transportation, financial, and agriculture and mining sectors.

There have been several benchmark studies specifically directed at identifying best practices for worksite health promotion programming (8,10,18,29). In the most recent of these studies, Goetzel and colleagues (10) came up with a list of elements that is not that different from the list of objectives in *Healthy People 2010*. Their list included (1) integrating program features into the organization's operations; (2) simultaneously addressing individual, environmental, policy, and cultural needs; (3) targeting the most important health issues; (4) tailoring programs to meet specific needs; (5) attaining high participation and engagement; (6) rigorously evaluating programs; and (7) communicating successful outcomes to key stakeholders. This list of best practices reinforces the emphasis on comprehensiveness but also adds important process or programming elements related to needs assessment, evaluation, and communication.

Two additional considerations related to quality deserve mention. The first involves the process for selecting the specific health promotion interventions to be implemented in a particular organization. Besides conducting good needs assessments, employers should give priority to choosing evidence-based interventions, such as those detailed in the *Guide to Community Preventive Services* (the *Community Guide*). The *Community Guide,* which compiles peer-reviewed evidence and assesses the available evidence in terms of effectiveness concerning various intervention strategies for health promotion (3), may be the closest thing we have in terms of quality standards (see chapters 9, 10, 11, and 17 for more on the *Community Guide*). The other additional indicator of quality is to develop broad-spectrum programs. Such programs not only include health enhancement (improving and maintaining the status of essentially healthy employees) but also address risk management, demand management, disease management, and disability management (31). This is especially important given the aging U.S. workforce and the current distribution of expenditures for health care.

The Small-Business Conundrum

Small businesses are an important part of our economy and the source of employment for the majority of workers in the United States. Improving health promotion programming in small businesses is not an insignificant public health issue. Without question, small businesses face a number of obstacles in being able to develop and implement high-quality health promotion programs for their employees. On the other hand, some of these challenges may be viewed as potential opportunities. Table 5.2 describes some of these issues.

Strategies for Expanding Health Promotion in Small Businesses

It seems quite apparent that any substantial expansion of health promotion programs within small, and many midsize, businesses is going to require creative solutions and, in all likelihood, the involvement of both governmental and nongovernmental organizations. Most businesses in this size range are not able to fund or staff their own self-contained, in-house program—nor are they likely to be able to hire outside vendors to develop and implement a customized and comprehensive program. The need to expand prevention and health promotion programming within small businesses is not just a private-sector issue. Many of these workers come from underserved and underrepresented groups that mirror the health disparities that exist in American society. From the perspective of economic development, many large national corporations started as small businesses, and small businesses have long been effective incubators for new ideas and technological innovations.

Private-public partnerships may provide an important mechanism for expanding health promotion programming among small and midsize businesses. As envisioned, such partnerships would bring together state and local health departments, hospitals, voluntary health organizations, business councils, public or private economic development agencies, small-business assistance programs, and other community resources. The direct participation of insurers would also benefit these partnerships. Many of these organizations already have formalized community outreach

Table 5.2   Worksite Health Promotion Obstacles and Opportunities for Small Businesses

Challenges	Opportunities
Small businesses typically offer fewer health promotion activities and services to their employees.	Small businesses tend to have more low-wage earners, more part-time employees, and more employees with lower levels of education. On the positive side, small businesses also possess some attributes that may be advantageous in terms of developing high-quality health promotion programs for their employees.
Small businesses are less likely to offer programs that meet current recommendations for comprehensiveness or high quality. Small businesses are increasingly less able to provide health insurance and other related benefits to their employees.	Small businesses often have closer and more supportive social environments than larger organizations have, and there is usually less formality and administrative distance between supervisors and employees.
Small businesses typically have more limited budgets, more immediate competing needs and priorities, and less staff expertise related to health promotion.	Small businesses are often more integrated into their local communities and have greater knowledge of, and access to, local institutions, resources, and policy makers.
Small businesses are overrepresented in some of the industrial sectors that have traditionally had the least amount of health promotion programming available; many small businesses also are in industries that pose substantial health and safety risks to employees.	Employees in small businesses appear to be as interested in health promotion activities and services as their counterparts in large businesses, and they may be more likely to participate in the programs that are available.
	Small businesses provide many Americans with their first work opportunities and are entry points for a diverse array of people, including young workers, old workers, workers resuming employment after rearing families, part-time workers, immigrants, and workers with limited job skills and formal education.
	Small businesses also provide important entrepreneurial opportunities for women and minorities.

missions, so their involvement in a partnership for worksite health promotion would involve refocusing current activities rather than adding entirely new programs or obligations. Community coalitions are not a new strategy in public health (4,16), but their potential has not been exploited in the context of worksite programming.

In essence, the purpose of these partnerships would be to overcome the obstacles small businesses face. The major goal would be to bring together a coordinated set of evidence-based health promotion programs and services and to make them readily available to small employers. Participating small or midsize businesses would then publicize the availability of the programs and facilitate the participation of their employees through flexible work scheduling, incentives, or other means. Depending on the funding or resources available, employers would pay a per-employee fee or otherwise contribute to the costs of the programs and services offered. Certain economies of scale could be created that would keep costs at a modest level and support consistent, high-quality programming.

A key task of these partnerships would be to establish a method whereby small-business owners and managers could be informed and educated about the benefits of disease prevention and health promotion programming (22,30). The objective here would not be to convert these owners and managers into health promotion specialists but to raise their consciousness and make them more aware of the available programs and services and the ways such programs and services could help both their employees and their businesses. This educational and awareness effort would also provide useful networking opportunities for small-business owners and managers. Arguably, a healthy and productive workforce is especially critical to small businesses, as absences, major illnesses, and other disruptions to production can have immediate and severe consequences in operations where every employee counts, where specialized skills are difficult to replace, and where business competition is severe and profit margins are small.

Most small-business owners in the United States are more familiar with occupational safety and health (OSH) programs than they are with health promotion programs. This is largely because OSH programs are mandated by federal occupational safety and health legislation and by state workers' compensation laws. With very few exceptions, small businesses are not exempt from these requirements. Some of the same barriers that small businesses confront when implementing health promotion programs, such as lack of time and in-house expertise, apply equally to implementing OSH programs (2). Yet, despite these limitations, most small businesses are able to comply with the requirements for OSH programs (2).

Some researchers have argued that the effort required to comply with OSH requirements actually undermines the ability of small businesses to implement health promotion programs (22). However, we know that health promotion activities in smaller businesses already tend to favor safety-related offerings (2,15,33). The point here is that workplace safety and health may serve as the rallying point for expanding health promotion programming in small businesses. The required transformation is to view OSH and health promotion as complementary rather than competing endeavors. Nationally, there is a trend toward program integration (NIOSH WorkLife Initiative), and accumulating evidence is showing linkages between lifestyle factors and workplace safety and health risks—for example, linkages between excess weight and occupational injury (19). It follows that health promotion initiatives involving weight management, nutrition, physical activity, smoking cessation, and stress management may all contribute to reducing injury rates, workers' compensation claims, and lost work time; they may also hasten return to work after injury and improve overall worker productivity.

American small businesses nearly always have to provide workers' compensation insurance. Although workers' compensation legislation varies from state to state, there are very few exceptions to this requirement. Many states require insurers to provide credits to organizations that have established drug-testing programs. The notion behind this incentive is to reduce exposure and incidents. Why then do governing bodies not require insurers to provide incentives for health promotion programming, allowing for improvement in availability and access? From the employer's point of view, evidence is growing showing that it is difficult, if not impossible, to separate the effects and costs associated with work-related and lifestyle-related injuries and illnesses (9).

Although insurance company underwriters are not mandated to provide credits for health promotion programs, credits may be negotiated through a direct agent or through an independent agent representing the small business. Although definitive proof of program initiatives and accomplishments remains elusive, it behooves the small-business organization to take on this task. Interestingly, major insurance carriers of workers' compensation do not yet appear to be addressing health promotion. Typically, major insurance carriers provide consulting services on loss control, safety, and health or risk management. These services have focused—and continue to focus—on occupational safety, injury prevention, industrial hygiene and occupational illness prevention, fire safety, liability minimization, and the like. They have not yet begun to address workplace health promotion despite the potential benefits. Small-business organizations, as the insured, should therefore be asking for assistance and services from these insurers to create change. Small businesses might also benefit from taking a similar position with their health insurance provider. More immediate opportunities may exist in this arena, but it is still important to ask for assistance. Furthermore, increasing bargaining power by joining in employer coalitions may be another method small employers can use to increase access to heath promotion resources through insurance carrier and employer collaborations.

Finally, a third strategy for expanding health promotion in small businesses is to take advantage of simple actions that can have positive effects on employee health and that represent the building blocks of a positive health culture within the organization. The following list presents a number of such actions.

Simple Strategies for Worksite Health Promotion

- Enact and enforce a no-smoking policy at the worksite.
- Decide to hire only nonsmokers.
- Enact and enforce a drug-free workplace policy.
- Lay out a walking path at the worksite or in the surrounding area.
- Allow employees a little longer lunch or break if they are using the time to exercise.
- Request that vending machine operators include healthy choices, including healthy beverages.
- Post health- and safety-related signs, posters, table tents, and so on around the workplace.

- Encourage employees to use their personal protective equipment and provide them with feedback.
- Develop a written policy on the importance of a safe work environment.
- Include breaks for stretching before and during work.
- Provide sunscreen to employees working outdoors.
- Enforce seat belt usage on the job and in company vehicles.
- Talk to employees about some aspect of their health each day.

Conclusion

The number of worksites offering health promotion services has increased significantly over the past couple of decades; however, small businesses lag behind larger businesses in the number of activities and comprehensive health programs offered. Considering the large number of persons working for small businesses and their importance to the American economy as well as the mounting evidence of the benefits of worksite health promotion, it is important that we identify creative ways to not only increase the health promotion programs in small businesses but also work with these businesses to develop effective comprehensive programs. This chapter identified both the strengths and the weaknesses of small businesses and offered several strategies for expanding health promotion in small businesses. The first step to achieving this expansion is the education of small-business owners and manag-

ers about the benefits of disease prevention and health promotion programming. Private-public partnerships can provide this awareness and be the mechanism whereby effective comprehensive health promotion programs are developed.

Chapter Review Questions

1. Assume you are a small-business owner. Create a plan for a health promotion program that provides all five elements of a comprehensive program.

2. Interview a small-business owner in your area to determine if this person offers a health promotion program. If not, why? If so, what are the components of the program and what strengths and challenges has the business encountered?

3. Identify three organizations in your community that a business could collaborate with to expand its health promotion program. List at least one service that each organization would provide.

4. Small employers cite numerous reasons for their inability to offer workplace health promotion. Yet, these same small businesses are addressing workplace safety and health. What linkages exist between these two fields? How can workplace health promotion capitalize on or play off of existing safety and health programming?

5. Compare and contrast how small, medium, and large businesses can facilitate participation in health promotion programs offered in the community or at the worksite.

6

Employee Health Promotion
A Legal Perspective

Alison Cline Earles, Esq., and LuAnn Heinen, MPP

A truly effective health improvement program uses a variety of available levers to help employees and their families maintain health-promoting habits and manage health conditions effectively. Worksite approaches may include peer support, health challenges, environmental design (such as well-lit, prominent staircases), on-site medical staffing, health fairs, employee health education, health plans that cover preventive care and offer health coaching, company cafeterias that provide healthy fare, and tax-qualified plans that reinforce healthy behaviors and results.

This chapter discusses the legal issues that U.S. employers face when they employ these resources to achieve the following:

- Obtaining information needed to design a health promotion program that meets enrollee needs (often through health risk assessments, health plan claims analysis, screening results, and surveys)

- Obtaining information needed to determine the effectiveness of a health promotion program in terms of health improvement and cost reduction (often through health plan claims analysis, surveys, screening results, analysis of absenteeism, and workers' compensation and disability claims)

- Obtaining information needed to inform participants of their risks of developing medical conditions and their need to take specific actions (often through health risk and behavior assessments with informational reporting provided to the participant)

- Obtaining information needed for disease management providers or health coaches to focus time and resources on appropriate

participants (often through provision of health plan claims analysis, proof of healthy behavior, and screening results to health coaches or case managers)

- Disseminating information about health promotion and getting enrollees to read and understand this information (often through newsletters, disease management coaches, cafeteria table tents, fitness center challenges, phone calls, e-mails, lunch and learns, internal training on productivity and energy management, and training on benefits)

- Providing diagnostic screening services, nutritionist services, or routine medical care through on-site medical clinics or health fairs

- Helping and motivating enrollees to comply with recommended standards of care for their health conditions, maintain appropriate levels of physical activity, eat a healthy diet, maintain normal body weight, avoid tobacco use, manage personal stress, avoid abuse of alcohol or drugs, and use seat belts and take other safety precautions (often through financial and social incentives provided through the health plan, other tax-qualified plans, hiring policies, cafeteria design and offerings, on-site automated screening kiosks, and worksite weight management and walking programs)

Employers must ensure that their health promotion programs comply with U.S. federal and state law as designed and as implemented. This chapter discusses briefly how the U.S. Health Insurance Portability and Accountability Act (HIPAA), American with Disabilities Act, state lifestyle discrimination laws, and tax laws affect common program features.

Summary of Relevant U.S. Laws and Their Effects on Health Promotion Programs

HIPAA privacy and security rules (1) affect who may see, store, share, and use protected health information from a health plan or health care provider to promote the goals of the program; how the information must be protected; and what agreements must be in place with business associates that operate the program.

HIPAA nondiscrimination rules affect how incentives for healthy behavior and results must be structured and communicated if offered through a health plan subject to HIPAA.

The *Americans with Disabilities Act (ADA)* affects how businesses hire employees and terminate employment, how health plan benefits may be designed to further the goals of a health improvement program, how health risk assessments and screenings may be used, and how on-site challenges and wellness campaigns should be delivered.

State lifestyle discrimination laws protect employees' rights to engage in lawful activity outside of work and therefore may affect health promotion programs that reinforce certain behaviors.

Tax laws affect the extent to which the employer may deduct the cost of health promotion programs incorporated into tax-qualified health plans, on-site medical clinics and fitness centers, free or discounted weight loss programs, and incentives or prizes offered in relation to these; the extent to which the employer must withhold from employees' income the value of these services and awards; and the extent to which vendors are responsible for issuing 1099 forms related to prizes and incentives paid directly to employees.

HIPAA Privacy and Security Rules and Health Promotion Programs

The goal of this section is to identify which components of a typical health promotion program are subject to HIPAA privacy and security rules and to determine how employers may limit the applicability of the rules. The U.S. Department of Health and Human Services implemented the HIPAA privacy and security rules by publishing extensive regulations. An employer must comply with HIPAA when it acts as a health care provider or when it acts on behalf of a health plan (2).

HIPAA Definitions and Applications to Components of Health Promotion Programs

Which components of a health promotion program are considered covered entities that must comply with HIPAA privacy and nondiscrimination rules?

The following are covered entities subject to the privacy rules: medical, dental, vision, and prescription drug plans; medical spending accounts; health reimbursement accounts; long-term care plans; EAPs that offer counseling; off-site medical clinics; and wellness fairs, medical clinics, doctors, nurses, and nutritionists providing medical care and engaging in standard electronic transactions with a group health plan.

Although many of the following may be incorporated into a HIPAA-covered group health plan or offered by a HIPAA-covered entity, they generally are not subject to HIPAA on a stand-alone basis: on-site medical clinics, health screenings, wellness fairs, and support groups; fitness centers; on-site doctors and nurses that do not provide medical care but rather administer workers' compensation or disability claims and provide first aid (3); 24 h health education lines; health risk assessment tools that provide information only to the participant; EAPs that offer referrals only; U.S. Code Section 125 cafeteria plans that offer employer contributions as incentives for healthy behaviors or results; employer contributions to health savings accounts as incentives for healthy behaviors or results; hiring practices (policy against hiring tobacco users, for example); and voluntary physical activity, tobacco cessation, or weight loss challenges that do not meet the definition of an *Employee Retirement Income Security Act* (ERISA) health plan (4).

What is a business associate to a covered entity?

The companies hired to process health plan claims, perform disease management or health coaching, offer EAP counseling, offer and analyze health and behavior risk assessments, operate tailored educational programming, adjudicate incentive eligibility, analyze health claim data, and assess the effectiveness of health plan benefits are considered to be business associates to HIPAA-covered entities because they need access to individually identifiable health information (protected health information, or PHI) from the covered entity in order to perform these services. A business associate contract as mandated by HIPAA requires the business associate to protect the PHI and honor patients' and enrollees' privacy rights.

What is an organized health care arrangement?

HIPAA allows all members of an organized health care arrangement (OHCA) to share PHI with other members of the OHCA as needed to carry out health care operations relating to the OHCA (5). The preamble to the regulations clarifies that OHCA members may share PHI with the business associates of other members in order to carry out health care operations of the OHCA (6). HIPAA defines an OHCA to include all health plan–covered entities sponsored by the same employer (7).

Effects of HIPAA Privacy and Security Rules

HIPAA-covered entities must fulfill many obligations outlined in the HIPAA regulations, including the development of comprehensive HIPAA privacy and security policies and procedures that specify how PHI is used, shared, and protected. Many employers incorporate health promotion programs into their health plans so that state lifestyle discrimination laws do not apply and so that they can ensure the health plan may use the information obtained through risk assessments and screenings for purposes of health coaching, risk analysis, plan design, and funding. For each stand-alone program (such as an on-site health fair), the employer must weigh the benefits associated with data sharing and integration of the program into the health plan against the additional costs of ensuring HIPAA compliance.

Employers with on-site medical services or staffed fitness centers that offer health screenings may choose to limit HIPAA obligations by clarifying that the staff members are not health care providers subject to HIPAA and do not act on behalf of the health plan. Alternatively, employers may consider the medical staff as working on behalf of the health plan. If so, the health plan must clarify this in its HIPAA privacy notice and in an amendment stating the appropriate uses of health

information obtained by the medical staff. In addition, the employer must establish the necessary internal firewalls and take all the steps outlined in the HIPAA privacy and security rules with respect to the staff members and the information they obtain. If on-site screening results are provided automatically to the health plan, this fact must be communicated in both the plan documents and the HIPAA privacy notice.

The following checklists provide an overview to addressing HIPAA-related obligations, data use, and data sharing.

HIPAA Nondiscrimination Rules and Incentive-Based Health Promotion Programs

The goal of this section is to clarify how employers may provide financial incentives and rewards for healthy lifestyles through a health plan without violating the HIPAA nondiscrimination rules. HIPAA regulates health plan–covered entities and prohibits them from discriminating against individuals on the basis of health status. The nondiscrimination rules set important limits but also clarify how plan sponsors may provide financial incentives for maintaining a healthy weight or for participating in a lifestyle change program.

Do the HIPAA Nondiscrimination Rules Apply?

If compliance with a health improvement initiative is not linked to eligibility for a health plan, benefits under the plan, premium discounts, rebates, reduced co-payments, or deductibles, the HIPAA nondiscrimination rules do not apply. Therefore, programs that do not relate to the group health plan or provide medical care or reimbursement for medical care and that are designed to support good health and healthy habits for all employees do not need to comply with the HIPAA nondiscrimination rules. The HIPAA nondiscrimination rules also do not apply to supplemental plans similar to Medicare or Tricare supplemental plans.

Summary of the Nondiscrimination Rules and the Health Promotion Program Exception

The nondiscrimination rules cover both *eligibility* and *premiums and contributions*. The rules state that health plans may not discriminate against

Checklist to *Limit* HIPAA Obligations and Correspondingly *Limit* Data Use and Analysis

☐ Offer wellness fairs or health clinics only at on-site locations. Prepare and distribute communication materials explaining that on-site wellness fairs and health clinics, on-site medical staff, on-site support groups, and on-site fitness centers are not part of any company health plan.

☐ Clearly state that health risk assessments are not a benefit under the plan and that individual results will be shared only with the employee.

☐ Meet with vendors and staff to ensure that only deidentified, aggregate information is sent from the on-site wellness fairs and clinics and fitness centers to the health plan or the company or that the vendor has a completed request from the participant to send the results on his or her behalf to the health plan.

☐ Train employees who might provide medical care to other employees to never use electronic media to perform a transaction for which there is a HIPAA electronic standard.

Checklist to *Increase* HIPAA Obligations and Correspondingly *Increase* the Ability to Share, Analyze, and Use Data

☐ Amend the health plan to clarify that health promotion program offerings are part of the health plan and are operated by business associates to the health plan.

☐ Interview disease management companies, data analysis vendors, and outsourced on-site medical clinics to make sure they will be able to comply with business associate agreements.

☐ Negotiate and finalize business associate agreements.

☐ When preparing HIPAA policies and procedures for the health plan, designate all health plans as members of an OHCA in order to ease the flow of health information among them for purposes of operating the OHCA.

☐ Draft the HIPAA privacy notice in a manner that explains that all company health plans, on-site clinics, and health promotion programs (including those administering health risk assessments) may share protected health information with each other in order to perform health care operations for any of the company health plans.

☐ Ensure that only deidentified data are used if the effects of the health promotion programs on disability and workers' compensation programs will be determined.

☐ Ensure that on-site medical clinics do not share individual health information with administrators of disability and workers' compensation programs.

similarly situated individuals on the basis of factors related to health status with respect to (1) eligibility for the plan or (2) premiums or contributions under the plan (8). However, a health plan could make distinctions on the basis of activities unrelated to health status, as long as the rule applies to all similarly situated enrollees, regardless of health status, and the rule is properly enforced. Moreover, the health plan may make

distinctions based on an enrollee's compliance with a medical professional's recommendations as long as there is no prescribed goal stated by the health plan. Note that compliance with the HIPAA nondiscrimination rules does not guarantee compliance with the ADA, the Age Discrimination in Employment Act, or other laws.

Is there any discrimination on the basis of health status? If the answer to this is *no,* then it is not necessary to comply with the five requirements outlined in the following list. However, if the plan does discriminate on the basis of factors related to health status, it will violate HIPAA nondiscrimination rules unless it complies with each of the five parts of the health promotion or wellness program exception:

1. The total reward for the plan's health promotion or wellness programs that require satisfaction of a standard related to a health factor must be limited—generally, it must not exceed 20% of the cost of employee-only coverage under the plan. If dependents (such as spouses or dependent children) may participate in the wellness program, the reward must not exceed 20% of the cost of the coverage in which an employee and any dependents are enrolled.

2. The program must be reasonably designed to promote health and prevent disease.

3. The program must give individuals eligible to participate the opportunity to qualify for the reward at least once per year.

4. The reward must be available to all similarly situated individuals. The program must allow a reasonable alternative standard (or waiver of initial standard) for obtaining the reward to any individual for whom the initial standard is unreasonably difficult to obtain due to a medical condition or for whom the initial standard is medically inadvisable to satisfy.

5. The plan must disclose in all materials describing the terms of the program the availability of a reasonable alternative standard or the possibility of a waiver of the initial standard (9).

Increasingly, employers are recognizing the effect of lifestyle choices on the health plan's costs and are seeking to provide financial incentives to employees who maintain a healthy weight and exercise regularly. Very often employers also want enrollees (enrollees are defined as all those enrolled in the health plan, including dependents) to participate in coaching, disease management, and possibly other health improvement offerings. The following questions and answers will help employers meet their objectives while complying with the law.

Application of the Rules: Eligibility to Participate in the Plan

Q: May the company require enrollees to pass a physical examination or prove that they maintain a normal BMI before they are eligible to participate in the health plan?

A: No. This practice discriminates against individuals, with respect to eligibility for the health plan, on the basis of a factor related to health status.

Q: May the company require all enrollees to complete and submit a health risk assessment to the disease management or health promotion company by the end of the initial enrollment period in order to receive coverage? May it make continued enrollment contingent on completing and submitting the assessment every year before the end of the open enrollment period?

A: Yes, but see Section IV on the implications of doing this under the ADA. Completing a health risk assessment is a health awareness activity and a health plan risk administration activity, and requiring that all enrollees engage in this activity does not discriminate on the basis of health status. The plan materials should state that eligibility for the plan is not affected by the answers on the health risk assessment—just by the timely completion and submission of the questionnaire.

Q: May the company require only the enrollees who have diabetes, heart disease, high cholesterol, high blood pressure, or depression to complete these health risk assessments in order to enroll in the plan or maintain coverage?

A: No. In this case the plan would be imposing an additional eligibility requirement on individuals who have poor health status. This would violate the eligibility rule.

Q: May the company require all enrollees (including spouses and children, with parental assistance) to complete a 2 wk food intake and exercise log before open enrollment each year as a condition of continued eligibility for the health plan?

A: Yes. Again, as long as the requirement applies equally to all enrollees and is enforced in a nondiscriminatory fashion, it would be permissible because the log is a health awareness activity that does not discriminate on the basis of health status.

Q: May the company require all enrollees to engage in health awareness activities as a condition of continued eligibility but only enforce the rule for individuals with health problems?

A: No. Even though the plan would be drafted in a manner that complies with the law, the practice of imposing the condition only on unhealthy individuals would cause the plan to violate the eligibility rule. The company should make engaging in health awareness activities a condition of enrollment only if it is prepared to enforce the requirement for all enrollees.

Q: What if the company is not prepared to enforce this requirement for its overseas enrollees or for senior management enrollees? Could the company require only the enrollees in the United States to perform the health awareness activities as a condition of eligibility?

A: Yes. The company could impose the health awareness activity requirement on some but not all enrollees without violating the nondiscrimination rules. (The rules apply only if the plan makes distinctions on the basis of health status, not on participation in a health awareness activity.) Treating various locations or various business classifications differently is generally acceptable. But health plans must be careful to avoid violating other nondiscrimination rules, such as the U.S. Code Section 105(h) and Code Section 125 rules prohibiting discrimination against nonhighly compensated employees. In addition, requiring only the enrollees 40 y or older to participate in the health awareness activities as a condition of enrollment would violate age discrimination laws.

Q: Could the company set lifetime limits on benefits for lifestyle-influenced illnesses?

A: Yes. The company may exclude or limit benefits without violating the nondiscrimination rules (10). However, when setting these limits, the company should be careful that such exclusions apply equally to disabled and nondisabled enrollees so they do not violate the ADA.

Q: Could the company exclude coverage or apply a lifetime limit for coverage of any kind of treatment for being overweight (including nutritional counseling, gastric bypass surgery, weight loss clinics, hospitals, or camps) without violating the nondiscrimination rules or the ADA?

A: Yes. As long as the limit applies to all similarly situated individuals and is not targeted at any particular individual, it does not violate the nondiscrimination rules. Such an exclusion or limit would apply equally to disabled and nondisabled enrollees. Therefore, it would not violate the ADA.

Application of the Premiums and Contributions Rule

Q: May the company offer any kind of premium discount, deductible waiver, or health plan cost reduction in exchange for proof that an enrollee

attended weight loss or weight maintenance meetings regularly (no outcome required), wore a pedometer and reported daily steps on a regular basis (no specific activity required), participated in regular telephone consultations with a disease management program representative, completed annual health risk assessments, completed all treatment and activities recommended by a physician, or did any combination of these activities?

A: Yes. None of these activities requires satisfaction of a health standard set forth by the health plan. Rather, these are incentives for participation. Therefore, there is no limit on the kind of health plan discount the employer could provide.

Q: May the company offer premium discounts or deductible waivers only to the enrollees who prove that they maintain a normal BMI, maintain a normal cholesterol level, maintain a normal blood pressure, maintain a normal blood sugar level, or complete an aerobic exercise class at an on-site gym 30 min 5 times a week?

A: Yes. However, the wellness program would need to satisfy the five requirements for the wellness program exception.

What Is a Reasonable Alternative?

Final rulings indicate that it is reasonable for the health plan to require that the enrollee comply with his or her doctor's recommendations. This compliance could be monitored by a disease management company, automated screening kiosks, self-report, or submission of a note from the doctor regarding completion. It is permissible for the health plan to require the enrollee to pay a reasonable amount to satisfy the alternative. There is no set rule as to what is a reasonable amount. This determination should be made in light of the value of the incentive award.

Amending the Plan to Provide Financial Incentives

The nondiscrimination rules apply only within a group of individuals who are treated as similarly situated individuals. In addition, the rules allow plans to discriminate in favor of individuals with adverse health conditions. The safe harbor specified in the nondiscrimination rules advises that any amendments limiting benefits should be effective in the first plan year following the decision to amend the plan (11).

Americans With Disabilities Act

The Americans with Disabilities Act (ADA) prohibits employers from discriminating against qualified individuals with disabilities with respect to compensation or access to benefits programs (12). ADA applies to various components of employee health improvement programs including the benefits plan and health risk appraisal activity. These two components are discussed below.

ADA and Benefits Plan Design

According to the ADA, distinctions in benefits terms and conditions may not be based on disability alone. If there is a distinction based on disability in benefits terms, the employer must show that (1) the plan is a bona fide benefits plan because it exists, pays benefits, and has been accurately communicated to eligible employees and (2) the plan is not a subterfuge to evade the ADA rules and the distinctions are justified by the risks or costs of the disability.

An exclusion or cap on coverage must affect disabled and nondisabled enrollees alike. Put another way, any requirements imposed by the health plan must be examined to ensure that the benefits are available on an equal basis to employees with and without disabilities (13). Therefore, it is permissible to place a limit on all weight loss and obesity-related treatments, regardless of medical necessity, because the limit affects those who are not disabled by their weight (14). However, it would not be permissible to exclude or limit coverage for gastric bypass surgery if it is performed only on individuals with morbid obesity and all or substantially all individuals with morbid obesity are substantially limited in a major life activity.

ADA and Health and Behavior Risk Assessments

The ADA specifically states that its rules do not prevent an insurer, hospital, or medical service company; HMO, agent or entity that administers benefits plans; or similar organizations from underwriting risks, classifying risks, or administering such risks that are based on or not inconsistent with state law (15). (Therefore, an insurance company could require medical examinations and inquiries in order to underwrite a fully insured health plan.) Similar provisions indicate that an employer that sponsors a bona fide self-insured plan may make such inquiries in order to underwrite, classify, or administer risks (16). Such inquiries are permissible as long as they are not used as a subterfuge to evade the provisions of the ADA. The U.S. Equal Employment Opportunity Commission (EEOC) has not specifically addressed the question of whether the insurance underwriting exemption from the ADA applies to health risk assessments and screenings required by a self-insured health plan. There is a strong argument that such assessments are a form of financial risk management when the information is used to reduce the health plan's financial exposure through focused counseling, education, and case management of individuals with certain medical conditions or health risks exemption.

The ADA prohibits employers from making medical inquiries or examinations of current employees regarding the existence, nature, or severity of a disability unless it is related to the job and consistent with business necessity (17). The ADA prohibition applies only to medical examinations and inquiries, so it is important to determine whether a health or behavior assessment meets the ADA definition (18). In 2000 enforcement guidance, the EEOC defined a medical examination as "a procedure or test that seeks information about an individual's physical or mental impairments or health. . . . [T]he following factors should be considered to determine whether a test (or procedure) is a medical examination: (1) whether the test is administered by a health care professional; (2) whether the test is interpreted by a health care professional; (3) whether the test is designed to reveal an impairment of physical or mental health; (4) whether the test is invasive; (5) whether the test measures an employee's performance of a task or measures his/her physiological responses to performing the task; (6) whether the test normally is given in a medical setting; and, (7) whether medical equipment is used."

In its list of medical examinations, the EEOC does not include weight screenings. The EEOC specifically states that physical agility tests and physical fitness tests are not medical examinations as long as they do not include measuring heart rate or blood pressure.

If an employer does perform health risk assessments or screenings that meet the definition of a medical inquiry or examination, it may do so as part of a voluntary health promotion program, as long as any medical records acquired as part of the wellness program are kept confidential and separate from personnel records (19). A health promotion program is voluntary as long as an employer neither requires participation nor penalizes employees who do not participate. It is unclear whether a program that provides incentives for certain health achievements (as measured through a screening or questionnaire) penalizes those who do not participate in the program at all. Those who do participate but do not earn incentives have been treated the same as those who did not participate at all. Moreover, the employer has not required any employee to participate in the program. Informal, nonbinding comments of the EEOC indicate that requiring an employee to complete a health risk assessment in order to be eligible for a health plan would render the program involuntary.

The medical inquiry and medical examination rules of the ADA anticipate that the employer is conducting the medical inquiry or has hired an outside party to conduct the inquiry on its behalf and that the employer will obtain the results of the inquiry. However, in most cases the employer is prohibited by contract from receiving any individual information from the health risk assessments. Given the ADA's exception for risk-management inquiries by self-insured health plans, there is a good argument that the ADA prohibition against medical inquiries does not apply to health risk assessments and health screenings offered by the health plan as long as the employer is contractually prohibited from receiving individually identifiable results.

State Lifestyle Discrimination Laws

Lifestyle discrimination laws are laws that prohibit employers from discriminating against employees or prospective employees on the basis of their activities outside of work or off the employer's premises (Colorado, North Dakota, California, and New York) or laws that protect the rights of employees to use lawful products such as tobacco outside of work or off the employer's premises (Illinois, North Carolina, Montana, Minnesota, Nevada, Tennessee, and Wisconsin). New Hampshire's lifestyle discrimination law applies only if an employer requires abstinence from tobacco products as a condition of employment. Nineteen other states and the District of Columbia prohibit discrimination based on tobacco use away from work.

When a self-insured health plan requires that tobacco users pay a higher premium for health insurance (in conjunction with a health promotion program that satisfies the five-part exception

from the HIPAA nondiscrimination rules), the health plan (and by extension, some would argue, the employer) is discriminating against employees on the basis of their personal use of a legal product. Section 514 of ERISA states that any U.S. state laws are void to the extent they relate to an employee benefits plan. Therefore, such a health plan design should be permissible even in a state that protects an employee's right to use tobacco outside of work. However, rewarding tobacco-free status outside of an employee benefits plan would violate state lifestyle discrimination laws. *For multistate employers, integration of health promotion programming with the health plan protects against having to comply with different state lifestyle discrimination laws.*

Tax Laws

Tax laws affect health promotion programs with respect to (1) the employer's ability to treat costs associated with the health promotion program as deductible expenses, (2) the employer's obligation to treat the value of the health promotion program as taxable income subject to withholding requirements, (3) the employer's obligation to treat incentives paid directly to employees by a health promotion program vendor as taxable income subject to withholding requirements, and (4) the health promotion program vendor responsibility to issue 1099 reports to recipients of incentives more than $600 U.S. in value.

When a health promotion program is incorporated into a tax-qualified health plan, incentives for compliance or goal achievement may be offered through premium rebates, co-payment reductions, and contributions to flexible spending accounts. Reasonable expenses for operating the program and communicating it to employees may be included as deductible expenses. Tax-qualified health plans may offer any components of health promotion programs, as long as these meet the definition of medical care under U.S. Code Section 213(d). Expenses for weight loss, tobacco cessation, and physical activity programs recommended by a medical professional may meet this definition if they are amounts paid for the diagnosis, cure, mitigation, treatment, or prevention of disease. Furthermore, benefits received by employees under the tax-qualified programs are not includible in income (or subject to withholding).

When a health promotion program is not incorporated into a tax-qualified health plan, an employer has to evaluate many possible tax consequences (as well as state law issues), an undertaking for which there is no clear written guidance. Moreover, traditional applications of tax law to employee-provided benefits directly conflict with the goal of preventing the employer from knowing which employee or dependent is enrolled in a health promotion program and whether or not that individual has achieved a goal.

Conclusion

Health improvement initiatives in the workplace must comply with appropriate U.S. federal and state laws. By incorporating such initiatives into their self-insured health plans, employers may limit the application of some of these laws. However, this approach requires compliance with health plan regulations. Designing health promotion programs that meet employer objectives and comply with all laws and regulations requires careful planning and legal review from an employee benefits, employment, and tax law perspective.

Chapter Review Questions

1. How can employers collect and use employee health information to support employee health promotion without violating HIPAA privacy rules?

2. What are the key legal considerations when designing incentives for employee health improvement programs?

3. What is the relevance of the distinction between satisfaction of a health outcome goal and completion of a health awareness activity?

4. What practices may be viewed as discriminatory under the ADA, and how can employers avoid such discrimination?

5. How might state lifestyle discrimination laws affect employer efforts to recruit and retain a healthy workforce?

7

Health Care Policy and Health Promotion

John M. Clymer, AB; Garry M. Lindsay, MPH, CHES; Jennifer M. Childress, MS, CHES; and George J. Pfeiffer MSE, FAWHP

To many worksite health promotion practitioners, health policy may appear as an abstract concept that pertains primarily to the implementation and administration of regulatory rules applying to health and safety and health benefits eligibility. Yet, as this chapter discusses, health policy within an occupational setting is more than complying with regulatory guidelines. It can in fact be viewed and leveraged as an integrated system that guides human capital managers (e.g., human resources, benefits, health promotion, employee assistance, work and life, occupational health, and safety) in protecting, enhancing, and supporting the health, safety, and productivity of their human assets.

As such, human capital managers are encouraged to address health-related policies not as silos of responsibility but as opportunities to define, create, and support an integrated culture of health within their respective organizations. Being involved in health policy decisions provides programming opportunities and aligns the function of health promotion practitioners with the broader business goals of the organization.

What Is Policy?

According to Merriam-Webster, a policy is "a definite course or method of action selected from among alternatives and in light of given conditions to guide and determine present and future" (7).

Types of Policy

Within organizations, policy can be classified as either *external compliant* or *internal compliant*. External-compliant policies are an organization's efforts through written protocols that interpret, monitor, and enforce the regulations of governmental or other outside regulatory agencies. Complying with minimum wage requirements, privacy of health information (HIPAA), safety regulations (OSHA), and the ADA are examples of external-compliant policy functions. In other cases, external-compliant policies are administered to conform to local or state ordinances and professional trade or watchdog organizations.

Internal-compliant policies are created and enforced by the organization in order to achieve desired company goals. They may include compensation and benefits policies to attract and retain employees, alcohol and drug policies to protect the health and safety of the workforce, policies for mandatory seat belt use in company vehicles to reduce the risk of injury, and policies for smoke-free worksites as part of a broader strategy for tobacco control. Another function of internal-compliant policy formulation pertains to its role as a lever in articulating an organization's guiding principles regarding its mission and business goals and, from a human capital perspective, the role and value of its employees in fulfilling these goals. Internal-compliant policies can also be influenced by legislation. For example, the Healthy Workforce Act, which was introduced by U.S. Senators Tom Harkin (D-IA) and Gordon Smith (R-MI) on July 9, 2007, proposes a tax credit to employers for the costs of implementing worksite health promotion programs (2). If the Healthy Workforce Act becomes law, it will offer an incentive to employers to develop internal-compliant policies that are consistent with those outlined in the bill. Information on legislative policies that affect worksite health is available on Web sites such as those of Partnership for Prevention (www.prevent.org) and Health Promotion Advocates (www.health-promotionadvocates.org).

Policy and Outcomes

As discussed, policy is intended to guide the achievement of desired outcomes (present and future) that benefit the organization as a whole. In policy study there are two primary effects that a standing policy creates: intended and unintended (17).

Intended Effects

Within intended effects, policies are developed to achieve desired outcomes such as reducing workers' compensation claims through adherence to safety procedures and mandatory safety meetings or increasing health risk assessment participation by implementing an incentive program. In policy design, decision makers need to first define the intended effects that a policy would hope to achieve in relation to the existing issue. Within worksite health management policy, intended effects can include the following:

- Reducing direct medical costs
- Reducing indirect costs such as those due to sick days, absenteeism, disability, workers' compensation, and presenteeism
- Reducing inappropriate medical utilization
- Eliminating or reducing tobacco use
- Improving health status of the covered population
- Increasing participation rates of sponsored programs
- Adding greater value to health benefits investments
- Improving compliance and adherence to health interventions
- Recruiting and retaining valuable employees
- Being considered an employer of choice
- Creating a culture of health throughout the organization

Unintended Effects

Corporate policies often produce unintended effects—adverse consequences to the intended goal or outcome (16). The reason for this is that policies do not function within a vacuum; they work within a complex, dynamic environment with many levers that may produce results that are contrary to the intended effect. A common example within worksite health management programs pertains to health benefits policies that intend to manage health care costs (intended effect) by shifting a greater cost burden to employees and their dependents. The unintended effects of cost shifting can lead to the following scenarios and consequences to the employer and to the employee:

Scenario 1

- *Intended effect:* Reduce the company's contribution to employee health care costs by requiring co-payments or coinsurance for preventive screenings.

- *Unintended effects:* Because of cost barriers, employees and dependents are not compliant with recommended screening schedules. Because health problems are not detected in the preclinical stage or early onset of disease, consequences include increased medical, absenteeism, disability, and productivity-related costs to the organization and illness to the individual (10).

Scenario 2

- *Intended effect:* Reduce the company's contribution to prescription drugs by creating tiered reimbursement schedules with escalating co-payments and coinsurance.

- *Unintended effects:* Because of cost barriers, patients reduce or stop taking medications for managing chronic health conditions such as diabetes, hypertension, and asthma. Consequences may include increased hospitalizations and disability costs to the organization because of poor medication adherence and adverse clinical outcomes to the individual (6).

Scenario 3

- *Intended effect:* Reduce the company's contribution to employee health premiums by implementing a high-deductible health plan.

- *Unintended effects:* Patients ignore symptoms or delay treatment because of higher out-of-pocket expenses or wish to save the cash balance in their company contributed health savings account (4).

Scenario 4

- *Intended effect:* To keep employees engaged in their work, all wellness programs are scheduled off the clock—before work, after work, or during lunch breaks.

- *Unintended effects:* The timing of programming creates access barriers that lead to lower participation rates in company-sponsored health activities and negatively affect overall participation rates and related health outcomes (3).

Maximizing Intended Outcomes and Reducing Risks

To minimize the unintended effects of proposed employee health-related policies and to maximize desired outcomes, it's important for organizations that are in the planning process to identify and assess the potential effects that the proposed policy may have on factors such as health status, total costs, participation, liability, and productivity. For more information, refer to page 64, Policy Development Process.

Common Health-Related Policies and Application to Health Promotion Professionals

Tables 7.1 and 7.2 summarize common external- and internal-compliant policies, their intended effects, and opportunities for health promotion practitioners to leverage programming to either comply with or enhance policy decisions (8).

Table 7.1 External-Compliant Policies

Policy initiative	Intended effects	Health promotion practitioner opportunities
HIPAA: privacy of health information (11)	Protect the privacy of health-related information of employees and family members.	Provide privacy statement with health risk assessments, health screenings, health fairs, and health coaching. Assure that privacy procedures regarding personal health information from coaching sessions are in secure place. Be transparent and present aggregate health risk assessment data through group orientations and periodic state of health reports.
OSHA: Omnibus Transportation Employee Testing Act (16)	Assure a drug- and alcohol-free workplace for transportation workers. Reduce the risk of on-the-job injury due to impairment or abuse. Begin random drug and alcohol testing.	Provide drug and alcohol abuse education. Provide stress management programs. Provide better sleep programs. Provide energy and alertness management programs.
Family and Medical Leave Act (14)	Grant an eligible employee up to 12 workweeks of unpaid leave during any 12 mo. Support caregiving responsibilities without penalty of termination. Take medical leave when the employee is unable to work because of a serious health condition.	Provide well-baby programs. Provide elder-care information and support services and seminars. Reinforce self-care skills for the management of health problems. Provide stress management for caregivers.
OSHA: industry and job-specific guidelines (15)	Decrease on-the-job accidents. Reduce workers' compensation claims. Train employees on safety procedures specific to their industry or job.	Assist health and safety department on industrial athlete programs. Provide ergonomic coaching at workstations. Develop on-the-job exercise and stretching programs. Develop and lead healthy back programs.
OSHA: blood-borne pathogen guidelines (13)	Protect workers in such professions as health care, fire and rescue, police, and housekeeping who have increased risk of exposure to blood and other bodily fluids. Reduce the transmission of HIV and hepatitis B and C.	Be sure that third-party vendors responsible for on-site health screenings and health fairs comply with needlestick and biohazard procedures. Provide periodic education on HIV and AIDS and hepatitis through company communications.
ADA (12)	Protect job applicants from discrimination due to physical or mental impairments. Protect employees from discrimination due to physical or mental impairments.	Through health coaching provide adaptive programming based on individual needs. Within on-site fitness centers provide adaptive exercise programs based on individual needs.

Based on Partnership for Prevention. Healthy workforce 2010: An Essential Health Promotion Sourcebook for Employers, Large and Small. 2008 Partnership for Prevention, Washington, D.C. Available at: www.prevent.org/images/stories/files/publications/Healthy_workforce_2010.pdf.

Table 7.2 Internal-Compliant Policies

Policy initiative	Intended effects	Health promotion practitioner opportunities
Free preventive screenings	Lower cost and access barriers. Increase compliance. Increase participation rates.	Organize on-site health fairs and screenings. Use demographics to organize periodic targeted on-site screenings (e.g., mammography, prostate-specific antigen (PSA) tests) coordinated with national health events.
Workplace violence	Protect employees from on-site violence, verbal abuse, and threats from fellow employees. Protect the employee from the threat of an abusive partner as well as other employees. Enact zero-tolerance policy.	Workplace violence issues are primarily the responsibility of corporate security and employee assistance in larger organizations. Health promotion practitioners can assist in offering: Education on domestic violence and outside resources (e.g., hotlines and shelters). Self-defense courses through the fitness center or other programs. Reinforce buddy programs in walking to parking lots at night.
Seat belt use	Require full compliance when using or traveling in company vehicles. Reduce the risk of on-the-job injury due to motor vehicle accidents. Reinforce full compliance during personal use.	Include seat belt use within health risk assessment. Sponsor defensive driving classes. Post buckle-up signs in company parking lots. Reinforce messages within company publications.
Health risk appraisal (HRA) with benefits credit	Increase HRA participation. Promote lifestyle management. Lower health risks and associated costs.	Develop and coordinate communication campaigns that promote and explain HRAs. Defuse privacy concerns. Coordinate work group presentations on aggregate results. Develop contest that rewards highest percentage of participants per work group.
High-deductible health plan	Decrease employer costs. Guide appropriate medical utilization. Teach employees about the true cost of health care.	Implement a medical self-care program. Provide lunch-and-learns on making better-informed medical decisions. Leverage existing and custom communications (e.g., health newsletter or health Web site). Reinforce medical consumer resources and benefits information.
Incentive programs	Improve participation within targeted programs such as HRAs, health screenings, and risk reduction programs (e.g., smoking, weight management).	Depending on level of incentives, promote programs through company communications. Work with benefits department to coordinate initiative when incentives are related to health benefits credits or other benefits-related programs.
Value-based pharmacy design for selected chronic health conditions	Reduce cost and access barriers (e.g., lower co-payments or coinsurance) to selective medications for managing conditions such as diabetes, asthma, and hypertension. Increase medication adherence. Improve clinical outcomes. Reduce direct and indirect costs.	Reinforce and market company-sponsored disease management and health coaching services. Develop information and support programs on improving adherence to medications, self-care, and lifestyle-related practices in managing chronic health problems.

(continued)

Table 7.2 *Continued*

Policy initiative	Intended effects	Health promotion practitioner opportunities
Health management and wellness aligned with business goals	Reinforce to all levels of management that employee health is inextricably linked to productivity. Hold management accountable for supporting employee health goals.	As part of a cross-functional team, provide on an ongoing basis aggregate reports regarding measures such as participation rates and aggregate risk profiles. Develop programming that is targeted to address the business needs of the organization.
Smoke-free workplace	Eliminate tobacco use from company buildings and premises or allow tobacco use only in designated locations (outside). Reduce the risks of tobacco use to the user. Reduce the risks of secondhand smoke. Reduce health- and productivity-related costs.	Coordinate smoking cessation programs to coincide with the smoke-free date. For example, begin programs 6 to 12 mo before implementation. With health benefits support and in conjunction with behavioral strategies, include pharmaceutical interventions and counseling for free or reduced cost. Reinforce the benefits of smoking cessation through communications.
Higher pricing of unhealthy foods and subsidizing of healthier selections in company cafeterias and vending machines and during company functions	Encourage healthier food selections. Reduce risk of obesity. Promote a healthier work culture.	Provide communications and workshops on healthier food selection. Provide tips on healthy brown bagging. Sponsor healthy food preparation through cooking demonstrations. Combine food-related communication with messaging related to physical activity and behavior change.
Drug and alcohol policy	Created a drug-free workplace. Reduce alcohol and substance abuse within the population. Encourage responsible drinking practices.	Include questions regarding alcohol use and illegal and prescription drug use within health risk assessment. Provide targeted resources in personal report. Promote responsible drinking practices through health communications. With EAP, promote guidelines for alcohol use during company-sponsored meetings. Sponsor ongoing stress management programs. Provide periodic self-assessment for alcohol, drug abuse, and depression within company communications.

Based on Partnership for Prevention. Healthy workforce 2010: An Essential Health Promotion Sourcebook for Employers, Large and Small. 2008 Partnership for Prevention, Washington, D.C. Available at: www.prevent.org/images/stories/files/publications/Healthy_workforce_2010.pdf.

Policy as a Cultural Catalyst

Beyond regulatory policy compliance and internal health-specific policies related to areas such as health benefits design, personal health data, tobacco, alcohol and drugs, and occupational health and safety, there is a broader aspect of policy development—policy as a cultural catalyst. Policy formulation can be used to help define and push forward a broader agenda of employee health as a productivity strategy that is aligned with the business goals of the organization.

Today, a number of organizations are articulating their vision of employee health through written policies and mission statements that start from senior management and are disseminated to middle management and to the rest of the workforce. A successful example of this model is the Leading by Example (LBE) CEO round table created by Partnership for Prevention in 2005 (9).

The LBE round table is designed as a CEO-to-CEO initiative that requires participating organizations to sign a statement acknowledging their commitment to three key principles:

1. Assuring that senior management is committed to health promotion as an important investment in human capital

2. Aligning health and productivity strategies with business goals

3. Educating all levels of management about the link between employee health and productivity and total economic value

In addition, participating companies are required to complete the Health Management Initiative Assessment, which in part verifies senior management's commitment to policies and practices that support employee health through increased investments in prevention and health promotion and provides organizations with an idea of what areas they can develop in making their program more comprehensive.

By having the CEO commit to these practices, the organization de facto agrees to take steps in achieving the LBE guidelines as a matter of corporate policy. The Dow Chemical Company, International Truck and Engine, GlaxoSmithKline, Pitney Bowes, Intel, and Pfizer are examples of the more than 40 organizations that have joined the LBE round table.

Noncompliance With Policy

The ramifications of not complying with established policies can be detrimental to both the organization and the individual. Noncompliance with established safety rules and regulations can lead to injury and death not only among employees but also among the public at large. Beyond bodily harm, consequences can range from fines and litigation for the organization to loss of pay and final dismissal for the employee.

Within health promotion, noncompliance with programming in the past has usually had no repercussions to the individual. However, today some organizations are taking a stick rather than a carrot approach to employee health through the imposition of policies that punish noncompliance with specific health practices or punish nonparticipation.

Such policies are most common in the area of tobacco use. Some companies (usually small employers) are requiring employees, and in some cases covered spouses, to be smoke free within a specific time frame. Noncompliance leads to automatic dismissal of the employee or noncoverage of health benefits. A more controversial policy being considered by some organizations is the inclusion of a BMI limit as a criterion for health coverage. The legality of these types of policies under the ADA is currently being questioned and most likely will be decided within a court of law in the near future (19).

Another example of noncompliance policies relates to mandatory participation within company-sponsored health programs—in this case—a health risk assessment or health screening program. Some organizations now require all employees (and covered spouses) to participate in periodic health risk assessments and health screening programs in order to be covered under the company's health benefits program. Noncompliance leads to no health benefits coverage.

Though most health incentive programs within the worksite pertain to awards such as benefits credits and other financial arrangements, negative incentives (pay or play) are gaining greater traction. The reasoning is that since the company bears the greatest cost and financial risk of health benefits, greater employee accountability is required. This can place the health promotion practitioner in an awkward position where program compliance becomes more of an enforcement function than an empowering function.

Planning and Implementing Health Policy

The development of health policy requires careful consideration when taking into account the number of stakeholders responsible for human capital management and, as discussed earlier, the issue of unintended effects. The following sections provide general guidelines for developing health-related policies within the worksite.

Creating a Cross-Functional Team

Depending on the comprehensiveness of the proposed policy and functions affected, a cross-functional policy planning team is recommended. This team should represent key stakeholders responsible for developing, implementing, managing, and evaluating the policy initiative. This is especially important in larger organizations that have a variety of in-house health management

Does Your Proposed Policy FIT?

A simple litmus test that can be applied during the initial planning process is the FIT Design model outlined by Mahoney and Hom in their book *BeneFIT Design. Seven Steps for Creating Value-Based Benefit Decisions* (5). In the case of policy development, organizations are encouraged to consider whether their policy is the following:

• **Fact-based.** Is a policy recommendation required to change or direct an intended outcome? Is a policy recommendation based on data that are credible and does it reflect (as much as possible) the total picture? Given the data, have the policy makers taken into consideration the intended effects as well as the potential negative implications (unintended effects) that this policy may create?

• **Integrated.** Are all primary stakeholders involved in the planning process? Have stakeholders identified their roles in implementing and administering the proposed policy? Within the organization, are communications integrated across media channels (e.g., print, online communication, group meetings) with consistent and reliable messages?

• **Targeted.** Given the data and the consensus of primary stakeholders, is the proposed policy targeted to an organizational need and intended to achieve stated goals and objectives?

functions such as human resources, benefits, corporate medical, health promotion and wellness, health and safety, employee assistance, and work and life initiatives.

Policy Development Process

The process for policy development varies from organization to organization, but in most instances it incorporates the following steps (1,18):

1. Issue identification
2. Review of options
3. Decision making
4. Policy formation and implementation plan
5. Policy approval
6. Implementation
7. Evaluation

Issue Identification

Within this step, key stakeholders identify the key issues or problems that need to be addressed through a policy and the intended effects (outcomes) that the policy is assumed to influence. Here data analysis is a necessary component by which a selected issue is viewed objectively and an argument for enacting a policy is built on solid, measurable facts.

Review of Options

Once a key issue has been defined, viable policy options are identified within the context of the following factors:

• Ability to maximize intended effects (desired outcomes)

• Minimization of unintended effects by identifying potential adverse consequences

• Corporate functions affected in implementing, administering, and evaluating the proposed policy

• Complexity and length of implementation

• Ease of measuring compliance and policy effects

• Total costs of policy implementation, administration, and evaluation

Decision Making

Using the analysis of potential options, key stakeholders select the most viable option that addresses the issue and its intended effects.

Policy Formation and Implementation Plan

Once selected, the option is drafted into a policy statement with appropriate addendums and an implementation plan is formulated. The implementation plan includes a comprehensive schedule, communication plan, and evaluation plan.

Policy Approval

Depending on the scope of the proposed policy and an organization's management process, the policy may be vetted through a review board or presented directly to senior management. Here the proposal may be accepted, rejected, or sent back for further revision.

Implementation

If approved, the policy is implemented according to the implementation plan submitted. At this stage, appropriate communications are developed that describe the new policy and, depending on the initiative, promote and reinforce its enactment.

Evaluation

Depending on the initiative, management is apprised of the policy's effect on targeted outcomes through periodic reports. Once its results are known, the policy may be reevaluated and revised so that it is better aligned with intended outcomes.

Conclusion

As discussed, health-related policies can help leverage the fulfillment of an organization's health goals while complying with regulatory guidelines. In addition, internal-compliant policies provide the opportunity to articulate and guide health- and productivity-related initiatives that are aligned with the organization's short- and long-term business goals. To the health promotion practitioner, health policies and the development of health policies afford the opportunity to enrich program offerings, further align health promotion with other business functions, and increase the value of worksite health as a viable business strategy.

Chapter Review Questions

1. Define the term *policy*.
2. Define, compare, and contrast internal-compliant and external-compliant policies.
3. What kind of effects does a policy create? Explain both effects.
4. Outline and discuss the policy development process.

The Case for Change
From Segregated to Integrated Employee Health Management

Ann L. Yaktine, PhD, and Mike D. Parkinson, MD, MPH, FACPM

In 2005, the U.S. Institute of Medicine (IOM) of the National Academies published *Integrating Employee Health: A Model Program for NASA* (18). The report was the culmination of the work of 12 experts* from areas relevant to health and wellness. The findings of the committee are summarized here. This chapter also examines ways that an integrated approach to health and wellness can improve the lives of employees regardless of the setting in which they work.

Identifying the Problem

The American workforce is changing and as a result, employers increasingly face new challenges in their quest to maintain high productivity standards and affordable health care expenditures. Traditional approaches to health and productivity program implementation have typically followed a non-integrated model. Occupational health services, health and wellness programs, disease management programs, onsite educational services and workplace health centers, and benefit plans have been implemented in a siloed approach and typically have focused on condition-specific intervention models with lesser emphasis on prevention. Changes in workforce characteristics and tension induced by soaring health care costs and health-related productivity losses are steering employers to more innovative approaches to population health management principles applied to the workforce.

A Changing American Workforce

The American workforce is in transition, moving away from manufacturing and other industry toward more knowledge-centered types of work and services. There is also increased demographic diversity within the workforce, an evolving work climate that includes multidisciplinary job assignments, more sophisticated technology, greater time demands on workers, and more collaborative efforts. The result is a workforce that is different from that of earlier generations of workers. Such changes in the way Americans work and the climate in which they work have influenced workers' health as well as the type of health concerns that are prevalent today. Success in such a rapidly changing work environment requires workers to be mentally and physically prepared to manage increased demands, and it requires them to be adaptable to change as well as resilient to impediments.

Why Isn't a Traditional Approach to Employee Health Working?

Many organizations have programs to promote wellness and support preventive health for their employees, but many of these programs aren't working as they were intended. To understand why requires examining the workplace setting and identifying ways to adjust health and wellness services to better meet the changing needs of the workforce. When new health and wellness

*The report was authored by the Committee to Assess Worksite Preventive Health Program Needs for NASA Employees: James A. Merchant (chair), Martin J. Sepulveda, Ann M. Coulston, Dee W. Edington, Pamela Ann Hymel, J. Richard Jennings, Tom B. Leamon, Rebecca M. Mullis, Michael D. Parkinson, Claudia Probart, Nicolaas P. Pronk, and Glorian Sorensen with support from IOM staff members Ann L. Yaktine (study director), Crystal Rasnake, Cara James, and Sandra Amamoo-Kakra.

programs are introduced through a traditional occupational health or health insurance benefits approach, the objectives of the programs often cannot be met. This is because success depends upon adapting the approach to meeting the health and wellness needs of employees to interface with the primary objectives of the organization. Key components to a successful employee health program are the following:

- Aligning the mission of the health program with that of the company
- Moving away from traditional models that are limited in program options, less focused on prevention, and more focused on management of specific health conditions
- Adapting health programs to change with the workforce, such as addressing increased diversity and flexible and globalized technology
- Making a policy-based commitment backed by managed data

Table 8.1 summarizes the changes in perspectives and emphases that have been shown to lead to a more healthy and productive workforce.

A traditional occupational health approach focuses on treating a disease after it has been diagnosed. The importance of changing the direction of employee health away from treatment of disease and toward integrated promotion of health and prevention of disease is underscored by the cost of health benefits and lost productivity (7). High stress levels, excess body weight, and multiple health risk factors are positively correlated with increased health care costs and higher absentee-

ism (1). Decreasing the risk factors, such as stress, that negatively affect employee health increases productivity and decreases medical care costs (10). Goetzel and colleagues (13) demonstrated that 26% in savings could be realized annually for each employee when a traditional approach to health programming was changed to an integrated approach.

Raising the Bar

As the need for a different approach is identified, integration is certainly emerging as a major area of focus. Additionally, programs need to achieve specific outcomes and work toward a healthy, productive, ready, and resilient workforce.

Goals of Wellness Programs

Keeping pace with rapidly changing workplace demands requires a motivated and productive workforce. The challenge lies in dealing not only with elements within the workplace but also with elements outside the workplace that can affect an individual's health decisions and with ways those elements can be modified to support health.

Behaviors and health choices that can directly affect worker health and productivity include use of tobacco, drugs, or alcohol; sedentary lifestyle; poor dietary choices; exposure to stressors; and risky reproductive behavior (9,23,34,38). The primary goal of a health promotion or wellness program is to promote health through the maintenance of healthy behaviors, the reduction of unhealthy or risky behaviors and poor health

Table 8.1 Current Trends Toward a Healthy and Productive Workforce

In recent years, some private employers and federal agencies have demonstrated that multifactorial determinants of health and productivity must be dealt with using new perspectives, metrics, and models.

Perspective	Current state	Desired state
Function	Absenteeism	Performance
Cost metrics	Medical costs	Economic outcomes
Care model	Treatment	Prevention
Medical model	Individual	Population
Health metrics	Disease status	Health status
Interventions	Single-risk focused	Multiple-risk focused
Framework	Program centric	Systems oriented
Management systems	Siloed (segregated)	Integrated

choices, and the prevention of chronic disease. In short, an integrated wellness program should

- reduce stress,
- increase activity,
- reduce blood pressure and cholesterol,
- reduce excess weight,
- improve nutritional heath,
- reduce substance use or abuse, and
- optimize workplace safety.

The effectiveness of these approaches to employee health and wellness is well documented (7,24,31).

Beyond Stovepipes

The changing American workplace that is no longer dominated by predictable shifts and a standard 40 h workweek requires employers to move beyond the traditional stovepipe approaches targeted to single risk factors or work-specific concerns. Employers must provide an integrated approach to providing workplace safety programs, occupational and environmental health services, and health insurance and other related benefits (workers' compensation, disability, EAPs, and so on). Stovepipe, employer-defined, and employer-centric (versus employee-defined and employee-centric) approaches cannot serve the needs of employees of the 21st century. Employers must now consider how work and life issues, health behaviors, and social factors influence the provision of health needs in the workplace.

In order for employees and the organization they work for to be successful and competitive in the 21st century, they need to be the following:

- Healthy—engaged in positive health behaviors such as minimizing modifiable risk factors, preventable illness, chronic disease, and injuries
- Productive—functioning at a level of productivity that maximizes their potential to achieve both personal goals and organizational goals
- Ready—able to respond to changing demands of an increasing work pace and unpredictable circumstances
- Resilient—prepared for setbacks, changing demands, and challenges and able to regain optimal well-being and performance without severe detriment to functionality

Each of these sentinel characteristics of an optimally healthy and productive workforce can be measured and improved. Doing so is critical if organizations, managers, and employees are to understand, own, and achieve better health and performance. Occupational health programs that support these attributes integrate health and safety at the workplace and include strategies that strengthen workers' psychological skills and health behaviors. Such programs also provide support for achieving health goals.

Revisioning the Role of Health Benefits

Health insurance benefits and related health benefits programs (workers' compensation, disability, EAPs, and so on) are critical components of an integrated employee health strategy that seeks to optimize health and performance. Historically, however, employers, consultants, and health plans have not designed or implemented benefits that clearly articulate, incentivize, and integrate health, wellness, and evidence-based care management practices. Traditionally, health insurance has focused on reducing both the number of units and the unit price of physician and hospital treatment services rather than offering preventive services or rewarding healthy behaviors (4). With growing evidence for the primary role of health behaviors as causative agents of unnecessary morbidity and mortality from heart disease, cancers, diabetes, stroke, and other chronic conditions, innovative employers are building or demanding comprehensive and integrated benefits designs from their brokers, consultants, and health plan partners (17).

The growing movement toward consumer-directed health plans and value-based benefits design (which can be applied to PPO or HMO plans) enables employers and consumers alike to better understand the relationships among health behaviors, the true cost of health care, and the difference in clinical effectiveness of types of medical services (5). For example, health reimbursement arrangement (HRA) or health savings account (HSA) insurance plans allow employers to pay 100%, without employee co-payment or deductible, for preventive services (screening tests, counseling, immunizations) and behavior change programs (tobacco cessation, weight management).

Employers can also offer financial incentives for employees with chronic disease to enroll in a health improvement or care management program. Employers can couple a proactive health insurance benefits approach that incentivizes prevention and healthy behaviors with on-site programs, primary care clinics, traditional occupational medicine services, fitness centers or benefits, and healthy nutrition options to create a comprehensive employee-centric, supportive, and high-performance corporate culture and environment. See chapter 28 for a discussion on the role of health benefits.

Determining the Health of the Workforce

Through the effective use of a series of tools available to employers, a health profile may be constructed of the entire workforce, created by aggregating employee health data collected at the individual level. Such tools include health assessments and productivity surveys.

Assessment Tools

Today's employer has many options in choosing tools to assess the health and wellness of the workforce. In selecting these tools, employers should follow standard guidance on the reliability and validity of the instruments and should periodically reevaluate the instruments used.

- *The basic tool: the health risk appraisal or health assessment.* One of the most commonly used instruments in workplace preventive health is the health risk appraisal or health assessment. This tool, which comprises a questionnaire, a risk estimate formula, and an educational component, can help predict an individual worker's risk for developing a chronic disease as well as assess the health status of and need for interventions within a group of employees. However, the health assessment cannot effectively reduce an employee's health risks when used as a stand-alone tool; it serves employers best when it is integrated into a comprehensive health strategy that also includes appropriate educational and behavioral intervention (2,10,16,28,37). Health assessments are often integrated into medical benefits plans to provide employers with data to develop disease management programs and coordinate health promotion efforts (12,16,35).

- *Tools to assess productivity.* The term *presenteeism* is used to describe reduced productivity in the workplace that occurs when employees are present at their jobs but because of physical or mental disease or impairment are not functioning at a fully productive level. Reduced worker productivity is a major source of economic loss to employers. Goetzel and colleagues (14) evaluated the cost of the top 10 physical and mental health conditions affecting productivity and found chronic disease conditions and depression-related illnesses to be among the most prevalent and expensive contributors to productivity loss.

Burton and colleagues (7) evaluated the cost of decreased on-the-job productivity using the Work Limitation Questionnaire incorporated into the health assessment of a large national company. Analysis of responses to the questionnaire revealed that 10 of 12 identified health risk factors were significantly associated with self-reported work limitations and that the cost of lost productivity in the company surveyed was $1,392 to $2,592 U.S. per employee per year.

Another analysis of responses to a health assessment demonstrated directional associations between changes in health risks and changes in presenteeism (6). Importantly, this study showed that when employees reduced their health risks they realized an improvement in productivity. When estimated as a cost to employers, an increased or a decreased risk was associated with a 1.9% change in productivity, translating to approximately $950 U.S. per year for each change in risk.

Stress and mental health assessment can be part of the health assessment, along with additional physical data such as elevated blood pressure. Instruments to assess stress, such as the Perceived Stress Scale and the Hassles Scale, focus on individual stressors (3,20,22). Assessment of stressors that arise at the worksite is an important component of a complete mental health assessment.

The Job Content Questionnaire is an instrument designed to assess job-related stressors such as psychological demands, decision latitude, social support, physical demands, and job insecurity (21). This instrument has been used in conjunction with other mental and physical health assessment instruments to identify relationships between job-related stressors and employee health and productivity (11,26).

Public Health Resources

A number of health and wellness programs are available from U.S. federal agencies such as the Department of Health and Human Services. Examples of programs from federal agencies are described in the following paragraphs.

- *Healthy People 2010.* The goals and objectives of *Healthy People 2010* (36) are the result of a collaborative effort among federal, state, and territorial governments and private, public, and nonprofit organizations. The two overarching goals for *Healthy People 2010* are

    1. to increase quality and years of healthy life and
    2. to eliminate health disparities.

Within the overarching goals are 28 focus areas, each with a concise goal statement, as well as 467 specific objectives. The focus areas include issues such as access to quality health services and occupational safety and health, specific chronic diseases, physical activity, and nutrition. The objectives of *Healthy People 2010* serve as a guide to better health for the U.S. population and are designed to be used at all levels of government and by public and private organizations.

The specific objectives of *Healthy People 2010* are implemented through various mechanisms, including the Healthy People Consortium. This consortium is an alliance of organizations that support the goals of *Healthy People 2010.* The membership consists of state and territorial public health, mental health, substance abuse, and environmental agencies and national organizations representing professional, advocacy, and business sectors. At present, there are more than 400 national membership organizations that have joined the Healthy People Consortium and that work together with federal and state agencies to advance health.

Members of the Healthy People Consortium assist in developing the *Healthy People 2010* objectives and play an important role in implementing, monitoring, and reporting on the United States' successes and challenges in health. Many consortium members have developed health promotion and disease prevention programs using *Healthy People 2010* objectives and have adopted *Healthy People 2010* objectives as part of their missions.

- *U.S. Task Force on Community Preventive Services.* The U.S. Task Force on Community Preventive Services issues recommendations regarding the use of specific interventions and population health improvement strategies. These recommendations are based on systematic reviews conducted by the scientists of the CDC in collaboration with other subject matter experts from academia, research, and practice settings as well as other federal agencies. The recommendations are published in the peer-reviewed literature and are assembled in the

Guide to Community Preventive Services (the Community Guide; 8). Reviews for the *Community Guide* focus on population-based strategies appropriate for communities such as worksites and health care systems. Chapters 9 and 10 offer excellent examples of a *Community Guide* systematic review and an overview of the importance of using evidence in the workplace health promotion field. Recommendations from the Task Force on Community Preventive Services specific to worksite settings may guide solid decisions for investment of resources. Other completed reviews and recommendations can be found on the *Community Guide* Web site (www.thecommunityguide.org).

- *NIOSH Steps to a Healthier US Workforce.* The Steps to a Healthier US Workforce initiative was developed to encourage workplace safety and health programs that focus on both preventing work-related illness, injury, and disability and promoting healthy living to reduce and prevent chronic disease. The Steps to a Healthier US Cooperative Agreement Program, of which the workforce component is a part, is coordinated by the U.S. Department of Health and Human Services and the CDC. This is a national, multilevel program focused on preventing chronic disease in communities across the United States (25).

The primary objective of the overall Steps program is to improve lives by helping Americans reduce their risk of chronic disease and enjoy longer, better, and healthier lives. This objective is implemented by providing funding to communities to implement disease prevention and health promotion programs that target three major chronic diseases—diabetes, obesity, and asthma—and their underlying risk factors of physical inactivity, poor nutrition, and tobacco use. The Steps program was designed to create an opportunity for the occupational safety and health community and the health promotion community to work together to develop and implement workplace programs aimed at preventing workplace illness and injury and optimizing the health of the U.S. workforce.

Implementing an Integrated Program

The actual integration of various program components is not an easy task. This process needs to benefit from both strategic and tactical planning and start at the highest level of the organization. Several aspects of implementation of an integrated program are discussed here.

Integrating Across Program Components

Key actions needed to join together health programs and create an integrated health system are breaking down a stovepipe approach to health programs and moving toward programs that integrate across organizational functions and changing from employer- to employee-centric health priorities. Integration strategies have been described in the research literature (18,32). Crucial to the success of these programs is targeting integration strategies at both organizational and individual levels.

At the organizational level, health promotion traditionally is separated from occupational health and safety. In a traditional system, programs are administered as separate entitites in separate offices with different training and education for program administrators. In an integrated system, these two entities work in tandem, providing employees with a comprehensive program that can help them plan health strategies that are complementary and thus more effective in meeting their needs at a lower cost to employers.

At the individual level, health programs can be enhanced through integration of program content. For example, providing employees with preventive health messages, such as smoking cessation, can be linked to messages about reducing hazardous workplace exposures, thereby reducing overall risk for adverse health outcomes inside and outside the workplace. A schematic view of integrated health management is shown in figure 8.1.

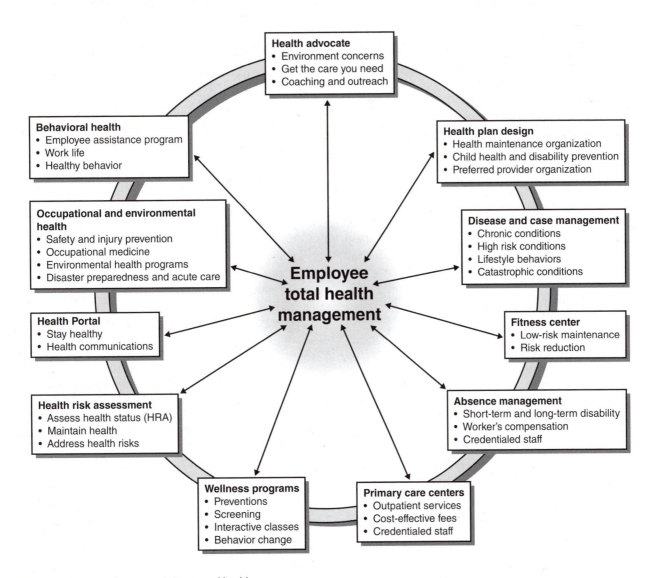

Figure 8.1 Employee-centric integrated health.

Reprinted with permission from Integrating Employee Health: A Model Program for NASA ©2005 by the National Academy of Sciences. Courtesy of the National Academies Press, Washington, D.C.

Transitioning From Health Promotion to Integrated Design

Successful implementation of an integrated health program requires careful planning that is based on appropriate needs assessments. In addition, program integration should be based on an employee-centric approach that responds to employee needs, readiness, workplace culture, and priorities. Avenues for employee input into integrated health program planning vary by organization.

Wellness committees that include employees working with management help to ensure that programs are developed in accordance with empolyee needs, readiness for change, worksite culture, and workplace priorities. Health and wellness committees should crosscut and be inclusive across organizations. However, workers whose job schedules have less flexibility or whose jobs may be at lower levels in the organization may not be motivated to contribute in a meeting that includes representatives from management (30). Thus, providing management-level support for participation in health and wellness committees is an important step in the process of transitioning to integrated health programs.

Options to Improve Productivity and Reduce Labor Costs

• *Include incentives for participation.* Incentives such as cash, spending account credits, gifts, or reduced premiums on medical plans can be used to increase employees' motivation to participate in health promotion programs. Financial incentives have been shown to increase program participation over other types of incentives (19), although incentives may not consistently improve outcomes (15,33). See chapter 28 for more information.

• *Overcome barriers to obtaining desired outcomes.* Several barriers that are significant challenges in the implementation of integrated programs should be considered (17). Health disparity, or the uneven distribution of health risk across the employee population, is one of the major barriers to consider. Disparities may exist among different occupational groups or racial or ethnic groups. There may also be disparities between regular and contract workers or English and non-English-speaking workers. See chapter 25 for more on addressing diversity and health literacy at the worksite.

Other barriers to consider include those related to organizational culture, the built worksite environment, and challenges employees face in balancing work and life. The organizational culture can significantly impede progress on implementation, as making change is difficult in a context that is not conducive to change initiatives. In such cases, organizational leadership becomes a critical element in turning the tide in favor of the change efforts (see chapter 26 for more on creating a culture of health). The built environment can substantially support change efforts, but in many cases it acts as a barrier. Promoting increased use of the stairs to support a physical activity program, for example, may be complicated when elevators are centrally located and stairs are difficult to locate, poorly lit, and unsafe. Issues in balancing work and life may pose significant barriers to implementating an integrated health program, as the family-related needs of workers may distract their attention away from participation. The consideration of family-responsive policies is a crucial component of a supportive health-oriented culture.

Data Integration and Management

Integrated health management relies on a systematic approach to data collection and management. Edington (10) noted that an integrated data management approach offers an advantage to employers by generating data reports that provide

• statistical information on program use and effectiveness,
• accountability measures on program performance,
• assessment and analysis information on program changes, and
• performance measures for future program research and development.

Organizational Framework

An effective data management and measurement system supports organizational objectives such as decision making, accountability, improvement, and surveillance. These four faces of measurement can be utilized in developing an organizational framework to achieve data management objectives (18,27).

1. Measurement for decision making requires that responsible managers with decision-making authority have appropriate access to information needed to achieve specific objectives. In addition, these managers must be provided with the highest quality data that are accurate, reliable, and up to date.

2. Measurement for accountability comes into play when measurements are used to report on progress toward stated objectives. These

measures may include process measures but most likely will be outcome measures.

3. Measurement for improvement involves data collection and measurement strategies that identify potential problems, barriers, or opportunities for improvement and facilitate the implementation of initiatives. It involves data collection (often in short cycles) to measure the improvement and to verify that change has taken place. Good examples of this strategy include Continuous Quality Improvement (CQI) and the Plan-Do-Study-Act (PDSA) cycle.

4. Measurement for surveillance supports the need for uncovering unanticipated problems, longitudinal analyses, and knowledge discovery related to integrated health programs. This strategy also allows for retrospective analyses of specific data sets that may support the need to understand concerns and provide critical insights.

Program Evaluation

Program evaluation is a critical component of a successful program since it allows for the quantification and documentation of experiences and the presentation of those results to the key stakeholders for continued program support. Program evaluation is described in detail in chapter 15 and should be in itself an integrated strategy. The ability to use data for purposes of documenting progress and driving strategy is central to continued success of the program.

Ongoing improvement efforts should also be driven by a recognized structure and process, which are driven by the organization's integrated health policies. Figure 8.2 presents this approach.

Conclusion

The case for change toward an increasingly integrated, employee-centered, prevention- and systems-oriented, data-driven population health strategy for organizations and worksites calls for a shift from the traditionally reactive and segregated employee health strategies to one that is aligned with company mission and organized around employee health needs while being driven by data. Integrated across a variety of organizational functions, this type of strategy provides a company culture and environment that support employees in their individual change efforts and creates a continuous feedback mechanism that provides ongoing data for use in improvement initiatives. Public health resources for health improvement easily accessible in the public

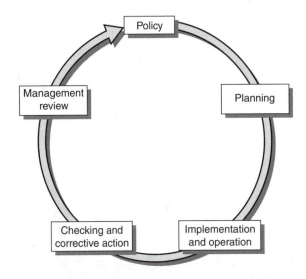

Figure 8.2 The cycle of continuous improvement.
Reprinted with permission from Integrating Employee Health: A Model Program for NASA ©2005 by the National Academy of Sciences. Courtesy of the National Academies Press, Washington, D.C.

domain and linked to major health objectives for the nation provide important information that may support the company in addressing health risks and concerns that are highly dependent upon community collaboration in order to generate successful outcomes.

Chapter Review Questions

1. Name several of the major shifts in philosophy and approach that must be achieved in order to create a healthy and productive workforce.

2. What are the characteristics of a healthy and productive workforce?

3. What evidence supports an integrated approach to employee health versus traditional approaches to wellness, human resources training, occupational health, health insurance, disability, and workers' compensation?

4. What health behaviors and risk factors should be addressed in a comprehensive, integrated employee health program?

5. Name several federal efforts and models that can be used to build an integrated approach to employee health using best practices.

6. Describe the importance and potential use of health and performance or productivity assessments in defining, implementing, and evaluating an integrated employee health program.

Part

II

The Evidence for Employer-Sponsored Health Programs

How confident can employers be that investments made in worksite health promotion are a wise use of company resources? What should be the type of evidence an employer ought to look for prior to making decisions regarding the allocation of resources to worksite health promotion programs? How should specific programs be connected to available scientific research findings that clearly establish an evidence-based foundation for such programs? How should evidence of effectiveness be considered in the context of a changing work environment and how health may be impacted by the changing organization of work? What should be the process and what concepts and strategies should be considered when solutions to health and productivity management are implemented at the worksite? These questions are central to the chapters presented in Part II of this book.

Chapter 9 presents a thoughtfully balanced introduction to the role of evidence in worksite health promotion. It sets the tone upon which the remaining five chapters in Part II build their message. Those chapters present a specific example of a systematic review that generates clear recommendations of effectiveness, a method to translate evidence into practical solutions and to inform research through practice-based learnings, an outline of best practices as a form of evidence of effectiveness, a consideration of the organization of work and how it affects the health of the worker, and an overview of health and productivity management processes and strategies that are couched in emerging evidence of effectiveness. Part II of this book presents an opportunity to deepen your understanding of evidence of effectiveness and how to consider such evidence in the context of practice-based realities.

9

An Introduction to Evidence on Worksite Health Promotion

Jonathan E. Fielding, MD, MPH, MBA, and David P. Hopkins, MD, MPH

Employers or health promotion planners intent on improving the health and safety of their workforce must efficiently find answers to difficult questions. What are possible approaches to improving the health of this working population? What should be done given the current resources? What types of evidence should be considered in choosing among different alternatives? And, of particular interest, what evidence exists on the effectiveness of different approaches, and how should this evidence be utilized in the decision-making process?

The first step for those interested in finding evidence is to define it. "The available facts, circumstances, etc. indicating whether or not a thing is valid or true" is how one dictionary defines evidence (19, p. 277). As discussed later, defining evidence within a decision-making process requires an effort to search for appropriate facts, to evaluate the validity of this information, and to draw a conclusion regarding truth across the available data.

What most decision makers want to know is whether there are facts that validate a particular type of approach and the choice of alternative ways to implement that approach. However, there are many different types of evidence that may be considered in the process, and a decision may depend not only on the evidence but also on the specific priorities and concerns of the sponsoring organization. For example, a health plan may decide to sponsor a worksite health promotion program for the workforce it covers simply to obtain a competitive edge in the group health insurance market. An employer may offer such

a program because it believes the program can enhance recruitment and retention in a tight labor market. In these decision-making situations, the major type of evidence considered (and sought) is the short-term effect on the sponsor's top and bottom lines of the profit and loss statement.

When the sponsor's goal is to improve the health and safety of a specific working population, an important form of information is evidence on effectiveness. The basic question is simple: Does a particular type of worksite health promotion activity or policy result in improvements in health or in risk factors that strongly influence future health? In addition, however, there are many subsidiary questions that need to be answered to inform program planning and implementation. Many of these questions can be answered through a careful review of the evidence on effectiveness. In what types of industries, settings, or working populations has a particular intervention been shown to work? What is the expected magnitude of effect? Does the effect of the intervention differ by gender, age, job classification, or ethnic or racial group? What are the characteristics of the activity or policy that are associated with effectiveness? How long is the effect likely to last?

Before delving deeper into evidence on effectiveness and the process of evidence-based decision making, it is helpful to review the range of objectives that demonstrate an effect on the health of a working population. An overall improvement in health will result from the combination of the following events within the workforce: (1) a reduction in unhealthy behaviors (such as smoking or binge alcohol consumption), (2) an

The findings and conclusions in this chapter are those of the authors and the Task Force on Community Preventive Services and do not necessarily represent the views of the Centers for Disease Control and Prevention.

increase in behaviors that promote health (such as regularly performed aerobic physical activity or better nutritional choices), (3) an improvement in the detection of modifiable or treatable health conditions (such as high blood pressure), and (4) an improvement in managing workers' existing health conditions (such as diabetes). The program planner considers implementing activities or policies to promote individual health action for one or more of these objectives. While the ideal program would address all of these goals, most health promotion programs lack sufficient resources to start with a comprehensive approach, and so the program must be built up over time.

Public health action occurs through the selection, adaptation, and implementation of interventions with the potential to affect the health or the health-related behaviors of some, many, or all individuals within a targeted population (many practitioners would add additional steps to this list, such as baseline needs assessment and ongoing monitoring with quality improvement; 17). These population-based interventions are implemented to change one or more behaviors in a group of individuals by utilizing basic strategies to motivate individual health action (with potential application to other settings, populations, and targeted outcomes).

Population change may occur when, for example, policies or regulations (such as the adoption of policies for a smoke-free worksite) alter the background environment and establish a new behavior norm (21). Change may also occur in response to the dissemination of educational or motivational information (such as posters or brochures promoting annual influenza vaccination). Finally, change may occur when opportunities for individual health action are created, provided, or enhanced through a variety of distinct approaches (such as providing facilities, instruction, or time at work for employees to be physically active).

Why is the search for evidence to inform these decisions so important? The best reason to search for evidence is to avoid wasting money. In most cases, population-based interventions require significant resources (staff, time, money, and social capital). An ineffective program not only wastes money up front but also delays the adoption of an effective program that actually improves worker health and provides a return on the investment.

Incorporating some or all of the evidence on effectiveness into the decision-making process provides guidance on the range of options for addressing each specific health issue or health-related behavior and provides an opportunity to learn from both the success and the failures of others who have tried to implement and evaluate a specific intervention.

Another critical reason to make evidence a part of the decision-making process is to build the foundation of support for the intervention proposal itself. In for-profit organizations, investment in employee health and well-being competes with other possible investments, such as acquisitions, with the ultimate goal being to maximize shareholder value. In nonprofit and governmental organizations, there is a responsibility to the public to spend resources wisely. In all organizations, the people who are responsible for the planning and implementation of any program are accountable to their superiors. Documenting the evidence base for a specific approach to improve employee health provides a much more powerful argument to support the final selection and implementation of that program.

Evidence-Based Worksite Health Promotion

Public health practitioners have long considered the worksite to be an essential setting for public health action, beginning with the identification and recognition of occupational diseases (see *De Morbis Artificum Diatriba* by Bernardino Ramazzini, 1700 [22]) and continuing into the modern age with efforts to reduce and prevent work-related illness, injury, and death. Although attention to occupation-specific health risks remains important in preserving the health of the working population, efforts to improve worker health have expanded in the last several decades to include efforts to address the chronic health behaviors and conditions that increasingly contribute to the actual causes of death in American society (15). This expanding perspective makes perfect sense from the standpoints of the employer, the employee, and society at large. First, the amount of time spent at work is significant. Second, important behaviors contributing to ill health (such as physical inactivity) are extremely prevalent in working populations. Third, employers who provide health care coverage to their employees are increasingly and appropriately interested in the overall health of their workforce (8). Fourth, basic changes to promote healthy or healthier behaviors (such as instituting smoke-free policies) can be readily implemented or adopted by employers and can influence the behaviors of employees both immediately and throughout the entire duration of employment. Taken together, these factors make it increasingly important that health promotion efforts in communities include the worksite as a setting for action and reinforce the need for establishing partnerships between worksites and their larger communities.

It is therefore logical and useful to apply definitions and standards regarding evidence described within public health directly to our understanding of evidence on the effectiveness of interventions to improve the health of workers. We can adopt, for example, a recent definition of evidence-based public health as "the process of integrating science-based interventions with community preferences to improve the health of populations" (14). We can also adopt the classification scheme for scientific evidence that was recently proposed by Lucy Rychetnik and colleagues (16) and expanded on earlier work by Ross Brownson and colleagues (5), in which each type of evidence provides information to one stage of evidence-based decision making and health promotion planning.

Type 1 evidence helps to identify and explain the relationships among the cause of disease, the development of disease, and the effect of disease on the population. This form of evidence contributes to the decision that something should be done and can provide direction as to the important health-related behaviors to target and approaches to consider. For example, literally thousands of studies published over the last 50 years provide conclusive information on the direct relationship between tobacco use and health, identifying diseases specifically associated with smoking and the population effect of death, illness, and disability attributable to smoking (20). Tobacco use remains the number one preventable cause of morbidity and mortality (20), and the wealth of available evidence firmly documents that any comprehensive worksite health promotion effort should do something about tobacco use (3,18).

Type 2 evidence informs the decision maker as to the effectiveness of a specific intervention in improving health. Evidence on the effectiveness or ineffectiveness of a specific intervention provides extremely useful information to program planners, who frequently need to choose between two (or more) potential approaches to address the targeted health condition or health-related behavior (and then advocate for that selection).

Type 3 evidence provides information regarding the implementation of a policy or intervention. This evidence helps the planner decide on the how-to aspects of the selected intervention. This part of the intervention process frequently requires the greatest input from the decision makers, as almost all settings have both common and unique barriers to address in the application and conduction of the intervention.

All three types of evidence play an important role in health promotion planning. Type 1 evidence provides a mandate for action and helps to provide the health behavior targets. Type 2 evidence provides the planner with a list of potential interventions and the evidence on their effectiveness. Type 3 evidence provides guidance for successfully implementing a potentially effective program. Although the remainder of this chapter focuses on type 2 evidence, all three forms of information should be considered in making program decisions. Even with a clear mandate for action and evidence of intervention effectiveness, the program results may still depend on the ability of implementers to translate the successful experiences of others into an approach that is effective in their own worksite and for their own workforce.

Sources of Evidence on Effectiveness for Worksite Health Promotion

There is no complete source of evidence, much less evidence on effectiveness, to aid in program planning and implementation. The evidence guiding the selection of which behaviors and conditions to target, which interventions to adopt, and which ways to implement these interventions must come from a variety of available sources. Useful information can be obtained from the shared experiences of others in the same field, from the opinion of an experienced or expert group, from a single formally designed and executed scientific study, or from a formal process of combining findings from a group of related studies. A sound decision-making process, however, should involve the differential consideration of evidence based on the strengths and limitations of the source and content of the information.

Finding sufficient evidence to inform any program decision is not always easy, but the scope of the search can be efficiently narrowed depending on the objectives of those who are developing the program. How comprehensive is the initial health promotion program going to be? What health or health behavior outcomes are the targets for change? Trying to change knowledge, for example, requires much less intensive programming than that required for changing most behaviors, but it may not, in the end, have a significant effect on worker health. Targeting health care utilization or health care costs for change involves a narrower search for evidence, as there are fewer studies that have addressed these outcomes. Only a small percentage of the published studies have as their objectives to bring about change in selected measures of productivity, either directly or by using more easily assessed indicators such as absenteeism.

The types of evidence sought also depend on the constraints imposed on the program planners. The worksites of the targeted employees may limit the range of intervention options and thus the search for evidence. For example, a widely dispersed workforce cannot use a centralized delivery model, such as a company gym. Technology constraints should also be considered. Web-based program delivery (and collection of evidence on effectiveness) is more feasible in settings in which employees routinely use a computer as part of their work. In most cases, financial constraints limit the types of health promotion programs that can be established. An intensive program can cost hundreds of dollars per year per employee.

Once the range of feasible program options has been determined, how can reliable and valid information be found on what has worked for others and what are the costs to implement each option in a particular workforce? As noted previously, there are a variety of sources of evidence, each with a set of strengths and limitations. Given the investment of time and other financial resources required for health promotion efforts, it makes sense to always consider the standardized and reliable information typically provided through scientific studies and the increasingly available summaries of findings across a body of scientific studies conducted according to systematic review methods.

Scientific Studies and Evidence-Based Decision Making

In general, evaluations that are subjected to peer review as part of the submission for publication have been assessed for the appropriateness of the research question, the study design and execution, the data analysis, and the degree to which specific conclusions are supported. This form of evidence (the scientific study) is commonly considered to be appropriate for an assessment of effectiveness. Nevertheless, peer review and publication do not guarantee the quality of the study or the validity of the study findings and conclusions. Incorporat-

ing scientific evidence on effectiveness into the decision-making process still requires a degree of critical evaluation (and baseline skepticism). In addition, there are likely to be significant differences between the content of any one scientific study and the specific information needs of the program planner or decision maker.

Those who are reviewing the evidentiary base should ask themselves several questions. Do I understand the specifics of the intervention described in this study? Is the study population similar to our workforce? Are the outcomes evaluated in this study relevant to our own health promotion objectives? Are the results presented in a manner in which I can determine the health effect attributable to the intervention? Does the information help me to judge whether the results justify the investment?

Systematic Reviews in Support of Evidence-Based Decision Making

A systematic review is a formal process conducted to identify all of the relevant scientific studies on a topic and to provide a concise evaluation of the findings across the body of evidence. The hallmarks of systematic evidence reviews are (1) an effort to find all of the available evidence; (2) an attempt to evaluate the quality of the available evidence, both individually and collectively; and (3) an attempt to acknowledge or to summarize the outcomes across the body of evidence (9). Each process follows explicit methods with the goal of providing a clear and defensible presentation of the included evidence. As scientific efforts, systematic reviews include a detailed methods description of the research questions, the interventions considered within the review, the outcomes considered in the assessment of effectiveness, the search strategy and yield of included studies, the analytic methods and results, and the basis for the conclusion. In most cases, these elements are tailored to provide information that is both useful and understandable to practitioners. Systematic reviews make it easier for planners and decision makers to appreciate all of the relevant information as well as how it was collected and summarized and how the conclusions relate to the information that was reviewed (9). Systematic reviews can also provide direct support for official or expert panel recommendations regarding the use of that intervention (12). Linking the systematic review process and findings directly to the recommendation regarding use provides a more transparent, understandable, and credible recommendation (9).

Evidence from systematic reviews provides several advantages for program planning compared with the contributions of a single scientific study. First, a consistent display of effect size across a number of similar studies can strengthen confidence that the observed effect was due to the intervention and not to other factors such as the specific study setting or target population, the presence of one or more confounders or forms of bias, or the role of chance. Second, evidence from a number of studies is more likely to include one or more studies in which approaches and results are more directly applicable to the target workforce and circumstances. Third, the distribution of results across the body of evidence provides a more useful (realistic) range of likely effects for the outcomes of interest (and also a pooled summary estimate when it can be calculated appropriately). Finally, a systematic review provides some protection against inadvertently or purposefully including or excluding evidence from certain scientific studies and thus strengthens the resulting decision or position proposal.

Nonetheless, there are important limitations in systematic reviews of which program planners and decision makers should be aware. First, systematic reviews do not protect against publication bias—the exclusion of relevant evidence because authors won't submit or journals won't accept completed scientific studies with negative, small, weak, and inconsistent findings (13). Second, differences in methods across systematic reviews may result in differences in what evidence is eligible for inclusion and can directly influence the findings and conclusions. Third, most systematic reviews depend on a body of evidence (generally from more than one study) to support a consolidated assessment and conclusion. As a result, they summarize existing findings rather than lead scientific investigation or innovation. Finally, because conducting a systematic review is labor intensive, some types of interventions have not yet been subject to systematic reviews or the available reviews are old, leading to significant gaps in published review literature. Thus, the reader must always consider the systematic review critically.

A number of systematic reviews and review organizations provide information regarding the effectiveness of interventions specifically evaluated in or generally applicable to worksite settings. The Cochrane Collaboration, for one, was created in 1993. In 1999 it expanded from the primary consideration of systematic reviews of health care interventions to address issues of health promotion and public health as well (6). The Cochrane Library provides a searchable database of Cochrane reviews for topics or interventions, other related systematic reviews, economic evaluations, and clinical trials (7).

The *Guide to Community Preventive Services* provides systematic reviews on population-based interventions to address a wide range of health topics (11,18). The reviews for the *Community Guide* focus on strategies appropriate for communities (including worksites) and health care systems. Using the findings of the systematic review, the U.S. Task Force on Community Preventive Services (Task Force)—a nonfederal, independent body of nationally renowned experts in public health research, practice, and policy—issues recommendations regarding the use of interventions. An example of a *Community Guide* systematic review and a recommendation from the Task Force specific to worksite settings is provided later in this book (see chapter 10), while other completed reviews and recommendations can be found on the *Community Guide* Web site (www. thecommunityguide.org).

Task Force conclusions and recommendations regarding the use of an intervention are based primarily on the evidence of effectiveness across a body of studies. Evidence of effectiveness across the studies evaluating an intervention typically requires a consistent demonstration of a meaningful effect on one or more health outcomes or behaviors directly related to health outcomes (such as quitting smoking). The Task Force also considers the applicability of the findings across the body of evidence to important target populations (such as worksites, schools, broader communities, and populations with recognized health disparities). Finally, the Task Force considers findings regarding other benefits, potential harms, and barriers to the implementation of the intervention (such as concerns about infrastructure requirements or threats to employee confidentiality).

Since its inception in 1996, the Task Force has conducted intervention reviews for a number of topics directly related to health improvement and promotion efforts for working-aged adults. Sets of intervention reviews are available for the following objectives:

- Reducing tobacco use and exposure to secondhand tobacco smoke
- Increasing physical activity
- Improving nutrition
- Improving cancer screening

- Reducing excessive consumption of alcohol
- Reducing drinking and driving
- Increasing the use of seat belts
- Improving condition management among persons with diabetes
- Increasing vaccination coverage for influenza, pneumococcus, and hepatitis B in adults at increased risk of infection or complications

A complete list of the intervention reviews and recommendations currently available can be located at www.thecommunityguide.org.

The Cochrane Collaboration and the *Guide to Community Preventive Services* are by no means the only sources of systematic reviews of evidence on effectiveness of interventions appropriate for consideration within a worksite health promotion program. A recent systematic review on the effectiveness of using pedometers to increase physical activity and improve health, with potential application to worksite health promotion efforts, was conducted by one of many academic and clinical research centers invested in the production of systematic reviews to address a wide range of topics and interventions (2).

Insufficient Evidence

With even the most thorough effort to find and consider the available information, the program planner will commonly face situations in which the available evidence regarding a new or promising health promotion approach is insufficient to fully inform a decision. In our experience of systematic review, finding insufficient evidence on whether an intervention works is most commonly the result of too few scientific studies (18). Other factors contributing to a finding of insufficient evidence include summary results across the evidence that are so small in magnitude that a planner might consider them too small to justify the investment and findings across the included studies that are inconsistent (so the planner is not sure what is going on). In some cases, most or all of the studies included in the review used different methods and measurements to evaluate health outcomes, complicating an overall assessment of effect. In other cases, the settings or populations included in the evidence are significantly different from the setting and population under consideration for a health promotion program.

When considering a systematic review as evidence on effectiveness, it is important to understand that insufficient evidence does not mean

that an intervention doesn't work (though this should not imply that an intervention is effective until proven otherwise). Given insufficient evidence regarding the intervention or health promotion approach under consideration, planners and decision makers are faced with several choices. One option is to select a different intervention or approach that has a stronger body of studies to support its effectiveness and a decision regarding its use. A second option is to reinforce a proposal for an insufficiently evaluated intervention by investing adequate resources to ensure a high-quality evaluation of its effectiveness. Careful evaluation is helpful not only to the sponsoring organization but also to the entire field, as it should become part of the body of studies with sufficient design and execution to be considered in future systematic reviews guiding future decisions. As noted previously, systematic reviews are not conducted to lead scientific inquiry or innovation. New approaches to worksite health promotion with a strong conceptual rationale or promising results in an initial study may be worth strong consideration for use in a given worksite and workforce.

Specific Issues Regarding Worksite Health Promotion Literature

There are some limitations in the conduct of scientific evaluations in worksite settings, and these limitations influence the kind of studies conducted and the types of data available to help in the decision-making process. First, although basic principles of public health and responsible organizational stewardship militate for evaluating the effect of every intervention and policy, conduction of the evaluation requires expertise and resources (which in many cases come out of the intervention budget itself). In the decision-making tug-of-war between allocating more programmatic resources and doing careful evaluations, the former often wins. This is unfortunate given the benefits of determining (sooner rather than later) whether an expensive health promotion program is having the desired effect on the targeted workforce (and is worth continuing or needs to be changed).

Second, regardless of the setting and study population, scientific evaluations are expensive, and the importance of measuring change in relation to an unexposed comparison population (costs for which can exceed the costs of the intervention itself) is underappreciated. From an employee relations perspective, it may not be tenable or logistically feasible to have a control group that does not receive (or has to wait years to receive) the touted health promotion program being provided to coworkers. As a result, in reviews of worksite health promotion the predominant form of evidence available to understand intervention effect remains the uncontrolled pre- and poststudy design in which it is difficult to determine if the observed change can be attributed entirely to the intervention or program. For most worksite health promotion approaches, there is a paucity of evidence from evaluations in which change is based on the observed difference between an intervention group and a concurrent comparison group. These study designs provide some protection against the influence of study participation, observation, loss to follow-up, and confounding of the measurements of health and health behavior change.

Additional Considerations on Evidence Regarding Worksite Health Promotion

Although peer-reviewed studies have some limitations, other sources of evidence are likely to have more. One source of evidence, for example, comes from companies that sell products and services for use in health promotion efforts. Their claims about their products should be considered critically.

Outside evaluation can help employers to determine whether their programs and policies are effective. However, there are potential sources of bias even when an outside, independent group is hired to perform evaluations. It is important to know the group's terms of engagement. Was the evaluation its only relationship with the funding entity? Does the outside group hope for continued business with the employer? In the evaluation, was the independent group free to develop research protocols, to determine the outcomes assessed, and to publish whatever it felt was appropriate to the field?

The value of asking these questions has been increasingly recognized. Issues raised with respect to research on pharmaceutical and medical devices have highlighted the need for greater scrutiny of companies that pay for independent research (1,10). Concerns about the objectives of the research and its conclusions have led to greater disclosure of the relationships between researchers and funders as part of articles published in many peer-reviewed journals (4). Similar issues deserve scrutiny in publications of original research on worksite health promotion programs or program components.

However, many of the peer-reviewed articles contributing to current evidence-based decisions were published before these types of disclosure were routinely required.

Reports of employer-conducted research also warrant critical consideration for potential sources of bias. The same individuals who planned and implemented these programs directed many of these evaluations. The inherent incentives in these evaluations are to demonstrate program success. In some cases, especially in private industry, demonstration of success can affect these individuals' (or their managers') base compensation, yearly bonuses, or likelihood of promotion.

Conclusion

Decision makers within the field of worksite health promotion must efficiently consider evidence, in its many forms, when selecting, implementing, evaluating, and modifying interventions to improve the health and safety of the workforce. Although information on the effectiveness of a specific intervention or health promotion program can be obtained in a number of ways, a decision-making process should always include an effort to appreciate the scientific literature. Systematic reviews provide an efficient and concise evaluation of a body of scientific studies and increasingly address specific questions regarding the effectiveness of population-based strategies appropriate for consideration by program planners and funders. Although the peer-reviewed scientific literature provides some protection, there remain limitations in the conduction, reporting, and publication of evidence on the effectiveness of approaches to worksite health promotion.

Chapter Review Questions

1. Describe the relationship between and the potential importance of worksite health promotion and public health.

2. Discuss the factors involved in evidence-based decision making regarding worksite health promotion.

3. Consider how types 1, 2, and 3 evidence might shape the decision-making process.

4. Consider the advantages and disadvantages of using evidence derived from a systematic review process compared with a single scientific study.

5. How can decisions regarding worksite health promotion be improved? What kinds of evidence might contribute to better decisions?

The Assessment of Health Risks With Feedback

Results of a Systematic Review

Robin E. Soler, PhD; Matt Griffith, MPH; David P. Hopkins, MD, MPH; and Kimberly D. Leeks, PhD, MPH

As described in previous chapters, improving the health of most workers depends on reducing risky behaviors and increasing healthy behaviors. One avenue designed to motivate individual behavior change involves providing information on personal health risk based on current health behaviors and physiological measurements. Identifying a person's risky behaviors may constitute an important step toward leading a healthier life.

Worksite health promotion programs often include a health risk assessment to identify risky behaviors of workers. A 2004 national survey of worksite health promotion found that nearly 50% of companies with more than 750 employees reported having offered a health risk assessment (9). Health risk assessments are easy to administer (computerized versions are available), obtain a lot of information quickly, permit access to large populations, provide health estimates across the workforce, and can be used to recommend employees for follow-up intervention. These attributes make assessments attractive to worksite health promotion planners. Additionally, since contributors to worker morbidity and mortality tend to cluster, these types of population-based assessments that identify multiple risk factors at once can be a time- and resource-saving intervention.

The *Guide to Community Preventive Services* (*Community Guide*) recently conducted systematic reviews of the published literature on health risk assessments. Because the terms *health risk appraisal* and *health risk assessment* as well as the acronym *HRA* have been used interchangeably in the field and in published literature, this chapter refers to the assessment under discussion as *assessment of health risks with feedback (AHRF)*. Systematic reviews for the *Community Guide* employ a standardized methodology for identifying, including, evaluating, and summarizing evidence on prioritized population-based interventions (3,13). After reviewing the evidence, the nonfederal and independent Task Force on Community Preventive Services (Task Force) issues an evidence-based recommendation for or against the use of the reviewed intervention or concludes that insufficient evidence exists to determine an intervention's effectiveness. The *Community Guide* also identifies research gaps related to all interventions and assesses cost efficiency for all recommended interventions.

This chapter discusses two systematic reviews of the *Community Guide:* one on the effectiveness of the AHRF when used alone and one on its effectiveness when it is used in combination with other interventions (AHRF Plus). In it, we provide summaries of the evidence for the effectiveness of this approach and its influence on the health and productivity of workers. For AHRF Plus we also summarize the economic evidence on the cost efficiency of the approach. Finally, we present the Task Force recommendations for using AHRF and AHRF Plus in worksite settings. Detailed

---

This entire review included 69 studies and excluded 13 studies. The reference list for this chapter is limited to those appropriate for the chapter itself. However, a full reference list of included and excluded studies is available at www.thecommunityguide.org/worksite.

findings of the systematic reviews, including summary evidence tables and the full conclusions of the Task Force, have been submitted for journal publication and are also available online at www.thecommunityguide.org/worksite.

The AHRF Intervention

Though health risk assessments have been conducted for more than two decades, there is no consensus definition of what they are. The HRA has been described as a tool, a technique, and, more recently, a process (1,2,5). The HRA was initially used to reduce the incidence of death by making individuals aware of their risks with the intention of motivating them to change their behaviors (15).

Most researchers in the field agree that there are common elements in the HRA process. These elements include an assessment of personal health habits and risk factors (which may be supplemented by physiological measurements), a quantitative estimation or qualitative assessment of future health risk, and feedback via educational messages or counseling describing how behavior change might reduce disease or delay death (1,2,5). The content of the intervention can vary among programs and can include different combinations of physiological and behavioral indicators, risk calculation methods, and feedback mechanisms.

The assessment portion of this intervention uses a tool to gather information about an individual's health behaviors or physiological indicators. It can vary in format and may consist of person-to-person interviews, Web-based data collection, phone interviews, or self-administered questionnaires. It can also vary in content, including, for instance, blood pressure measurements, cholesterol levels, weight, BMI, smoking status, alcohol use, and seat belt use.

The next step of the AHRF intervention includes some type of calculation of an individual's health risks or risks of death or disease. The calculation might be a health risk score, a health age, or some other summary risk result. However, all calculations are tailored to the information gathered in the individual's assessment. The various algorithms and thresholds used each have different strengths and challenges.

Feedback takes the information gathered by the assessment tool and the calculated health risks and attempts to motivate individual action. Feedback can vary in form and function but typically involves presenting a letter or report to the employee that includes the generated health risk estimate. The estimate may be accompanied by more detailed information regarding individual responses to assessment items or by information regarding behavior change, tailored to the employee's risk or focusing on behaviors or chronic diseases of interest to the employer. Delivery of the feedback can also differ among programs (e.g., delivery can be by mail, one-on-one counseling, or a group session for individuals in the same risk category).

Evaluation of Effectiveness Across the Qualifying Body of Evidence

The first review described in this chapter includes only studies that examined the effectiveness of the AHRF process when conducted alone. The subsequent review includes all studies of AHRF that also used health education and may have included additional intervention components (e.g., enhanced access to settings for physical activity, smoke-free policies, or reduction of out-of-pocket costs for health care services). Multiple outcomes were assessed in this literature, which we classified into three categories of outcomes most frequently examined in the studies reviewed: health behaviors, physiological indicators, and a group of other variables that are important indicators of overall health in a worksite setting. This group of other variables included summary variables of health risk estimates that are typically obtained from the intervention assessment tool itself (such as an HRA) and that are designed to capture the combined effects of change across targeted behaviors and conditions. Although summary health risk estimates measure change across a wide range of health behaviors and indicators, they are based on the specific set of measurements included in each assessment tool. Effects of the intervention on the use of health care services by individual workers were also assessed to capture the combined effects of change across multiple health behaviors and conditions. Finally, measurements of worker productivity (typically days absent from work due to illness or injury) provided another opportunity to capture the combined effects of changes in health outcomes.

We calculated summary effect estimates when the included studies provided a sufficient number of similar (if not identical) outcome measurements. The summary effect estimates provided in this chapter include the median measurement of change across the qualifying evidence and the interquartile interval (IQI). For bodies of evidence whose measurements of change numbered fewer than seven but more than one, we did not generate an IQI and instead provide the median measurement of change and the simple range of values (minimum and maximum). For single indicators, we provide qualitative findings. Graphic depictions of the evidence are available at www.thecommunityguide.org/worksite.

Results: Intervention Effectiveness

This next section provides an overview of the results in terms of effectiveness of the AHRF and AHRF Plus interventions. Several case studies representing either of these two interventions have been provided as well.

Review of Evidence on AHRF

Our search identified 36 studies within 50 published articles evaluating the effectiveness of the AHRF. We assessed these studies and scored them on nine criteria for quality of execution; these criteria were described by Briss (3) and are available at www.thecommunityguide.org/methods. Of the 36 studies, 5 had six or more limitations in quality of execution (were limited studies) and therefore were not included in the body of evidence. For the 31 qualifying studies, information regarding study design, sample size, basic intervention characteristics, and results for outcomes considered in the review is available at www.thecommunityguide.org/worksite.

The 31 qualifying studies each reported on somewhat different iterations of an AHRF intervention, and no two studies reported on the same group of outcomes. Study samples varied in size (40 to 9,845 participants), though in all cases, employees who participated did so on a voluntary basis. In the following case study of Merrill Lynch, we provide one example of a randomized controlled design with results that are fairly representative of the overall body of evidence in terms of both the implementation of the intervention and the resulting health outcomes.

After careful review of the results of the Merrill Lynch and other studies, the Task Force found insufficient evidence to determine the effectiveness of using the AHRF alone to achieve improvements in one or more health behaviors and conditions among participating workers. Evidence was considered insufficient because positive findings were often small in magnitude and most

Case Study: Merrill Lynch, New York City

Merrill Lynch offered on-site physical examinations to employees who had at least 1 y of uninterrupted service with the company and who were at least 30 y of age. Gemson and Sloan (6) evaluated the effectiveness of integrating an AHRF intervention into this process. The intervention included the following:

- A physical exam conducted by a board-certified physician
- A biometric assessment (including blood pressure, weight, and fasting lipid profile and blood sugar) directed by a registered nurse
- Completion of the 1984 version of the CDC's HRA (no longer in circulation)
- Provision of a two-page written report with a computerized appraised age
- Review of the two-page report with a physician (counseling)

The comparison group participated in the physical exam, underwent a biometric screening, and completed the HRA but did not receive a report or receive counseling from the physician (though they did receive counseling if abnormalities were detected in their exam or biometric screen). Study participants were asked to return to complete a follow-up HRA in 6 mo. At baseline, 161 employees participated in the study, while 90 completed the follow-up HRA (42 in the HRA group and 48 in the comparison group).

The AHRF intervention participants reported significantly greater increases in the amount of physical activity they engaged in each week and also showed a more favorable decrease in the HRA-generated appraised age. The AHRF and comparison groups did not differ significantly in their total cholesterol or systolic blood pressure results, change in weight, or self-reported seat belt use. The authors of the study concluded that though the changes were modest, "even small reductions in major risk factors may result in significant improvements in health for many people" (6, p. 465).

of the studies did not include comparison groups to control for potential confounding factors. In addition, studies were not consistently in support of the AHRF intervention for most outcomes examined. So while Gemson and Sloan and others might conclude that small reductions in major risk factors may result in significant overall improvements, the science base available for the AHRF intervention does not support a conclusion that small reductions in risk factors were attributable to the intervention.

In addition to the broader concerns just described, the Task Force finding that there was insufficient evidence to determine AHRF effectiveness was based on concerns with recurring combinations of flaws in individual studies across the body of evidence. Many of the studies identified in the review provided the intervention of interest (AHRF alone) to the control arm of the trial and focused on the question of the effectiveness of the combined intervention (these results were considered in the multicomponent intervention review described in the next section). Due to the absence of measurements from a concurrent comparison population, the Task Force noted a potential for bias in the reliance on self-report for most measured changes in behavior. Additionally, most studies analyzed only a small subset of participants whose follow-up data were complete (baseline data from participants who did not return for follow-up were not included in the reported baseline measurements). Because follow-up rates across this body of evidence were generally low, the analytic focus may have favored the inclusion of results from individuals who had changed their health behaviors in the interval.

Review of Evidence on AHRF Plus

Though AHRF can be offered as an independent intervention, it is often applied as a gateway intervention to a broader worksite health promotion program that may be risk specific or broad in scope, may be of limited duration and intensity, or may occur over many months or years (with few or multiple contacts). When used as a gateway intervention, the assessment is typically conducted one or more times and the feedback is offered along with information about the identified health risks, information about programs directed toward the prevention or treatment of the identified health risks, or referrals to programs or providers related to the identified health risks. The use of AHRF varies from program to program, and

AHRF may serve as (1) a screening tool whereby people with certain risks are identified and directed toward a tailored program, (2) a general assessment tool to track employee progress over time (with or without program goals and related incentives), (3) a tool used by a health specialist to guide employees toward specific program offerings, or (4) a tool for employees to use as self-guidance. All studies included in this review assessed the effectiveness of unique combinations of interventions of which AHRF was a component, used AHRF in different ways, and had varying degrees of program intensity and duration. The overall heterogeneity in the way interventions were implemented led to the creation of a very broad category of interventions called the *assessment of health risks with feedback when combined with additional interventions (AHRF Plus)*.

Our search identified 59 studies within 90 papers evaluating the effectiveness of the AHRF Plus. Of the 59 studies, 8 were not included because they had six or more limitations in their quality of execution. Details of the 51 qualifying studies, including intervention components, brief sample characteristics, outcome measures, and study effect sizes, are available in summary evidence tables at www.thecommunityguide.org/worksite. Examples of the qualifying studies evaluating AHRF Plus are described by Shi (11,12) of Pacific Gas and Electric's HealthWise Stepped Intervention Study and by Goetzel and colleagues (7) of Johnson & Johnson's Health and Wellness Program.

The HealthWise program has elements and results that represent the broader group of studies included in the AHRF and AHRF Plus reviews. Levels 1 and 2 are pre- and poststudy arms for AHRF and were included in the AHRF review as such. Levels 3 and 4 are worksite health promotion programs that are broad and able to respond to a range of health risks that might be identified in the AHRF process. Level 4 also offers focused attention to employees who present with certain chronic conditions. The evaluation of Johnson & Johnson's Health and Wellness Program used a pre- and poststudy design for health outcomes and a time-series study design for cost outcomes. It also included a program for employees with health risks. Both of these examples are drawn from evaluations of complex programs offered by large companies.

After reviewing the evidence included in the 51 qualifying studies, the Task Force recommended the use of the AHRF when combined with health education programs, with or without additional

Case Study: Pacific Gas and Electric's HealthWise Stepped Intervention Study

The HealthWise intervention was designed to test the hypothesis that providing information to employees about the relationship between lifestyle and health outcomes would help the employees see the threats that their lifestyle choices posed to their health. Provision of information and opportunities to act—in the form of case management and reinforcement of past accomplishments—were each represented by specific components of the HealthWise program and were included to address aspects of Bandura's social learning theory (see http://en.wikipedia.org/wiki/Social_learning_theory). The intervention included four levels:

- Level 1 consisted of an HRA with biometric screens followed by provision of feedback and a health newsletter.
- Level 2 consisted of the HRA and newsletter, an on-site resource center, and self-care books.
- Level 3 included level 2 components plus lifestyle workshops, behavior change classes, and a social support function coordinated by the division HealthWise team.
- Level 4 included level 3 components plus a focus on environmental change with provision of on-site exercise space, implementation of smoke-free policies, use of incentives to participate, and sponsorship of health fairs. Level 4 also included a case management program for high-risk employees.

The HealthWise stepped intervention was conducted in nine Pacific Gas and Electric divisions located in northern California. The nine divisions were randomly assigned to 1 of 4 study conditions (levels 1-4). Each study condition, or level, was a step in the HealthWise intervention. The first two levels fit the AHRF intervention category and the second two fit the AHRF Plus (plus health education plus additional interventions) category. A no-treatment condition was not included. Participation was voluntary. To assure confidentiality, individuals were not tracked; analyses were conducted at the group level. As in other studies included in the review of evidence on AHRF Plus, the authors did not report participation rates for the various intervention components. However, because of the nature of the study and the typical ordering of study components, it can be assumed that all employees completed at least one HRA. No mandatory level of contact with the program was stipulated. Thus, the results likely reflect the full range of employees: those who participated only in the HRA and those who used all available components.

Though broad in scope, all levels of the intervention were successful in reducing tobacco use and heavy alcohol use, total cholesterol readings, and blood pressure levels, but they were not successful in motivating participating employees to lose significant amounts of weight. These changes varied by outcome and by intervention level (see the following table). The HealthWise program was evaluated for economic efficiency. The authors concluded that "the results of this study demonstrate strong associations between health promotion interventions and subsequent reduction in medical costs related to hospital days, doctor visits, and sick days based on different cost estimates. . . . The extent of the benefits seems to be associated with the level of intervention programs." Level 3 of this intervention showed the greatest economic ROI.

Comparison of HealthWise Levels 1 Through 4 and Percent Change From Baseline for Selected Outcomes

Level	Components	Smoking	Heavy drinking	Overweight	High cholesterol	High blood pressure
1 AHRF	HRA, biometric screens, feedback, and health newsletter	−34% $p < .01$	−22% $p < .01$	−1% $p > .1$	−29% $p < .01$	−14% $p < .05$
2 AHRF	Level 1 components plus on-site resource center and self-care books	−18% $p < .1$	−20% $p < .01$	3% $p > .1$	−34% $p < .01$	−3% $p > .1$
3 AHRF Plus	Level 2 components plus lifestyle workshops, behavior change classes, and social support function coordinated by the division HealthWise team	−35% $p < .01$	−11% $p > .1$	−2% $p > .1$	−41% $p < .01$	−17% $p < .05$
4 AHRF Plus	Level 3 components plus on-site exercise space, smoke-free policies, incentives to participate, health fairs, and case management program for high-risk employees	−44% $p < .01$	−17% $p < .05$	−12% $p > .1$	−49% $p < .01$	−28% $p < .05$

Case Study: Johnson & Johnson's Health and Wellness Program

The Health and Wellness Program was the result of a series of planned modifications of Johnson & Johnson's earlier Live for Life program. The earlier program was modified to incorporate a shared services initiative integrating programs for health, wellness, disability management, employee assistance, and occupational medicine. The program aspired to provide services designed to address health events before, during, and after they occurred in order to "maximize employee function and rapid return to work" (7, p. 419). In addition, the Health and Wellness Program included special services, or Pathways to Change (PTC), for employees found to be at high risk through the health risk assessment. All employees had access to the following intervention components:

Pre–Health Event Management

- HRAs, referrals to high-risk intervention programs, and risk-specific feedback mailed to all participants
- Incentives (financial rewards for completion of HRA and $500 U.S. medical benefits plan credit for HRA and participation in referrals to PTC)
- Client education programs including the following:
  - General education mailings and health and safety education and trainings
  - Workplace drug and alcohol awareness training
- Ergonomic assessment and job conditioning

Health Event Management

- Emergency care
- Limited nonoccupational care and occupational injuries and illness care
- Medical case management
- Modified work assignments
- Medical surveillance and regulatory compliance
- Programs managing health risk
- Critical incident response
- EAP
- Substance abuse management and referrals

Post–Health Event Management

- Return-to-wellness programs
- Monitoring of functional assessment, substance abuse rehabilitation, and modified work assignments

More than 4,000 employees participated in the Health and Wellness Program during the study, and about half of these took part in some aspect of PTC. Changes in the percent of employees with high health risk indicators for 10 different outcomes (for example, the percent of employees with BMI of >30 kg/m^2 or the percent of employees with total cholesterol of $\geq$200 mg/dL) were used as indicators of success for the overall program. Results for all program participants are listed in the following table.

Significant reductions in percent at risk	Significant increases in percent at risk	No significant change
High serum cholesterol (66% to 43%)	High body weight (76% to 78%)	Pipe smoking
Low dietary fiber intake (50% to 41%)	Risk for diabetes (49% to 52%)	
Poor exercise habits (46% to 35%)	High dietary fat intake (22% to 25%)	
Cigarette smoking (33% to 24%)	Cigar smoking (1% to 2%)	
High blood pressure (10% to 1%)		
Lack of seat belt use (5% to 3%)		
Drinking and driving (4% to 3%)		
Snuff use (1% to <1%)		

(continued) ▶

► Case Study: Johnson & Johnson's Health and Wellness Program *(continued)*

Ozminkowski and colleagues (10) looked for potential cost savings from this program. They examined medical benefits records for the 5 y before and the 4 y after the program implementation and found that the program saved Johnson & Johnson approximately $225 U.S. per employee per year over 4 y. The combination of health and cost savings outcomes led the authors to conclude that "integration of occupational health disability, wellness, and medical benefits may have substantial health and economic benefits in later years" (10, p. 21).

interventions. This recommendation was made on the basis of strong evidence of effectiveness in improving one or more health behaviors or conditions in populations of workers. Additionally, the Task Force recommended the use of the AHRF when combined with health education programs to improve specific outcomes among program participants; in this case the strength of the evidence varied by outcome. See table 10.1 for the detailed Task Force recommendations.

Results for high-risk subgroups within the AHRF Plus review sample were analyzed for all outcomes with adequate data. Results for diastolic blood pressure, systolic blood pressure, and total cholesterol indicate greater effectiveness for high-risk individuals than for the overall review sample. Results for weight and BMI among high-risk individuals were similar to those for all participants, showing only small changes.

The interventions evaluated in the review of evidence on AHRF Plus were conducted in diverse industry sectors including manufacturing plants, health care facilities, health insurance companies, government offices, field settings, banks, schools, and one ambulance service. Most studies were conducted in companies or worksites that had more than 500 employees and were located in urban or suburban settings. The average age of participants was about 40 y, and a range of educational levels and job positions was represented. The majority of the studies were conducted in the United States, and Whites and African Americans were well represented in the studies reporting information on race and ethnicity. Adequate information regarding other ethnic groups was not available, and data were not available to determine if the AHRF Plus intervention had different effects for different racial or ethnic groups. Because so many lifestyle and genetic characteristics associated with health outcomes are also correlated with racial and ethnic group membership, conclusions on applicability for different racial or ethnic groups should take these factors into account. More study on effects in racial and ethnic groups is warranted.

Table 10.1 U.S. Task Force for Community Preventive Services Findings for Improving Individual Health Outcomes Based on Strong, Sufficient, or Insufficient Evidence

Due to *strong* evidence of effectiveness, the Task Force recommends using AHRF combined with health education programs to reduce:	High blood pressure
	High cholesterol
	Number of days lost from work due to illness or disability
	Tobacco use (cessation)
	Dietary fat intake
Due to *sufficient* evidence of effectiveness, the Task Force recommends using AHRF combined with health education programs to reduce:	Nonuse of seat belts
	Unsatisfactory summary health risk estimates
	Nonpreventive health care service use
	Excessive alcohol consumption
	Physical inactivity
Due to *insufficient* evidence of effectiveness, the Task Force could not determine the effectiveness of using AHRF combined with health education programs to alter:	Body composition (e.g., BMI, weight, percent body fat)
	Fitness
	Dietary fruit and vegetable consumption

Potential Adverse Effects and Barriers to Implementation of AHRF Plus

Studies were reviewed for information on adverse effects of the AHRF Plus intervention. This information was presented to the Task Force and taken into consideration during the formulation of recommendations. Though no study provided empirical data on adverse effects, studies did suggest a number of possible effects, including the following: information received in the feedback portion of AHRF may cause anxiety for the recipient; false positives are likely, particularly with the biometric screenings; some employees may experience white-coat hypertension when their blood pressure is being checked and other employees may not follow guidelines for fasting before cholesterol checks; and, finally, breach of confidentiality may occur and is a significant concern in worksite settings. If breach of confidentiality occurs, it may influence decision making not just about programs to offer but also about benefits to provide. Wagner (14), in an early discussion of health risk assessments, cautioned readers to consider other potential harms that might result from the receipt of feedback from the assessment: anxiety, depression, hypochondriasis, payment of unnecessary medical expenses due to use of unnecessary treatment, confusion, guilt, and possibly being provided with misinformation.

The fear of breach of confidentiality may also serve as a barrier to implementation of AHRF Plus. Employees who think or know that they have significant health risks may be the least likely to participate. Some experts have argued that interventions such as this attract the worried well—people who seek out medical information on a regular basis (8)—even though workers who are less healthy might benefit more from these programs. Some employers may initiate a program but decide to reduce its scope or cancel it because of low participation in health education or other components. However, the results presented in the review of AHRF Plus suggest that even with low rates of participation, employees reap benefits.

An economics review team conducted a search for evidence on the economic efficiency (cost benefits and cost savings) of AHRF Plus. The economics review was conducted subsequent to the previously described review of AHRF Plus. Studies evaluating AHRF Plus were evaluated with established *Community Guide* standards (4) to determine their eligibility for economic assessment. Broadly speaking, these eligibility requirements state that studies need to be published in English, be implemented in a country with a high-income economy as defined by the World Bank, and have utilized an economic evaluation method (4).

Nine studies with economic outcome data met inclusion criteria based on abstraction and quality scoring. Economic benefits were derived from direct medical costs averted or indirect productivity losses averted. Whereas most studies included in this review considered only disability days averted as indirect benefits, one study measured both disability days and days missed due to illness along with direct medical benefits. All program costs and economic benefit data from the qualifying studies were adjusted to 2005 U.S. dollar values by using inflation factors from the consumer price index, available at www.bls.gov.

Program costs in studies ranged from $73 to $285 U.S. per participant per year. Two studies were based on a single group pre- and poststudy design that involved all employees at the particular workplaces. Costs were $60 and $195 U.S. per employee per year respectively for these two studies. Most studies did not report detailed costs for implementation of the intervention being evaluated. Economic benefits from the intervention ranged from $92 to $695 U.S. per participant or per employee.

Eight studies that included a cost-benefit analysis reported ROI ratios, and one study reported a cost-effectiveness ratio (CEA; the cost per 1% reduction or prevention in cardiovascular disease risk). The range of ROI ratios for the eight studies was 1.4:1 to 4.7:1 per year, with a median of 2.4:1 per year. The interpretation of the range of ratios provided would be an annual gain of $1.40 to $4.70 U.S. for every dollar invested into the program. The CEA for high-risk participants in the final study varied from $13.86 to $72.85 U.S. per 1% reduction in cardiovascular disease risk for the three more-intensive intervention groups compared with the less-intensive or comparison group (to which the equivalent of AHRF Plus was also offered); for moderate-risk participants, the range varied from $10.94 to $72.85 U.S. Lacking any benchmark values in terms of risk reduction for other diseases or interventions, it is difficult to interpret the economic efficiency of these particular estimates. A final conclusion regarding the economic efficiency of this intervention is not possible due to the variance of method and heterogeneity of data.

Additionally, studies in this review did not consider presenteeism, a significant economic cost to employers. Despite the nonconsideration of presenteeism-related productivity losses, all studies reported a positive ROI. In the case of the one study reporting CEA, all cost-effectiveness ratios were found to be less than $100 U.S. However, due to the lack of a standard cost-effectiveness ratio based on a percentage reduction in health risk, it is difficult to interpret the economic efficiency. Conclusive economic effectiveness for using AHRF Plus cannot be determined until more economists research the intervention using standardized econometrics. Future cost-effectiveness studies in this area should include comprehensive information from both sides of the equation (program costs and program benefits related to worker productivity and health cost savings).

Methodological Challenges of the Review

The heterogeneity of intervention components, outcomes, and settings examined in this review provided many methodological challenges for the study review team. All worksite health evaluations confront challenges in terms of cost and participation. For example, establishing a group or individual randomized trial requires a large number of sites or participants, and the strength of that research design is compromised if voluntary participation is used and is inadequate. In turn, mandatory participation presents many ethical challenges. One of the strengths of the review, therefore, was that effectiveness was assessed across different types of study designs with different types and rates of participation.

Evaluating the AHRF intervention itself presented a challenge. The intervention is multicomponent in nature, but the main component—the assessment—serves as both the baseline and a follow-up tool along with biometric screening. Thus, participants who dropped out of the process could not be evaluated sufficiently. Important questions arise when one considers that a population with less-than-favorable results may have inhibitions about returning for a follow-up assessment. Those interested in using AHRF Plus therefore need to pay careful attention to implementation, minimizing attrition, and ensuring adequate follow-up.

Many of the studies included in this review had potential bias in their reporting of outcomes. In more than a few studies, the authors reported that they assessed multiple outcomes, but they presented only a few. In one extreme case, the authors reported only one outcome out of several that were assessed. In many other cases, the authors merely reported that the findings for a particular outcome were not statistically significant and did not provide any data. The Task Force therefore assessed the strength of evidence separately for each outcome, and the *Community Guide* suggests that future studies pay greater attention to reporting results for all outcomes.

Conclusion

Despite these methodological challenges, the systematic reviews of the use of AHRF in worksite settings was able to answer important questions that earlier reviews were unable to address: Does an AHRF, when used alone, lead to behavior change or change in health outcomes among employees? Does this type of assessment, when used with education and other worksite-based intervention components, result in change? What types of behaviors or health outcomes does the intervention affect?

The results of these worksite-specific reviews (AHRF and AHRF Plus) and the related recommendations made by the Task Force on Community Preventive Services indicate that the AHRF plays an important role as part of a broader worksite health promotion program that includes health education and potentially other components as well. The health education, as defined in the AHRF Plus review, should last at least an hour or be repeated multiple times during a year and may include multiple health promotion activities. The specific magnitude of effect an employer might expect from implementing different types of health promotion programs including AHRF and health education will vary and may be influenced by the type and duration of intervention components offered, the type and rate of participation, the participant characteristics (evidence suggests that high-risk participants will experience greater health gains), and other contextual factors.

Though these reviews answered important questions, they also raised two additional questions: Are worksite health promotion programs with a health education component effective in the absence of AHRF? Does AHRF add value to worksite health promotion programs with regard to behavior change and improvement in health outcomes (i.e., is it a necessary component of these programs)? These, and other outstanding questions identified earlier in this chapter, will require substantial resources to address. As the field of worksite health promotion continues to develop, program funders and researchers should carefully consider the importance of ensuring sufficient resources for evaluation, of using consistent measures or reporting data that will allow the calculation of common metrics in future systematic reviews, of reporting data by race and ethnicity, of collaborating across sites within companies or across companies to increase sample sizes, and of ensuring generalizability to different populations of workers.

Chapter Review Questions

1. Briefly describe the process employed by the Task Force on Community Preventive Services to issue evidence-based, intervention-specific recommendations.

2. Describe the overall intervention and the individual components associated with the label "assessment of health risks with feedback" (AHRF).

3. Discuss the differences between "strong," "sufficient," and "insufficient" evidence of effectiveness.

4. Discuss why despite the availability of a sufficient number of studies, no final conclusion regarding the economic efficiency of the AHRF intervention could be reached.

5. Describe the reasons why systematic reviews suffer from the different methodologies employed in research studies in reaching clear and thorough conclusions. Also, describe why such methodological variability may be a strength when conclusions are reached.

11

Practice and Research Connected
A Synergistic Process of Translation Through Knowledge Transfer

Nicolaas P. Pronk, PhD, FACSM

Public or population health issues and concerns can have a significant effect on regional, national, and global economic considerations. Because of their rapidly increasing trends, high prevalence, and associated treatment costs, conditions such as obesity, diabetes, cardiovascular disease, hypertension, certain cancers, and other related disorders negatively affect the overall health of populations, escalate health care expenditures, add significant health and financial burdens to individuals and organizations, and strain the resources supporting the health care system in many countries (3). Efforts to help reduce risk factors for such major public health concerns include public health policies, evidence-based medical and public or population health interventions, and increasing focus on the promotion of healthful lifestyles.

Underneath such broad health policy issues are concerns that more directly relate to the worksite setting and involve the challenges of finding effective practical solutions for many health-related excess expenditures, whether medical or productivity related. Such challenges include individual factors such as lifestyle (health behaviors), care-seeking behavior, and self-management as well as organizational factors such as preventive-oriented health care benefits, a health-conscious company culture, and access to health-generating resources. To address these challenges and close the gap between research and practice, a broad-based conceptual model or framework is needed to provide a solid foundation for the creation of effective solutions (5). It is the purpose of this chapter to provide a framework that allows for multilevel solutions to be generated as well as recognizes the importance of the practice setting in which programs are implemented (such as worksites, clinical care delivery settings, community settings, or other locations), integrates business principles into the design of programs so as to optimize implementation success, and acknowledges that practice-based learnings are an important input to research efforts in this domain.

Whereas much is known about what works to improve the health of large populations, too little of this knowledge is being applied. Consider, for example, that research conducted as early as 1981 conclusively demonstrated the benefits that beta-blockers provide to patients recovering from a heart attack (6). Yet, 15 y after the conclusive results of the Beta-Blocker Heart Attack Trial, beta-blockers were being administered to only 62.5% of heart attack patients in the United States. In 1996, when the National Committee for Quality Assurance (NCQA) translated the use of evidence-based best practices into a model of action and accountability by introducing the beta-blocker-after-heart-attack measure into its Health Plan Employer Data and Information Set (HEDIS), this changed. As a result of broad acceptance and application of this model among managed care plans, the rate of beta-blocker administration

Acknowledgments: The constructive feedback and critical reviews of earlier versions of this manuscript by Dr. Lawrence W. Green and Dr. Thomas Kottke are very much appreciated.

after heart attack improved from 62.5% in 1996 to 92.5% in 2001 (20). Whereas beta-blocker use is an example of a biomedical intervention, many other examples exist that describe the often slow application of research-based knowledge into scalable and sustainable practical solutions in areas of individual behavior change (in clinical settings related to patients or providers or community settings such as worksites). Examples include the use of aspirin as a short-term therapy for acute myocardial infarction (7), physicians providing advice to obese patients to lose weight (11), or community health promotion interventions (39).

Despite best efforts, it appears to be remarkably difficult to turn research-based knowledge into actionable, effective, and affordable programmatic health improvement solutions. This may be especially true when the research-based knowledge involves health behaviors, regardless of whether a behavior is that of patients, employees, service providers, administrators, policy makers, or others. Making decisions about what initiatives to fund or invest in should be based at least in part on the degree to which such programs are effective in generating positive effects. Preferably, decisions on resource allocation should be based on a consideration of all the evidence of effectiveness—in other words, summarized as a result of systematic reviews of all available research (such as those reviews conducted by the Task Force on Community Preventive Services; see www.thecommunityguide.org; 34). Systematic reviews currently provide the best, least-biased, and rational way to organize, cull, evaluate, and integrate the available research evidence. Yet, to facilitate the adoption of practical applications of programs supported by research, the opinions, advice, and even active participation by practitioners should be considered in the research plan—arguably, if a practice-informed research path were followed, the adoption rate of research-based evidence would benefit.

Employers are directly affected by both these health concerns and the lack of effective solutions. They struggle in their efforts to manage increases in health care costs and excess productivity losses. As a result, an increasing number of employers, vendors, health plans, and coalitions are engaging in dialogue around benchmarking and best practices with the intent to generate more programmatic solutions that can support employee health and productivity management and can address overall financial concerns.

To optimize efforts toward evidence-based practice, a process, framework, or model is needed to provide a path to conceptualization and drafting of a practical solution that will generate positive effects. Obviously, various models may be proposed, and one model may not be particularly superior or inferior to any other providing that it helps the user improve the chances of success, it can be improved based on experience, and the process of modification improves its predictive capabilities. Regardless, central to any model ought to be an explicit recognition that research-based learnings of interventions need to be considered in the context of practice-based realities that allow the solutions to be accepted and utilized. This, in effect, means that in our efforts to generate practical solutions, science-based learnings are only one component of the overall effort to bring about the solution. Other components include, but are not limited to, program design based on current knowledge of health-related interventions and business principles, the inclusion of continuous quality improvement principles as part of day-to-day operations in order to facilitate an integrated process improvement method, and action research (27).

This chapter describes a framework that combines scientific research findings with business principles to optimize the likelihood that resulting programmatic solutions will be applicable to the settings in which they will be implemented. Furthermore, it extends the traditional model of translating research into practice (1) through a focus on optimizing practice through research (16,17) into a synergistic interplay between practice and research called the *practice and research connected model*. It also delineates a specific role for action research in the identification of practice-informed research needs through hypotheses generation to be tested in efficacy and effectiveness trials. Finally, it recognizes the important objective of organizational learning (31) by placing a translation curve centrally in the framework. This translation curve allows for a deeper and more explicit recognition of the tasks associated with the generation of new solutions that go beyond the notion of *what* (structure) needs to be created to *how* (process) solutions will be crafted and *from where* (thought) the commitment, intent, and purpose of shaping those solutions will come (31,28). Overall, the practice and research connected model is based on the notion of knowledge transfer among multiple stakeholders and collaborative teams made up of researchers and practitioners (26,22). Together, these teams are intentionally focused on creating solutions and as a result achieve more together than they could when working apart. This synergy that is established through a closed-loop process between practice and research allows for a research-informed practice path and cycles around to providing a practice-informed research path. Hence it provides a foundational structure for a learning organization (31) and at least partially addresses the question of how systems science can aid population health in generating more practice-based evidence of effectiveness (13).

Translation as a Knowledge Transfer

Translation of research into practice, or vice versa, may be considered in the context of a knowledge transfer. The idea centers on the notion that a transfer of knowledge allows for continued progress to take place even if such progress is not generated by the same individual or group of people. The discussion of knowledge transfer is framed around a definition of knowledge in the context of evidence-based and evidence-informed program development and bridges the hand-offs between research and practice.

Definition of Knowledge

Any discussion of knowledge transfer should include a definition of the term *knowledge*. It has been broadly accepted that in order for a statement to be counted as knowledge, it must be justified, true, and believed (24). Thus, the traditional definition of knowledge is justified true belief. Western epistemology (the theory of knowledge) has mainly focused on truthfulness as the essential attribute of knowledge that is considered absolute and static. However, when considering the process of knowledge transfer, knowledge itself is considered to be dynamic and context specific, as it depends on a particular time and space (36). It is also considered to be humanistic because it inherently relates to human action. Knowledge is deeply rooted in human belief and value systems and is relational, as is exemplified by things such as beauty and goodness that are in the eye of the beholder. In the context of this chapter, the definition of knowledge as proposed by Nonaka and Takeuchi is adopted: "Knowledge is the dynamic human process of justifying personal belief toward the 'truth'" (22; p. 21).

Types of Knowledge

There are two types of knowledge: explicit knowledge and tacit knowledge (23). Explicit knowledge is visible and can be expressed in formal and systematic language and shared in the form of data, scientific formulas, protocols, specifications, manuals, and so on. It is based on an external reality experienced through observation. Tacit knowledge, on the other hand, is much more difficult to describe and formalize, and it is highly personal—it resides deep inside the individual and thus is difficult to communicate to others. Furthermore, as proposed by Scharmer (29), we may consider two forms of tacit knowledge: tacit (embodied) knowledge and tacit, self-transcending (not-yet-embodied) knowledge. The difference between these two forms of tacit knowledge centers on the notion that tacit, embodied knowledge reflects on knowledge about things we do whereas tacit, self-transcending, not-yet-embodied knowledge reflects on knowledge about the thought conditions that give rise to the things we do. As an example, consider a car. Certain things about the car—such as its wheels, shape, color, and doors—are examples of explicit knowledge. The work factory workers put in to build the car is an example of tacit, embodied knowledge. The knowledge that enabled an automobile designer to invent the car in the first place, before bringing it forth into the world (i.e., to sense and actualize an emergent reality), is an example of tacit, not-yet-embodied knowledge. Figure 11.1 depicts these epistemologies as parts of a whole. In this figure, explicit knowledge is open and visible to the world; tacit, embodied knowledge is knowledge in use but not visible; and tacit, self-transcending, not-yet-embodied knowledge is knowledge about a not-yet-enacted reality (23,28,29).

Moving Beyond Science

Generally speaking, it is recognized that there are an art and a science to health promotion; however, it may not be intuitively clear how art and science are actually represented in the health promotion work we do. The process outlined in figure 11.1 shows that it is important to focus not only on *what* we do (structure) but also on *how* we do it (process) and *from where* we operate when we do it (thought; 30). As Aristotle outlined two and a half centuries ago (2), science is limited to things that cannot be otherwise than they are and refers to *what* knowledge. However, Aristotle also went on to argue that there are four other ways to grasp the truth besides science that apply to other contexts of reality and life. The second and third ways are art and technology

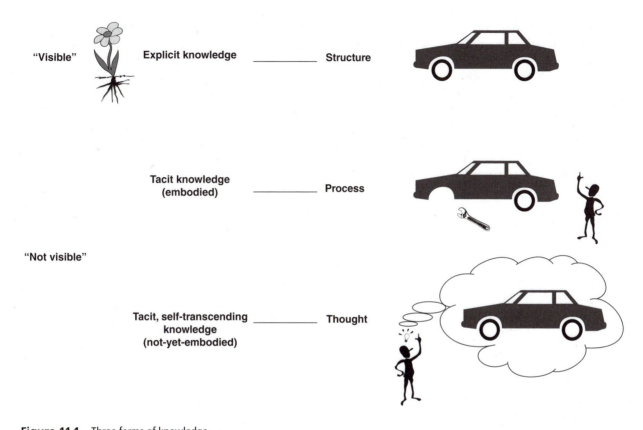

Figure 11.1 Three forms of knowledge.

Adapted, by permission, from HealthPartners, 2007, Practice and research connected: A synergistic process of translation through knowledge transfer.

that refer to *how* knowledge. Finally, the fourth and fifth ways are awareness and wisdom that refer to *thought* knowledge giving rise to primary knowing. Thus, Aristotle provides us with a method to consider how to use inputs from science, art, and technology as well as intuitions, hunches, and a deeper understanding of our own theoretical wisdom to shape programs, products, and services that have the highest likelihood of being effective, scalable, and sustainable and not merely a shallow reactive response to an expressed need for solutions.

Practice and Research Connected

The previous section on knowledge and knowledge transfer may seem too theoretical in the context of a chapter focused on creating practical solutions. However, it provides a solid foundation upon which to build a robust model with a clearly outlined path toward creating such practical solutions. The context in which this work is conducted is also highly important. First, we should base the building of new practical solutions on the evidence of what we know to be effective in

research settings. Next, we should consider how to translate such knowledge into programs that fit into practice settings, are scalable to reach the populations of interest, and are sustainable through positive effects. Furthermore, we should evaluate the programs in the context of their real-life applications so they may be improved upon and new questions may be formalized that can inform the research community about what issues need to be addressed.

The NIH has proposed a road map with the intent to transform new scientific knowledge into tangible benefits for people (21). The Agency for Healthcare Research and Quality (AHRQ) has introduced a funding stream to promote Translating Research into Practice and Policy (TRIPP), which also shares the objective of finding more efficient means to apply research findings toward improvement of population health (1). The HealthPartners Research Foundation (HPRF) has proposed a process called *optimizing practice through research* that focuses on the incorporation of research into practice and explicitly recognizes the role of creating a supportive environment for the delivery of research products (16,17). Yet, in total, a need remains for an inclusive, synergistic model that recognizes the need to conduct quality research, systematically review the evidence, systematically translate findings into practical applications that incorporate business principles, apply new programs into practice with integrated improvement processes, incorporate practice-based research and evaluation to understand the effects, and inform research funding agencies of practice-based needs that may be formulated as new research hypotheses.

The Practice and Research Connected Model

The practice and research connected model is depicted in figure 11.2. It has two pathways that connect process and activity between practice and research—the research-informed practice path and the practice-informed research path. The connections between research and practice that allow for a two-way synergistic model are the

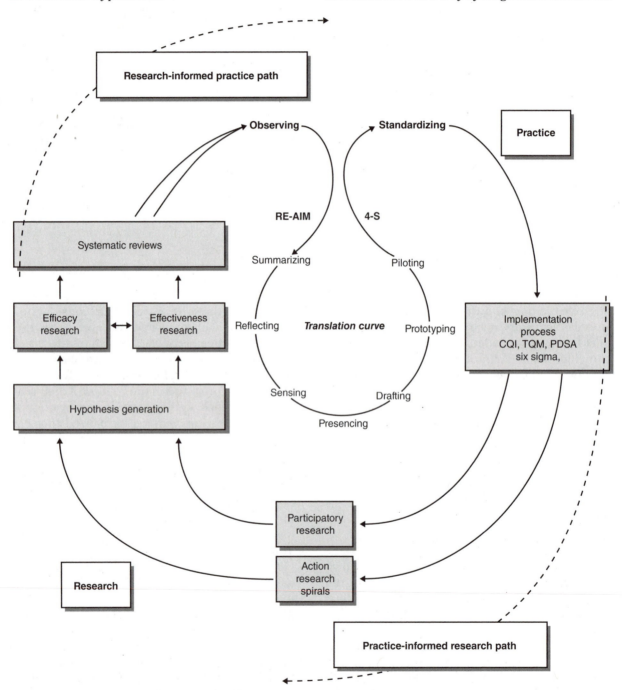

Figure 11.2   The practice and research connected model. RE-AIM = Reach, efficacy and effectiveness, adoption, implementation, and maintenance; 4-S = size of the effect, scope of services, scalability, and sustainability; CQI = Continuous Quality Improvement; TQM = Total Quality Management; PDSA = Plan-Do-Study-Act cycle.

Adapted, by permission, from HealthPartners, 2007, Practice and research connected: A synergistic process of translation through knowledge transfer.

translation curve and the action research transition processes. Both these processes are learning oriented, but they are positioned in opposite directions. The major components of the model can be outlined as (1) the research component, (2) the translation curve, (3) the practice component, and (4) the action research component. Descriptions of these model components follow.

The Research Component

The research component comprises efficacy and effectiveness research. While certainly other research methodologies, such as qualitative research, surveillance, and other preexperimental design research, are important in their own right and provide additional input to the process in the translation curve, most of the evidence of effectiveness of interventions is derived from these two types of research. Efficacy research has high internal validity that provides strong assurance that the outcome observed is attributable to the intervention. Effectiveness research is designed to generalize the findings by positioning the research into a context that is less controlled and more typical and that more closely resembles real-world conditions (14).

A systematic review is a technique that provides scientific evidence of the effectiveness of interventions (33). Based on the available evidence that stems from such systematic reviews, recommendations may be crafted that inform decision makers regarding appropriate allocation of (scarce) health-related resources. Systematic reviews summarize information on the effectiveness of public health and population health interventions and allow for identification of gaps in the scientific literature. They are also frequently accompanied by additional information on cost-effectiveness, cost benefit, or applicability across a variety of settings. Systematic reviews in areas that apply directly to health promotion at the worksite appear more and more frequently in the literature (10,35). Additionally, several highly accessible review resources have been made available by initiatives including, but not limited to, the Task Force on Community Preventive Services (www.thecommunityguide. org), the Cochrane Collaboration (www.cochrane. org), the National Institute for Health and Clinical Excellence (www.nice.org.uk), and the U.S. Preventive Services Task Force (USPSTF; www.ahrq.gov/clinic/uspstfix.htm).

The Translation Curve

Following the process designed to create systematic reviews, the model enters the *translation curve*. The curve is best described as an adaptation of several social, ecological, organizational, and behavior change processes outlined by Lewin (19), Green and Glasgow (14), Best and coworkers (5), Glasgow and colleagues (12), Kottke and Pronk (16), Senge (31,32), Wilbur (37,38), Scharmer (28,30), and Nonaka and Teece (23), among others. The *translation curve* allows for a transfer of knowledge across the three forms of knowledge (outlined previously in this chapter) through a process that prevents program design and development efforts from merely reacting to a set of inputs at a shallow level. The curve does this by intentionally probing into a deeper level that allows for more profound innovation. As a result, research-based knowledge can be transformed into evidence-informed practical solutions by following the series of stages in the translation curve. Whereas these stages are presented in figure 11.2 and defined in this discussion sequentially, they are actually all part of a complex matrix that is operational at all times (30). The individual stages are all important, and while they can be considered individually, as pairs, or as clusters, in reality, going through the stages is more like dancing with all of them simultaneously (32). The stages in the translation curve include observing, summarizing, reflecting, sensing, presencing, drafting, prototyping, piloting, and standardizing.

- Observing: The first step and access point into the translation curve is to observe. Observation is a cornerstone concept in science and allows for interpretation of what is happening factually. The idea is to take in information while suspending judgment and to remain open to receive the information for the purpose of gathering input. Observing relates to seeing reality with a new set of eyes. It is objectively accessing what is known by using tools and techniques that reflect current evidence rather than merely gathering information that confirms preexisting assumptions.

- Summarizing: Summarizing is taking stock of what is known about a specific topic in the context of program structures, processes, and outcomes. This step includes the identification of knowledge gaps.

- Reflecting: Reflecting is contemplating and uncovering the meaning of what has been observed and, in so doing, uncovering the possibilities and intentions of what may need to be done in order to generate new solutions.

- Sensing: Considering the potential solution as part of a new mental model (rather than reflecting in the context of mental models that are solely based on past experience) that allows for innovations that stem from emerging futures (or not-yet-embodied knowledge) uncovers an emerging new purpose and will to generate solutions.

• Presencing: Presencing is the process that starts at the point when team members recognize and realize what the solution will be. The vision of what needs to be created presents itself, and clarity of purpose initiates the emergence of the new reality—the practical solution. This bringing forth of the new solution reflects the notion of departure from the old way of doing things to bringing the new solution into current reality and building toward the future—a process Scharmer termed *presencing* (30).

• Drafting: Drafting is the first step in building the practical solution as the team members create the new program by sharing their plans, thoughts, and ideas. This step generates the blueprint for the new application.

• Prototyping: Prototyping is the first attempt at building the solution so it can be tested, improved upon, and prepared for initial market readiness. Lots of customer and consumer insights are gathered at this stage.

• Piloting: Piloting is testing the most promising prototype in a real-world situation that is highly reflective of the marketplace in which this practical solution has to perform. This stage allows for final adjustments to the product solution before full production.

• Standardizing: Standardizing is the full implementation of the solution in the market according to a newly created or established method and process that are routinely followed to optimize performance and reduce variance in outcomes.

Tools to Generate, Transfer, and Apply Knowledge

Several tools are well suited to support the journey through the translation curve. In the observing stage, the systematic review is an important input. It is, however, by no means the only input. Other information related to the task should be gathered from other fields beyond health promotion. For example, business principles, case studies (the gold standard for business research), promising practices, benchmarking, and process reports are all important inputs at this stage.

In the move from the observing to the presencing stage, the RE-AIM model may be particularly helpful. RE-AIM (*r*each, *e*fficacy and effectiveness, *a*doption, *i*mplementation, and *m*aintenance) is an evaluation (i.e., observation and analysis) framework designed by Glasgow and colleagues (and available at www.re-aim.org) to expand the assessment of interventions beyond efficacy to multiple criteria that may better identify the translatability and public health effect of health promotion interventions (12). As a result it appears on the left-hand side of the translation curve.

For the move from presencing to standardizing, the 4-S model has proved insightful (25). This model identifies four simple rules for program design that optimize the chances that the practical solution will be successful once implemented in the field, particularly since these rules add business rules to the program operations and implementation. As a result, the 4-S model is positioned on the right-hand side of the translation curve. The name *4-S* represents (1) the *s*ize of the effect of the intervention, (2) the *s*cope of services that make up the program, (3) the *s*calability of the intervention, and (4) the *s*ustainability of the program. These factors, added to the learning brought about by the RE-AIM model, connect the health-related critical features of the program with the operational realities of implementing an intervention as part of a business plan that needs to be successful in the context of economic realities.

The Practice Component

The practice component involves implementing the intervention with an eye toward optimal performance, exceptional experience, and sustained effectiveness. To facilitate this type of ongoing implementation, the practice component should include processes that allow for evaluation cycles that are ongoing and as close to real time as possible. These cycles should provide critical information to the administrators, front-line staff members, and practitioners of the programs. Examples of such processes include, but are not limited to, Continuous Quality Improvement (CQI; 4), Total Quality Management (TQM; 8), Six Sigma (9), and Plan-Do-Study-Act (PDSA) cycles (8).

Action Research

Action research may be best described as a participatory and voluntary process that seeks to bring together action, reflection, theory, and practice, in participation with others, in the pursuit of practical solutions to issues of pressing concern to people and the flourishing nature of individuals and their communities (27). In effect, action research may be implemented as a regular part of ongoing day-to-day practice with the purpose of integrating a systematic approach to development of knowing and knowledge. Action research is based in a different form than that of traditional research. It has different purposes, involves different relationships among its stakeholders, and has different ways of conceiving knowledge, especially in its relation to the practice setting (27,2,19). Of particular interest is the application of action research in the workplace. Since the workplace is central to human existence, it is not surprising that many social scientists have spent significant efforts on the study of this setting. Action research approaches are directly applicable to addressing a variety of issues pertaining to workplace considerations that may have a dramatic effect on worker health and organizational performance, either separately or in combination. In 1951, Kurt Lewin introduced his field theory, which states that the behavior of an individual is a function of both personality and environment (18). He went on to provide evidence for this premise by showing that leadership styles directly influence productivity and conflict among groups of employees. By using an action research model, he was able to initiate positive changes (18). Hence, applying action research on the practice side of the practice and research connected model makes intuitive sense, as the issues of individual behaviors, workplace productivity, physical and social environment, organizational culture, and leadership are all central to the overall value proposition of worksite health promotion.

Participatory Research

A way to generate a better understanding of the relevance of research conducted is to engage practitioners in the research projects themselves—that is, to make practitioners true partners in the design, implementation, analysis, and reporting of the research. Such an approach is central to integrating translational issues into the research by design and will certainly support a better fit between science and practice (15). Whereas community development projects and health promotion programs have experienced some support for funding for

participatory research, calls for a more explicit recognition of the value of this approach continue to be heard (15,16,17). Participatory research can address the need to recognize the complexity of contexts in which people live, work, and play. This complexity is multilevel and multifactorial and is readily found in the real-world setting. Controlling for variables that are central to the reality in which the programs will be implemented may hinder the observation of valuable learnings.

As a result of new knowledge gained by using action research and participatory research, new hypotheses may be generated that address major gaps in knowledge. Those newly generated hypotheses will represent important issues, as they will be directly based upon or influenced by challenges in the practice setting. Furthermore, action research and participatory research (just as the translation curve), will provide paths to collaboration among researchers and practitioners, one of the four principles of success identified in the efforts to optimize practice through research (16,17). Finally, closing the loop, the new hypotheses may be tested in efficacy or effectiveness trials so the research efforts may continue to feed the systematic review process as one of the key inputs to the overall process of translating knowledge into action.

Conclusion

This chapter has outlined a robust model to support the development of new innovations in the health promotion industry. The practice and research connected model is heavily couched in research support across a variety of fields. Arguably, much of what has been presented in this chapter is theoretical or even philosophical; however, research is an activity based on intellectual investigation aimed at discovering, interpreting, and revising knowledge about things. As a result, research can use the scientific method but need not do so. Research couched in the social sciences, business research perspectives, or practice-based insights using nontraditional research approaches such as focus groups or case studies may be used to derive a more robust model closely aligned with research and practice.

The practice and research connected model is designed in a closed loop that allows for a synergistic relationship between practice and research and that includes process steps that support transitions between the two. A central component of the model is a translation curve that incorporates a systematic transfer of knowledge. The introduction of action research and participatory research as explicit components in the model provides paths to practice-informed research. Such paths create bridges between practitioners and researchers that may initiate collaborative projects and constitute important access points for funding agencies into practice-based insights that address issues that matter and are worthy of research funding.

Chapter Review Questions

1. Describe differences between efficacy and effectiveness research on the one hand and action research on the other.

2. Define knowledge and its various types.

3. What are systematic reviews, what insights do they contribute, and what are examples of organizations that conduct such reviews?

Benchmarking and Best Practices in Worksite Health Promotion

Jessica Grossmeier, MPH; LaVaughn Palma-Davis, MA; K. Andrew Crighton, MD, CPE; Margaret Sabin, MHSA; and David R. Anderson, PhD

Although substantial evidence demonstrates that comprehensive worksite health promotion programs are effective in improving employee health and cost outcomes (12), limited evidence exists in the peer-reviewed literature to identify the optimal combination of program components and tactics to achieve such outcomes (5). Additionally, while one national survey of U.S. employers indicates that 63% offer worksite health promotion programs (10), another such survey indicates that only 7% offer comprehensive programs (9). In the absence of published evidence on the specific practices that yield superior health and financial outcomes, many employers have turned to benchmarking initiatives. This chapter introduces the concept of benchmarking and explains how it can be used to identify best practices in worksite health promotion. Additionally, several benchmarking and best-practice tools are reviewed and case studies are presented illustrating the use of benchmarking to create best-practice programs.

Benchmarking

A review of the history of benchmarking reveals that the concept is relatively young. Although it is difficult to identify conclusively an emergent event or source of benchmarking, credit is often given to the Xerox Corporation (14), which introduced the concept to others via publications and training events beginning in the early 1980s. Benchmarking can be described as an ongoing, systematic process of evaluating the products, services, or processes associated with superior results (2,14). This general description can be adapted for the worksite health promotion field by defining it as an ongoing, systematic process of identifying the programs, services, and implementation procedures companies use to achieve superior health and health-related financial outcomes in their benefits-eligible population. The American Productivity and Quality Center (APQC; 6) offers an alternative definition of benchmarking, stating that it is "the process of identifying, understanding, and adapting outstanding practices from target organizations to help other organizations improve performance" (6, p. 8). In the absence of empirical evidence about the specific practices or combinations of programs that yield the best outcomes, employers can use benchmarking approaches to guide their selection or design of a comprehensive worksite health promotion program. Partnership for Prevention recommends benchmarking for this purpose, claiming that "effective worksite health promotion programs begin with benchmarking" (3, p. 10). Once programs have been implemented, an organization can compare its outcomes against those achieved by other employers using similar or different practices.

There are three main types of benchmarking activities employers can use to identify best practices in worksite health promotion: internal, competitive, and functional or general (14). These activities are discussed in the following sections.

Acknowledgments: The authors would like to acknowledge the following colleagues for their contributions to the case studies reported here: Keith Winick, Wellness Coordinator, Prudential Financial; Mary Anna Weklar, MHSA, Director of Business Development; and Kris Baldwin, Director of Operations, Sutter Health Partners.

Internal Benchmarking

The focus of *internal benchmarking* is to use data that exist within segments of the organization to differentiate the most-effective strategies from the least-effective strategies. The value of doing this is to disseminate the practices proven to be effective in one part of the organization to other parts of the organization. For example, one company location or business unit may have piloted a health improvement program that yielded results that are desirable to other areas of the company. Internal benchmarking can help identify such practices and build a business case for implementing them company wide.

Competitive Benchmarking

Competitive benchmarking activities take an external focus by examining the practices of an employer's direct competitors. This type of benchmarking may be less focused on identifying superior practices than on determining how similar or different the organization's practices are from those of other organizations with similar characteristics and operational functions. In the worksite health promotion field, this type of benchmarking might be supported by a third-party vendor that serves numerous companies in the same industry. In exchange for sharing information about their own practices, employers are given access to information about what others are doing. One variation on competitive benchmarking is to go beyond direct competitors to get information about noncompetitors in similar or related industries. For example, instead of limiting data collection to automotive manufacturers, an employer in this industry might also include manufacturers of home appliances or heavy equipment.

Functional or General Benchmarking

Similarly to competitive benchmarking, *functional benchmarking* relies on information about other organizations. The distinction is that functional benchmarking expands the purview beyond competitors to other organizations with similar functions. This activity allows comparisons to be made across a large body of employers based on the functions they have in common. For example, benchmarking might be done to determine how other companies have integrated their health promotion programs into the benefits function or health and safety initiatives. Another variation is *general benchmarking,* which observes the practices of a wide variety of companies regardless of industry or function. This type of benchmarking

activity is multidisciplinary because it identifies promising practices and programs across many industries and types of organizations and seeks to apply these practices to the organization, industry, or discipline of interest. For example, practices observed in the disciplines of benefits, human resources, business, public health, or health care might be applied to worksite health promotion. Readers wanting more information about the different types of benchmarking or the process of benchmarking are referred to chapter 15 of an earlier ACSM reference book edited by Carolyn Cox (4).

Best Practices

Inherent in benchmarking activities is the goal of doing the right things and doing those things right. In this way, benchmarking activities drive the identification of best practices. Through the process of creating standard definitions for the purposes of comparison, a set of superior processes or outcomes is identified. In the worksite health promotion field there have been several benchmarking initiatives undertaken to identify best practices. These studies are reviewed and summarized in an article by Goetzel and colleagues (7). Generally speaking, these studies have relied on a functional approach to benchmarking because they consider employers of different sizes across different industries using different approaches to worksite health promotion.

There are two main approaches to identifying best practices as part of a benchmarking initiative—deductive methods and inductive methods. Deductive methods are most familiar to people in research or academic settings who are well versed in hypothesis testing. Deductive methods start with a defined hypothesis or statement about what is believed to be true and then use research methods to test that hypothesis. Such methods are also characterized as a top-down approach. Conversely, inductive methods take a bottom-up approach by starting with the desired outcomes and working backward to determine what factors influence the achievement of those results. Many of the best-practice initiatives in the worksite health promotion field have relied on inductive approaches, starting with a list of companies that were already considered to be best-practice organizations and then comparing them in order to identify the practices they had in common. A variety of approaches have been used to identify best-practice organizations, including conducting searches of the peer-reviewed literature and industry or trade journals; interviewing experts in the field, including respected researchers; and reviewing lists of best-practice award winners recognized via a standardized award process such as the C. Everett Koop National Health Award and the WELCOA Well Workplace Award. Goetzel and colleagues concluded in their review of these efforts (7) that the existing best-practice initiatives are complementary rather than definitive in their identification of best practices in the field of health promotion. There is a great deal of overlap in the practices identified as exemplary by these various initiatives, but more work is needed to tie specific practices to measurable outcomes. Additionally, more work must be done to standardize the measurement of best practices so outcomes can be generalized to a diversity of organizations (11). In the worksite health promotion field these outcomes might include program participation and completion rates, participant satisfaction rates, and beneficial changes in health, clinical, and health-related financial outcomes.

Application of Benchmarking Approaches

Any organization can benefit from benchmarking if a consistent set of procedures is used to make comparisons among organizations. The published literature on benchmarking and best practices provides a foundational list of promising practices in the field. Comparing an organization against this list can help identify gaps in its program elements or the implementation of its program elements. If an organization is interested in obtaining third-party assessment of its practices, applying for one of several existing best-practice awards can provide an excellent option for collecting information on the extent to which recommended practices have been implemented. Additionally, an organization can reach out to worksite health promotion vendors or consultants to find out how it compares with other clients of these firms in implementing best practices or achieving superior program performance. Table 12.1

Table 12.1 Tools to Identify Best Practices in Worksite Health Promotion

Name	Description	Sponsoring organization
APQC Best Practice Study Methodology	An overview of a four-step general methodology for benchmarking used to identify best practices in a broad range of endeavors including health and productivity management initiatives	APQC (www.apqc.org)
C. Everett Koop National Health Award criteria	Criteria for an award that recognizes organizations and programs that can demonstrate health improvement and reduction in health care costs	The Health Project, a nonprofit consortium chaired by C. Everett Koop (http://healthproject.stanford.edu)
Employer Measures of Productivity, Absence and Quality (EMPAQ)	A set of precisely defined and standardized benchmarking measures that can be used to measure and evaluate programs that aim to affect health, absence, and productivity	National Business Group on Health (www.empaq.org/empaq)
Healthy Workforce 2010: An Essential Health Promotion Sourcebook for Employers	A resource guide that provides an overview of the U.S. Department of Health and Human Services' Healthy People 2010 objectives for worksites and establishes criteria for a comprehensive worksite health promotion program	Partnership for Prevention (www.prevent.org)
HERO EHM Best Practice Scorecard	An inventory of best-practice elements and outcomes to promote employee health management	HERO (www.the-hero.org)
Health Management Initiative Assessment	An assessment to identify gaps in current approaches to employee health management	Partnership for Prevention's Leading by Example initiative (www.prevent.org)
WELCOA Seven Benchmarks of Success and Well Workplace Platinum Award	Benchmarks of quality wellness programs that have been implemented in well workplaces and benchmarks that serve as the criteria for the Well Workplace Platinum Award	WELCOA (www.welcoa.org/wellworkplace)

From the Historical Archives of The Prudential Insurance Company of America, *The Prudential,* 1916 publication.

provides a list of tools available to assess an organization's use of practices recommended by experts in the worksite health promotion field. This list includes a promising new initiative by HERO that is described in the following section along with examples of how two organizations used a best-practice assessment tool that HERO developed for benchmarking purposes.

HERO Employee Health Management Best Practice Scorecard

HERO is a national nonprofit coalition of corporate and provider members committed to facilitating research and dissemination on the value of prevention in employee health management (EHM). As part of its strategy to create, test, and distribute best-practice measures useful to corporate decision makers, HERO developed the EHM Best Practice Scorecard (Scorecard). The Scorecard identifies nine broad categories of best practices that are generally recognized as essential components of the most successful EHM programs. These categories are corporate culture and leadership commitment; strategic planning; communications, marketing, and promotion; comprehensive program components; benefits design; incentives; program coordination; data management and program evaluation; and achievement of program outcomes. Development of the Scorecard included a review of the criteria used in several reputable award programs, including the Health Project's C. Everett Koop National Health Award and the WELCOA Well Workplace Platinum Award, as well as the U.S. Department of Health and Human Services' *Healthy Workforce 2010* criteria, the Partnership for Prevention's Health Management Initiative Assessment, and the peer-reviewed published literature. The Scorecard was subjected to rigorous review by HERO members as well as other national experts in the field of worksite health promotion. The Scorecard is in its second revision and will continue to undergo testing and revision as more evidence emerges on the outcomes associated with best practices.

The Scorecard can guide the identification or development of best-practice programs by serving as an inventory of best-practice components. It can also be used to compare programs based on the number of program components that have been fully implemented in an organization or based on the program outcomes achieved. The complete Scorecard can be downloaded from the HERO Web site (www.the-hero.org).

The University of Michigan is a HERO member that used the Scorecard in a benchmarking process supporting the development of a 5 y strategic plan for the university's Michigan Healthy Community Initiative. The tool was used initially as a resource for educating university leaders and other key constituents about what best-practice organizations were doing. It was then refined and customized into two tools for the following purposes: (1) to perform a gap analysis by major university location or campus and by population (e.g., employees, dependents, retirees) and (2) to create a prioritization matrix showing what level of resources needed to be invested according to the Scorecard's best-practice components across each of the 5 y in the strategic plan. This was translated into specific recommended actions in the strategic plan and the associated budget to achieve the recommendations. The Scorecard was extremely helpful in communicating the breadth of what needed to be accomplished to move the University of Michigan to best-practice levels and to achieve the desired health and health-related financial outcomes. The gap analysis and prioritization matrix that were informed by the Scorecard were also helpful in garnering support for the 5 y strategic plan. This case study demonstrates how one tool was used to guide the development of a comprehensive worksite health promotion program. The following additional case studies provide information on how benchmarking activities can shape a best-practice approach to worksite health promotion programs (see pp. 105-108).

Conclusion

As evidenced by these case studies, benchmarking strategies provide practitioners and decision makers with valuable guidance on how to plan and improve worksite health promotion in their organizations. There are numerous tools available to assist organizations in benchmarking and identifying best practices, including established awards programs, peer-reviewed studies, and inventories such as the HERO EHM Scorecard. These tools can help identify the elements that should be included in new worksite health promotion programs, identify gaps in existing programs, and offer guidelines for the kinds of outcomes that can be achieved by

Case Study on Using Benchmarking to Guide Integration: Prudential Financial

Prudential Financial (Prudential) has a history of promoting health and fitness that dates as far back as the late 1890s, when insurance agents distributed brochures on well-being to their customers (see figure 12.1). Today, Prudential offers many worksite health promotion programs and services to its employees, including on-site fitness centers and medical clinics, EAPs, work–life programs, safety and workplace accommodations, and Web-based personal health management. Whereas Prudential is proud to have created a workplace culture that supports good health and wellness for its employees and their families, it took time to evolve to this point. In the past, health-related services that were provided operated independently of one another and competed for the attention of the employee population. Through internal and external benchmarking, Prudential has developed an integrated approach to providing health and wellness programming that is referred to as *total health management*.

Prudential makes it a practice to benchmark not only against other companies in its business sector (i.e., competitive benchmarking) but also against organizations considered to be the best in the specific areas being compared (i.e., functional benchmarking). This dual approach requires more work, but it allows the company to present a comprehensive business case to senior management, which is important for garnering ongoing support. For example, in 2006, Prudential introduced a Web-based health risk assessment tool that allows the organization to track aggregate information related to health risks of the population. This enables the company to tailor its suite of health and wellness programs and provide relevant communications to employees and their dependents. Benchmarking results indicated that the typical utilization rate for this type of tool without an incentive is only 5% to 10%. With a goal of achieving higher utilization of the Web-based tool, Prudential-specific and benchmark data were used to build a business case for offering a cash incentive for employees to complete the health risk assessment. This led to senior management approval and support to offer a $150 U.S. incentive for completion of a health risk assessment on an annual basis beginning in January 2008.

Benchmarking also helped Prudential identify a need to move from independently operating departments to a more integrated approach to health management. A review of the best practices in the industry identified a need to better integrate programs, services, communications, and data to improve the health and well-being of the benefits-eligible population. For example, Prudential initiated a hypertension management program in 2001 through its on-site clinics. Under the total health management approach, Prudential integrated the services provided by the fitness, medical, and EAP staff to address factors affecting individuals identified in hypertension screenings. Other examples of integration include

- integrating EAPs and work–life programs with return-to-work programs to help employees on disability leave return to work faster,
- combining the efforts of employee assistance professionals and Prudential's on-site nurses to foster chronic condition management, and
- integrating communications across Web-based and on-site health management service providers and Prudential's employee benefits department to encourage employees to take a more active role in their health.

Effective vendor management is a large component of total health management and is critical to successful integration, which is identified as a best practice on the HERO Scorecard. Prudential spends many hours training and providing feedback to its vendors to ensure that employees obtain the maximum results from the extensive benefits offerings available to them. For example, a partnership with a Web-based tool vendor offers the opportunity to assess the health of Prudential's population and to disseminate health information through an easy-to-use online interface. In addition, a partnership with a data integrator allows Prudential to review aggregate health claim data and gain a clearer picture of employee health. Data integration revealed that employees who use Prudential's on-site fitness centers cost $500 U.S. less in health care claims than employees who do not use the centers. This type of integrated reporting is often used in combination with benchmarking data to guide ongoing decision making on program design.

(continued) ▶

In summary, the total health management concept enables Prudential to create an environment offering seamless entry into any of its health management programs and offerings. Prudential's goal is to increase the likelihood that employees participating in any of its total health management programs will identify and engage in other needed programs. With improved integration, more employees will use a care counselor or health coaching program, attend a medical clinic, become a member at one of Prudential's fitness centers, receive a return-to-work or ergonomic intervention, or participate in a disease management screening or health seminar. The goal of total health management is to meet the needs of the entire employee population, whether employees choose to enroll in one of Prudential's health benefit programs or not.

The company's long-term goal is to continue to assess the health risks of its population, provide appropriate programming to reduce those risks, and to sustain a workplace culture that supports this vision.

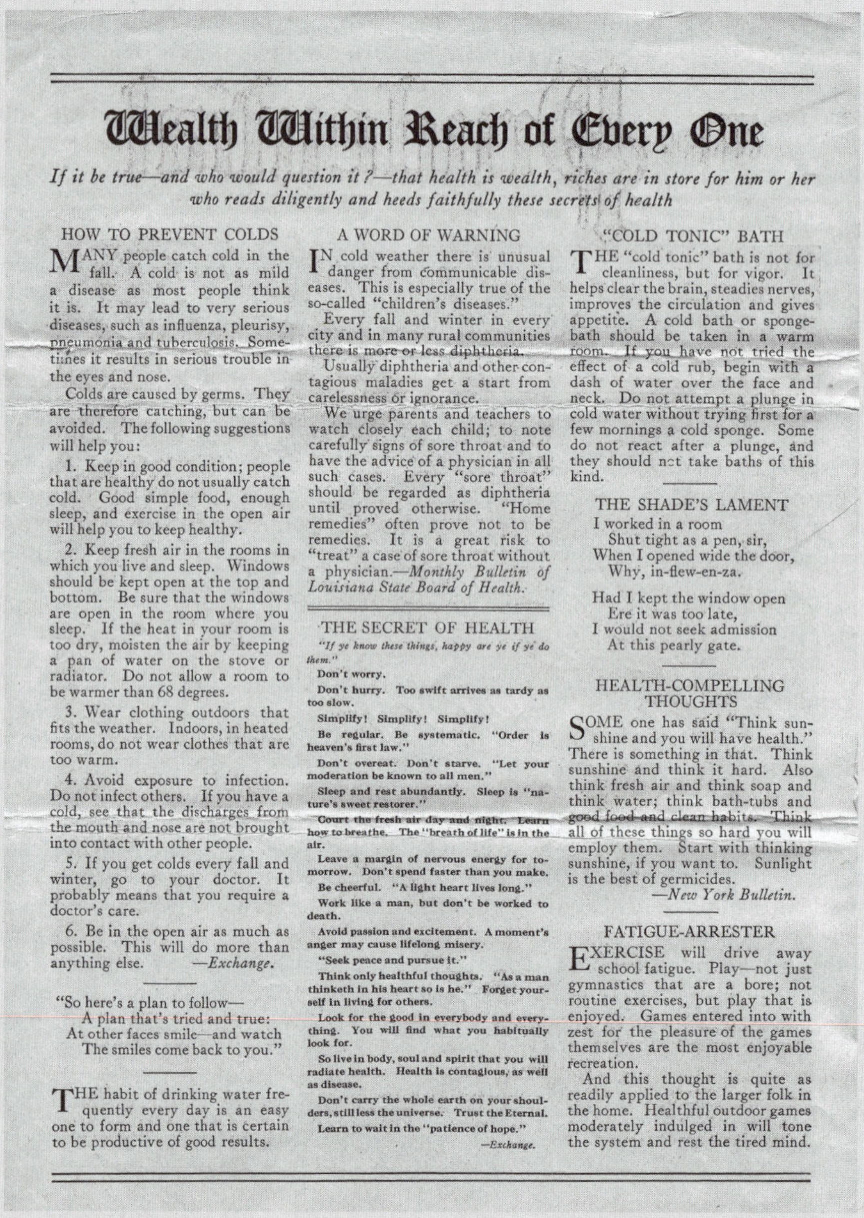

𝕎ealth 𝕎ithin Reach of 𝔼very 𝕆ne

If it be true—and who would question it?—that health is wealth, riches are in store for him or her who reads diligently and heeds faithfully these secrets of health

HOW TO PREVENT COLDS

MANY people catch cold in the fall. A cold is not as mild a disease as most people think it is. It may lead to very serious diseases, such as influenza, pleurisy, pneumonia and tuberculosis. Sometimes it results in serious trouble in the eyes and nose.

Colds are caused by germs. They are therefore catching, but can be avoided. The following suggestions will help you:

1. Keep in good condition; people that are healthy do not usually catch cold. Good simple food, enough sleep, and exercise in the open air will help you to keep healthy.

2. Keep fresh air in the rooms in which you live and sleep. Windows should be kept open at the top and bottom. Be sure that the windows are open in the room where you sleep. If the heat in your room is too dry, moisten the air by keeping a pan of water on the stove or radiator. Do not allow a room to be warmer than 68 degrees.

3. Wear clothing outdoors that fits the weather. Indoors, in heated rooms, do not wear clothes that are too warm.

4. Avoid exposure to infection. Do not infect others. If you have a cold, see that the discharges from the mouth and nose are not brought into contact with other people.

5. If you get colds every fall and winter, go to your doctor. It probably means that you require a doctor's care.

6. Be in the open air as much as possible. This will do more than anything else. —*Exchange.*

"So here's a plan to follow—
A plan that's tried and true:
At other faces smile—and watch
The smiles come back to you."

THE habit of drinking water frequently every day is an easy one to form and one that is certain to be productive of good results.

A WORD OF WARNING

IN cold weather there is unusual danger from communicable diseases. This is especially true of the so-called "children's diseases."

Every fall and winter in every city and in many rural communities there is more or less diphtheria.

Usually diphtheria and other contagious maladies get a start from carelessness or ignorance.

We urge parents and teachers to watch closely each child; to note carefully signs of sore throat and to have the advice of a physician in all such cases. Every "sore throat" should be regarded as diphtheria until proved otherwise. "Home remedies" often prove not to be remedies. It is a great risk to "treat" a case of sore throat without a physician.—*Monthly Bulletin of Louisiana State Board of Health.*

THE SECRET OF HEALTH

"If ye know these things, happy are ye if ye do them."

Don't worry.

Don't hurry. Too swift arrives as tardy as too slow.

Simplify! Simplify! Simplify!

Be regular. Be systematic. "Order is heaven's first law."

Don't overeat. Don't starve. "Let your moderation be known to all men."

Sleep and rest abundantly. Sleep is "nature's sweet restorer."

Court the fresh air day and night. Learn how to breathe. The "breath of life" is in the air.

Leave a margin of nervous energy for to-morrow. Don't spend faster than you make.

Be cheerful. "A light heart lives long."

Work like a man, but don't be worked to death.

Avoid passion and excitement. A moment's anger may cause lifelong misery.

"Seek peace and pursue it."

Think only healthful thoughts. "As a man thinketh in his heart so is he." Forget yourself in living for others.

Look for the good in everybody and everything. You will find what you habitually look for.

So live in body, soul and spirit that you will radiate health. Health is contagious, as well as disease.

Don't carry the whole earth on your shoulders, still less the universe. Trust the Eternal.

Learn to wait in the "patience of hope."
—*Exchange.*

"COLD TONIC" BATH

THE "cold tonic" bath is not for cleanliness, but for vigor. It helps clear the brain, steadies nerves, improves the circulation and gives appetite. A cold bath or sponge-bath should be taken in a warm room. If you have not tried the effect of a cold rub, begin with a dash of water over the face and neck. Do not attempt a plunge in cold water without trying first for a few mornings a cold sponge. Some do not react after a plunge, and they should not take baths of this kind.

THE SHADE'S LAMENT

I worked in a room
Shut tight as a pen, sir,
When I opened wide the door,
Why, in-flew-en-za.

Had I kept the window open
Ere it was too late,
I would not seek admission
At this pearly gate.

HEALTH-COMPELLING THOUGHTS

SOME one has said "Think sunshine and you will have health." There is something in that. Think sunshine and think it hard. Also think fresh air and think soap and think water; think bath-tubs and good food and clean habits. Think all of these things so hard you will employ them. Start with thinking sunshine, if you want to. Sunlight is the best of germicides.
—*New York Bulletin.*

FATIGUE-ARRESTER

EXERCISE will drive away school fatigue. Play—not just gymnastics that are a bore; not routine exercises, but play that is enjoyed. Games entered into with zest for the pleasure of the games themselves are the most enjoyable recreation.

And this thought is quite as readily applied to the larger folk in the home. Healthful outdoor games moderately indulged in will tone the system and rest the tired mind.

Figure 12.1   Historic newspaper article.

Example of an early publication on the benefits of a healthy lifestyle. From the Historical Archives of The Prudential Insurance Company of America, "The Prudential," 1916 publication. Reprinted with permission.

Case Study on Best Practices in Coaching: Sutter Health Partners

Sutter Health is a health care system of hospitals, health centers, and physician organizations serving more than 100 communities in northern California. Sutter Health Partners (SHP) is the employee health enhancement program of Sutter Health and has been providing personalized lifestyle management and wellness coaching services to employees within the system since 2001. In 2007, SHP introduced its best-practice program, Live Well For Life, to the employer market to assist employers in improving the health status of their employees and in reducing overall health care costs. One of the unique differentiators of the Live Well For Life program is that this program was developed within a major U.S. health care system and was implemented within a number of its site affiliates for its own employees first. In 2001, when SHP began development of its program, there were few face-to-face wellness coaching programs with widespread or publicized success. A benchmarking effort identified a similar program that inspired the formation of SHP. Exorbitant increases in health care costs, rising obesity-related workers' compensation claims, and a desire to improve employee morale and retention supported the business case for developing the program.

The Live Well For Life program is comprehensive and combines many of the best-practice approaches identified in the HERO Scorecard, including personal health assessment, biometric health screenings, and personal wellness coaching for all participants regardless of risk level. The entry point to participation is completion of a personal health assessment. All participants are provided a coupon for a biometric health screening that can be completed at a local medical facility; on-site testing is also available. If a participant has had lab work done within the last 12 mo, those lab results are used. Employees who complete the personal health assessment are then assigned to an individual wellness coach. They meet face to face, and the coach completes additional screenings, including blood pressure, weight, body fat, and waist-to-hip ratio. At the same meeting, the coach reviews the personal health report and screening results with each participant and establishes goals to lower identified risk factors. The coach and participant agree on subsequent follow-up meetings, which are intended to provide the participant with support and accountability to facilitate lifestyle behavior changes toward identified wellness goals. Additional core components of the program include on-site education classes, ongoing health campaigns, and group exercise classes. All of these elements are identified as best practices in the HERO Scorecard.

Use of James Prochaska's transtheoretical model and its associated stages of change framework (13) is a recognized best practice in long-term health behavior change. Dr. Prochaska has applied these techniques with great success in his work with cancer patients and people with addiction. This model, along with Albert Bandura's concept of self-efficacy (1), provided a foundation for the coaching model at SHP. These foundational principles are personalized by the coaches as they work with individuals to identify specific health risks, develop goals, and overcome challenges in making positive health changes.

Another best-practice component of the program is its use of incentives to promote employee motivation and engagement. In 2001, incentives started with a waiver of a portion of the health insurance premium. The value of this incentive was $600 U.S. per year for an individual and $1,200 U.S. per year for a family. Cash incentives were introduced in 2005, and in 2007 cash incentives amounted to $500 U.S. per year. One of the challenges of using cash-based incentives is sustaining their effectiveness over time. Thus, along with cash incentives, SHP introduced sequential progressive incentives to continue to engage and motivate participants to meet their goals. Overall, SHP participation rates within its site affiliates reach nearly 60% for cash incentives and nearly 80% for premium waivers. Incentives would potentially be higher in a nonunion environment. The type of incentive system implemented takes into account culture, environment, and financial status among other factors that are unique to each organization. Future incentive program development will further integrate incentives into the benefits structure, which is a recommended best practice on the HERO Scorecard.

In keeping with the other best-practice criteria identified in the HERO Scorecard, the SHP programs have been linked to projected financial outcomes through a third-party study of the program's effectiveness. Researchers at a consulting firm were engaged to conduct a third-party economic analysis of the SHP program. The researchers analyzed SHP data and projected savings for medical and pharmacy costs, absenteeism (including short-term disability), and presenteeism (on-the-job productivity loss). Cost savings estimates were developed from a wide variety of published studies and information available through the consulting firm. The general savings estimates were then applied to the specific program design and

(continued) ▶

▶ Case Study on Best Practices in Coaching: Sutter Health Partners *(continued)*

personal coaching delivery of the SHP program. Based on a projected average employer medical cost of $8,796 U.S. per employee in 2007, the medical savings were estimated at about 2.5% of medical costs. In addition, absenteeism and presenteeism savings were estimated at 1.9% of employee pay.

The use of comprehensive data analysis and reporting to measure program effect is another best practice identified in the HERO Scorecard. SHP is contracting with a large third-party data analysis vendor to integrate health care utilization and specific wellness results to determine ROI for the wellness program. This effort is an integral part of the development of a total health and productivity data platform that will involve merging the full range of health-related data, including absence, workers' compensation, sick time, disability, and medical claims. These data will be used along with the SHP program participation data to measure the full effectiveness of the program.

a best-practice program. Still, there is a need for much more research on best practices in worksite health promotion. As worksite health promotion programs continue to evolve, new innovations must continue to be evaluated according to their contribution to health, productivity, and financial outcomes. Such evaluation of today's promising approaches to employee health management provides the foundation for the best practices of tomorrow.

Chapter Review Questions

1. Identify and briefly explain three organizational strategies or practices that may be supported by benchmarking.

2. List and describe the various forms of benchmarking.

3. What sources of information have been used in identifying best practice companies in worksite health promotion?

4. Compare and contrast inductive and deductive approaches for identification of best practices as part of benchmarking projects.

5. Based on what is currently available in the literature, discuss what research endeavors will most likely advance the field of worksite health promotion best practices and benchmarking.

Health and the Organization of Work

David Gimeno, PhD, and Benjamin C. Amick III, PhD

As Cappelli and Sherer explain, "what is unique about behavior in organization is presumably that being in the organization—the context of the organization—somehow shapes behavior, and it is impossible to explore that uniqueness without an explicit consideration of the context" (16).

Work (and jobs) can be created, destroyed, and transformed. While business performance and productivity are typically the outcomes of interest, how work is organized has a tremendous effect on worker health. Whether the health outcome is beneficial or harmful will depend on many factors. Although abundant research considers how work influences health, much of it focuses exclusively on the individual worker or on populations of workers (3). Few researchers consider the organization and how it structures work, creates the context for individual behavior, or affects the formation and maintenance of social groups and behavioral norms. Moreover, the theoretical models of work organization and health were proposed in the 1960s and 1970s. Given the continuously changing nature of work and the development of a global economy, the old models may be growing less relevant (55). Modifications to psychosocial work organization models have recently been suggested (22,73). The geography of business has changed, requiring those who are interested in making changes within worksites to consider a broader integrative perspective linking multiple contextual levels to explain how work organization influences health and what can be done to prevent potential harmful effects.

Contextual Levels Shaping the Organization of Work

Figure 13.1 guides our perspective on the contextual levels shaping the effect of work organization on the individual. The global, societal, and labor market levels are distal factors shaping the organization, groups, and jobs (proximal factors) that more directly shape work organization. In this section, we briefly review all six levels and then focus on the health effects of organizational, group, and job factors, as these are where a change in the work organization can exert the most effective actions to create a healthier workplace and promote a healthier workforce.

Global Factors

The nature of work, especially in economically and industrially developed societies, has undergone significant change over the past three decades due in part to globalization and three related tendencies: (1) trade liberalization (i.e., removal of trade barriers such as tariffs and quotas), privatization (i.e., sale of state-owned assets to private owners), and deregulation (i.e., removal of government restrictions and interventions on capital flow; 87); (2) the rise of the service economy and knowledge-based industries; and (3) the penetration of technology into everyday work. While these changes are not novel, each has dramatically accelerated significantly changing labor market structures and work organization. Concurrently, the nature of the workforce is also changing. For example, the aging workforce is a demographic trend that many, if not all, workplaces are facing.

Societal Factors

Not all societies are affected equally by the global trends. For instance, economically developed societies retain a core set of jobs while hazardous manual and labor-intensive jobs are transferred to less-developed societies that exert less, if any, control over working conditions (and presumably have low wages, low security, low social protection, and so on). Other important features of this

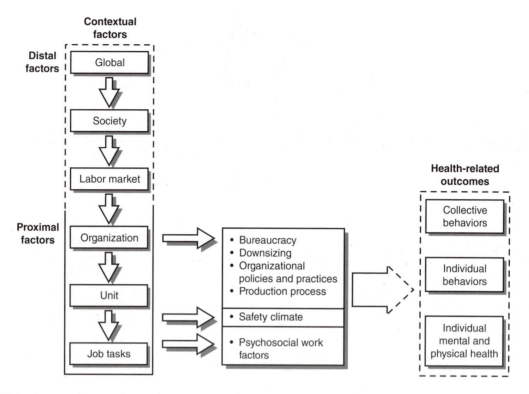

Figure 13.1 Contextual factors shaping the organization of work and their relation to health.

context are historical, cultural, and economic factors.

Labor Market Factors

The labor market affects work organization through both the industrial and occupational mix and the regional economic development, which directly affects the type of industries and occupations that are available or offered and the economic and work-related policies and regulations (e.g., absenteeism and workers' compensation regulations). Although this context can traditionally be seen as nested within societies, given today's global economy, labor markets can also be characterized by the loss of geographical linkage.

Organizational Factors

Organizations (whether workplaces, firms, or companies) are instrumental in how they organize their workforce (in terms of both structure and function) and what jobs they require their workforce to perform. The organizational environment consists of the structural organizational and business characteristics of the firm, such as size, industry type, unionization, and bureaucra-

tization, as well as the managerial style and firm culture that shape policies and practices, work climate, and orientation toward employees. The production process (e.g., lean production) determines the way workers are organized, the workers' schedules and shifts, the way workers work with others (whether they work in teams or alone), and the level of technical involvement required in the jobs to achieve the organizational goals. In the era of globalization, it is common for firms to restructure, downsize, merge, unmerge, centralize, and decentralize, and thus organizational features are subject to change over time.

Unit Factors

At this level, the social environment emerges with interactions among unit (or group or team) members and between workers and leadership (i.e., managers and supervisors). This environment creates both formal and informal workplace social support networks and social norms (i.e., shared assessments of policies, procedures, and practices and expectations employees have in their workplace). Groups define standards of appropriate behavior, which are based on shared assessments, and create social controls that regulate employee behaviors.

Job Task Factors

Job tasks are specific job demands, duties, and responsibilities workers are required to perform, including physical and psychological job requirements. Health research has focused on psychosocial work factors (e.g., demand and effort, control, rewards, and justice).

Toward a Multilevel Perspective on Work Organization

Researchers focusing on only organizational, group, or job or task levels may conduct more in-depth investigations, but a multilevel approach would enrich the available evidence and provide a more realistic picture of the complex nature of the organization of work. As figure 13.1 illustrates, no level can be considered to be totally independent of another. There is a constant complex interplay across levels. For instance, employment arrangements or contracts (36), work schedules or hours, and the role of managers and supervisors are some of these factors. Alternative work arrangements (arrangements that are nonfixed and highly flexible both in working time and in place of work), although not new, are becoming predominant in today's workplaces (7). The types of work arrangements used in a specific workplace are influenced by the global economic trends, the societal development, the regional labor market, and the organizational production and managerial styles of an employer. Also, length and structure of work time and work content are fundamentally linked, and long working hours interact with irregular schedules and shifts in their potentially damaging health effects (45). Despite the connectedness of organizational life, the following summary of the research evidence comports to figure 13.1. The evidence is not comprehensive, as the literatures are diverse and deep; rather, our summary is intended to give the reader a sense of perspective on the levels and important concepts and approaches.

The Health Effects of the Organization of Work: What Do We Know?

In considering the impact of the organization of work on health, several topics may be considered. Here we discuss the following: bureaucracy, downsizing, organizational policies and practices, production process, safety climate, and psychosocial work factors.

Bureaucracy

Organizations influence workers by how they structure production flows and the jobs in those production flows. Organizational structures are designed to allow management to coordinate and control the production process and the employee (8) and aim to improve efficiency and maximize productivity through division of labor and standardization of procedures (20,88). Bureaucratic systems are characterized by explicit rules and institutional norms (i.e., formalization) with clearly defined authority levels (i.e., verticalization), tasks (i.e., departmentalization), and responsibilities over decision making (i.e., decentralization; 63,64). Although bureaucracy may provide guidance and clarify work roles, thus lowering stress and increasing efficiency (1,32), it may also constrain workers' decision latitude and participatory and self-actualization opportunities, generating boredom, listlessness, alienation, and resistance (13,63).

What is known about the direct effect of organizational structure on workers' well-being is scarce, cross-sectional, and mixed. Among U.S. and Japanese companies, high verticalization, departmentalization, and formalization are associated with low levels of commitment and satisfaction, while decentralization and participatory decision making are associated with high commitment and satisfaction (63). Among U.S. nurses, vertical and horizontal participation (i.e., the degree to which decisions are taken in agreement with superiors and peers) but not formalization is positively associated with satisfaction (15). U.S. salespeople in organizations with less verticalization reported lower satisfaction, less anxiety and stress, and more efficiency than reported by salespeople in organizations with more verticalization (42).

Downsizing

In response to the increased competitiveness in global markets, the aspiration for improved financial performance, and the concentration of power in owners of large companies (i.e., corporations; 17,65), organizational restructuring has become a central mechanism to reduce human costs and intensify production efficiency systems (14). Although restructuring may occur by means of several organizational actions, such as downsizing, merging or unmerging, and centralization or decentralization, downsizing is the main "strategy designed to improve financial standing of a firm by reducing and changing the structure of the workforce in order to improve operational results" (65, p. 40).

Longitudinal research on the health effects of downsizing suggests it exerts a direct negative influence over workers' well-being. Workers with multiple exposures to downsizing report higher levels of job insecurity, depression, intention to quit, and health problems (66). Among the workers who remain employed (i.e., the stayers), health effects occur between pre- and postdownsizing. The greater the degree of downsizing, the greater the increases in sickness absences (85), musculoskeletal problems (53), consumption of psychotropic drugs (52), early retirement (before 55 y of age) as granted, permanent disability pension because of medical reasons (84), and even mortality due to cardiovascular diseases (85). Downsizing effects appear to be mediated by changes in physical demands, opportunities for control, and feelings of job insecurity (53,54). The consequent job insecurity of a major organizational downsizing increases minor psychiatric disorders, blood pressure, and weight (31).

Organizational Policies and Practices

Organizational policies and practices allow the organization to prevent and manage health problems and the associated high costs of injury and disability. Organizational policies and practices are designed for prevention (before the health problem occurs) and management (once the health problem has occurred) as well as for the managerial style and the organizational culture (that is, the commitment of the organization to its employees). Specifically, organizational policies and practices include safety and ergonomic practices, health and safety committees, disability case management, and return-to-work policies, as well as whether the organization has a people-oriented culture.

One of the first attempts to evaluate the effect of organizational policies and practices on workers' health was the Michigan studies conducted during the late 1980s and early 1990s (41). These studies showed that organizational policies and practices predict better health performance. These findings have been recently confirmed among carpal tunnel syndrome patients in Maine (2) and in educational, health care, and hospitality facilities in Ontario, Canada (2,19).

Production Process

Lean production is a generic term referring to the Japanese system of work organization, production, and management. It was first developed by the automobile manufacturer Toyota Motor Corporation as a reform of the Fordism and Taylorism mass production systems (48,60,74). Small, multiskilled cells or teams complete the entire product. Production is supported by just-in-time engineering systems, elimination of inefficient (wasted) steps and time, and continuous improvement through the systematic recording and standardization of work procedures (62). The ultimate goal is increased productivity, quality, and responsiveness to customers.

Whether lean production has positive or negative health effects remains uncertain. Team empowerment, enhanced participation in decision making, shared problem solving, rotating jobs, and skill development and training opportunities are considered to be health promoting. Alternatively, lean production intensifies labor (i.e., a neo-Taylorism) through peer pressure in meeting team incentives, simplified job tasks, shorter and more repetitive cycle times needed to be just in time, and limited decision-making authority, all of which leave the old hierarchy and the assembly line essentially intact (9). Lean production may also have complex consequences by mixing hazardous exposures to industrial processes formerly separated in distinct areas (11). Lean production has been linked to significantly greater perceived stress, fatigue, and tension; a higher rate of musculoskeletal injuries (60); and depressive symptoms (71). These effects seem to be provoked by the increase of workload, the reduction of autonomy and skill utilization, and the deception of unfulfilled greater empowerment and participation (60,71).

Safety Climate

Safety climate is a feature of organizational groups (e.g., departments or teams) and not of the individual, but it is measured by asking individual workers. It captures shared perceptions guiding safe behaviors. The perceptions result from unequivocal and consistently enforced safety policies (i.e., strategic goals), procedures (i.e., tactical guidelines), and practices (i.e., execution of policies and procedures) rather than formally declared policies (77,89). Top managers establish the policies and strategic goals that supervisors execute. Differences in the execution of the same policies are expected between groups within an organization (90). Safety climate has been studied in chemical, nuclear, manufacturing, health and service, and construction industries (18,33,46). It is hypothesized that safety climate increases compliance with safety practices, which, in turn, reduces work-related accidents and injuries. A recent meta-analysis found strong support for the suggestion that safety climate influences safety practices but, due to scarce prospective research, found weak support for the suggestion that it influences accidents and injuries (18).

Psychosocial Work Factors

Two models are frequently used when discussing psychosocial work factors: the demand-control model (also known as the *job strain model;* 47) and the effort-reward imbalance model (79). More recently a third model, the organizational justice model, has been introduced (27). All three psychosocial work organization models, despite their different conceptual foci (job strain focuses on job tasks, effort-reward imbalance connects the labor market and the job tasks levels, and organizational justice connects the labor market and the organization or unit), propose prolonged stress as the causal mechanism affecting health. We separate the evidence, but theoretical and empirical studies testing the degree of overlap among the three models would deepen our knowledge and improve our ability to effectively change psychosocial work environments to improve health.

The job strain model suggests that the highest health risk occurs in high-strain situations, when psychological demands are high and control, a combination of skill discretion and decision authority over the demands, is low. A variation of the model adds social support from colleagues and supervisors. The highest health risk results from high demands, low control, and low social support (44). The effort-reward imbalance model identifies the highest risk jobs as those having a negative imbalance in the rewards (i.e., money, esteem, promotion, and security) received for the efforts (both mental and physical) performed to do the job—that is, jobs involving low rewards and high efforts (79). The organizational justice model proposes that unfair treatment of employees by supervisors affects employee health (27). Two components of justice are considered: one

procedural (i.e., decision-making procedures are applied consistently, suppress bias, and are accurate, correctable, and ethical; 61) and one interactional (i.e., the supervisor considers the workers' viewpoints, shares information concerning decision making, and treats people fairly and truthfully; 67).

The body of prospective evidence for health consequences of job strain and effort-reward imbalance is large and covers many health outcomes (21,23,80,86). High job strain and low reward for high effort are prospective risk factors for common mental disorders (82), health risk behaviors (e.g., cigarette smoking, alcohol consumption; 81), obesity (12), and heart disease risk factors (6,72). There is inconclusive evidence for musculoskeletal problems (10,70). Only one study found that effort-reward imbalance predicts compensated low-back and neck injury incidence in a 7.5 y follow-up (76). In addition, there is limited prospective evidence that high demands, low leader support, and high strain influence the development or maintenance of insomnia (43) and that high effort with low rewards and a high effort-to-reward ratio influence sleep disturbances (29). High strain has also been shown to affect return to work (35).

Evidence for organizational justice is less extensive. Organizational injustice has been found to predict health risk behaviors (58), minor psychiatric disorders (27,49,50), sickness absence (30,49), reduced heart rate variability and altered systolic arterial pressure variability (26), incident coronary heart disease (CHD; 51), and CHD mortality (28). Finally, all three approaches to psychosocial work exposures have been found to be important determinants of sickness absence (24,39,83).

Methodological Issues to Consider in Moving Forward

Controversy over the validity of having workers report job and organizational factors and how to measure both has persisted for two decades (37). When workers report, it is assumed their reporting is valid and reliable. There is limited evidence testing the assumption (34). Ossmann and colleagues examined the agreement between manager and employee reports of organizational policies and practices (69). Moderate agreement was found for a combined index of organizational support and strong agreement was found for a people-oriented culture. However, agreement ratings may not be the best way to prove reliability since discrepancy among managers, supervisors, and employees in the assessment of the same situation may capture, for instance, valid differences in the design and implementation of policies at each level (e.g., managerial, supervisory, and employee). The questions of reliability and validity of self-reports remain unresolved.

For unit-level factors (e.g., safety climate, support networks, and norms), researchers should identify the natural (i.e., functional) social units in which the group members interact rather than the structurally defined units (e.g., section or department) in which members may or may not interact (89). For instance, peer group reports to a supervisor may more accurately reflect the social group even if the reporting relationships are not recognized in organizational charts (5). Data from only formally defined groups may be too heterogeneous, hiding true relationships between social exposures and health.

Time is needed for an organizational exposure to work through the pathways required to affect a worker's health. Still today, the research literature is dominated by cross-sectional studies over well-designed longitudinal studies, limiting our ability to present strong evidence. While prospective studies have investigated many factors, restricted observational times that do not coincide with the latency time between an exposure and its effects further limit the strength of the evidence. Researches should consider the feasibility of longer follow-ups as well as the availability of long-term repeated measurement data of both exposure and outcome, as both change in a complex labor market and global economy.

Threats to external validity (i.e., generalizability) of research come from research conducted in a limited number of workplaces and the use of labels to refer to work organization without describing specific features of the unique organization. For instance, a variety of studies may be performed on factors such as lean production. However, the concept of lean production may be difficult to study since in practice companies adapt the original design of lean production to their local needs and particular conditions, creating mixed lean production systems incorporating elements from other production systems. Therefore, labels are not enough to compare results across studies; the clear description of the particular organizational context is required to allow synthesis of findings.

Interventions on the Organization of Work With Health Outcomes: What Can We Learn?

Intervention studies that attempted to change the way in which work is organized may provide valuable insight into health impact associated with such changes. This section reviews what is known on this topic and what learnings may be generated from it.

What Has Been Done?

Interventions may target workers (e.g., increasing their coping capability) or work organization (e.g., improving organizational policies and practices or the psychosocial work environment) or both. Many interventions use the worksite to reach the workers rather than treat it as an environment to be changed. Thus, available literature on individual stress management and behavioral interventions is large while the literature on work organization interventions is small (68). In the following discussion we summarize work organization interventions rather than interventions focused on the individual worker. Figure 13.1 highlights the complexities involved in work organization interventions. The multiple levels where different interventions have been applied, the designs used, and the various outcomes investigated make any summary challenging.

Job enrichment has been used since the 1960s to increase employee satisfaction and work motivation and to retain workers by reducing turnover and absenteeism (75). While many job enrichment theories have been developed, they all focus on changing the work content to augment employees' decision authority, task variety, and opportunities for learning skills and social interaction (40). Literature exists on job redesign interventions not captured in the health literature, but our aim is to review only those work organization interventions for which health outcomes were used to evaluate effectiveness.

Recent systematic reviews have assessed the literature on work organization interventions (4,25,59). To date, most work organization interventions have focused on reducing work stress, and the majority of the findings come from interventions based on the job strain model. By and large, evidence shows the effectiveness of organizational-level interventions by means of enhancing employee participation and, thus, increasing control, decreasing demands and improving social support. Of 18 interventions designed to increase employee participation or control, 8 showed that, overall, reducing demands and improving workplace control or support improved health, a finding that is in line with the hypotheses of the job strain model. The most effective participatory actions were based on (1) employee committees to identify workplace stressors and ways to reduce them and (2) committees including employees, managers, and external agents (e.g., researchers) to discuss changes and how to improve team communication and resolve conflicts. The observation of a beneficial health effect of increasing recognition for good work supports the effort-reward imbalance model (25).

An evaluation of 19 studies on task restructuring interventions concluded that improving the psychosocial work environment by increasing task variety had at most a modest positive health effect; teamwork, as a method to address collective coping and decision making, changed the psychosocial environment for some, but not all, of the workers and thus translated into little apparent health effects. The evaluation also concluded that the introduction of autonomous production groups (such as those of lean production) mainly worsens the psychosocial environment and, consequently, adversely affects health. In sum, increasing worker empowerment appears to be more important than reducing demands or increasing support. However, some of the psychosocial environment changes were negligible, and so health effects were not measurable.

In short, despite some methodological concerns (56), evidence of the health benefits of interventions tackling the organization of work is highly promising. Particularly, findings from interventions based on the job strain model provide very strong evidence that health can be improved by changing harmful work organization features.

What Are the Challenges?

Designing and implementing successful interventions to change work organization are challenging (78). We discuss three key elements to success; namely, intervention assessment, contextual issues, and organizational-level versus individual-level interventions.

Intervention Assessment

Evaluation of the intervention is needed at different stages. A careful initial appraisal of the work environment before the intervention, which is rarely done, is essential. Changing the organization of the work may cause previously good jobs to deteriorate as a consequence of the changes, outweighing the potential benefits of the intervention. So, before beginning the intervention, ask who the work organization changes will affect, where the changes could be most usefully applied, and who will benefit the most from the changes. Also ask if other interventions are being planned at the same time that could interact with the planned changes. A change agent should be confident that the intervention implementation, duration, and intensity will elicit the expected health improvements. Additionally, it is necessary to closely monitor how the changes are being implemented and to document the implementation process, since waiting until the end of the intervention to assess its effects may miss informative changes that occur during the process of the implementation. Finally, evaluation of the effects at the end of the intervention should consider that some changes may take more time than others to work through the pathways required to affect a worker's health. Some health effects may be noticeable right after the implementation, some may dissipate shortly after, and some may take a longer time to be apparent.

Qualitative assessment should be carried out in addition to quantitative analysis in order to generate a clear understanding of the full effect of an intervention. Subtle changes in the social environment, supervisory styles, or communication channels may have large long-term effects in either supporting or diluting the intervention effectiveness.

Context Matters

The organizational context into which an intervention is implemented is critical to the intervention success. Sometimes interventions don't work because of a lack of management commitment to the work. External factors such as outsourcing or downsizing may occur at the time of the intervention, and technological constraints may cause the intervention to not be as feasible as wanted. Even in the best-designed system a management policy could incite unintended behaviors. Berggren documents an increase in neck and shoulder problems among workers in the newly designed assembly production systems in which the work occurs in autonomous groups and is supported by advanced dock assembly technologies. But the production quotas set in labor management negotiations were quite high, and thus the speed of production overwhelmed the engineering of the production system (9).

Organizational Versus Individual Interventions

Not surprisingly, reviews have shown the superiority of organizational-level interventions to address organizational factors compared with interventions targeting individual factors. However, these reviews have also shown that integrating individual components into organizational-level interventions may be an essential complement to a successful and generalizable intervention (59). The role of moderating individual psychological characteristics and job experiences and circumstances is known (38). For example, workers are at different stages of change and may benefit more or less from the intervention depending on their need and capacity to adapt to the changes. Simply put, individuals must be motivated to change.

What Works?

If one characteristic of successful interventions should be highlighted, it is the need for participatory approaches to change. Employee participation and empowerment appear to improve employee health. Top-down organizational interventions, implemented and controlled by management without including the workers (the people who will be most affected by the changes) in the decision process, tend to produce negligible or even negative health effects. Those interested in work organization interventions should be heartened by the consistent findings of the job strain interventions supporting the importance of psychosocial work organization in worker health.

Conclusion

The organization of work has a significant impact on the health of the employee. Factors that impact whether the outcome is harmful or beneficial are many but include such contextual factors as the ageing of the workforce, control over work conditions, the type of occupations that are available or offered, size of the company, managerial style, work unit social culture, and the specific job task performed (physical or psychological requirements of the job). Whereas most research is conducted at the individual level, research conducted at the organizational level shows much promise. It appears that participatory approaches to change the context of the work environment generate positive health outcomes. On the other hand, management-controlled types of intervention tend to produce negligible or even negative health outcomes. The importance of considering the psychosocial work organization in worker health can not be overstated.

Chapter Review Questions

1. What are the contextual levels shaping the organization of work where an organization can be most effective?

2. What are the criticisms to our current knowledge?

3. What are the most common interventions, and what works?

4. What are the challenges for future research and practice?

14

Health and Productivity Management
An Overview

Joseph A. Leutzinger, PhD

Health and productivity management (HPM), sometimes described as the *integrated health management model,* has emerged as a major strategy to support corporate solutions in the fields of health improvement and organizational performance. As the field of health improvement (promotion) evolves into a more integrated approach to employee health management, the HPM model will become increasingly important to health service providers (vendors) and organizations such as health plans and corporations. The intent of this chapter is to provide an overview of the HPM model and to discuss how to implement it within an organization.

What Is Health and Productivity Management?

HPM is a relatively new and emerging construct. As of today, there is no universally accepted definition of HPM. However, there is broad-based acceptance of a working definition from the Academy for Health and Productivity Management (AHPM), which is the teaching division of the Institute for Health and Productivity Management (IHPM), that will be used in this chapter: HPM is "the integration of all organizational Human Capital/Resource-related departments designed to accomplish a comprehensive approach for reducing or eliminating health and injury risks while enhancing the portion of personal performance that is related to health." (see www.ahpm.org/info/definition.html) In addition, HPM involves the integrated management of health and injury risks, chronic illness, and disability to reduce employees' total health-related costs, including medical expenditures, unnecessary absence from work, and lost performance at work (presenteeism; 6).

The major emphasis within the definition from IHPM is placed on health problems or health concerns that are preventable, including both chronic and acute conditions, which have economic, medical, and productivity financial implications for employers. Additionally, reducing or eliminating prospective risks to enhance personal functionality, which leads to improved organizational performance, is an important emphasis of the model.

While numerous factors such as supervisor relations, skills, and training influence productivity, this discussion of HPM considers the productivity portion to be specific to health-related productivity. Productivity in general may be viewed as the relationship of inputs (e.g., resources and time) to outputs (e.g., products, services, and knowledge) and can be considered at the macro level (revenues and profits) or at the micro level (the amount an employee generates per hour of work).

Health-Related Productivity

Health-related productivity is the component of productivity that takes into account personal health strategies as well as chronic and acute conditions that influence an individual's ability to perform at work. While health has a significant influence on productivity, there are several other factors that are also important. Yet health affects virtually all other factors related to productivity. As a result, health clearly affects human performance and functionality. The largest source of productivity loss is attributed to common diseases that are comparatively inexpensive to treat medically (e.g., migraines, depression, and back conditions). One recent finding in the HPM literature is that inexpensive and common diseases have a greater effect on productivity than more expensive conditions such as heart disease, diabetes, and cancers have on productivity (6).

Presenteeism and absenteeism are two main components of health-related productivity. Presenteeism describes how productive an employee is while at work and is related to the quality and quantity of work done by the employee (i.e., number of errors or mistakes made at work, low work quality, and unrelated tasks performed at work; 7). It has been determined that presenteeism is the largest single component of productivity losses in the workplace. Costs associated with presenteeism, when measured with valid instruments, have been found to be significantly higher than absenteeism costs (6). An example of a serious disease that has a significant effect on presenteeism is depression. In 2003, 478 million workdays were lost across the United States due to 55 million employees reporting they were unable to concentrate at work or generate desired work output due to personal depression or an episode of a family member (2).

Absenteeism is the amount of missed work time or a paid absence. Absenteeism causes the organization to lose what would have been the employee's contribution for the length of the absence; depending on the position, another employee has to take the place and be paid to do the work of the employee who is absent. In 2003, missed workdays due to illness among U.S. workers totaled 407 million (2).

Absenteeism and presenteeism can be broken down further into disability, lifestyle risks, and chronic conditions. Disability is a subcomponent of absenteeism. Typically, disability occurs when employees are away from the workforce due to health reasons and cannot do their jobs. For an absence to be classified as a disability, typically it must be an absence of 3 or more consecutive days. Disability results in the loss of the employee's contribution to the workforce.

Lifestyle risks refer to the behavioral choices made by the employee that ultimately result in absenteeism or presenteeism. Various behavioral choices affecting personal health can result in the employee missing work time, the employee not getting work completed on time, or the complete loss of the employee from the workforce. Personal lifestyle choices account for a portion of the total absenteeism and presenteeism experienced by the employee.

Chronic conditions such as heart disease, diabetes, stroke, and cancer can also lead to presenteeism and absenteeism among the workforce. In 2003, 18 million Americans between the ages of 19 and 64 y were not working due to a chronic disease, health reason, or disability (2).

Figure 14.1 depicts a combination of productivity influences and determinants of health. This chart of productivity influences reveals the factors related to personal performance (5). Note that health-related productivity loss does not totally explain productivity loss. Furthermore, there is a portion of the variance in productivity that is not explained. The HPM model mainly attempts to address the health-related productivity factors. However, expansion of the model within other segments of the organization could start to affect other areas that influence productivity.

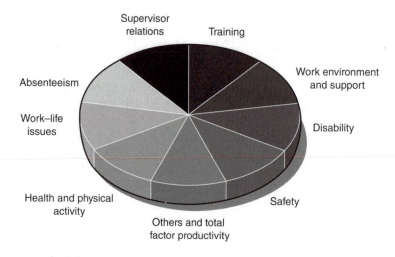

Figure 14.1   Influences on productivity.

In addition to identifying the factors that influence productivity, it is important to identify the factors that influence health. Evans and colleagues, in the book *Why Are Some People Healthy and Others Not? The Determinants of Health of Populations,* attempted to identify such factors, which they termed the *determinants of health* (3). Figure 14.2 depicts the determinants of health as a pie chart. This pie chart provides an integrated view of all identified determinants, but it does not attempt to quantify the individual contribution of each determinant to overall health—that is, the size of each slice does not reflect a determinant's contribution to the size of the overall pie. Regardless, understanding the various components of health and productivity provides guidance for structuring interventions to address the prevalent health issues of the population.

HPM Model

The HPM model is a structured approach for planning, implementing, and evaluating the integrated health management model. The HPM model consists of two parts; the first describes the four verticals mentioned shortly, and the second describes planning components such as individual elements, organizational components, and workplace culture.

HPM Model Part 1

Larry Chapman describes four major stages, or verticals, that make up the first part of the HPM model (6):

1. Needs assessment
2. HPM interventions
3. Intermediate effects
4. Outcomes expected

The needs assessment stage of the HPM model is the starting point for identifying and assessing the needs of individuals within the organization. Employee health and productivity are directly related to the seven subcomponents that fall within the needs assessment vertical. The seven subcomponents are health risks, injury risks, chronic illness, disabilities, absenteeism, medical costs, and presenteeism. The subcomponents are measurable through various metrics designed to evaluate each subcomponent.

The next stage within the schematic represents the interventions, which fall into seven categories: policy changes, education, plan design changes, individual intervention, incentives, administrative changes, and cultural changes. Each is a different intervention within the HPM model and will be briefly discussed. *Policy changes* are initiatives

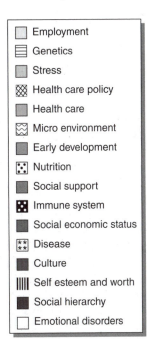

Figure 14.2 Determinants of health.

aimed at modifying organizational policies so that they have a positive effect on the health of employees and families. *Education* involves interventions that inform employees on their benefits and the health improvement program, injury prevention, consumer health, and other health-related topics. *Plan design changes* that enhance and incent the overall program offerings are very effective integration strategies. *Individual interventions* are typically mail, Internet, or telephone interventions and generally have an outreach feature. They are designed to address lifestyle risks and chronic diseases. *Incentives* are used to encourage employee participation and are beginning to be tied to outcomes. *Administrative changes* are designed to affect the application and administration of benefits and policies that affect health. *Cultural changes* include interventions that influence norms, values, beliefs, and attitudes that drive health behaviors.

The third stage of the schematic represents the intermediate effects of HPM. The intermediate effects are positive outcomes that occur after the implementation of the HPM interventions. They are organized into three sections: behavior change, health outcomes, and enhanced productivity. The first section, behavior change, may be observed among employees, family members, and coworkers. Behavior change is an expected outcome from HPM intervention strategies. Behavior changes include directly observable metrics such as quitting smoking or increasing physical activity. However, they may also consist of outcomes such as preventive screening practices, appropriate health care use, improved safety, and compliance with rehabilitation practices that may be less readily observable in the worksite.

The second section of intermediate effects involves health outcomes. Screening tests are typically used to measure health outcomes. Screenings used within the HPM framework include basic biometric tests as well as self-efficacy levels, depression scale scores, and strength and flexibility results.

The third section of intermediate effects, enhanced productivity, refers to self-reported productivity measures such as those obtained through presenteeism assessment instruments as well as objective measures of productivity that are unique to the job or organization. Hence, this section is usually measured through self-report feedback from interviews, health risk appraisals (HRAs), or other survey instruments.

The ultimate stage of the HPM model, outcomes expected, defines the expected macro-outcomes from the HPM initiative and provides the justifica-

tion for the investment in the HPM model. These outcomes are the measurable improvements in both economic and noneconomic dimensions of productivity. Economic gains include savings in health plan and sick leave costs, workers' compensation, and disability costs as well as costs associated with presenteeism. Noneconomic costs or costs that are more difficult to measure involve decision quality, stamina and resilience, interpersonal skills, positive attitude, strength and flexibility, company loyalty, morale, recruitment, retention, turnover, and overall employee. Figure 14.3 depicts this set of interrelated set of needs, interventions, effects, and outcomes.

HPM Model Part 2

Figure 14.4 presents a schematic that serves as the planning framework for the second part of the HPM model (4). Individual elements, organizational components, and workplace culture influence program design to yield desirable and expected outcomes. Each of these important planning components will be discussed in more detail.

Individual elements influence the program and outcomes by targeting health-related behaviors among employees and management. Program design elements may incorporate health enhancement initiatives, injury prevention initiatives, and program requests or may ensure that the interests of the workplace are met through individualized programming. Informal leaders and opinion makers can be used for gathering input as well as can be among the first to participate in the individual-based offerings. The individual elements also include the involvement and input of employees and management as well as the baseline data measures (health care costs, absenteeism, and presenteeism, along with other organizational health indicators).

Organizational components comprise health promotion, disability management, occupational health, regulations, incentives, benefits, needs assessments, and evaluation projects. In short, integrating the functions of the human resource department enhances the overall reach and effectiveness of the programs. This particular aspect of the model sets it apart from traditional approaches.

Workplace culture may be regarded as the most important factor for accomplishing sustained behavior change as well as ensuring the program is integrated and maintained throughout the organization. This component focuses on policy enhancement, workplace and job satisfaction,

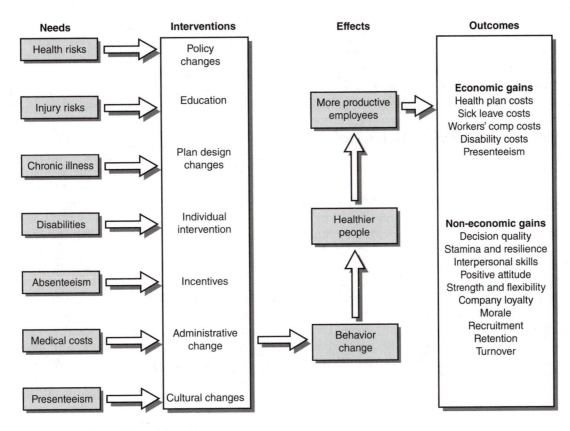

Figure 14.3 Part 1 of the HPM model.

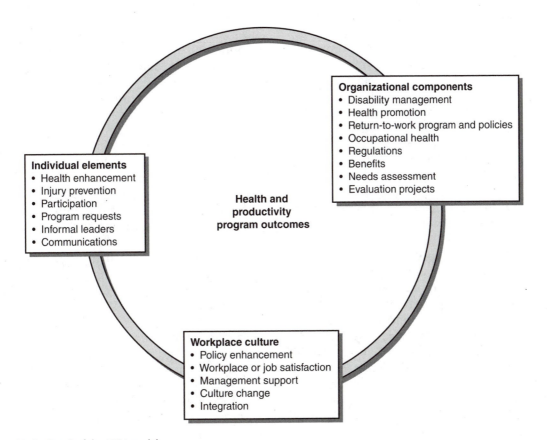

Figure 14.4 Part 2 of the HPM model.

management support, and cross-department cooperation. It is important for the HPM model to become part of the organization's culture instead of acting as a stand-alone initiative. This topic is revisited at the end of this chapter in order to highlight its importance.

What Makes HPM Unique?

Conventional worksite health promotion is quite different from HPM. Typically, conventional programs are not coordinated or fully integrated within and throughout the organization. There are several other distinguishing features within the HPM approach that make this model unique and more effective.

One feature is the inclusion of a wide range of health issues within the worksite interventions. Another key feature focuses on avoiding fragmentation so that all interventions are compatible, linked, and aligned. This refers to intraorganizational programs as well as those provided by vendors. Additionally, HPM is a gauge for measuring the value of human capital. HPM has a strong proactive prevention orientation that helps to distinguish it from traditional practices and interventions. Passive recruitment is typically used in the traditional health promotion model. Within the HPM model, techniques such as strong positive incentives, personalization, tailored programs, and high levels of integration to create a proactive outreach approach are used effectively. By incorporating the three HPM model components of individual elements, organizational components, and workplace culture into the overall approach, there is a greater probability of reaching those employees who typically would not participate.

Another distinguishing factor is strategic alignment of the health and business goals of the organization. Having multiple interventions to address major health problems as well high productivity losses is another unique aspect. Some of the health issues addressed through the HPM model (e.g., migraines and sleep disorders) are not the common ailments or risks addressed by traditional health promotion programs. These conditions have been shown to negatively affect productivity and are often prevalent but unrecognized among populations within many organizations. The HPM model is a strategy designed to enhance personal performance, improve organizational productivity, and achieve positive health outcomes. In summary, the HPM model and its associated tactics evolve a traditional program approach toward a fully integrated health management approach (6).

Implementation of the HPM Model

When an organization decides to implement the HPM model there are at least three major considerations to take into account. First, both an organizational and an individual framework should be chosen. Second, there are three sequential components necessary for the implementation of the HPM model: (1) organizational health indicators, (2) program mix, and (3) evaluation outcomes. The last consideration is to account for current program offerings that exist within the organization. There are three possible organizational scenarios: no program, a program in need of revision, or a partially integrated HPM program already in place (4).

It is suggested that the individual and organizational frameworks be implemented together to ensure that all aspects important to both the employees and the organization are addressed. The individual framework focuses on knowledge, skills, attitudes, motivation, incentives, opportunities, and integration. The HPM model helps to address issues related to duplication of programs and resources. It is also a structured approach for addressing collaboration and ensuring that there is synergy between and among departments as well as internal and external resources. Even though there are multiple departments and vendor offerings included, the HPM program should appear seamless to participants. The organizational framework takes into account policies and regulations and organizational factors such as timing and ties to topics of interest as well as organizational and programmatic administration. Administration involves the feasibility of the program, the current atmosphere within the organization, and the middle management acceptance. Middle management buy-in is crucial to the overall success and tenure of the program.

The steps taken during the implementation process will depend on the program status that exists within the organization. As described previously, there may be no program in place, a program in place that needs revision, or a partial HPM program in place (4). If a program does not currently exist, it is recommended to first identify the organizational and individual health indicators of the organization. Organizational health indicators are the measures used to establish program success for the organization. Lifestyle-related health care costs, absenteeism, productivity, turnover, recruitment, and employee relations are examples of such indicators. If an organization identifies the top three organizational health indicators in descending order of importance, doing so will help guide the overall program offerings and effectiveness.

The individual health indicators are determined by examining health care data as well as aggregate HRA results. The most prevalent health risks within the population, coupled with the conditions mentioned previously that influence productivity, should be considered for programming. The organizational and individual health indicators will provide the rationale for the program offerings and any policy or wide-ranging cultural changes that are implemented as a result of the HPM initiative.

Identifying and establishing organizational and individual health indicators will assist with the strategic planning process. A detailed strategic plan helps ensure that the program stays on track and that the overall initiative does not become a program of the month in which the emphasis constantly shifts and there is no overall direction for the program.

Establishing a committee for review and input of the strategic plan is a recommended feature of the HPM model. The basic premise behind the book *The Wisdom of Crowds* (8) is that if diverse individuals with a common purpose and a framework for making decisions get together to discuss an issue the outcome is always superior to that of any decision made by a single person.

When there is an existing program within the organization and leaders or practitioners want to revise the current program to emulate the HPM model, the following guidelines are suggested. First, revisiting some of the accepted positions and decisions will assist with program evolution. For example, reexamining the organizational health indicators is important. If the organizational health indicators are not known, or if there is confusion concerning their descending order, then this topic should be resolved by senior management and program staff. For example, productivity may become one of the top three organizational health indicators, and therefore adjustments to the program design and options will need to be identified to fit this projected outcome. The program committee should be reviewed and possibly updated or expanded to reflect the revised program direction. Reviewing and revising the program goals, objectives, and strategic plan are also recommended. Once revised, the goals, objectives, and strategic plan should be shared with all stakeholders. The significant changes should be noted and, if approved, the rationale and movement toward the integrated HPM model should be highlighted. These changes will likely require an updated evaluation plan. An advantage to the HPM model is obtaining relative immediate outcomes by including productivity measures (e.g., presenteeism).

Partial HPM programs already encompass components of the HPM model but still require basic steps to be taken to become the fully integrated model. When the revised program has been in place for 12 to 18 mo, ask the question, "Is the program part of the culture?" This question helps the organization examine the program to determine if it is just a supplement to the previous organizational milieu or if the organization has truly adopted a new health-enhancing environment. Table 14.1 outlines each of the organizational scenarios and suggested implementation approaches.

Table 14.1 How to Implement the HPM Model

No current program	Current program needing revision	Partial HPM program
Identify health indicators of the organization.	Evaluate the current program.	Identify needed follow-up.
Determine baseline costs.	Revisit past goals.	Make your case.
Identify representative team of employees.	Identify representative team of employees.	Revise the plan.
Complete the strategic planning process.	Complete the strategic planning process.	Execute the HPM model.
Present the proposal.	Present the proposal.	Keep the program going and establish momentum.
Commit resources.	Commit resources.	Ask, "Is the program part of the culture?"
Execute the program.	Execute the program.	
Refine the program based on evaluation and outcomes.	Refine the program based on evaluation and outcomes.	

Based on J. Leutzinger, 2005, *Academy for health and productivity management,* presentation at the Annual IHPM conference, Scottsdale, AZ.

Trends in HPM

The recent emergence and continued evolution of HPM are associated with several trends in the marketplace. Five trends are summarized to conclude this chapter. In addition, a final word about the importance of evaluation is included. First, however, there is a brief discussion on the importance of culture.

Discussing the importance of culture in the early stages of implementation will help with the acceptance of this message. It is advantageous if all employees understand the difference between a one-program-at-a-time approach and a culture of health. If this approach and objective are clearly communicated and actively supported, the employees may decide to take an active part in the organizational efforts to transform the company. Ultimately, the goal is for the program to become a norm within the organization and not just a voluntary option, even though some program components will remain voluntary.

Changing an existing culture is not an easy task. However, employee buy-in, especially from upper and middle management, is necessary for the transformation to take place within the organization. For this change to take place it is necessary to plan, execute, and refine the HPM model to fit within the organization and its existing culture.

It is becoming increasingly evident that organizational culture is extremely important to adequately addressing health improvement in organizations. Once the HPM model is being implemented with an eye on integration, the organizational environment will be vital to the success of the program.

Value-based benefits are fast becoming the latest trend in HPM. The premise behind this trend is that the employee benefits package is viewed as an investment rather than an expense and that effort is taken to ensure that the value is achieved by paying attention to various components within the benefits structure. There are employers reviewing their existing benefits design to determine if appropriate prevention services are included in the package and that barriers such as high co-payments for preventive-oriented medications are reduced or eliminated. Another component is reduced co-payments for pharmaceuticals such as asthma and diabetes drugs that are recommended for practicing prevention and lower-cost treatment.

Another trend being brought about through the HPM model is a renewed focus on community health. Employer groups are acknowledging the value in recognizing and including community health groups within their organizational programming efforts. It is the opinion of many health professionals that for lasting behavior change, the community initiatives need to be coordinated with employer efforts. The community focus is also related to the previously mentioned trend involving culture change.

The classification of multiple risks into a condition called *metabolic syndrome* and the recognition of risks that affect productivity, such as migraines, sleep disorders, chronic fatigue, headaches, and anxiety, are changing the offerings of HPM programs. The focus on other, nontraditional risks as well as the explicit recognition that risks occur simultaneously within an individual will need to be addressed with innovations in the menu of interventions and solutions. This trend is likely to continue as productivity measurement of these conditions is further refined.

The last trend to address is the creation of megavendors within the field of health improvement and HPM. Before this phenomenon, employers moving toward an integrated model attempted to select the best niche vendors from each program offering. Now several vendors are consolidating in an attempt to be the single solution of HPM products and services to employer and community customers. Undoubtedly, some employers may opt to bring together all aspects of the integrated HPM solution under one contract with a single vendor. On the other hand, other employers may continue to look for best-in-class vendors and may contract with an organization for the role of integrating all of those different companies providing programs and services. Either way, employers should consider the most effective means to get the outcomes they want and to achieve those outcomes through a process that generates an exceptional experience for employees. Such a context will prove optimal for all parties.

Evaluation

Evaluation is a key component of the HPM model. Evaluation outcomes verify whether the predicted and expected outcomes occurred. Evaluation also provides a barometer for program acceptance. Lastly, evaluation helps to decide what further adjustments need to be made.

There are three levels of evaluation that apply to the HPM model: process, effect, and outcome. Process evaluation provides feedback on the quality of the program, program acceptance, and implementation issues. The process evaluation component refers to participation and health improvement among employees and can be measured through self-reports such as surveys or interviews with employees after the program has been implemented. Effect evaluation includes changes in behaviors, attitudes, skills, beliefs, and knowledge. It is important that employees begin to alter their view of these factors to reflect the changing culture of the organization. The outcome evaluation helps to determine the effect of the program on organizational health indicators mentioned earlier in this chapter. This level of evaluation will assist in identifying organizational benefits and health status of employees and is important in determining the success of the program.

Conclusion

The basis of HPM is to design a fully integrated and coordinated approach to enhance workplace productivity and to preserve and improve the health of employees. The HPM model outlines the key components needed to implement an effective HPM initiative. HPM should become part of the organization's culture and not just another program offered to those who want to participate. Ultimately, the success of HPM comes down to planning, execution, and refinement.

Chapter Review Questions

1. Define HPM and its key components.
2. List some benefits of an organization using the HPM model.
3. How does the HPM model differ from traditional practices?
4. List some components an organization, under the HPM model, could use to evaluate the program.
5. How could your organization best implement an HPM program within the workplace?

Part

III

Assessing Worker and Organizational Health

Starting with the end in mind is good advice. And when such advice is heeded, making sure that you have guideposts along the way is a good idea as well. However, how can you ensure that information becomes available in a timely manner so as to update and report to key stakeholders on progress made? How can you be sure that necessary programmatic changes are based on data? If you are not able to regularly report on program status, it will be difficult to continue to receive the appropriate support to maintain quality and performance standards and, subsequently, outcomes may suffer. The adage "what gets measured gets done" rings true and may be regarded the central message of Part III.

Part III is all about measurement and evaluation. Chapter 15 provides an overview of how to organize a practice-oriented, realistic, and actionable evaluation plan specific to the worksite setting. The remaining chapters discuss other important

but separate and more focused aspects of assessment, measurement, and evaluation. Chapter 16 presents an in-depth discussion of health assessment tools, their proper use, and suggestions for implementation. Chapter 17 addresses the tools needed to assess the organizational status to act as a supportive environment for health. Productivity assessment tools are considered in Chapter 18. Chapter 19 presents an in-depth discussion of appropriate methodology and various considerations related to the calculation of economic return of health and productivity management programs. The use of claims data to support program strategy and planning is described in Chapter 20. Whereas other chapters throughout the book reiterate the importance of integrated approaches to assessment and evaluation, Part III is focused on data-driven preparation for rollout, ongoing evaluation of program implementation, and overall evidence of success for worksite health programs.

15

Practical Program Evaluation
Ensuring Findings Are Used for Program Improvement

Thomas J. Chapel, MA, MBA, and Jason E. Lang, MPH, MS

Although program evaluation is widely recognized as a core function of public health, it might not be as widely practiced by businesses with respect to their workplace health programs. Differences in the definition of what constitutes an optimal evaluation practice often lead to evaluations that are time consuming and expensive and, most importantly, produce findings not employed for program improvement. This chapter offers simple, systematic guidelines to maximize the likelihood that the time and effort to evaluate will result in program improvements that are likely to achieve intended outcomes. Based on the CDC's Framework for Program Evaluation in Public Health (2), the central premise of this chapter is utilization-focused evaluation—that no evaluation is optimal unless its results are used and that matching evaluation design with the purpose and the potential user in each evaluation situation is the way to ensure use. This chapter emphasizes how the early steps of the CDC's framework build conceptual clarity about the program that is needed to choose the right evaluation focus, and it uses two crosscutting workplace health promotion examples to illustrate these points.

Multiple reasons, both internal and external, provide the impetus for evaluation. Although external mandates are effective in motivating organizations to evaluate, use of findings is enhanced when programs are moved by the internally perceived need or desire to evaluate, even when not required. For U.S. organizations sponsoring workplace health promotion, OSHA guidelines on tracking injuries at worksites or union or stakeholder requirements for proven interventions are examples of external mandates that might compel an organization to evaluate. However, equally motivating might be internal concerns regarding increases in health risks among the workforce, which in time are likely to have a negative effect on health status and health costs at the workplace, aging of the workforce, and a competitive environment that demands increased productivity. Often, they may also create a general skepticism about the efficacy or ROI of health promotion efforts on the part of unions, management, and stockholders. Strong program evaluation can be of value in

- helping prioritize activities and guide resource allocation,
- informing program funders whether their dollars are being used effectively,
- informing stakeholders of the program's value (in either economic or health terms), and
- providing information that can be useful in the design or improvement of similar programs.

The findings and conclusions in this report are those of the authors and do not necessarily represent the views of the Centers for Disease Control and Prevention.

As will be discussed, different evaluation designs can provide this value. Although certain evaluation designs resemble research designs, and indeed research studies might be necessary to answer with rigor why programs are working or not working, program evaluation and research differ in intent and orientation.* Research aspires to generalizable knowledge, whereas program evaluation is case specific, generating information about an identifiable problem, population, and beneficiary, and has a specific use or user of evaluation findings in mind. Perhaps an old adage says it best: Research seeks to prove, whereas evaluation seeks to improve.

CDC's Framework for Program Evaluation in Public Health

In formulating its framework, the CDC intentionally employed broad definitions of both evaluation—examination of merit, worth, or significance of an object (4)—and program—any set of intentional, interrelated activities that aim for a common outcome (2). The aim was to ensure that practitioners at all levels saw program evaluation as something they needed and had the capacity to undertake.

The six steps that make up the framework are (see figure 15.1) engage stakeholders, describe the program, focus the evaluation and its design, gather credible evidence, justify conclusions, and use findings and share lessons learned. The underlying logic of these steps is as follows: (1) No evaluation is optimal just because the methods and analysis are valid and reliable—rather, it is optimal because the results are used. (2) Having the evaluation used means paying attention to creating a market before creating the product or the evaluation itself. (3) The evaluation focus is central to developing this market by ensuring that the evaluation includes questions that are relevant, salient, and useful to those who will use the findings. (4) Determining the right focus requires identifying key stakeholders (others who care about program efforts and success) and understanding the program in all its complexity.

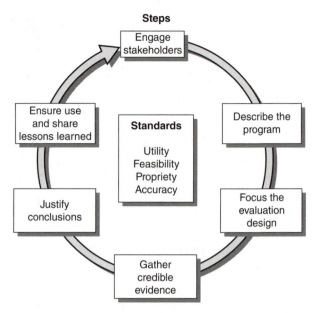

Figure 15.1 CDC evaluation framework.

At the center of the circle graphic in figure 15.1 are four evaluation standards (3). These help guide practitioners at any of the six steps by prompting them to ask the following questions: (1) Who will use the information and how will they use it (utility)? (2) How many resources are available for evaluation (feasibility)? (3) What must be done to be correct and ethical (propriety)? (4) What approaches will produce the most accurate results, given the intended use (accuracy)?

This chapter is intended to provide those who implement or evaluate workplace health promotion programs with general guidance on why and how to do program evaluation, practical approaches to steps in the CDC framework, and application of the steps to two hypothetical examples of workplace health promotion.

Applying the Framework Steps

The two hypothetical case studies provided will be referred to throughout the discussion of the individual steps in the framework. A description of each step and the important components within each step are discussed next.

---

*For elaboration of the contrast of evaluation and research, see U.S. Department of Health and Human Services. *Introduction to program evaluation for comprehensive tobacco control programs*. Atlanta, GA: U.S. Department of Health and Human Services, Centers for Disease Control and Prevention, Office on Smoking and Health; 2001:7-8.

Two Hypothetical Case Studies Illustrating Program Evaluation Steps

Whereas outlining and describing the individual steps of the evaluation framework is important in itself, bringing it to life through the use of case study examples will provide clear examples of how such a framework may be applied in practice. The two case study examples provided here are hypothetical cases but they illustrate how and through what process the framework can support and enhance overall program implementation.

Case 1

Company A is a small, privately owned, office-based professional and business services employer with its own office space; a young, nonunionized, white-collar workforce; and a small management team. The company has limited financial resources and space to dedicate to employee health promotion activities but is concerned with certain emerging problems in which health is a factor (e.g., high turnover rates and absenteeism rates that are higher than normal). The workforce's single most pressing health concern is the high rate of tobacco use, which management fears is related to the absenteeism rate and will lead to other health problems and future high health care costs. To address this problem, the company formed an employee-led health promotion committee, which conducted a survey to determine staff interest in and barriers to health promotion activities related to tobacco use. On the basis of the survey results, the committee and management decided to implement the following interrelated interventions: (1) creating a tobacco-free policy that prohibits tobacco use in the office building, (2) providing training for employees and managers on the new tobacco-free policy, (3) holding a seminar series inviting local health experts to talk about tobacco concerns, (4) providing support for those who want to quit (e.g., providing referrals to cessation programs or quit lines and self-help materials and allowing employees to organize a support group), (5) creating competitions with low-cost incentive prizes (e.g., a stop smoking challenge with management). A desktop tracking system will be implemented to allow employees to record progress and encourage each other and to help the committee monitor the competitions. The management team has agreed to participate actively in these activities, enforce the policy, and implement environmental changes, including posting signs on the tobacco-free policy and health effects of smoking and removing ashtrays and tobacco vending machines from the building. The company hopes that these interventions will lead to less smoking by staff members and thus create a healthier workplace for all that demonstrates that the company cares about the health of its employees. The company expects this action to lead to reductions in absenteeism and employee turnover and to increased productivity in the short term and to reduced health care costs and insurance costs, among other benefits, in the long term.

Case 2

Company B is a large, publicly traded manufacturing company with multiple U.S. worksites. Its blue-collar, unionized workforce is aging, and according to the results of a health risk assessment, its workforce has overweight and obesity and physical inactivity rates that are higher than average. The poor health habits are starting to manifest as an increased incidence of heart disease, diabetes, and cancer. The company self-insures for health benefits and has invested considerable resources in health promotion, including on-site occupational clinics and disease management programs. Previous health promotion activities have met with mixed success, in part because standard approaches do not account for the diversity and culture of the local sites. In addition, lack of trust exists between labor and management and between staff members at headquarters and staff members at remote sites, who seek local autonomy in decisions related to employee health. The company wants to pilot a new approach that

(continued) ▶

> ▶ Two Hypothetical Case Studies Illustrating Program Evaluation Steps *(continued)*
>
> combines company-wide goals and system and policy changes with local flexibility in developing programs to meet the company-wide goal. It has chosen overweight and obesity as the focus of the pilot effort. The company-wide goal is to double the number of employees who are at a healthy weight within 2 y. Company-wide policy changes include a healthy foods policy for employer-sponsored meetings, vending machines, and cafeterias. In addition, site progress on company-wide performance goals will be part of the site managers' performance plans. Employee benefits already include full coverage for recommended clinical preventive services; the company will actively promote use of these benefits, in part with on-site screening days at each site. To assist sites, the company will compile an inventory of effective physical activity and nutrition approaches and provide seed money to each site to implement an inclusive planning process for selecting site-specific approaches to meeting the company-wide goal of reducing overweight and obesity. The company expects that reduced obesity rates will help contain health care costs by slowing the incidence and progression of chronic illnesses being experienced by the workforce and the retirees whose health benefits the company continues to fund. The company also hopes that the local autonomy and inclusive planning approaches will increase trust between management and labor and that workforce health programs will help the company be regarded as an employer of choice in a competitive marketplace.

Step 1: Engage Stakeholders

Rarely are evaluators or even program practitioners able, independently, to ensure that evaluation findings are put to use. Programs that want use of evaluation findings should be committed to engaging stakeholders (i.e., the persons and organizations with an interest in the program and its performance). Stakeholders for the typical health promotion program include (1) those who are involved in program operations (e.g., wellness committees or wellness managers), (2) those who are affected by the program (e.g., employees), and (3) those who will use evaluation results (e.g., people in leadership and management, who might also be part of the first two groups). Embedded in these categories are a program's most important stakeholders—those whose support and involvement are needed to enhance the credibility of the evaluation or its results, to implement the evaluation's recommendations for program improvement, or to continue authorization or funding of the program.

Keeping these stakeholders engaged requires identifying the activities and outcomes they believe must be achieved to judge the program a success and being attentive to the values and preferences they bring to data collection, analysis, and interpretation. Engaging them at the outset of the evaluation helps ensure that program descriptions, evaluation questions, data collection and analyses, and reports are relevant, responsive, and likely to be used.

In the two workplace cases, the chief authorizers or funders are the members of senior management, who hope that workplace health promotion efforts will lead to certain ambitious or long-term outcomes—reduction in health problems, health care costs, and turnover and increases in productivity and even profitability.* In case 1, implementers include not only the management team members but also the employees themselves, who, desirably, will participate in activities and adopt the recommended behaviors. However, employees might have multiple motivations to participate instead. Employees might not necessarily be motivated to participate by management's desire for increased healthy behaviors; yet, they may have reasons of their own (e.g., the prospect of time off or building relationships with colleagues). Effectively engaging employees will help identify these motivations and thus enhance

---

*The fact that stakeholders want those outcomes does not mean that the program is able to achieve them. This conflict will be discussed in more detail in a later section on setting an evaluation focus.

the chances of program success. In case 2, key implementers include the company's multiple sites; members of these sites are being granted autonomy to customize approaches, and they desire to perform well on company goals. Unions are also an implementation stakeholder because they lend necessary credibility to the effort, advocate for improvements in employee health and safety at the workplace, and work to protect workers' interests (e.g., privacy).

Knowing stakeholder needs and preferences at the outset can provide information for the design and implementation of the intervention as well as its evaluation. Whether it occurs before or after the intervention is underway, stakeholder engagement identifies the program activities and outcomes that must be included in the evaluation to keep stakeholders involved and supportive. Multiple stakeholders might be identified, but only a limited number might be essential for credibility, implementation, or continuation of the program. Determining the needs, opinions, and preferences of the limited number of stakeholders need not require extensive or scientifically rigorous data collection; often key informant interviews or superficial data collection can suffice. Finally, stakeholders might choose to be involved in only selected steps of the evaluation.

Step 2: Describe the Program

To ensure that evaluations are focused on what matters most, a need exists to understand the whole program, including the following:

- Need: The problem on which the program hopes to make an effect
- Target or priority groups: Those persons or organizations who must change in a way that achieves the intended effect
- Outcomes: The ways in which these target groups need to change
- Activities: The actions of the program and its staff that are intended to achieve the outcomes
- Inputs: The resources necessary to mount the activities effectively (e.g., staffing, funds, and legal authority)
- Context: The trends and forces in the larger environment that might affect program success or failure (e.g., politics, economics, social and demographic factors, and technology)

When programs are complex or multifaceted, a visual depiction of the program—often called a *logic model*—can make program components and their interrelationships clearer. To construct logic models, evaluators or program staff members start by listing program activities—actions taken by the program and its staff—and intended outcomes—ways in which persons or organizations other than the program will change. Next, any logical sequencing within the list of activities or outcomes (early or short-term, intermediate or midterm, or later or long-term) is depicted (i.e., knowledge, attitude, and belief change would be presumed to precede behavior change; developing materials would be presumed to precede dissemination of materials). Finally, the inputs or resources necessary to implement the activities are added. What results is a four- to six-column table, which might be the necessary level of clarity. Often, simple logic model tables are formatted as flowcharts by adding arrows to connect activities to their intended outcomes or to connect early outcomes to later outcomes. The following are high-level logic models for case 1 and case 2 (figures 15.2 and 15.3).

The activities and outcomes in the two logic models are drawn directly from the narrative, but the inputs are generated by asking what resources, typically from others, are necessary to implement the activities successfully. Staff and budget are obvious resources, but others also exist. In case 1, activities rest on a foundation of the following inputs: workforce survey results, recommendations from the staff committee to management, and a network of local experts and the services they offer. Activities in case 2 draw on inputs from health risk assessment data, information and access to a network of occupational clinics, the company's existing benefits program, and an understanding of the site-specific culture and facilities.

Two final components complete our program description, even though they are not always depicted in the logic model. Outputs are the direct products or services that are expected to result from program activities. They serve as documentary evidence that program activities have been implemented as intended. In case 1, selected outputs might include the number of seminars held or the number of referrals made to community cessation programs. Case 2 outputs might include the number of advertisements or announcements related to on-site screening days or the number of manager performance reviews

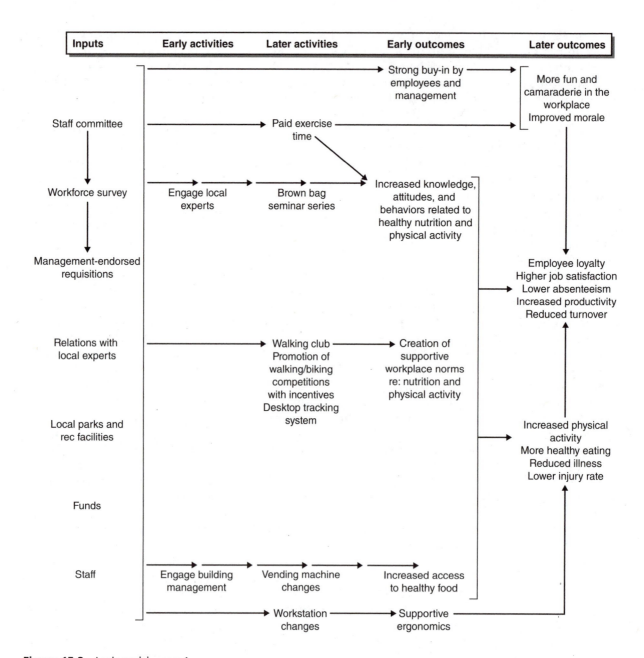

Figure 15.2 Logic model—case 1.

that include performance goals. Note that outputs do not prove that the activities worked as intended (i.e., that the knowledge of seminar participants increased, that the clients fulfilled their referrals, or that the employees showed up for screening days)—they prove only that the activities were implemented as intended.

Moderators, the other final component of our program description, are outside trends and factors (e.g., political, economic, social, or technological factors) that might influence program implementation or success. In our two cases, workforce demographics are an important social moderator. That the workforce is aging in case 2 and young in case 1 predisposes both companies toward certain outcomes and activities. The local job market is an economic moderator that interacts with the demographics in case 1; even the best-intended efforts to increase worker loyalty might be undone in a competitive labor market for young, mobile workers. Political moderators predominate in case 2. The culture of autonomy

| Inputs | Early activities | Later activities | Early outcomes | Later outcomes |

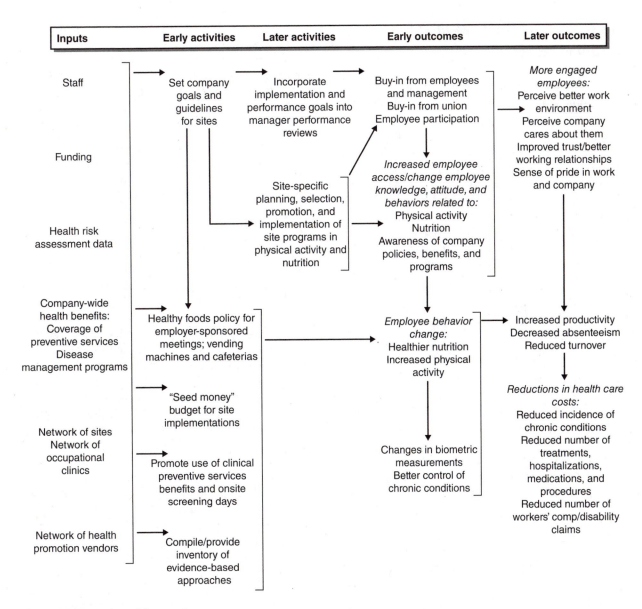

Figure 15.3 Logic model—case 2.

at remote worksites moderates the way in which company directives will be implemented; indeed, this culture was the motivation for the current approach. Moreover, although the company is giving seed money to each site, differences in infrastructure and resources at each site will moderate the nature of the approach.

As noted previously, the early framework steps yield benefits for program planning even before the program evaluation is implemented or even

if the program evaluation is never implemented. Clarifying program activities and outcomes, identifying potential flaws in the program logic, and acknowledging and resolving differences among stakeholders about the program outcomes of most importance are key benefits in their own right. Such benefits are called *process use* and are the payoffs from the use of an evaluation process as opposed to the payoffs from the use of evaluation findings.*

---

*Citation, the benefit of process use is further described in the nondestructive evaluation (NDE) literature. NDE is the technique of inspecting something without destroying or damaging it.

Step 3: Focus the Evaluation and Its Design

Any component of the program—inputs, activities or outputs, outcomes, or moderators—can be part of an evaluation. Step 3 narrows the evaluation's scope to those program components that need to be part of a specific evaluation at a specific point. This focus will reflect the purpose, use, and user of evaluation findings and, as such, will evolve over time. By being attentive to this evolution, the focus step ensures that each evaluation product has a ready market for its findings. A specific evaluation might include the following four types of questions, although a single evaluation rarely includes all four types:

- Implementation or process: Have the activities been put in place as intended?
- Effectiveness or outcome: Have the outcomes occurred as expected?
- Efficiency or cost-effectiveness: What level of resources was necessary to mount the activities and outputs? What level of resources was necessary to produce a change in any or all outcomes?
- Causal attribution: Were any observed changes in outcomes caused by the program and its efforts as opposed to other factors?

To determine which program components need to be part of the ongoing evaluation focus and which types of questions are most important, two of the four evaluation standards—utility and feasibility—come into play. As noted, utility asks the following questions:

- What is the purpose of the evaluation?
- Who will use the evaluation results?
- How will they use the evaluation results?
- What key stakeholder needs identified in step 1 must be addressed to keep the stakeholders engaged?

The answers to these questions help identify the program components that must be part of the evaluation if it is to be relevant (i.e., useful) to the intended users of the findings. By contrast, the feasibility standard acts as a reality check. It questions whether an evaluation that focuses on these program components is feasible at this point in time, given the following:

- Stage of development of the program: Is it too early in the program's life to expect the specific program component of interest to have occurred?
- Program intensity: Even at maturity, is the program intense or strong enough to produce the program outcomes of interest?
- Resources for measurement: Do easy-to-access data exist on the activities or outcomes of interest, or do adequate resources exist to collect these data?

The responses to these questions might affirm the initial evaluation focus or identify an inconsistency between what the users need or desire and what is feasible.

Both case 1 and case 2 involve relatively new efforts; the first intended users of evaluation findings might be program implementers who want to assess the quality of implementation—a classic process evaluation. In case 1, process evaluation questions might assess if the vending machine changes occurred, if seminars were held, or if referrals to outside agencies were made. Process evaluation in case 2 might assess if sites used their autonomy to develop customized health promotion programs (i.e., if program plans were developed), if screening days occurred as intended, or if company goals were translated into managers' performance plans. Process evaluation findings are important in helping to identify needed adjustments early in the program's life. They also help distinguish an optimal program from an inadequate program.

Both case 1 and case 2 have senior managers as key intended users. They want information on outcomes to determine program effectiveness, and in both cases their interest is in a selected ambitious long-term outcome. In case 1, the emphasis is on the adoption of healthy or safer behaviors (reduced tobacco consumption) by employees and a host of outcomes related to work life (e.g., increased morale and job satisfaction and reduced turnover). Senior management in case 2 wants these same outcomes but, because of the company's aging workforce, is more acutely interested in longer term outcomes (e.g., control of health care costs).

A good evaluation focus should balance utility and feasibility. Senior financial managers might want to see reduction in the company's health care costs or improved profitability, but both the stage of development of the program and the program intensity can cause difficulty for a health promotion program alone to generate those outcomes. Distinguishing attribution from contribution is sometimes helpful at this point. When short-term intended outcomes occur, attributing them to the program activities is plausible. By contrast, as we move out the logic model to intermediate- and long-term outcomes, often the program efforts contribute, along with the efforts of other programs, to the achievement of outcomes. Identifying early any disconnection between what senior managers want and what can plausibly be attributed to the program allows us to use the logic model to engage these managers. That discussion might identify other outcomes that are more feasible to accomplish and yet would still be considered critical milestones and markers. In contrast, everyone might conclude that the program cannot produce the outcomes of interest, and the program might be changed or refocused.

A final task in the evaluation focus step is to identify the appropriate evaluation design. Usually, evaluations employ one or more of the following three designs:

- **Experimental designs** use random assignment to compare the outcome of one or more groups that received an intervention with the outcome of an equivalent group or groups that did not receive the intervention. This design allows you to attribute change in outcomes to your program.

- **Quasi-experimental designs** make comparisons between nonequivalent groups and do not involve random assignment to intervention and control groups. Documenting that the intervention and comparison groups are similar on key factors such as population demographics and related current or historical events is important.

- **Observational designs** are common in program evaluation, including time-series analyses, cross-sectional surveys, and case studies.

The details of these designs are discussed elsewhere (1). The emphasis of this chapter is on presenting the options and the factors that enter into selecting an appropriate one. Choosing the best design for a specific evaluation—as with all aspects of evaluation focus—balances utility and feasibility. What is the purpose or use and who is the user of the evaluation? What amount of time, resources, and expertise can be brought to bear? In both case studies, proof is requested that progress on a long-term outcome is the result of the program. However, the rigor required to find that proof is likely to be substantially lower in case 1, since it involves a small company in which a limited number of other health promotion activities are occurring in the workplace and all parties are known to each other and hence improvements on desired outcomes are more likely to be attributed to the program. Case 2 involves a large, multinational organization in which multiple factors besides the health promotion effort might influence the distal outcomes. Senior managers in case 2 are likely to demand rigorous proof of success if the program is to continue. Also, because the company in case 2 grants its remote sites autonomy in selecting their efforts, senior management is likely to want rigorous documentation of best practices. Meeting both needs of senior management in case 2 may require experimental or quasi-experimental designs. As with the selection of the evaluation focus, such designs might or might not be feasible for program sites, and the design can be adjusted accordingly.

Although quasi-experimental and experimental designs might make the most sense for case 2, they are not always the most appropriate choice, even when feasible. As the WHO has noted, the use of randomized control trials to evaluate health promotion initiatives is, in most cases, inappropriate, misleading, and unnecessarily expensive (5).

Steps 4 and 5: Gather Credible Evidence and Justify Conclusions

After the evaluation focus, questions, and design have been chosen, the program evaluation proceeds as with any data collection effort: Identify indicators and data sources, collect and analyze the data, and issue the results in one or more reporting formats. The premise of utilization-focused evaluation is that clarity gained in steps 1 through 3 makes selection and implementation of data collection and analysis easier and ensures that findings will be used.

Indicators convert the components of programs—often expressed in global or abstract terms—into specific, measurable statements. Table 15.1 displays selected indicators for components from the logic model for case 1.

Outcome indicators such as those in table 15.1 make outcomes clearer and help guide selection of data collection methods and content of data collection instruments. In the same way, process indicators for activities in the logic model

Table 15.1 Indicators for Selected Program Outcomes—Case 1

Program intended outcome	Indicator
Enforcement of tobacco-free policy	Number of compliance checks conducted, number of responses to complaints regarding noncompliance, number of warnings or citations given
Strong buy-in from employees and management	Percentage of employees and management indicating support for creating and actively enforcing tobacco-free policy
Increased knowledge and supportive beliefs related to tobacco use and tobacco-free policy	Percentage of staff who think secondhand smoke is harmful and who are willing to ask someone not to smoke in their presence Percentage of smokers who think exposing others to secondhand smoke is unacceptable or who are aware of local cessation services
Increased use of community-based cessation and support services	Increase in number of people calling quit line, percentage of smokers using a cessation program, percentage of smokers who follow up on referrals
Creation of supportive norms regarding no tobacco use	Percentage of staff indicating support for smoking bans in work and public places Percentage of staff adopting no-smoking norms in homes and personal vehicles
Compliance with tobacco-free policy	Percentage of staff who indicate personal compliance with policy Percentage of staff who indicate perceived compliance by others Reductions in warnings or citations given and infractions reported
Reduced tobacco consumption	Percentage of staff smokers who report reduction in average number of cigarettes smoked per day Percentage of staff smokers who report sustained abstinence (successful attempts at quitting)
Increased productivity	Reduced number of days absent Fewer smoking breaks taken by staff Percentage of staff who indicate productivity increases
Reduced exposure to secondhand smoke	Reduction in percentage of staff reporting exposure to secondhand smoke in workplace
Reduced tobacco-related health problems	Reduced number of hospitalizations for selected tobacco-related conditions Reduced average dollars spent on health care for smokers Reduced number of days absent

state more clearly what constitutes optimal or strong implementation of the activities—not just making vending machine changes but making the right or best changes and not just implementing customized site programs but implementing strong or appropriate site programs.* For case 1, useful process indicators might include the complete removal of all tobacco products from vending machines in the building, the number or percentage of heavy smokers who attend the seminars on tobacco cessation, or the number of referrals made to community cessation services or tobacco quit lines. For case 2, indicators of strong customized site programs might be the number of site programs that have an inclusive or a participatory decision-making process, are actively marketed, are based on documented employee health problems at the site, and are aligned with the company's health goals. Again, indicators translate an abstract idea into a measurable, tangible statement. Final points in writing indicators include the following:

*If the program description included outputs, it is likely that many of them can serve as process indicators.

- An activity or outcome can have more than one indicator.
- Indicators should be clear and specific in terms of what they will measure.
- Indicators should measure an important dimension of the activity or outcome.

Programs might be able to draw on indicators developed by others for other purposes (3). For example, if a previously evaluated health promotion program is being implemented, perhaps the original developers provided inventories of indicators that were pretested for relevance and accuracy and specified the best data sources for collecting them. When different programs are using the same indicators, comparing performance across programs or summarizing national performance becomes possible. Programs can have existing information sources that are useful for indicator development. The worker survey in case 1 identified initial interests and barriers related to health promotion activities; these might serve as outcome indicators to monitor throughout the program. In case 2, the periodic health risk assessment offers a range of potential indicators of risk behavior outcomes, and occupational health clinic data, in aggregate form, might include indicators for injury or illness rates or selective biometric markers.

In choosing data collection methods and sources for indicators, programs might be able to draw on existing data sources—secondary data collection—or might need to collect their own data—primary data collection. For workplace health promotion programs such as those in case 1 and case 2, OSHA injury reports, time and attendance records, health risk assessment results, clinic records, or claims data are potential sources of secondary data.

The most common primary data collection methods fall into the following broad categories:

- Surveys, including personal interviews, telephone interviews, or instruments completed in person or received through the mail or e-mail
- Group discussions or focus groups
- Observation
- Document review, such as review of medical records, diaries, logs, minutes of meetings, time and attendance records, participant registries, and so forth

Certain methods yield qualitative data (e.g., employee attitudes or needs), and others yield quantitative data (e.g., absenteeism or biometrics). If the question involves an abstract concept or one where measurement is insufficient, using multiple methods is often helpful. The four evaluation standards provide a checklist for choosing the best data collection sources and methods from among the options.

- Utility: Who will use these data? Will certain methods make the data more credible with skeptics or key users? For example, senior leadership might be most interested in the program's economic results, human resources might be most interested in how to market the program to employees, and employees might be most interested in improvements in their own health. Do you seek a point-in-time determination of a behavior, seek to examine the range and variety of experiences, or seek to tell an in-depth story?
- Feasibility: What resources are available for data collection? How long until the results are needed? How often do you need to collect the data? Are there staff members who are trained in the data collection method or do you need to hire an outside consultant?
- Propriety: Given the characteristics of the respondents, will concerns such as literacy or spoken language make certain methods preferable to others? Will selected methods be observed as intrusive by participants? Are there concerns of confidentiality or safety of the respondent in seeking answers to questions?
- Accuracy: What is the nature of the question? Is it about a behavior that is observable? If not, will respondents respond honestly? Is the answer something the respondent is likely to know?

Our two cases offer multiple options and complexities. Both organizations already collect time and attendance data, turnover data, and so forth. In case 1, a worker preference survey and activity logs are also being used through a desktop tracking system, and in case 2, claims records and health risk assessments exist that might serve as data sources. Chief among the complexities are data questions related to healthy and risky behaviors that can lead to inaccuracies in self-reports if workers think they might be punished if they do not exercise or eat wholesome foods. In case 2, this concern is exacerbated by indications that a general lack of trust exists between management and workers. In case 1, workers might distort self-reports to win competitions. In neither case would we be likely to abandon the indicator; rather, these complexities remind us that self-reported surveys might need to be corroborated by other verifiable sources. For example, compliance with the tobacco cessation policy is measured through self-report by smokers but also through self-report by other employees. Self-reported use of community cessation services is validated by follow-up measures to ensure that referrals were fulfilled. Reported decreases in tobacco consumption might need to be validated by periodic urine screening.

Step 5 is called *justifying conclusions* and not *analyzing data* to emphasize that the evidence does not stand on its own but is judged and interpreted through the prism of (potentially different) values that each stakeholder brings to the evaluation. Fortunately, the identification of any significant differences in values and standards was a core part of step 1, and as a result the evaluation design should already reflect the stakeholders' priority outcomes and preferences for credible data collection. In this step, those values and priorities are used to interpret the evidence and judge the success of the program.

In case 2, for example, whereas all parties might agree that a 50% increase in employees routinely participating in physical activity is a significant achievement, supervisors might resent the time taken off from work to exercise unless the physical activity has resulted, as promised, in more productivity or higher morale. As noted previously, senior financial managers in case 2 should be persuaded that such increases are worthwhile even if in the short term they do not reduce company health care costs.

Step 6: Ensure Use and Share Lessons Learned

Because the evaluation has been based on the six steps of the CDC evaluation framework, the majority of the seeds for ensuring use were sown earlier and are ready for harvest at this step. Key actions in step 6 that ensure use are obvious and include the following:

- Recommendations
- Preparation: Giving early warning about themes and results to key evaluation audiences to prevent blindsiding them
- Feedback: Allowing for review and response to early versions of results to encourage buy-in and utility and to get a better sense of best format and emphasis
- Follow-up
- Dissemination: Sharing the results and the lessons learned from evaluation

Of these actions, dissemination has been most enhanced by the work already accomplished in earlier steps. Because the key users of the evaluation findings and their purposes and needs have already been identified, as have the key stakeholders who need to be engaged to implement program improvements, the market for the evaluation product is known. Hence, the dissemination decisions are simple ones of working from audience to emphasis and from audience to format. Asking the stakeholders what messages and delivery method would be of most value to them is important, although this should be part of the stakeholder engagement in step 1.

In both case 1 and case 2, senior leadership might be interested in receiving information such as such productivity and costs in a relatively brief and unobtrusive way (e.g., bulleted information or routine faxes or e-mails). Senior managers might also be interested in receiving feedback in a consolidated risk profile format through graphs or charts. The union might want more details to ensure equity across positions and sites, and employees might want to see information on their own health status or on the policy changes made as evidence that management has met its commitments.

Conclusion

The CDC evaluation framework offers simple guidance that is not intended to make program evaluation more onerous or time consuming. Rather, the intent is to offer simple, systematic insights that ensure that the time and energy spent on program evaluation are devoted to the part of the program that matters most and will result in the use of evaluation findings to make program improvements.

Chapter Review Questions

1. Describe some internal and external factors that might motivate evaluation for a workplace program. How might the motivating factors influence the content and design of the evaluation?

2. Describe some potential moderators (political, economic, social, and technological) that might act as barriers to success in the two cases provided in this chapter.

3. How do the evaluation standards of utility and feasibility inform a decision regarding which evaluation questions to ask and which design to use?

4. What would you, as a program developer or evaluator, do when an important stakeholder expects the program to make progress on long-term outcomes that are clearly infeasible for the program to achieve?

5. Describe the differences between attribution and contribution. Discuss examples from the cases provided in this chapter.

◀ **16** ▶

The Assessment of Health and Risk

Tools, Specific Uses, and Implementation Processes

Edward M. Framer, PhD, and Yosuke Chikamoto, PhD

You are a health promotion professional with a degree or even advanced degrees in health promotion, dietetics, psychology, exercise physiology, health education, human resource management, nursing, or any other of a half-dozen specialties including medicine. (That's right: No single specialty owns health promotion and disease prevention.) You now work for a corporation. There are anywhere from hundreds to hundreds of thousands of employees. You are part of the team or perhaps the only individual charged with developing a comprehensive, population-based health management process and procedures for your organization. And senior management, not to mention your direct supervisor, wants you to be able to project and then demonstrate the ability to improve the health of the workforce. They also want you to demonstrate ROI and prefer to see it within 2 y.

Are your feeling overwhelmed yet? Where do you start? Do you know exactly where you are taking your organization? Are you aware of the health strengths and the burdens of illness that characterize the organization's employees and dependents? Do you know what programs are needed and who within the population needs them? Perhaps you do, but the likelihood is that no matter your expertise, if the company hasn't already run an extensive claims analysis or health assessment, you don't. While this chapter won't support you with the information to accomplish everything, it will present or review, depending on your previous experience, much of the basic information you need to understand, plan, and deliver a functional health risk and health status survey.

Assessment of Health Risk and Health Status

The assessment of health risk and health status is nothing new. In one way or another it goes back to antiquity. For example, what do the bumps on your head mean (phrenology)? What do the lines on your hand have to say about your personality, social behaviors, or future health, including the length of your life (palmistry)? Phrenology and palmistry are a bit further back than the authors will take you. However, current intent and purposes are not all that different. Bumps on the head are out and reading your lifeline is out, but family history, personal health history, lifestyle behaviors, medical biometric measurements, and the ability to perform independent activities of daily living (IADLs) are in.

But why use measurement or assessment tools at all? Why palmistry in the past and health risk appraisal or health risk assessment now? Why care at all? The answer is simple. People want to know what the future holds. In a world that often appears random and capricious, people want an edge on understanding what's likely to come their way in the future. That is exactly what palmistry or phrenology appeared to do in the past, however poorly. It is also what scientists and clinicians try to do now with health risk appraisal, health risk assessment, health status assessment, and biometric measurements. We are trying to clarify likely connections between lifestyle behaviors, including the decision to use appropriate preventive services, and current or future illness, health, and mortality.

When contemplating where to start, and specifically where to start selecting your assessments, it is important to review typical assessment tools and terms that you are likely to encounter. First, we will briefly define the types of measurement instruments that are currently available—the ones likely to be considered for many comprehensive, population-based health management or health promotion intervention projects. Second, we will consider why and how they might be employed in health promotion, disease prevention, or wellness programs. Third and last will come an examination of the issues involved in installing and operating the health risks and health strengths assessment processes in a contemporary worksite. The term *health assessments* will be used to cover the entire range of instruments, both physical measurements and questionnaires, whose output is used to make one or more statements about current and predicted health or functioning.

Health Risk Appraisals

According to Alexander, health risk appraisal, as originally conceived, is a technique for estimating the odds that a person with certain characteristics will die from selected causes within a given time span (1). The certain characteristics included things such as age, gender, age at onset of menstruation for women, height, weight, total cholesterol, how much alcohol is typically consumed each week, what size car is usually driven, and how far the car is driven per year. The selected causes included death from many types of cancer, heart attack, stroke, motor vehicle accidents, and all causes lumped together into all-cause mortality. Earlier in time, Schoenbach, Wagner, and Berry (11) included other elements in this definition and presented the health risk appraisal as a procedure for using epidemiologic and vital statistics data to provide individuals with projections of their personalized mortality risk and with recommendations for reducing that risk, for the purpose of promoting desirable changes in health behavior. Health risk appraisal calculations are based on the risk of death (mortality estimates) that can result from various health-related behaviors, family history, life experiences, and the presence or absence of certain medical conditions. While these mortality estimations are certainly useful at the population level—for example, are good at predicting how many excess deaths from cancer are likely to occur in a workforce over the next 10 y—they are less useful for communicating health information to individuals with the hope of strongly motivating

healthy behavior change. Strecher and Kreuter (12) summarize it succinctly: "What little research we have found provides only limited, if any, support for behavior change effects resulting from the receipt of health risk appraisal feedback." (p. 75) There is little basis in the behavioral sciences for expecting that communicating these risk-of-death estimates to people will substantially change how the majority will choose to live their lives.

Health risk appraisal was initially developed by Lewis C. Robbins, MD. His goal was to have an educational tool that would assist physicians in communicating prevention information to their patients. In an ironic twist of fate, Dr. Robbins' chosen setting for health risk appraisal—during the patient's visit in a doctor's office—is actually one of the last places where health risk appraisal is regularly used. Health risk appraisal became far more likely to be used as a part of worksite health promotion programs, and health risk appraisals and health risk assessments (discussed next) are also increasingly used by health plans such as HMOs and preferred provider organizations (PPOs). Each environment has its own strengths and issues when it comes to driving high rates of assessment utilization and the delivery of follow-up programming for identified risks.

Health Risk Assessments

Unlike the health risk appraisal, health risk assessments focus less or not at all on multiple statistical risk estimates. Rather, they focus on whether individuals are meeting public health standards or good health recommendations. These standards and recommendations come from government agencies, consensus panels, and nationally and even internationally respected health organizations. See Common Sources for Good Health Standards and Recommendations for a partial listing of sources of good health recommendations. Harris and Fries (8) note, "The term 'health risk appraisal' is itself gradually being less utilized because it connotes a goal of quantitative overall health risk computation rather than triaging personalized interventions, assessing quality, measuring change, and meeting other goals. Newer terms include 'Health Assessment Questionnaire' and 'Health Improvement Questionnaire'. As such, the newer questionnaire instruments are an essential part of the most effective, comprehensive health promotion programs." (p. 15) And these comprehensive programs are generally, although not exclusively, delivered in work-related settings.

Common Sources for Good Health Standards and Recommendations

- American Heart Association (AHA)
- American Cancer Society (ACS)
- American Diabetes Association (ADA)
- American College of Sports Medicine (ACSM)
- American Dental Association (ADA)
- American Dietetic Association (ADA)
- American Public Health Association (APHA)
- American Academy of Family Physicians (AAFP)
- National Institutes of Health (NIH)
  - National Cancer Institute
  - National Eye Institute
  - National Heart, Lung, and Blood Institute (NHLBI)
  - National Cholesterol Education Program (NCEP; current standards are Adult Treatment Panel (ATP)-III)
  - Joint National Committee on Prevention, Detection, Evaluation, and Treatment of High Blood Pressure (within the NHLBI; current standards are The Seventh Report of the Joint National Committee on Prevention, Detection, Evaluation, and Treatment of High Blood Pressure [JNC 7])
  - National Institute on Alcohol Abuse and Alcoholism (NIAAA)
  - National Institute of Allergy and Infectious Diseases (NIAID)
  - National Institute of Arthritis and Musculoskeletal and Skin Diseases (NIAMS)
  - National Institute of Diabetes and Digestive and Kidney Diseases (NIDDK)
  - National Institute of Mental Health (NIMH)
  - National Center for Complementary and Alternative Medicine (NCCAM)
- Centers for Disease Control and Prevention (CDC)
  - National Institute for Occupational Safety and Health (NIOSH)
- Office of the Surgeon General
- U.S. Preventive Services Task Force (USPSTF) housed within the Agency for Healthcare Research and Quality (AHRQ)
- U.S. Task Force on Community Preventive Services (the Task Force) housed within the CDC
- U.S. Food and Drug Administration (FDA; for dietary guidelines)
- World Health Organization (WHO)

It is important to note that the use of good health recommendations in the typical health risk assessment is not more—but certainly not less—scientific than the use of the epidemiologically based death tables that form the underlying science for many health risk appraisals. Either type of instrument can have strong scientific underpinnings—or embarrassingly weak ones. The health risk appraisal and health risk assessment are two differing approaches to assessing the health and health risks of individuals and populations. Neither tool is inherently superior or inferior to the other. It is only that the approach each uses is different and the end points each is trying to represent can be different. Health risk appraisal frequently ties to mortality estimates, while health risk assessment often ties to morbidity estimates or even to general likelihood statements. A likelihood statement might be something such as, "People who eat a diet that is rich in saturated and trans fat, exercise little if at all, smoke, and are obese are more likely to experience chronic illness and premature death than are people who limit their intake of unhealthy fat, exercise 4 or 5 d most weeks, do not smoke, and maintain a BMI in the 18.5 to 24.99 kg/m^2 range."

When statistical projections are made by health risk assessments, they tend to include subject-specific projections such as the Gail equation for estimating breast cancer risk (5) or the Framingham equations (3,7) for projecting death from cardiovascular disease. The use of broad categories such as overall cancer risk or all-cause mortality are absent from the typical health risk assessment. Indeed, it is not unusual for health risk assessment instruments to eliminate questions that are needed to drive health risk appraisals based on epidemiology or vital statistics. Most vendors limit the questionnaire's scope and length in order to have an instrument that the average participant will complete. Health risk assessments might choose to devote several questions to your consumption of fish or fish oil supplements and other omega-3 sources while not asking which class of car (subcompact, compact, intermediate, or full sized) you usually drive. However, failure to ask about class of car means that a frequently used statistical appraisal of motor vehicle death risk no longer gives a useful answer. In order to find the proper assessment to meet their needs, users must decide what kind of information they want to know, what kind of format they want to offer to their participants, and what interventions they want to make available.

As noted previously, the questions included in a health risk assessment are less determined by mortality or even morbidity risk statistics than are the questions found in a health risk appraisal. Instead, the purpose of health risk assessment instruments is to pose questions that will elicit the most useful information for comparison with public health standards (e.g., questions about tobacco use, physical activity, or nutrition goals). They may also include questions that ask about

- quality of life issues,
- health care utilization,
- health care cost estimation,
- worker productivity,
- presenteeism,
- previous or current medical diagnoses,
- current prescription and over-the-counter medications, and
- family history of chronic diseases and conditions.

More and more often, health risk assessments also add questions that address

- depression,
- anxiety,
- anger,
- sleep,
- fatigue, and
- other psychosocial issues (which are typically absent in health risk appraisals).

It has become abundantly clear from the HERO study (6,15) and other recent studies (10) looking at the effect and ultimate cost of depression, anxiety, fatigue, and chronic disease in the workplace that psychological and psychosocial variables carry as much of the variance in lost productivity and increased medical care costs as physical problems such as arthritis or heart disease carry. They may sometimes carry even more.

Health risk assessments have also been expanding to include a range of behavioral theories, models, and tools, including

- readiness to change (stages of change),
- self-efficacy,
- outcome expectations,
- barriers and aids,
- health belief model,
- theory of planned behavior, and
- motivational interviewing.

Including questions driven by behavioral theory is intended to make the feedback messages more relevant, tailored, and potent. Proceeding from these theoretical perspectives can also result in population segmentation strategies that increase the efficiency and efficacy of health risk assessment reports and interventions (12). Health risk appraisals and health risk assessments are the forms most frequently used in worksite health promotion programs.

Condition-Specific or Condition-Targeted Appraisals and Assessments

These appraisals and assessments are somewhat specialized, and you are less likely to see them used in average worksite health promotion implementations. There are three basic approaches to these appraisals and assessments:

1. Adjusting health risk projections based on the knowledge of preexisting illness (usually chronic illness)
2. Focusing on providing information on other risks while tailoring the feedback to participants who have already developed a specific illness or condition
3. Asking questions that allow feedback based on history and lifestyle behaviors that look to be preventing the specific chronic disease or death from the disease

The first type, adjusting risk projections based on preexisting illness, and sometimes looking at how multiple lifestyle and physical measures affect a specific illness, is rare. The necessary science is difficult and expensive to do. Also, these instruments seem more applicable to health plans and the like than they are to worksite health assessment.

The second type, providing information on other risks while tailoring feedback to acknowledge a current or previous chronic disease, is easier to accomplish. It takes the communications approach that attempts to steer you toward good health behaviors while placing new recommendations in context with your previous chronic disease.

The last type of condition-specific health assessment focuses on good health behaviors, including appropriate preventive screenings that make a given disease more or less likely. It is condition specific in that it gives feedback on how your family history, personal history, biological measures, and lifestyle behaviors increase or decrease the likelihood that you will develop a given—and usually chronic—disease. Thus a heart health assessment in this framework is one whose questions and algorithms focus almost exclusively on heart disease.

Health Status Assessment

The health status assessment is also sometimes referred to as the *functional quality of life assessment*. Examples of health status assessment tools are the SF-36, SF-12, SF-8, and Dartmouth COOP. In the past, these tools were used mainly in health service research on the quality of life before and after medical treatments such as knee and hip replacements or after treatment for diabetes, asthma, or lupus. They are a standardized way for people to report on their self-perceived ability to function in a typically healthy manner. Health status assessments have seen very limited use with individuals in worksite health promotion settings. Rather, they have been used (especially the SF-8 and SF-12) to get a summary measure of the functional health of a population. The health status assessment is also useful when examining functional recovery after short-term or long-term disability due to injury or illness (14).

Biometric Measurements

The purpose of biometric testing in the workplace is for screening rather than diagnosis or treatment. This class of frequently used measurements is part of worksite health promotion. It includes measurements for total cholesterol, high-density lipoprotein (HDL), low-density lipoprotein (LDL), triglycerides, blood glucose, blood pressure, BMI, and waist-to-hip ratio. These measurements can help classify overweight and obesity and predict or detect cardiovascular problems and diabetes. They can also become part of the health risk assessment, which then triggers additional risk and health reporting. Other biometric measures that are sometimes collected in worksite health promotion programs include percent body fat (from skin calipers or electronic measurement units), hemoglobin A1c (Hb_{A1c}), and high-sensitivity C-reactive protein (hs-CRP). Not all measurements are generally recommended; in fact,

worksite biometric screening is one place where less is often more.

The more blood chemistries and other biometric measurements a program chooses to do, the more often the program will experience a false positive. A false positive is a test that says a participant who doesn't really have a problem has a problem. Since a dozen false positives can upset many people as well as eat up a lot of medical dollars while the test results are being disconfirmed, worksite programs should select their test metrics carefully. In short, if you don't intend to communicate aggressively with your workforce about the results of a test, perhaps setting up intervention programs or getting participants to their physicians for careful review, we recommend not including that test in your battery. See table 16.1 for additional information and recommendations on biometric measurements.

The most difficult portion of most biometric testing is the blood draw. Many people do not like needles. That aside, blood chemistry results often have great utility when assessing cardiovascular and diabetes risk. There are two ways to get the blood sample and do the analyses. The first is a venous draw. A venous draw is a standard acupuncture. The tubes of blood are sent off for analysis, and sometime between a couple of days and a week the participant usually receives a report. The second way to take a blood sample is the finger stick. A very sharp, sterile lancet nicks a finger and a tiny sample of blood is drawn into a capillary tube. Most often this sample is processed in a desktop blood chemistry unit that produces results in approximately 5 min. The beauty of this method is that the participant gets almost instantaneous reporting and a handsome computer-generated summary and can ask for explanations before the screening event draws to a close. Teachable moments are common when using the finger stick with a desktop analyzer.

Implementing Population Health Measurement Systems

No matter where you want your program to take you, the first steps are information gathering, goal setting, and goal sharing. Since health assessments were built for varying purposes, each has its own best uses and weaknesses. Therefore it is critical that you clearly define your program goals before beginning the assessment process. Goals sometimes come from senior leadership and sometimes come from the wellness committee; goals are

Table 16.1 Biometric Measurements and Worksite Screening

Measure	Recommendation[1]	Notes [3]
		This information is for worksite screening purposes only.
Total cholesterol	1	This test is accurate when drawn fasting or nonfasting.
HDL cholesterol	1	This test is accurate when drawn fasting or nonfasting. The ratio of total cholesterol to HDL predicts cardiovascular morbidity and mortality.
LDL cholesterol	2	The standard test for LDL requires 9 to 12 h of fasting before blood is drawn.
Triglycerides	2	The U.S. Preventive Services Task Force reports no empirical evidence for or against triglycerides measurement as part of routine screening for lipid disorders. Blood is drawn after fasting for 9 to 12 h.
Fasting plasma glucose	1	Screening is not diagnostic. Elevated measures should be confirmed by physician. Assumes an 8 to 12 h fast. [2,4]
Hb_{A1c}	2	Measure of average blood sugar levels over 60 to 90 d. If fasting plasma glucose is being tested, there is no need for concurrent Hb_{A1c} testing. [2]
BMI	1	This calculation requires height and weight.
Waist-to-hip ratio	2	This ratio requires waist and hip circumferences. Correct measurement technique is critical. This ratio seems to be as, or more, sensitive for predicting coronary heart disease as BMI is.
Percent body fat	2	This measurement is especially helpful in determining if heavily muscled participants are also too fat and for determining if participants who appear to be skinny carry too much body fat for the amount of muscle they have.
Blood pressure	1	Adults aged 18 y and over should have their blood pressure measured regularly.
hsCRP	3	In January 2003, the AHA and CDC issued a statement on hs-CRP. It is not to be considered a screening test for cardiovascular disease in general. It may have diagnostic utility in the hands of a physician. [2]
Liver enzymes	3	This measurement is frequently part of comprehensive blood test panels.
Electrolyte profile	3	This measurement is frequently part of comprehensive blood test panels.
Cell blood count (CBC)	3	This measurement is frequently part of comprehensive blood test panels.
Prostate specific antigen	3, 1	PSA measurement is only appropriate for men who are in their 50s or older or who are in their late 30s and 40s depending on their ethnic and racial background and family history of cancers.

[1]Authors' recommendations for broad-based worksite biometric screening: 1 = recommended, 2 = discretionary, and 3 = not recommended.

[2]Adapted from references 2, 4, 9, and 13.

[3]Screenings are not diagnostic. Their results are not appropriate for treatment purposes.

[4]Some tests, such as blood glucose, would not be recommended as a stand-alone test; however, if they are performed as part of the same finger stick used to test cholesterol and triglycerides, the incremental cost can be as little as $0.50 to $1.00 U.S. per screened participant.

sometimes focused and clear and sometimes not. Sometimes the direction given is sensitive and thoughtful; other times the direction is reactive and even punitive. Sometimes the worksite health professionals may be given a free hand to run their own process, to listen as they will to every level of the company, and sometimes not. But whatever the source, it is their responsibility to find an appropriate health assessment tool that meets the goals that are established. This task can be easy, or it can require a fair amount of effort. There is an important rule to remember. If you want to run

a successful program, get representation from both the workforce (and the union if applicable) and the management, to the greatest extent that you can. Management and labor are then more likely to work together, involving themselves in the process of determining program goals and implementation strategies. By having all parties involved, potential concerns as well as perceived benefits are more likely to be captured in this initial stage. To facilitate the decision process, worksite health professionals are expected to be competent in presenting and educating various levels of employees and management on the differing purposes of various health assessment tools. And all of this comes before you settle on a specific health appraisal or assessment. At the end of the goal setting, measurable metrics should be established. As the program goes forward, these metrics are then used to determine whether program goals have been met (see the following checklist).

Health Assessment (HA) Program Checklist

- Goals of HA Program

  Clearly Defined as They Are Aligned With the Mission of the Corporation

  Clearly Shared with:
  - ☐ the management
  - ☐ the union (if applicable)
  - ☐ employees
  - ☐ the vendor

- HA Program Review

  Questions/Screening Items
  - ☐ Does the HA capture metrics that are aligned with the goals of your program and company?
  - ☐ Relevance to your population
  - ☐ Sufficiently comprehensive coverage of risks/behaviors
  - ☐ Consider whether to include readiness-to-change questions
  - ☐ Examine the breadth of the readiness-to-change questions (e.g., stages of change, self-efficacy, outcome expectation, pros and cons)
  - ☐ Clear wordings
  - ☐ Pilot test to determine how long it takes to complete (should not take more than 20 minutes; 15 minutes is better; 7-10 minutes better yet)

  Personal Reports/Feedback
  - ☐ Up-to-date information
  - ☐ Risk presentation vs. public health recommendations
  - ☐ Use of collected readiness-to-change information
  - ☐ Consistency with and integration of available follow-up resources into the report or other follow-up services provided by your vendor
  - ☐ Appropriate reading level for your population
  - ☐ Visual appeal

Aggregate Reports
  - ☐ Determine whether metrics that are aligned with goals are included and evaluated
  - ☐ Capability to present comparisons against norms
  - ☐ Capability to compare results over time (Cross-sectional vs. Cohort)
  - ☐ Determine when and how (e.g., hard copy, electronically) aggregate reports are received

- HA Program Participation Eligibility Determination
  - ☐ Full-time and/or part-time
  - ☐ Employees and/or contractors
  - ☐ Employees and/or their dependents

- HA Program Delivery Methods
  - ☐ Determine on/off company time for HA participation
  - ☐ Assess computer access on and/or off company time
  - ☐ Determine online, pencil-and-paper, telephonic, kiosk, notebook computer or mixed delivery modes
  - ☐ Determine whether to offer on-site biometrics screenings
  - ☐ Determine how participants receive their results

- Marketing
  - ☐ Choose appropriate channels (e-mail, flyer, poster, bulletin board, announcement in meetings, etc.)
  - ☐ Craft effective messages (benefits of HA, easy participation, incentives, testimonials, contact information, etc.)
  - ☐ Consider the use of incentives to increase participation

- Biometric Screenings
  - ☐ Review the protocols for scientific validity and reliability
  - ☐ Communicate requirements for effective assessments (e.g., fasting) to employees
  - ☐ Set up the time conducive to employees' adherence to the requirements
  - ☐ Check the credentials and training of screening staff
  - ☐ Review the liability release form
  - ☐ Review the treatment of bio-hazardous materials
  - ☐ Reserve appropriate space

- Data Handling
  - ☐ Provide staff with training on personal health information handling
  - ☐ Provide a HA assessment environment where PHI is kept confidential and employees are clearly assured appropriate confidentiality.
  - ☐ Establish secure data transfer to and from the vendor
- Implementation Monitoring
  - ☐ Monitor program implementation
  - ☐ Monitor participation
  - ☐ Pre-establish appropriate protocols to handle emergencies or complaints
- Evaluation
  - ☐ Consider to whom and how you will present the aggregate reports
  - ☐ Consider repeated offerings for over time comparisons to understand trends and/ or program outcome evaluation
  - ☐ Determine what's next

Once the goals of your health assessment program are determined, the next step is to share them with the entire workforce. Discuss not only the benefits but also how you will deal with potential concerns.

Detailed Review

When selecting a health assessment, careful attention needs to go into the selection process and the review of specific aspects of the health assessment tool. Consider a review of such areas as the questions, ensuring the question and answer options are set automatically; the personal report every participant receives; and the aggregate report the company receives. A discussion of these areas follow.

Health Assessment Questions and Items

To select the specific health assessment instrument, prepare to pay careful attention to the details of each question or item as well as the health assessment as a whole. The first important question is whether an instrument collects the metrics your company deems important. Does the instrument make it easy for you to collect the information that helps you achieve your program goals? As a whole, does the health assessment cover enough of the health indicators and health behaviors that are relevant to your population?

If an assessment appears basically sound, then review it question by question, for both clarity and scientific sensibility. Pay attention to both the questions and the response options. Use your imagination. Examine whether all or most of the possible responses to a given question are accommodated by the answer options. Remember, if it is possible for someone to read the assessment questions or answer options in an odd or idiosyncratic way, someone will. You may also want to run a pilot test by administering the health assessment questionnaire to several people who are similar in demographic background to those in your population. Look for clarity of questioning and ease of use. The test drive could also provide a good idea about how long it would take for people in your group to complete the health assessment. Most ethical, professional vendors will be happy to accommodate your prepurchase explorations. Lengthy health assessments often reduce the participation and completion rates, whereas short health assessments encourage participation and completion but may not cover all of the information you would like. An excellent completion time for a health assessment is 7 to 10 min. Assessments lasting 15 to 20 min are still generally acceptable. Longer instruments are not recommended for general population health assessments.

Unless you are using a health assessment as a very preliminary survey of basic health risks in a population, you will most likely benefit from also assessing psychological and behavioral issues, as these frequently relate to health behavior change. The term *readiness for change* is often used to refer to such psychological and motivational issues. Readiness for change may include stages based on Prochaska's transtheoretical model and other psychological variables such as self-efficacy and outcome expectancy from social cognitive theory. Perceived benefits and costs of behavior change from the health belief model or decisional balance from the transtheoretical model can also be important. Such information makes it possible to tailor health education messages for each individual and provides clues to effective program offerings for a group.

Personal Reports and Feedback

Visual appeal or the lack of it is something people notice immediately. This appeal is important as people may decide whether to read the report depending on its visual appeal. If the participants decide to read on, then the reading level of the report also needs to be appropriate for your population. You will also need to look carefully at the details of the report contents. As described earlier, mortality risk information make up the core of reports in health risk appraisals whereas deviations from public health recommendations are the core of health risk assessments. Furthermore, reports from health risk assessments are often developed to use readiness-to-change information in order to help people change their behavior. It is worth some time to examine if message tailoring carries both a positive emotional tone and clearly delivered information

To maintain the credibility of your health assessment program, the health information provided in personal reports should be up to date and scientifically valid. You should ask vendors how often they do a systematic evaluation and update of the science in their instrument.

Furthermore, messages in personal reports should be consistent with available follow-up resources. For example, if a personal report recommends that people receive evaluation of their office ergonomics, it is important to see if any ergonomic help is available. Failure to be able to use a report's recommendations often frustrates the individual participants and eventually their bosses.

Aggregate Reports

Aggregate reports not only give worksite health professionals ideas for priority areas and effective programming (especially when readiness-to-change information is collected) but also play a significant role in presenting the results to employers. Due to legal and ethical concerns over tying each employee's health assessment results to health risk decisions, employers are provided the results only in an aggregate form. If even aggregated results seem to reveal the identity of specific individuals (e.g., when the workforce is small or very few employees are of a certain gender), seriously consider eliminating that information from the aggregate report. Your assessment vendor should have an automatic process to accomplish this protection.

Aggregate reports must contain the program's goal metrics. This is critical so that management and employee committees can see information that is important to them. Some health assessment aggregate reports compare the data from your population against norms. The norms may be derived from various sources such as published results on health assessment systematically conducted in worksites, governmental data such as *Healthy People 2010* baseline data, and the vendor's client database. Such comparisons

enable you to understand how well your population is doing and where the health improvement priorities should be.

When health assessment programs are offered more than once, say, annually, the capability for comparing aggregate health assessment results over time becomes critical. Given a potential change in the eligible workforce due to new hires, retirement, or turnover, it is critical that aggregate reports have the ability to track the same group of people as they move through time (i.e., track a cohort).

On a procedural matter, you need to know the timing of the delivery of an aggregate report from the vendor so that you can schedule a presentation to the management and other interested internal groups. How are the summary data delivered? Is the report in paper format or electronic format? Does it allow editing to include company logos, additional text, and so on? Some vendors will even send an individual to present the results to you and your management.

Health Assessment Program Participation Eligibility Determination

In addition to determining which health assessment program is offered, it is important to determine who is eligible to participate in the program. The eligibility determination must be made with a clear understanding of how it will affect your goals. The goal of health care cost containment would lead you to review all the lives covered by your company's health insurance, which probably include employees, spouses, children, and possibly retirees. When the goal of productivity enhancement is important, all employees regardless of their status (full-time, part-time, or contractor workers) would make up the eligible group. Medical cost reductions are not the only potential win for the organization.

Health Assessment Program Delivery Methods

Program delivery methods have direct effects on increasing participation in the health assessment program, and they are also a way to show that the company cares about its employees. Even though online delivery of health assessment programs is becoming more and more prevalent, a paper copy should be made available for employees with limited access to computers. In many cases, a mix of delivery methods may be needed to provide equal access to the program across various segments of your workforce.

In addition to data collection methods (how participants complete the health assessment), the delivery of health assessment programs affects how participants receive personal reports. Online delivery has the advantage of providing immediate feedback. Thus, it directly supports teachable moments. Many who do not have access to a printer may want to keep a hard copy of their assessments. As part of service with a smile, you need to support access to a printer where they will feel comfortable printing out their personal information if they want to.

Another important consideration is whether biometric screening is provided along with your health assessment programs. Almost all health risk assessments and appraisals include questions about biometrics. Unless you provide on-site biometric screenings, expect many missing values—missing values that will have a significant effect on the usefulness of the results.

Marketing

Even if you have chosen an attractive, effective health assessment program, full effectiveness will not be realized until the vast majority of those who are eligible choose to participate. Incentives are effective in increasing participation in a health assessment program. An increasing number of corporations are beginning to provide financial incentives for participating in health assessment. These can take the form of gift certificates, points at a company store, or even a reduction in health insurance premium.

Regardless of the specific incentives used, marketing efforts should be crafted with care. Ask yourself, "Which channels seem to reach the eligibles?" Are these channels e-mails, flyers, posters, bulletin boards, announcements in meetings, several channels combined, or something else? What messages should be communicated to the eligibles through the channels? Do they need to hear about the benefits of health assessment, the easy participation, the available incentives, the testimonials from previous participants, the endorsements from their leaders, the contact information for the program, and so on?

Biometric Screenings

Whether you decide to use your company's occupational health staff or a screening vendor, review the protocols for their scientific validity and reliability. Also, inquire about the credentials and training of screening staff members. Ask how they are going to treat biohazardous materials. It is surprising and somewhat appalling that not every vendor takes care with such elementary precautions.

In order for the assessments to be adequately performed, participants' collaboration is essential. If a blood draw for glucose testing requires fasting, for example, be sure to communicate the requirement to employees. Furthermore, schedule a time for screening that is conducive to employees' adherence to the requirements. If fasting is required, screening at the start of shifts is recommended.

Be prepared for unexpected events. Discuss liability issues with your company's lawyer. Demand that your vendor use a suitable liability release form in addition to making sure that emergency protocols are in place and that screening staff members are well informed.

Data Handling

Health assessment programs almost always collect personal health information. Therefore, it is essential that you familiarize yourself with HIPAA regulations. Provide training on data handling for staff members who will be involved with any phase of the health assessment program implementation in which they might gain access to personal health information. Most of the time, violations of appropriate data handling occur without evil intentions. Avoid casual transfer of personal health information by e-mail unless your e-mail connections are secure.

Secure handling of personal health data is important from a legal standpoint and also assures employees that their concerns or secrets stay safe. Dealing with privacy concerns should usually result in higher participation rates and more reliable responses. Provide a health assessment environment in which employees clearly feel that personal health information is being treated with respect and confidentiality.

Implementation Monitoring

Once a health assessment program is launched, continuously monitor the program implementation. Doing so is a part of process evaluation. Questions you should ask include, but are not limited to, whether the URL for the health assessment program is always up and running and whether screening staff members show up on time.

Do not wait until the end of the health assessment program to look into program participation. Conduct periodic reviews of participation and do more marketing if necessary.

Evaluation

What you do with the results of a health assessment program is as important as the implementation itself. Study an aggregate report very carefully to identify priority areas, trends, and potential issues. Consider the strategic implications of who should quickly see the results and how the results should be presented.

Take the time to reflect on the assessment results and lessons learned. When presenting the results to management, be ready to propose future steps. You may want to propose that the same health assessment program be offered each year or every other year so that over time comparisons can be made. Look carefully for trends and seek to understand them. Furthermore, if additional programs are offered during the next year, consider that T1-T2 comparisons could be used to evaluate the effectiveness of the program.

Conclusion

This chapter has focused on the health assessment tools, processes, and associated considerations that represent important factors in implementing a high quality health assessment process. From considering the appropriateness of a given health assessment tool for your company, to the inclusion of questions dealing with productivity, and the addition of biometric screening data, all aspects of this process should be considered carefully prior to making final decisions on tool selection and process implementation.

Chapter Review Questions

1. Compare and contrast health risk appraisals and health risk assessments.

2. What kind of information do health status assessments collect?

3. Outline the process and process components of a comprehensive health assessment with biometric screening.

17

Organizational Assessment for Health

Thomas Golaszewski, EdD

Organizational health assessment has been a key feature of the worksite health promotion movement since its earliest days (20). Other than safety inventories, evaluation has traditionally centered on the assessment of the employee, with the results pooled to reflect the health status of the workplace. Health risk appraisal has been most noted for this approach (4). Other common individual health measures, such as medical claims and absenteeism data, cultural norms surveys, and social support inventories, among other employee-focused measures, have formed the basis of determining the health of the organization.

However, as the science of worksite health promotion advanced, comprehensive intervention began to recognize that both assessment and intervention of the organization are fundamental to employee health behavior change (5,24). DeJoy and Wilson (6) recently introduced the phrase *organizational health promotion* (p. 337) to recognize this change in intervention emphasis. As a result, measuring both the organization and its employees has emerged as a trend in the industry (11).

Several factors in particular reinforce this thinking and give rise to the conceptualization of this chapter. One, as the worksite health promotion movement matured, greater attention was paid to establishing best practices and quality assurance in program delivery (12). As worksite health promotion transitioned from mostly art to science, a more defensible position emerged as to what strategies worked best and under what circumstances. Two, consistent with the development of best-practice guidelines, a movement arose to recognize companies of excellence—organizations that delivered programs best according to the accepted standards of the time. This factor led to the creation of a variety of program award mechanisms and, subsequently, a need to develop systems to evaluate organizations. Three, throughout much of its history, worksite intervention activity mainly focused on the individual. Programs were largely developed to address employee health knowledge, attitudes, beliefs, and skills. However, by the late 1980s, scholars began to argue for a more comprehensive approach of influencing employee health behavior (18). In particular, the social ecology movement began to highlight the effects of the larger social and physical environments on human behavior, including the influence of the workplace environment (22-24). Employee health behavior was considered a function of the workplace's health-supportive facilities, support services and policies, and social culture. Subsequently, the workplace environment became an object of intervention, and systems were needed to measure it. With respect to these factors, this chapter provides (1) a brief review of worksite health promotion best-practice standards and award and recognition mechanisms, (2) a review of current organizational assessment tools, and (3) a look at recommendations for future development.

Best-Practice Guidelines and Award Mechanisms in Worksite Health Promotion

The systematic identification of benchmarks for worksite health promotion has a limited history, as studies on the topic first appeared in the literature during the late 1990s. The most recent analysis culminated in the identification of promising practices in health and productivity management (HPM)—the current phrase to describe comprehensive worksite health promotion initiatives (12). A strategy consisting of literature review, discussions with subject matter experts, online inventory of 39 promising practice companies, and site visits to the nine highest scoring of these companies identified the following best practices: (1) integrating HPM programs into the organization's operations; (2) simultaneously addressing individual, environmental, policy, and cultural factors affecting health and productivity; (3) targeting several health issues; (4) tailoring programs to address specific needs; (5) attaining high participation; (6) rigorously evaluating programs; and (7) communicating successful outcomes to key stakeholders. These general topics were further delineated into more specific subcomponents, thus defining the state of the art in workplace health promotion delivery. The results of this effort both added to and supported earlier findings in benchmarking initiatives.

Later discussion will show the link between program standards of excellence (such as those just listed) and the emerging area of organizational assessment tools. However, these same criteria form the basis of multiple reward and recognition processes that have been and continue to be an important part of worksite health promotion. Several examples of these award and recognition processes are the former Johnson & Johnson Health Care Systems Quality Audit, the WELCOA Well Workplace Award (26), and the American Cancer Society CEO Cancer Gold Standard (2). Each in some way evaluates a company's health initiative using criteria perceived to represent ideal characteristics of a health-supportive company.

Organizational Assessment Tools

A recent effort by the Health Communication Unit at the Centre for Health Promotion at the University of Toronto resulted in a compilation of assessment tools that are suggested for use in worksite health promotion initiatives (16). The Health Communication Unit's rigorous process resulted in the identification of 21 instruments deemed recommended and an additional 8 instruments considered promising. One of the results of this effort was the categorization of assessment tools by type and focus, such as current practice surveys, health risk assessments, interest surveys, needs assessments, organizational culture surveys, and workplace audits. Though all of these tools have important uses in the worksite health promotion milieu and characterize an organization's health, the latter category, workplace audits, forms the basis of this section.

By definition, a workplace audit is "a type of situational assessment tool that provides a snapshot in time of what's happening in the workplace. [It] collects information about what the workplace offers employees" (4, p. 47). The previous section described systems that sought to identify characteristics of worksite health promotion initiatives that met established benchmarks and to use this information to grant recognition to sponsoring companies. This section borrows much from the same literature and evaluates largely the same criteria, but it approaches the issue from a more scientific perspective. Where the previously discussed assessments are largely driven by qualitative or judgment-based methods, workplace audits draw from the tenets of measurement science. This assessment group has structured protocols and numeric results and, as in any good measuring tool, provides empirical evidence on its metric properties. Listed in a somewhat chronological order of their development, organizational assessments, or more precisely workplace audits, are described in their current state in the following section.

Heart Check

The Heart Check may be the grandfather of systematic workplace audits as they are currently envisioned. Developed in 1994 as part of the New York State Department of Health's Healthy Heart Program, the Heart Check was conceived as a means of measuring the environmental characteristics of a workplace that support heart health (13).

The Heart Check is a 226-item survey divided into seven subscales, each representing a lifestyle component of heart health, program administration, or some other health-related factor. These subscales include tobacco use, nutrition, physical activity, stress, screening, administrative support (e.g., presence of a wellness committee), and organizational foundation (e.g., presence of subsidized health insurance). Items were constructed for these seven areas based on accepted best practices of the time and the project team's professional judgment. Measured constructs were observed as opposed to being opinionated responses. Therefore, quantitatively based operational definitions were written into items where needed—for example, "During the past 12 months, were at least two communication avenues used to promote . . . ?" Individuals with health promotion backgrounds were trained as raters by applying a standardized scoring protocol. Using a combination of site observations and interviews with key workplace managers, items were awarded

1 or 0 points based on their presence or absence. Item responses were simply summed by each subsection and totaled to create numeric scores that were also translated into percentages of optimum. A Heart Check evaluation typically required between 30 and 45 min to complete.

A number of studies have been performed to determine the instrument's metric properties (13). For example, internal consistency reliability assessments have rated within the good to excellent ranges. Interrater reliability assessment has also shown consistency among teams of raters observing the same worksites. Along with face and content validity established by review of external examiners, construct validity has been established by observing strong and predictable relationships among subscales as well as logical relationships between Heart Check subscale scores and individual employee health behaviors. Finally, criterion validity has been established through the observation of similar workplace rankings for program quality between Heart Check and an established organizational rating process.

Since the mid-1990s, the Healthy Heart Program has used the Heart Check within a number of research venues (13). With more than 1,000 companies tested to date, the presence of a large database allows for the development of statewide Heart Check norms, both by subscales and by total (see figure 17.1). The results of organization-based interventions using Heart Check scores as the dependent variable have also been encouraging. For example, within a sample of more than 200 companies across New York, total Heart Check scores before and after the intervention increased about 75% on average, with corresponding increases observed in most subsections, which were led by physical activity (143%), nutrition (114%), and administrative support (109%).

Other research has shown demographic predictors of high Heart Check scores (10). In general, company size (more than 250 employees), industry type (primarily manufacturing), and presence of unions were the strongest predictors of high

Label	Tobacco control	Nutrition	Physical activity	Stress	Screen	Adm. support	Org. support	Total HC
Excellent 2+ SD	>52	>38	>42	>75	>58	>41	>89	>40
Good 75th percentile	>27-52	>16-38	>20-42	>52-75	>21-58	>13-41	>67-89	>22-40
Above average 50th percentile	>23-27	>6-16	>10-20	>32-52	>4-21	>2-13	>56-67	>15-22
Below average 25th percentile	18-23	3-6	2-10	23-32	1-4	1-2	39-56	11-15
Poor <25th percentile	<18	<3	<2	<23	<1	<1	<39	<11

Figure 17.1 Heart Check preintervention standards (as percentages) based on New York state results (*n* = 1,000 worksites).

Reprinted, by permission, from T. Golaszewski and B. Fisher, 2002, "Heart check: The development and evolution of an organizational heart health assessment," *American Journal of Health Promotion* 1(3): 137.

scores. More recently, after controlling for age and gender, a cross-sectional analysis of 20 companies and more than 2,000 employees in western New York has shown an inverse relationship between Heart Check scores and selected employee risk factors (8). Finally, in the ongoing California Department of Health Services' worksite wellness project, preliminary analysis of an organization-based intervention has shown a decrease in 11 of 15 selected employee risk factors following a substantial increase in Heart Check scores (17).

The present Heart Check has its limitations; it is too lengthy, has some wording difficulties, and contains items that are not needed or lacks others that should be added. It also uses a hand-scored, paper-based system that makes analysis and reporting inefficient. Nevertheless, its history over the past dozen years supports early speculation on its utility as a needs assessment, evaluation, and research tool. Heart Check probably has the most extensive use and most comprehensive research history of any assessments in this category.

Checklist of Health Promotion Environments

In recognizing ecological factors in health behavior, the Australian National Workplace Health Project developed the Checklist of Health Promotion Environments at Worksites (CHEW; 19). CHEW is a 112-item inventory that assesses workplace environmental features believed to influence physical activity, healthy eating, alcohol consumption, and smoking. Three environmental domains of the workplace are analyzed: (1) physical characteristics, such as the availability of exercise facilities and healthy foods; (2) information environment, including health-related signs, newsletter articles, and program announcements; and (3) surrounding neighborhood, including food shops, fitness centers, and parks.

The instrument was developed by generating a checklist of items related to environmental factors that would be applicable to a wide range of workplaces. Developed as an observational rating system, operational definitions were identified for CHEW items to describe the presence of each characteristic. Observers were trained to standardize scoring; the characteristic either exists or does not exist. Some items were simply counted, such as the number of healthy or unhealthy foods in vending machines.

Observers toured the workplace, including lunchrooms, common areas, stairwells, and fit-ness facilities. For the physical environment, up to 17 subscales could be created to represent each subsection of investigation—one example is an exercise equipment subscale. Similarly, 12 sub-scales could be generated for the observance of features in the neighboring environment. Finally, scores consisting of simple counts were calculated for the observance of signage supporting each health content area. The assessment process took about 35 min to complete.

An analysis of 20 mostly blue-collar worksites in the Australian National Workplace Health Project helped establish evidence for interrater reliability of the physical and environmental sections of CHEW (19). Additionally, the instrument was prepared based on theoretical constructs defined in the literature and has high acceptance by users in program planning, thus offering evidence for face and content validity.

Although further metric testing of the instrument is necessary, CHEW is an important contribution to worksite health promotion assessment. It is unique because it extends assessment to the community surrounding the work environment. And as seen in later discussions, CHEW has served as a model for the development of a number of other assessment tools.

Workplace Physical Activity Assessment Tool

The Workplace Physical Activity Assessment Tool (WPAAT) was developed in response to objectives identified in the Active Living Strategy of Alberta, Canada (14), along with recommendations compiled from a comprehensive needs assessment undertaken in the province of Alberta (21). Borrowing considerably from the tenets of social ecology, a multilevel conceptualization of physical activity support formed the basis for the development of the workplace program standard. The program standard then became the starting point for the development of WPAAT.

The development of the program standard followed a strategy of literature review, identification of key physical activity recommendations from the review, and ratings of these recommendations by a panel of experts. Ratings were supportive of a 9-point framework for enhancing physical activity. This framework borrows components from diffusion theory, needs and environment assessment, and social ecology, particularly the linking of individual, social, organizational, and community factors, to form an integrated system supporting physical activity. The acceptance of the program standard led to the creation of items for the WPAAT. Using the CHEW as a model, 45 items were created and divided into 10 subsections, including, for example, management and employee commitment; individual level of knowledge, attitude, and skills; program administration; and safety and risk management.

The WPAAT is designed for use by in-house workplace managers, with detailed instructions provided to standardize assessment. A dichotomous scoring system is used—the characteristic either exists or does not exist. A positive response needs one or more of the following to establish its validity: personal observation, supportive documentation, or interview response from a workplace employee. Summing the positive responses creates scores for the total WPAAT and for each subsection.

Usability of the WPAAT was established by pilot testing. The reading level of items was also tested and adjusted to ensure comprehension at the grade 12 level. Content validity was established through multiple reviews by experts in workplace physical activity and through follow-up qualitative reviews by users after pilot testing. Finally, interrater reliability was established using paired raters at multiple worksites. High compatibility of scores was observed between raters, though scoring consistency varied by type of organization (e.g., multisite versus single-site workplace).

The current WPAAT has its limitations, including a lack of research results supporting its application and the use of in-house raters as opposed to trained external observers. Currently, research is ongoing to address the former issue. The latter issue may introduce rater bias in data collection since managers are judging their own workplaces. Subsequently, the current WPAAT may be best labeled as an internal awareness building and planning aid rather than a formal evaluation tool. However, a focus on a single topic, a comprehensive development strategy, a use of a sound theoretical framework to construct items and sections, and a relative ease of administration make the WPAAT an assessment tool of considerable promise. Furthermore, its structural format could serve as a model for assessments of health behaviors other than physical activity.

Heart Check Lite

Because of its length, the Heart Check was not practical for large-scale studies. Therefore, an empirically driven process was employed to create and then test a reduced-item version of Heart Check, which is referred to as the *Heart Check Lite (HCL;* 9).

A random set of 1,000 worksites located throughout New York that had previously completed a Heart Check was used as the target of study. A combination of Guttman and factor analysis and professional judgments was applied to identify two reduced-item versions of HCL, one containing 27 items (HCL-27) and one containing 55 items (HCL-55). The reduced-item versions were then assessed for their ability to similarly rank and detect changes in 255 different worksites participating in an intervention program and using the Heart Check.

Results indicated that the two new versions showed strong relationships to the full Heart Check. Similar findings were also noted for each subscale. Furthermore, both reduced-item versions demonstrated a moderate to strong ability to reproduce the intervention results observed with the full Heart Check.

These results indicate that both versions of the HCL can produce findings similar to those of the Heart Check and can offer assessment advantages over the original. Although the full Heart Check is the preferred method of assessment within comprehensive interventions, the shorter versions are particularly useful in, for example, large-scale surveillance studies.

An electronic version of the HCL is available at www.albany.edu/sph/prc/worksites. This source calculates the full Heart Check results based on weighted HCL scores established in this research.

Heart/Stroke Check

During 2006, the CDC initiated an effort to expand the Heart Check by developing the Heart/Stroke Check (1). An expert work group of U.S. federal, state, academic, and private-sector representatives was organized to develop the new instrument. Using the Heart Check as a model, the expert group conducted a literature review and contacted state health departments to identify other worksite surveys that addressed heart disease and stroke prevention. Through an iterative and collaborative process, the panel identified other domains to insert into the new instrument, such as risk reduction and secondary prevention, availability of communication that identifies signs and symptoms of a heart attack or stroke, and emergency response services at the worksite.

The Heart/Stroke Check is scored similarly to the original Heart Check, awarding 1 point or 0 points for the presence or absence of a characteristic. To date, the Heart/Stroke Check has been pilot tested among various work organizations and is undergoing refinement. Validity and reliability testing is slated for the near future.

Workplace Solutions Survey

The Workplace Solutions survey was developed by the American Cancer Society as an adaptation of the Heart Check (28). Overall, it was designed to address chronic conditions, including heart disease, but it contains a special emphasis on cancer. The survey went through several iterations during its development that eventually led to an assessment of the 15 best-practice guidelines of the U.S. Task Force on Community Preventive Services (as identified in their *Guide to Community Preventive Services;* 3). The current version contains 50 items and is administered online by a trained representative of the American Cancer Society using a focused interview process, though site visit assessments have also been used. Information is provided by key corporate professionals, usually the benefits or human resources manager. Figure 17.2 provides an example of survey items found under the heading of Health Insurance Benefits. The rater judges whether the company possesses the characteristic based on the information provided and its relationship to the item description. Qualitative comments can also be

captured, though they are not scored. Responses are then translated into a computer-generated report highlighting the company's needs. Generally, 3 to 5 recommendations are suggested for the company to address.

Though the survey is relatively new, a pilot test of its application within a comprehensive intervention has indicated a 67% increase in the use of best practices by subject companies (15). Currently, it is being integrated with other worksite health promotion services of the American Cancer Society. The survey is also undergoing testing to establish its metric properties, with preliminary results showing promise (unpublished).

With its focus on an established set of best practices, its electronic data collection and reporting ability, and its integration with the American Cancer Society's program marketing plan, the survey should have a strong effect on worksite health promotion activity across the United States. It may also represent the prototype workplace audit system of the future.

Environmental Assessment Tool

The Environmental Assessment Tool (EAT) is a by-product of an ongoing study addressing worker obesity from both an individual and an environmental perspective (27). EAT, an adaptation of both the CHEW and the Heart Check, contains three subscales (7): (1) physical activity,

Section 1. Health Benefits
Health Plan Availability

1.1.1 Yes No — Does your company pay for at least 50% of the total cost of personal health insurance for all full-time employees?

1.1.2 — Does your company health plan(s) offer individual prescription coverage with at least half of all health care plans?

1.1.3 — Does your company pay for at least 50% of the total cost for family coverage of all full-time employees?

1.1.4 — Does your company health plan(s) offer family prescription coverage with at least half of all health care plans?

Figure 17.2 Example of possible health benefits.

(2) nutrition and weight management, and (3) organizational characteristics and support (e.g., work rules, written policies, and existing health promotion programs and services).

EAT was developed through a structured process consisting of literature review, prototype development, and pilot testing. A team of health promotion, content area, and research experts was responsible for its development, and item construction was based on best-practice standards from the literature. Additionally, a relative value rating system was used to weight items according to their importance. Most items use a dichotomous scoring system; the characteristic either exists or does not exist.

After pilot testing, a final edition consisting of 100 items was identified. For scoring purposes, equal importance was assigned to the physical activity and nutrition subsections (32 points each), and relative value weights were assigned to items.

Data collection was eventually adapted to a computer-based system. Trained observers toured the test site and recorded their observations, including assessment of the social environment through interaction with employees. Afterward, observers met to achieve consensus in scoring for the total instrument and each subscale.

Interrater reliability for EAT was assessed by comparing scores between two trained observers. High percentages of agreement on item responses, as well as high and mostly significant correlations between total and subscale scores, have been observed.

An ambitious test of concurrent validity was also undertaken with the examination of EAT-generated scores for 1 y (the same year as the assessment) health care claim costs and absenteeism. Using multivariate statistical procedures and the worksite as the unit of analysis, significant relationships were identified for absenteeism but not consistently for health care claims. For example, as EAT scores increased, paid absenteeism decreased, as did emergency room payments using EAT subscales. A similar pattern emerged when the unit of analysis was at the employee level (with the employee's company EAT score included). Finally, the same multivariate analyses were conducted to predict postassessment absenteeism and health care costs as indicators of predictive validity. Associations were observed with absenteeism costs but not with medical payments. An additional analysis of concurrent validity showed significant correlations between EAT scores and the metrically tested Leading by Example (LBE) questionnaire, which is a measure of environmental supports for health.

With the use of a structured protocol during development, computer-linked data collection, and new strategies to determine reliability and validity, EAT is an advancement in workplace audits. In particular, its research examining workplace factors for both health care costs and absenteeism data establishes a valuable precedent for future study.

HERO EHM Best Practice Scorecard

HERO is a national, research-oriented coalition of organizations concerned with health promotion, disease prevention, and health-related productivity research (25). Founded in 1995 as a nonprofit, HERO has a mission to facilitate research to support a shift in health care policy toward a greater emphasis on disease prevention and health promotion. The development of the EHM Best Practice Scorecard (the Scorecard) is an extension of this research agenda.

As an understanding of best practices in worksite health promotion emerged, HERO undertook an initiative to develop a system to measure organizations against these criteria. A task force for metrics was appointed, and out of its efforts stemmed the development of the self-scored HERO Scorecard.

The task force, made up of corporate executives and program providers, first identified best-practice guidelines provided by many of the sources identified earlier in this chapter. Selected elements from these sources, along with judgment by the task force, went into the development of the Scorecard. At this writing, at least 23 drafts have been shared among the membership and various national authorities to develop the current version.

The Scorecard is organized along eight critical core components that are generally accepted as fundamental to a successful EHM program. These core components include corporate culture and leadership commitment, strategic planning, communications, comprehensive program components, incentives, supportive health benefits, data management and program evaluation, integrated program coordination, and documentation of outcomes. These core components are divided into 44 subcomponents representing program process elements (e.g., senior leadership commitment) and six outcomes (e.g., 80% or greater participation in health assessment during the most recent 3 y). Specific criteria are described and used to judge whether these subcomponents and outcomes are met.

The Scorecard rating uses a 4-point scale ranging from 0 (element not included) to 3 (element fully included). Scores can reach a maximum of 152 points (52 × 3). A four-tier ranking is used to rate companies. For programs in operation for 3 y or more, the ranking includes the HERO Best Practice Program (137-152 points) and the HERO Honorable Mention Program (122-136 points), and for programs in operation for less than 3 y, the ranking includes the HERO Emerging Best Practice Program (94-104 points) and the HERO Honorable Mention Program (83-93 points).

To date, the Scorecard is going through continued review and pilot testing. The instrument is currently considered to be an educational tool to assist employers and practitioners with program design, strategic planning, vendor selection, gap analysis, and program evaluation. However, its projected applications include descriptive studies, comparative research, and identification and recognition of exemplar EHM programs.

Future Recommendations

As discussed earlier, The Health Communication Unit at the Centre for Health Promotion identified a group of workplace audits in its 2006 report. This chapter reviewed three of its recommended workplace audit tools: the Heart Check, the CHEW, and the WPAAT. However, most of the workplace audits described in this chapter have come into existence since the Centre's very recent initiative. In fact, many tools, such as the EAT, the Workplace Solutions survey, and the HERO Scorecard, have yet to produce published findings at this writing. Even the more established tools are in various stages of redevelopment, as exemplified by the emergence of the Heart Check Lite and the Heart/Stroke Check. These observations highlight the rapid growth of the organizational assessment movement.

Because of the relative novelty of this type of assessment, there appear to be exciting opportunities for the future. The following suggestions are provided to define the continued development and use of the next generation of workplace audits:

- Continue to develop new tools based on the latest and most empirically generated standards of excellence in worksite health promotion delivery.
- Consider alternative item construction formats, such as a scaled rating system (versus an almost exclusive focus on dichotomous scoring systems), to better measure organizational support constructs and improve test sensitivity.
- Add organizational health culture components to assessment in order to better capture the social dynamics that are increasingly seen as important in the strategic mix of health promotion.
- Expand metric testing to further substantiate reliability and validity. Particularly, examine the validity of company-provided, self-reported data.
- Refine the automation of data collection, including placing such tools on the Internet for widespread access.
- Develop detailed summary reports to provide companies with how-to information that addresses their identified organizational weaknesses.
- Conduct large surveillance studies and use the findings to develop norms and standards of excellence based on organizational characteristics such as company size and industry type.
- Establish a research agenda similar to that of the health risk appraisal to determine the relationship of organizational characteristics to employee risk factors, absences, productivity, and health costs and to other organizational variables of interest.
- If the results of the recommended research agenda prove promising, identify workplace characteristics of a healthy company.
- Link a variety of reward and recognition mechanisms to organizations that meet standards.
- Develop alternative assessment tools that address various health topics (e.g., mental health) or that are specific to unique work environments (e.g., schools, heavy industry).

Conclusion

The use of formal workplace audits dates back to the mid-1990s with the publication of the first Heart Check papers. Over the past decade, this topic has grown substantially, resulting in its inclusion in this text—probably the first chapter of its kind in the worksite health promotion literature. Despite this limited history, the use of workplace audits should continue to grow and offer a new research and application outlet for scholars in the field. As the ability to measure the workplace improves, the likelihood of finding more sophisticated workplace-focused interventions should also increase.

Chapter Review Questions

1. What factors have led to the creation and use of worksite audit assessment tools?

2. What organizational features are generally measured in a worksite audit?

3. How are data collected and scored?

4. Describe several examples of promising research results using worksite audits.

5. Describe features of future worksite audit models.

18

Assessment Tools for Employee Productivity

Nicolaas P. Pronk, PhD, FACSM

The connection between health and productivity has long been recognized as a key ingredient of a healthy economy (3,8). Employers clearly recognize that health conditions influence the functional capacity of their employees while they are at work. Chronic health conditions certainly affect an employee's productivity due to the time spent away from work. Presenteeism, or working at a reduced capacity while being present at work, is increasingly recognized as another dimension of lost productivity that adds to an employer's indirect health-related costs (2). In fact, evidence is emerging that relates health improvement to improved performance on the job. For example, it has been found that as health risks reduce, presenteeism reduces as well (1).

Since the January 2001 *Health, Productivity, and Occupational Medicine* special issue of the *Journal of Occupational and Environmental Medicine* was published, a large body of research has been published that addresses productivity measurement and quantifies the effect of disease and health-related risk factors on productivity. The ability to assess overall productivity, which is defined as a combination of absenteeism and presenteeism, has improved significantly and continues to be a topic of considerable research interest. Self-report tools provide increasingly sensitive and specific information on health-related productivity loss and also inform us all that different health conditions, such as mental versus physical conditions, have different effects on various aspects of productivity (4).

This book includes several chapters that are devoted almost exclusively to health and productivity issues (see chapters 13 and 14) as well as many other chapters that include discussions of various aspects of the health and productivity relationship. The purpose of this chapter is to complement those chapters with a succinct overview of the actual tools being used—in other words, the self-report instruments being used to measure health-related work productivity. The intent is not to provide an exhaustive review of the literature or to compare and contrast the various instruments. Rather, the intent is to present an inventory of the available self-report tools that are designed to measure health-related productivity loss.

Approach

A search of the literature was conducted to identify review articles on self-report productivity assessment tools that provide insight into health-related losses due to absenteeism and presenteeism. The search focus was on generic instruments; the search was not designed to identify instruments that report on condition-specific productivity loss, such as loss due to migraine, allergy, or angina, among others. The objective of this search was to provide additional detail on already existing articles or reference sources in this area and also to create a summary table that provides easy information at a glance.

Research Reviews on Health-Related Productivity Instruments

Four reviews were identified in the literature, including one guide (6) and three articles (5,7,9). The IHPM produced the *Measuring Employee Productivity: A Guide to Self-Assessment Tools* booklet in 2001 (6). This guide, edited by Lynch and Riedel, presents an in-depth look at seven instruments that were actively being used in research projects or practice applications in 2001. It provides information on each individual instrument, compares the instruments, presents psychometric properties of the instruments, and presents the actual questionnaires themselves.

The three review articles on self-report instruments designed to measure health-related productivity loss take a similar approach to reviewing measurement instruments for health-related productivity loss, but do so in slightly differing ways. Lofland and colleagues (5) identify health-related productivity loss survey instruments and consider them in the context of metrics that are suitable for direct translation into a monetary figure. Prasad and coworkers (9) review the literature in this domain with an emphasis on patient-reported outcome measurement and the effect of illness on productivity in both work and nonwork activities. Lastly, Mattke's team of researchers (7) reviews the evidence on the availability of health-related productivity loss instruments and the validity and reliability of those currently used in research. Table 18.1 presents an overview of these resources.

Compilation of Individual Health-Related Productivity Instruments

Across the four reviews, a variety of health-related productivity instruments were identified. Lofland and colleagues (5), Lynch and Riedel (6), Mattke and coworkers (7), and Prasad and researchers (9) identified 11, 7, 20, and 6 survey instruments, respectively. Given the overlap among these resources and the goal of this review to identify generic (not condition-specific) tools, a subset of 13 instruments was selected. These instruments, along with several key characteristics, are outlined in table 18.2 to enable practitioners to identify a good fit for their program.

Psychometric Properties

In selecting a survey instrument, practitioners should consider the psychometric properties of the tool. Psychometrics refers to the validity and reliability of the assessment tools and provides a degree of confidence that the instrument in question consistently measures what it was intended to measure. Many of the health-related productivity instruments currently available are relatively new

in their design. As a result, data on their psychometric properties are generally lacking.

Three psychometric properties of self-reported health-related productivity instruments are of particular interest:

- *Reliability* (or reproducibility) refers to agreement among repeated measurements—in other words, the instrument yields the same results when applied multiple times. A good instrument should yield the same value if applied repeatedly under similar circumstances.

- *Validity* provides insight into the extent to which the instrument measures what it is intended to measure. A good instrument should yield the correct value; hence, being reliable is not good enough if the results are consistently wrong.

- *Responsiveness* indicates the extent to which the instrument can accurately measure change over time.

A fourth important feature is acceptability. *Acceptability* refers to the degree to which the intended users will accept the questions and agree to complete the survey. Especially when their work productivity is being documented, employees may not accept questions that are perceived as invasive or use wording not consistent with a corporate culture despite the fact that as a measurement tool these questions are valid and reliable. It is therefore advisable for any company to examine the actual wording of the instruments under consideration and perhaps even to run some focus groups or informal tests to feel comfortable with employee acceptance before making a final selection.

There are several types of statistical tests that may be applied to these measurement indicators. Basically, these tests all involve the amount of error in the measurement. Consider that there exists a true value of the health-related productivity for every employee. Every employee has a certain level of work performance during a certain time frame. The true value of that work performance for every employee is often unknown; only the measured value may be available, such as the value obtained via self-report (using one of the instruments in table 18.2). Any discrepancy between the true value and the measured value is measurement error. As a result, the more that is known about the psychometric (or measurement) properties of a specific instrument, the more

Table 18.1 Overview of Four Major Reviews on Health-Related Productivity Instruments

Year of publication	Comments on the identified resource
2004	Resource: Review article
	Reference: Lofland, J.H., Pizzi, L., and Frick, K.D. A review of health-related workplace productivity loss instruments. *Pharmacoeconomics.* 2004;22(3):165-84.
	Purpose of the resource: This article identifies health-related workplace productivity loss survey instruments, with particular emphasis on those that capture a metric suitable for direct translation into a monetary figure.
	Number of instruments discussed: 11
	Brief description of the resource: An in-depth literature search and telephone-based survey of business leaders and researchers were conducted to identify health-related workplace productivity measurement survey instruments. The review was conducted from a societal perspective (considering policy implications), and each identified instrument was reviewed for reliability, content validity, construct validity, criterion validity, productivity metrics, instrument scoring technique, suitability for direct translation into monetary figures, number of times, modes of administration, and disease states in which it had been tested.
2001	Resource: Review guide booklet
	Reference: Lynch, W., and Riedel, J.E., ed. *Measuring Employee Productivity: A Guide to Self-Assessment Tools.* Scottsdale, AZ: Institute of Health and Productivity Management; 2001.
	Purpose of the resource: This guide presents and reviews self-assessment instruments used in research settings that are designed to estimate work performance and detect the effects of health on performance and productivity.
	Number of instruments discussed: 7
	Brief description of the resource: This guide provides an overview and in-depth discussion of self-assessment tools designed to measure worker productivity. All tools reviewed qualified for inclusion by having been or by being in process of serious validations as of the spring of 2001. The tools were identified through literature searches, contact with researchers in the field, and discussion with employers. The authors found no previously published list of tools, so this guide may be regarded as the first available review on this topic. The guide presents detailed information on the tools, the general areas of productivity measured, and the psychometric properties and includes the actual questionnaires (some of the guidelines include directions for scoring, special versions of the tool, and requests from the authors of the tools about sharing of results).
2007	Resource: Review article
	Reference: Mattke, S., Balakrishnan, A., Bergamo, G., and Newberry, S.J. A review of methods to measure health-related productivity loss. *American Journal of Managed Care.* 2007;13:211-7.
	Purpose of the resource: This article systematically reviews the instruments used to measure productivity loss and its costs.
	Number of instruments discussed: 20
	Brief description of the resource: This article is a systematic review of the published and gray-market research literature from 1995 through 2005 on methods for estimating productivity loss and monetizing that loss. The identified survey instruments include some that have been validated. Conclusions recognize the challenges of measuring presenteeism, noting that these far exceed those associated with absenteeism primarily because many jobs do not have easily measurable output. Methods to estimate the costs of lost productivity were also identified, although none of these appear to have been validated according to the authors.
2004	Resource: Review article
	Reference: Prasad, M., Wahlquist, P., Shikiar, R., and Shih, Y.-C.T. A review of self-report instruments measuring health-related work productivity. *Pharmacoeconomics.* 2004;22(4):225-44.
	Purpose of the resource: This article provides a comprehensive assessment of productivity instruments available in the current literature that attempt to measure health-related work outcomes with an emphasis on patient-reported outcomes.
	Number of instruments discussed: 6
	Brief description of the resource: A review of the literature from 1990 through June 2002 was conducted to identify published articles focusing on instruments measuring health-related work impairment or productivity, including both presenteeism and absenteeism. Evidence of psychometric properties was found to a varying degree, informing the field of the need for additional research in this area.

Table 18.2 Health and Productivity Measurement Instruments

Instrument name	Number of items measured	Recall duration	Response burden	Access
American Productivity Audit (APA) and Work and Health Interview	9 (3 for absenteeism and 6 for presenteeism)	2 wk	Moderate	Proprietary
Endicott Work Productivity Scale (EWPS)	25	1 wk	Low	Proprietary
Health and Labor Questionnaire (HLQ)	30 (4 modules: absence from work, reduced productivity, unpaid labor production, and labor-related problems)	2 wk	Low to moderate	Proprietary
Health and Productivity Questionnaire (HPQ)	44	1 wk and 4 wk	Low to moderate	Proprietary
Health and Work Questionnaire (HWQ)	24 (6 modules: productivity, concentration and focus, supervisor relations, impatience and irritability, work satisfaction, and nonwork satisfaction)	1 wk	Low to moderate	Proprietary
Health-Related Productivity Questionnaire Diary (HRPQ-D)	9	1 wk	Low	Proprietary
SF-36	36 (8 items on the SF-12 are specifically related to productivity)	4 wk	Moderate	Proprietary
Stanford Presenteeism Scale (SPS)	35 (exclusive focus on presenteeism is often combined with questions on absenteeism)	4 wk	Low to moderate	Proprietary
Work Ability Index (WAI)	7	12 mo	Low	Proprietary
Work Limitations Questionnaire (WLQ)	25 (4 scales: time management, physical, mental, interpersonal, and output demands)	2 wk	Low	Proprietary
Work Productivity and Activity Impairment (WPAI) questionnaire	6 (4 scales: percentages of time missed due to health, impairment while working, overall work impairment, and activity impairment)	1 wk	Low	Public domain
Work Productivity Short Inventory (WPSI)	15 conditions and 20+ questions	2, 12, and 52 wk	Moderate	Proprietary
Worker Productivity Index (WPI)	~40	Unable to assess	Unable to assess; instrument is specific to customer service employees	Unable to assess

informed the decision will be to select it as the instrument of choice and the more confident the practitioner may be in accepting the measurement results as the true values of work performance.

For the 13 instruments presented in table 18.2, information on the psychometric properties is varied. Many of the instruments have been validated and used in research studies to some degree. Of all the instruments presented, the SF-36 and the WPAI questionnaire appear to have been tested the most extensively. These instruments have been used most frequently, are available in many languages, and have been validated against each other. Other instruments with extensive documentation and acceptable psychometric properties are the HPQ and the WLQ. In all, most instruments have some degree of established validity or reliability, although data on responsiveness over time are not available as often.

Practical Application

As the worksite health practitioner or program administrator, you will recognize the importance of selecting the right instrument. It has to fit with the overall goals and objectives of your program measurement strategy, and some instruments may fit better than others. Depending on what kind of additional information you may have on the productivity of your workforce, self-report of health-related productivity may be more or less important for measuring program effect. Considering response burden, you may need to select an instrument that is brief. Alternatively, if the objective is to gain a deeper level of understanding of this domain, an in-depth, comprehensive tool may be needed. Is there a need to integrate the productivity assessment instrument into the overall health assessment tool? Does your health assessment vendor already have this capability in place? Does the vendor provide a productivity scorecard for reporting purposes and does the vendor report change over time? Regardless of the answers to these questions, considerable thought will go into the selection of the most appropriate

instrument for your company. Tables 18.1 and 18.2 will provide initial guidance to help you consider available resources.

Conclusion

This chapter has provided an overview of several excellent resources in the literature that practitioners may use to familiarize themselves with various options for a self-report health-related productivity instrument. Important considerations in selecting the right tool for any organization include the psychometric properties of the instrument, the response burden (completion time and effort) acceptable to both the company and the employees, the nature in which the instrument is implemented (part of an overall health assessment process, integrated into a single tool, and so on), and the reporting capabilities that complement the overall measurement and evaluation strategy.

Chapter Review Questions

1. Define, compare, and contrast absenteeism and presenteeism.

2. Explain what psychometric properties tell us about a particular self-report survey instrument.

3. Why is it important for a given instrument to have both acceptable reliability and acceptable validity?

4. If you were responsible for implementing a productivity assessment at your company and had to recommend an assessment tool to your executive leadership, which instrument from table 18.2 would you select? Explain your rationale and include the following program considerations: assume a program duration of at least 5 y, assume that completion of the survey will be allowed during work time, connect the productivity loss information to health risk factors, and express the productivity loss in monetary terms.

◄ **19** ►

Calculating the Economic Return of Health and Productivity Management Programs

Seth Serxner, PhD, MPH, and Daniel B. Gold, PhD

Sponsors of health and productivity management (HPM) programs need to know whether their programs are having the intended effect; however, with the range of results presented in the literature and by providers of HPM programs, it is hard to know what to expect. Even the literature has published broad ranges of program effect (3,6,8) on economic ROI as well as productivity measures. In this chapter, we address calculating the economic return of HPM programs. In doing so, we also cover the broader topic of assessing program effect. The real question that evaluators should ask is, "What value are we getting for our investment?" This, in turn, helps set a broader context for understanding ROI. Our recommendation is to view ROI as only one part of a more comprehensive approach to program measurement and evaluation.

A key value proposition of the measurement process is the resulting recommendations. Recommendations based on the measurement results support data-driven decision making. Program design and ongoing enhancement need to be based on well-founded research that is tested in applied settings.

Ultimately, even if we have the best measurement possible with the most rigorous methodology and the best possible program elements, if there is little to no program participation, there will be no program effect and no ROI. While participation is critical to program effect, so is engagement in the actual behavior change initiatives. Participation in a health assessment is the foundation to many programs, and high levels of participation are correlated with high program effect. Engagement in targeted behavior modification programs and completion of the program goals, on the other

hand, are critical to reducing risks and mitigating the process of people becoming less healthy (i.e., risk migration). Finally, successful implementation of a comprehensive program is essential to achieving desired effects on health service utilization and related claims costs.

The discussion that follows is structured around a three-step process titled *measure, monitor, and modify*. This approach gives a comprehensive assessment of program effect that provides the context for an economic analysis. We will review each phase in detail. To support the discussion, table 19.3 defines a set of terms that are used throughout.

Approach

The *measure, monitor, and modify* process is a measurement approach to HPM programs. HPM programs are broadly defined as those programs that span the continuum of health from *well* to *at risk* to *chronic conditions* to *catastrophically ill*. Typical HPM programs include personal health assessments, prevention and risk reduction programs, and disease and case management programs as well as any number of other elements such as incentives, campaigns, communications, educational materials, and environmental and organizational initiatives (10). One important issue to understand when measuring these programs is that they take place in an applied setting and not in a controlled laboratory. Therefore, the usual cornerstones of valid and generalizable research are undermined since there is rarely the opportunity for random assignment, control groups, stable program implementation, or consistent populations across a study duration (1). However, there are a number of ways to strengthen the approach, all of which build the credibility of the analysis of overall program effect and ROI.

Measure

The first step in the measurement process is to create a comprehensive, multiyear evaluation plan. This plan covers both process and outcome measures; the emphasis starts on process measures in the early phase and moves toward effect and outcome metrics in the later phases (table 19.1).

Because of the long-term nature of financial analyses (which typically require at least a full year of claims data and runout, for example), short-term metrics are necessary. Short-term metrics involve program participation and satisfaction, which provide a strong sense of whether the program is on track to achieve the financial targets.

A comprehensive evaluation strategy supports the economic analysis and gives us confidence in the savings projections. To build the credibility required to present financial savings projections, it is necessary to explain results in the context of the program's causal chain of events. Theoretically

the process involves participation in a program, satisfaction with the program in order to continue participation, participation in risk-related programs, increased knowledge and positive behavior change, improvement in health risks, change in health service utilization, and claims reduction. Measuring details of program participation, such as program modality (delivered online, by mail, by telephone, or on-site), program type (seminars, campaigns, or individualized coaching), and program element (health assessment, lifestyle management, disease management, nurse line, or on-site clinics) as well as integration (program referrals), is critical to measuring the relationship between program effect and ROI.

HPM programs affect more than just direct medical costs. Productivity data can be incorporated into the financial analysis but should be conducted as a separate analysis in addition to the direct health care claims analysis. This way the audience members can make their own judgment on the value of incorporating productivity into the overall economic return to the organization. The details of productivity measurement are beyond the scope of this discussion, but it is worth noting that productivity encompasses a range of measures, including absence, disability (both

Table 19.1 Comprehensive Program Measurement Plan

Short-term measures (0-12 mo)	Intermediate-term measures (13-24 mo)	Long-term measures (2-5 y)
Program delivery Process flow Program cross-referrals	**Program delivery** See short-term measures	**Program delivery** See short-term measures
Participation Baseline utilization Participant characteristics	**Participation** Repeat program utilization Characteristics of repeat participants Completion rates	**Participation** See intermediate-term measures
Awareness Program awareness Name and brand recognition Program perception	**Awareness** See short-term measures	**Awareness** See short-term measures
Program satisfaction	**Program satisfaction**	**Program satisfaction**
Effects Knowledge, attitudes, beliefs Self-efficacy Behaviors	**Effects** Change in health Health status Health risks Clinical values	**Effects** See intermediate-term measures Effect on organizational culture
Baseline analyses Relationship between poor health and excess	**Outcomes** Health care utilization Lost work time Productivity Employee turnover Employee satisfaction and culture	**Outcomes** See intermediate-term measures Medical costs Trend ROI

List is of sample metrics and is not meant to be all inclusive.

occupational and nonoccupational), and presenteeism. Some of the measures are documented processes and others are self-reported.

Another way to think about these measures is to consider leading and lagging indicators. Leading indicators tend to be process measures, such as participation, that provide information as to whether the program will deliver effect in the future. The lagging indicators are those measures that occur some time following the behavior change. Lagging indicators tend to be outcome measures such as change in health status and health care costs. The financial indicators, which are examples of lagging indicators, involve claims data categorized by point of service (inpatient, outpatient, emergency room, and so on) and available at the individual level. This individual level data access enables the linking of participation data to claims. Clinical metrics are somewhere in between leading and lagging measures. Changes in biometric values (blood pressure, cholesterol levels, blood glucose, and so on) can occur within a short time after a behavior change occurs and translate into lower health care costs in the future.

In addition to leading and lagging indicators, you have operational measures, or measures that assess program delivery. Although there is an obvious connection between program delivery and the ability to deliver outcomes, monitoring these measures is an important piece in demonstrating the entire value proposition. Typical operational metrics include data such as call center statistics (data taken in or sent out, frequency, quantity, time to answer, dropped calls), member contact (number of attempted calls, outbound calls, inbound calls, mail-based contacts, e-mails), reporting, and account management. Member satisfaction often falls into this category and ideally should be based on not only members who are completing a program but also members who dropped out or declined participation.

The previous discussion on data implies a process and an infrastructure to integrate the data for analysis and reporting. While it is possible to rely on a single source for reporting, often that falls short on the organizational demand for measurement. A data warehouse or decision support system can facilitate the process. One of the main benefits of a data warehouse is the ability to generate individual-level integrated reporting across multiple carriers, programs, and outcome measures.

There are three broad data categories that make up the integrated data record. The first cat-egory, eligibility data, involves individual demographics such as age, gender, employee status, job location, job type, and tenure. This category can also include health risk status and chronic disease conditions. The second broad category of data is program participation and engagement. The participation data involve all potential program offerings, from health assessments, wellness campaigns, interventions, and on-site clinics to disease and case management. As the programs become more integrated, the participation data might also include disability management. In addition to knowing the actual program participation, it is valuable to understand the level of engagement. For example, is the individual participating in coaching or counseling sessions telephonically or participating in a self-directed module online? Finally, the third category encompasses the outcome measures. The outcome measures involve medical and drug claims at a level of detail allowing for an analysis of health service utilization categories. Health care claims data are often the primary measure of financial effect that will be linked to program participation, while adjusting for individual differences. However there are any number of other valuable outcome measures, such as those having to do with absence, disability, and safety. In some cases, the health assessment may have collected self-reported productivity data as well. Likewise, information on health status, gathered through claims analysis or self-reported health assessment, also provides important outcome measures. Table 19.2 describes these three categories of an integrated database.

Monitor

The monitoring process is the process in which the analysis of program effect occurs. This analysis and interpretation can consist of several levels of rigor, depending on the needs of the audience (sponsor), the maturity or evolution of the program, the access to data, and the availability of resources. Some organizations require a very detailed economic and data-driven business case to justify program investment, while others do not. Some organizations may also believe that conducting an analysis is difficult and expensive and are therefore more comfortable with strong reporting rather than strong analyses. As noted in the comprehensive evaluation plan presented in table 19.1, an outcome or ROI analysis is probably not worth conducting until well after the program has been implemented and has been meeting participation targets. There is little value

Table 19.2 HPM Integrated Database

Eligibility, individual	Participation, engagement	Outcomes, financial
Age	Health assessment	Medical claims
Gender	Lifestyle management	Drug claims
Employee status	Disease management	Behavioral health claims
Location	Case management	Disability
Job type	On-site clinics	Absence rate
Tenure	Nurse advise line	Productivity and presenteeism
Health risk and status	Wellness campaigns and seminars	

in assessing a program with low participation, poor implementation, missing components, or poor execution. Evaluation also requires access to historical data on health care claims and program participation. An evaluation may be limited based on the availability of this historical data. Merging data to create individual-level claims and participation records can be a challenge if eligibility files are not consistent and if individual identifiers have not been systematically protected.

There are numerous levels at which monitoring can take place. The first level of monitoring simply involves the review and understanding of the metrics and methodology used in the reporting of programs. For example, the definition of program participation can include those who were identified for a program, those who were eligible, those who were eligible and did not decline participation, or those who actively engaged in the program for a set duration. Understanding how participation is defined allows more appropriate comparison with benchmarks and helps build the causal chain toward outcomes. The causal chain, or value proposition, is the underlying process by which the intervention has an effect on outcomes. Understanding the level of program participation and delivery is also an important factor in setting the context for reviewing the reported ROI, which is why assessment of program effect requires a broad understanding of the entire causal chain. For example, scorecards or dashboards allow for the identification of key metrics to build the case for the reported outcomes. Scorecard metrics can involve participation, satisfaction, health risk, health status, and disease stratification data, all compared with a benchmark such as a relevant previous time frame, performance goals, and client-defined targets or industry-based best-practice standards.

The second level of monitoring involves an aggregate claims analysis. This is a process of

reviewing the selected methodology, confirming that the data used are appropriate, and checking that the analysis complies with expectations (e.g., with a contractual methodology). In a sense this is a third-party peer-review process of checking the math and confirming whether the results are consistent with other metrics of engagement, risk migration, and change in utilization. Often this process involves working to provide more transparency to the methodology and the definition of metrics used in an analysis. As part of this process the reviewer might decide to change some of the assumptions used in the model, thereby changing the results substantially. For example, a national trend may have originally been used in the review of a disease management financial reconciliation. However, the reviewer might find that this trend is significantly different from the experience of the given organization. By changing the trend to a client-specific trend in order to align the analysis with the experience of the organization, the results are likely to change dramatically. In this case, the lower the trend used, the lower the projected savings and the lower the ROI, which may have implications for performance targets.

The third level of monitoring is an individual-level claims analysis or outcomes study. This is the most resource-intensive and rigorous level of analysis. The process involves having access to individual-level claims data and linking those claims to eligibility files and participation data as described in table 19.2. Any meaningful analysis will require several years of data (ideally, at least 2 y of data before program implementation to establish a baseline and at least 1 y of data post-implementation, operations, or reporting time frame). Individual-level analyses that compare program participation of different groups over time require enough members in each group to make the analysis meaningful. Currently there are no standardized cutoffs to the sample size requirements. Sample size requirements can be calculated using statistical power analyses, but even those analyses need to be considered within the context of what is statistically meaningful in an applied setting.

Regardless of which level of review is being conducted, much consideration should be given to the ROI methodology used in a given report. This area of HPM program evaluation has drawn considerable attention as of late, given the increase in program adoption and the promise of significant program effect via ROI. Skepticism of reported ROI often has come from the absence of reporting information on the causal chain as well as from methods lacking scientific rigor, particularly in the disease management arena (4). The following is a description of the key areas of consideration in a review of ROI methodology. The first issue is to determine what is being evaluated. This may seem obvious, but if a program is limited to a questionnaire and education materials, it may not be worth conducting an individual-level claims analysis. On the other extreme, if the intervention is comprehensive, involving multiple programs, it is probably well suited for an equally comprehensive individual-level claims analysis.

In terms of determining the financial effect of HPM programs, two broad categories of methodology have been described: *population based* and *individual level* (9). The population-based approach is most common in disease management and applies actuarial modeling to create a health care cost trend for what would have happened in the absence of a program. A trend is applied to a baseline chronic group experience before program implementation. That application of trend to baseline creates a projected cost for the program year, which is then compared with the actual cost. The difference between the projected and the actual costs in the chronic population is considered to be the savings generated by the program. The Disease Management Association of America (DMAA) has recently published a set of guidelines that describes its recommendations regarding the population-based approach (5). While the population-based approach has been the standard in disease management, there are a number of concerns about the methodology. One major concern is that there is a heavy reliance on using a trend to project what future costs would have been had there been no program, and the ability to determine an accurate trend can be a challenge. The most common approach is to use the trend of the nonmanaged (nonchronic) population and apply it to the managed or chronic group. Depend-

ing on how the managed and nonmanaged groups are defined, their trends can differ significantly (2). In addition to the issue of trend, there is the issue of how to attribute savings when more than one program is being implemented. For example, if an organization has implemented a disease management program and a health management program (health assessments, lifestyle management, educational campaigns, and so on), it may be misrepresentative to attribute all the savings to the disease management program. Therefore, while a population-based approach has some appeal in terms of its practicality and feasibility, there are serious concerns among sponsors about accuracy and sensitivity.

In comparison to the population-based approach, an individual-level approach provides greater accuracy, including confidence intervals and statistical significance around the findings, as well as the ability to attribute specific results to each program component while statistically controlling for demographics such as age, gender, and comorbidity. The individual-level approach uses a quasi-experimental design and multivariate statistics to determine program effect. Worth noting is that the individual-level approach requires more integrated data than the population-based approach requires and that the statistical analysis may be less intuitive than a trend-based model. Regardless of which approach is used, both methods address some common themes.

One of the most important themes to address within the methodology is the time frame for the baseline as well as the definition of the baseline. In many disease management financial reconciliations the baseline (preprogram implementation) is only 1 y. This is problematic due to concerns around regression to the mean and the variability in claims data. Disease management programs in particular are highly susceptible to this issue due to the natural progression of disease. For example, the typical disease management program identifies individuals with appropriate conditions through medical and drug claims analysis that looks for triggering events such as hospital admissions that indicate an individual has a given condition. The common utilization and cost cycle is that following the high-cost events the member costs decrease due to the standard care process. Therefore, regardless of any program intervention, the year (or months) following a trigger event generally demonstrates significantly lower utilization and costs. The bias that regression to lower cost introduces can be mitigated by introducing new high-cost members into the analysis in the program year to offset the low costs. This is still not enough to fully address the bias; rather, it is the standard population-based approach in disease management. However, extending the baseline an additional 12 mo in order to include claims before the trigger event is another way to address the issue. For disease management, a retrospective cohort for the baseline can be created by identifying those individuals in the 24 mo before the program launch. By using 12 mo of identification and 24 mo of claims, the low-cost claims before the trigger event average with the high-cost claims to produce an overall cost that is lower per member per month. When conducting HPM analysis on the individual level the methodology is not dependent on the identification of certain individuals, and therefore the baseline can be enhanced by averaging the member experience over the 24 mo before the program launch.

A recent study conducted by the RAND Corporation and Mercer (7) revealed that baseline length and trend adjustment had the greatest effect on results when holding all other parameters constant. As indicated earlier, the use of a population-specific trend is critical when conducting a population-based analysis. That specific trend can be determined using actuarial adjustments for age, gender, and plan design. There also needs to be an understanding as to whether the trend is for the total population or for the nonmanaged and nonchronic population. The effect of trend is less dramatic but still important in a statistical model. In the individual statistical model the trend, or inflation factor, is used only to normalize the baseline U.S. dollars to the program-year value. Once the baseline dollars have been brought up to the value of the program-year dollars, any differences between baseline and program year or between participants and nonparticipants cannot be attributed to general changes in health care costs. Ideally, the client-specific factor is used to inflate baseline dollars to program year, but if necessary the medical CPI supplied by the U.S. Bureau of Labor Statistics will suffice (11).

Another important issue to address while conducting an economic effect analysis is the eligibility and definition of the study population. This issue involves specifying the number of months an individual has to be in the medical plan to be considered for the analysis. The study population will change substantially between an eligibility requirement of 12 mo and a requirement of 1 mo. The rationale for requiring a certain level of eligibility has to do with making certain there has been enough program exposure or opportunity for

exposure as well as with providing a stable basis for creating an average claims cost. Typically, individuals who are new to the organization tend to have lower claims than those of individuals who have been with the organization longer. While there is some variation on approach to this issue, our recommendation is to use an eligibility of 6 mo with no gaps in coverage greater than 30 d depending on how the data are collected. An eligibility of 6 mo allows for enough opportunity for program exposure while not biasing the study group to look differently from the majority of the participants. Furthermore, the definition of a chronic member may not be consistent across programs. As discussed earlier, the trends between identified and nonidentified disease members can differ significantly or can be similar depending on this definition. Using an annual requalification methodology is most consistent with using a nonidentified group trend for comparison and is currently the recommendation of the DMAA (5).

Excluding certain high-cost conditions, such as trauma and organ transplants, is a common practice in program evaluation. Likewise, capping high-cost claims (i.e., truncating claims greater than a certain value) is a common practice. Both exclusions and capping affect the outcome of an analysis. The difficulty with excluding certain conditions is determining which conditions to exclude and whether to exclude the member or just the claims related to the condition. Our recommendation is to not exclude high-cost conditions such as traumatic automobile crashes or organ transplants and, if there are exclusions, to conduct the analysis both with and without those exclusions to understand their relative effect. There are several sources listing key conditions for exclusions (5,9). One important condition that is often excluded is pregnancy. We do not recommend excluding pregnant members. Excluding costs related to pregnancy may possibly be appropriate, but in many cases interventions are supposed to help improve the pregnancy experience, and therefore pregnancy costs should not be removed.

We recommend a similar approach to claims capping. In general, we prefer not to cap high-cost claims since they are a true reflection of the payer's experience and many interventions are aimed at reducing the number and absolute value of high-cost claims. However, high-cost claims can simply reflect random outliers that can bias an analysis. This may be particularly true in smaller sample sizes. Therefore, we recommend conducting the analysis with and without capping to determine the relative effect of capping as well as the value of the capping for the baseline and program year for participants and nonparticipants. In terms of the specific process of capping, we recommend that rather than using an arbitrary value such as $100,000 U.S., capping be performed at 99.9% of all claims.

Finally, one of the most difficult issues to deal with in conducting economic analyses of HPM programs is determining the degree to which program costs are influenced by the program versus other factors such as network discounts or carrier changes. To address this issue we recommend a utilization-based analysis. In this approach the focus is on understanding the program effect on health care utilization in points of service such as inpatient hospitalization, outpatient visits, emergency department visits, office visits, and prescription drug use. The process involves taking the utilization statistics and multiplying them by a unit cost specific to the point of service in order to derive a cost by point of service for a given individual. Those utilization-based claims costs are then used in the statistical or population-based analyses.

After focusing on this rigorous methodology for determining the economic effect of HPM programs, it is important to remember that financial effect is a function of reduced utilization, which in turn is a product of improved health status and reduced health risks. Therefore, in addition to conducting a financial analysis, it is important to have some measure of risk or health status effect that can be used to confirm that the changes in costs are consistent with the changes in health status. There are many clinical risk tools that can be applied to a population to understand the health and risk trends in the population accounting for demographic characteristics (12).

Modify

The result of the monitoring process is a better understanding of the effect of the overall program and the program components and of the opportunities for improvement. Often the key opportunity lies with improving engagement, targeting a given condition, or modifying a given protocol to better meet the needs of the population. Measurement and evaluation should be an act of continual process improvement. Data-driven identification of opportunities for program improvements need to be understood and acted upon appropriately.

The key to the monitoring phase is to interpret the raw data and analysis in meaningful and actionable ways. The real value of the process comes from providing context for the findings and providing the ability to make specific recommendations for modifications that can be implemented to improve outcomes. In some cases these recommendations may be to terminate a given program. Not all programs will work for all populations at all times. There may be important reasons why a given program should be halted and another should be promoted more aggressively. Neither action can be taken without having a data-driven process to inform the decision making.

Measurement and Evaluation Activities

There are several additional applications of measurement and evaluation that follow from the previous discussion and may be relevant to sponsors of HPM programs. The first is selecting a program provider. Provider reporting and measurement methodology can provide differentiation between providers and create a basis for comparison. This also applies to how providers might project savings. Ultimately, requiring a specific and consistent methodology for financial performance guarantees also takes the ambiguity out of the process as well as guides the reporting requirements.

Provider assessments are another by-product of a clearly established measurement and savings methodology. Conducting an independent third-party review of the provider reports can be a way to establish credibility of reported results and to confirm that the provider is meeting service obligations. There are three levels of review that range in resource requirements and rigor. The first level involves a simple review of the provider reports that focuses on consistency and comprehensiveness. Observations and recommendations should be part of the review output. A second level of review involves confirming that the provider used the appropriate methodology, that the provider calculations were correct, and that the vendor provided aggregate data so that the evaluation can replicate the analysis. In some cases, adjustments may also need to be made to the analysis. For example, a client-specific trend might replace a national trend or a 2 y baseline might replace a 1 y baseline. The third level of independent third-party review involves merging individual-level health care and HPM participation data to conduct an analysis in addition to any provider analysis. This claims-based analysis would generate the economic savings based on the specified methodology to establish an additional point of reference to the reported savings.

General Discussion

This chapter addressed the assessment of the economic effect of HPM programs from a comprehensive framework. Across the industry, measurement is affected by different terminology and associated definitions of terms. Sometimes, differing terminology creates confusion as assumptions may be incorrectly linked to definitions of terms that are not what is expected. For purposes of providing clarity, we have outlined a series of key terms associated with economic analysis and ROI calculations. These terms are presented in table 19.3, which is a list of terms that are commonly used in the economic evaluation of HPM programs. It is important to note that some of these terms may be defined differently in different settings or by different organizations, but for the purposes of this chapter, the following definitions are used.

One key message in this chapter was that the economic analysis is a subcomponent of the overall program evaluation, and without the supporting context the economic results have less credibility. When reviewing the economic outcomes of a program, one of the first things to understand is where the results come from. For example, how many people participated in the intervention and what was the intervention? Does it make sense that the number of people participating in the type of intervention implemented can generate the savings indicated?

The second message was that ROI analyses are a subcomponent of the economic analysis and likewise need to be viewed in context. The chapter discussed the issues surrounding the calculation of savings or of the return portion of the ROI. Of note is that while much of the focus of ROI is on the *R,* or savings, the calculation of the investment is just as important since ROI is a ratio of costs and savings. For example, to engage most programs requires staffing, communications, incentives, and participant time, which often is on company time. These cost factors are inconsistently used as part of the analysis. Most reported figures include only the vendor fees in the ROI calculations. Even many published studies don't provide a comprehensive accounting of all costs, making comparisons among reported program results difficult.

Another theme in this chapter was that a significant data infrastructure is required to conduct measurement and evaluation. In most cases managing data can be challenging in that there are usually several data sources being combined over multiple years. Add to that the complexity of a dynamic study environment that includes plan and carrier changes, employee turnover, and program design modifications, and data management becomes even more challenging. One approach is to be very focused on the question being addressed. If the question involves the effect of program participation on health care costs, then there may be no need to collect biometric data or program satisfaction measures. Knowing the audience members and their required level of rigor in the analysis can also help guide the data management. However, in most cases there will be a need to integrate data into one analytic set for either a one-time study or an ongoing evaluation.

Another point made in this chapter was that methodological approaches can be at the population or individual level. Population-level analyses have the advantage of using readily available aggregate data. Individual-level analyses, on the other hand, offer several advantages over the population approach. The most important advantage is that the analysis can more accurately demonstrate the relationship between program participation and outcomes (e.g., financial, behavioral, or clinical outcomes) while accounting for individual-level characteristics such as age, gender, and job tenure. Controlling for the double-counting savings by categorizing the participant results to specific programs, using a trend to project savings, and not accounting for person-level factors are significant trade-offs in using the population-level approach.

The last significant theme throughout this chapter had to do with the sensitivity of evaluation methodologies. There are a number of methodological parameters that significantly affect the outcome of an economic analysis. These include the length of the baseline, the calculation of a trend or an inflation factor, the member eligibility, the exclusion of selected medical conditions, and the handling of high-cost outliers. We have made recommendations on these issues in this chapter and elsewhere (9) and continue to review data to determine the best approach for each specific circumstance. Our recommendation is to conduct analyses with and without some of these design constraints in order to determine the relative effect on the outcomes of excluding select medical conditions or capping high-cost claims. This approach provides a range of savings, and then, given the context, the evaluator can focus on a given methodology.

Table 19.3 Terms Commonly Used in HPM Programs

Term	Definition
Participation	Participation in HPM programs such as health risk assessments, lifestyle coaching, and disease and case management.
Engagement	A broad term that encompasses any form of individual involvement in behavior that is consistent with health and productivity initiatives. The primary form of engagement is program participation, but engagement could also include supporting others in participation, communicating about the programs, referring to programs or resources, using tools and resources, or being involved in related activities.
Return on investment (ROI)	ROI is a financial metric that involves the ratio of the financial benefits or savings to the costs of the program or services that generated the savings. For example, a 1:1 ROI means that for every $1 U.S. invested there was a $1 U.S. return (a cost neutral effect), whereas a 2:1 ROI means that for every $1 U.S. invested there was a $2 U.S. return (a positive ROI).
Absenteeism	The act of not being physically present at work. This is measured in hours or days, and the definition of absenteeism may vary by organization.
Presenteeism	The act of being physically present at work, but not necessarily being productive. Different levels of presenteeism are measured in terms of how productive an individual is while being physically present. Presenteeism is expressed as the loss of productivity while being present at work. For example, a person with a terrible headache may be present at work but not be very productive and therefore is considered to a higher level of presenteeism as compared to another person who feels healthy, is focused and on-task.
Lagging indicators	Indicators or measures that take a longer time to result from a given action. An example is effect on utilization, which may lag a year or longer behind a positive change in behavior such as improving eating habits.
Leading indicators	Measures that occur shortly after a behavior takes place and that have a strong relationship with lagging indicators. Participation in a health risk assessment and lifestyle management program are leading indicators. Change in health risk is a leading indicator when compared with change in utilization, which lags health risk.
Measure, monitor, and modify Phase 1 Phase 2 Phase 3	An evaluation process that involves three phases: *measure* involves identification of metrics, targets, and data collection. *monitor* involves the analysis of the data. There are varying levels of rigor regarding the monitoring; these are described as levels 1, 2, and 3. *modify* refers to insights and recommendations yielded from the interpretation of the previous phases.
Population-level claims analysis	Analysis that is conducted on group or population levels. An example is comparing the average change in total costs of a group from one year to another.
Individual-level claims analysis	Analysis that compares changes or characteristics of individuals as opposed to changes or characteristics of groups. An example is comparing the change in average cost per member per month for individuals who participated in a health assessment with the change in the same cost of those individuals who did not participate.
Claims capping or truncating	A process in which health care claims included in an analysis are assigned a value or cap, which if exceeded will be assigned the cap value. For example, if the cap is $100,000 U.S. and an individual has claims of $125,000 U.S., the individual's claims would be transformed or capped at $100,000 U.S. for the analysis.
Trend	Generally, this term refers to the health care cost difference in at least two points in time. An example of a common usage is, "The trend increase between 2006 and 2007 was 10%."
Confidence intervals	Statistical values that represent the probability of a result occurring within a specified range.
Quasi-experimental design	An experimental design that does not have random assignment but does have pre- and post-intervention measures as well as a comparison group.

(continued)

Table 19.3 *Continued*

Term	Definition
Regression to the mean	A statistical phenomenon occurring during repeated measurements of the same individuals in which subsequent scores tend to shift toward the group average. For example, high-cost claimants in one year will typically have lower cost claims in subsequent years that look more like the average claims of the group regardless of any external intervention.
Medical consumer price index (CPI)	An index that represents medical cost inflation as a subset of a broad CPI.
Utilization-based analysis	An evaluation methodology that applies a standard unit of service cost to the quantity of services used to determine individual costs. Individual costs are then used in the individual-level claims analysis.

Conclusion

The bottom line is that measurement and evaluation are conducted to provide actionable data-driven recommendations regarding program continuation, termination, or enhancement. Sponsors want to understand what they are getting for their investment. While we would like to have one simple metric, such as ROI, judge program performance, the reality is that HPM programs are complicated strategies implemented in dynamic environments with inconsistent data. The best we can do is to apply multiple measurement points and rigorous methodologies in order to provide a range of economic savings within a broader business context.

Chapter Review Questions

1. What is the real question evaluators are asking when they want to know the ROI?

2. What is the three-phase approach proposed for economic evaluation?

3. Name the key differences between the individual-based and the aggregate or population-based analyses.

4. What information beyond financial information can be used to build the context for ROI results?

5. What are some of the key parameters that affect the sensitivity of economic analysis?

20

Using Claims Analysis to Support Intervention Planning, Design, and Measurement

David H. Chenoweth, PhD, and Jeff A. Hochberg, MS

As the issue of cost justification has intensified at most worksites, so has the use of health care claims data as a tool for health management planning and evaluation. When used to its fullest extent, claims data analysis can be applied to all levels of health management, ranging from primary prevention to secondary prevention and treatment (3). The purpose of this chapter is to describe various opportunities and challenges associated with claims analysis and various ways to optimize the use of claims data to support employee health management initiatives.

Do It Yourself or Hire It Done

When program planners and administrators consider the use of claims analysis in the planning, design, and evaluation of their employee health management program, one of the first decisions to consider is whether to use in-house or external resources to conduct the analysis. Almost without exception, claims-based analyses are complex and time consuming and require expertise. Furthermore, employers must protect individual employee privacy and confidentiality when it comes to health-related and personal information and will certainly want to maintain a strong sense of integrity when it comes to these issues of employee relations. As a result, organizations planning to do in-house claims data analysis should first assess their resources to determine if it is operationally and financially feasible for them to do so. The major prerequisites for doing an in-house analysis include the following:

- Personnel members who are knowledgeable in risk identification and appraisal techniques
- Adequate time for personnel to request, acquire, review, and analyze the data
- Access to appropriate and complete claims data from insurers, third-party claims administrators (TPAs), and health care providers
- A teamwork approach in which personnel members from key departments (benefits, medical, safety, human resources, risk management, and so on) work together in reviewing and analyzing appropriate data in order to produce an objective report that has universal value
- A framework that guides analysts through a systematic and methodical step-by-step process to effectively conduct an analysis
- A process and set of safeguards that address any and all legal and regulatory requirements to ensure employee confidentiality and protection of personal health information

Requesting Appropriate Data

Although most midsize and large organizations receive *some* type of annual report on health care claims data from their insurers or TPAs, much of today's health care claims and cost data are long on numbers and short on information. This may be due, in part, to the company not asking questions that allow for the appropriate data and information to be analyzed and presented. On the other hand, insurers and TPAs may tend to limit their reports to those that meet standard requirements and not address unique issues related to the company specifically. Furthermore, little or no education is provided to the employers to help them understand how to properly interpret claims data reports (6). Whatever the circumstances, an organization is legally entitled to *request* and *receive* this important report card from their insurer or TPA in order to determine whether the insurer or TPA *is* processing and paying claims within the parameters of their contract. Moreover, all parties should understand that these reports are aggregate (group) reports that represent the entire population rather than identify individual workers or dependents.

To obtain useful data from the insurer or claims administrator, the employee health management staff should develop a corporate health care data analysis strategy consisting of the following phases and procedures (which are described in more detail later in this chapter):

Phase I: Cracking the Code

- Access and review any existing on-site claims reports.
- Determine what types of data are missing in existing reports.
- Develop goals for an analysis.
- Formulate questions for requesting data.

Phase II: Requesting the Right Information

- Request data from your insurer or claims administrator.
- Obtain data.
- Review data.
- Prioritize data of value.

Phase III: Thinking Strategically

- Analyze data.
- Identify key trends and challenges.
- Generate findings.
- Develop a report for key decision makers.

Defining the Types of Data to Consider

Unfortunately, many claims data reports provided to employers are generically formatted and provide little, if any, strategic planning value. Thus,

it is essential to request and obtain *several types* of claims and costs data to fully reveal the scope and specificity of an organization's real health care utilization and cost patterns.

Traditionally, organizations have asked only basic assessment questions when requesting claims data reports (4), such as the following:

- What are the most common types of claims?
- What are the most expensive types of claims?
- What is the average length of stay for the most common (inpatient) conditions?
- How did this year's overall cost compare with last year's?

Although the preceding questions may provide decision makers with information, they are confined primarily to the employer and offer no opportunity for external comparisons. In contrast, the following *problem-focused* questions are more likely to help identify specific problems and trends on a much broader spectrum:

- What are the most common claims by Major Diagnostic Category (MDC), Diagnostic-Related Group (DRG), and International Classification of Diseases (ICD) (5)?
- What are the most expensive types of claims by DRG or ICD?
- How does the outpatient utilization rate compare with local, regional, and national norms?
- What have been the fastest-growing outpatient claims in the past 5 y?
- What percentage of total health care charges for the top five outpatient MDCs were incurred by employees? Spouses? Dependent children?
- What percentage of charges for the top five inpatient DRGs are linked to lifestyle, environmental or occupational factors, genetics, and poor health care?
- If current trends continue, what will the organization's health costs be in the next 3 to 5 y?

As employers seek to gain more information from their claims data, they must request and obtain data beyond the scope of general MDCs. They must obtain *DRGs or ICDs within each MDC* in order to address important problem-focused questions (1).

Table 20.1 Percentages of Specific Groups by Enrollment, Number of Claims Filed, and Total Charges

Enrollee group	% of enrollees	% of health care claims	% of health care costs
Employees	40%	30%	25%
Dependents	50%	50%	45%
Retirees	10%	20%	30%

Early in the data request phase, it is important to know the composition of the organization's enrollee population (all persons enrolled in the company's health plans). If the organization provides health care benefits to dependents and retirees, be sure to request claims data reports that include (and hopefully differentiate) all enrolled groups. Essentially, this level of specificity reveals differences between and within each of the respective enrollee groups. For example, a typical profile may reveal differences such as those shown in table 20.1.

Given the profile of the organization, specific differences may be identified. It can then be determined if disproportionately more health care resources and dollars are being used by a certain group and what, if any, interventions or changes are necessary or may be warranted.

Making Sense of Medical Claims

Just as the overall success of any worthwhile endeavor is directly linked to the quality of the up-front planning process, successful analysis and application of medical claims data depend on a predefined strategy. For many practitioners, it is helpful to divide the process of medical claims analysis into three distinct phases. These phases address understanding the types of data already available, understanding the new data to be requested and obtained, and the culmination of turning the analytical work into a report to inform decision makers in the company.

Phase I: Cracking the Code

The first phase in making sense of the company's medical claims data is a general assessment of the health care claims information that is currently available to the organization. This means that you will have to identify and seek out the individual who serves as the keeper of the reports. Once the right individual is found, the existing claims reports need to be gathered, and then you need to roll up your sleeves and dive into the paperwork. As you'll soon see, the reports will be filled with all sorts of strange codes and numbers. To make matters worse, you will soon discover that few medical claims reports provide all the information that you need to conduct an accurate analysis. As a result, you'll not only have to wade through the existing data but also have to identify any additional information that will be required in helping you to gain a more accurate picture of your company's health care concerns. In fact, as important as medical claims reports are, you will soon see that the vast majority provide precious little information that is of any real value.

The big question looming is whether your program may benefit from the application of medical claims data. Chances are, if the program is anything like the majority of programs across the United States, meaningful medical claims data could be of great value. The problem is, deciphering the code that will reveal the value of this strategy can be more than a little tricky.

In order to begin phase I, you'll have to know and understand the differences among the standard types of medical claims provided to employers. In essence, there are three major classifications of medical claims—MDCs, DRGs, and ICDs. While the language can be a bit confusing, there is no need to be intimidated by these classifications. For clarification, a detailed description of each follows.

1. Major Diagnostic Categories (MDCs). MDCs make up a broad category that reflects various conditions, illnesses, or disabilities related to a particular body system (e.g., circulatory system, respiratory system, or musculoskeletal system). A complete listing of MDCs follows.

Major Diagnostic Categories

- Blood related
- Burns
- Infectious and parasitic
- Circulatory
- Mental
- Congenital
- Musculoskeletal
- Digestive
- Neoplasm (cancer)

- Ear, nose, and throat
- Nervous
- Endocrine, nutrition, and metabolic
- Pregnancy and childbirth
- Factors influencing health status
- Respiratory
- Female reproductive
- Male reproductive
- Genitourinary
- Signs, symptoms, and ill defined
- Injury and poisoning
- Skin and subcutaneous
- Hepatobiliary and pancreas

2. Diagnostic Related Groups (DRGs). Each MDC comprises 20 to 25 DRGs. Each DRG represents a *group* of similar diagnostic conditions, illnesses, or disabilities relevant to a particular MDC. One of the most common musculoskeletal DRGs is *medical back problems,* which, by its designation, includes a wide variety of back-specific conditions.

3. International Classification of Diseases (ICD). ICDs represent specific types of medical conditions, illnesses, or disabilities within a particular DRG (5) (see figure 20.1). For example, the DRG known as *medical back problems* contains numerous ICDs. Collectively, there are more than several thousand ICDs across the full spectrum of DRGs. Thus, it's not uncommon for a particular DRG to contain several hundred ICDs.

So there you have it—MDCs, DRGs, and ICDs. Understanding the three classifications that are used to formulate medical claims reports will enable you to confidently review any existing on-site claims data and understand what they represent. While the language is somewhat cumber-

some, it's important that you get comfortable with these codes if you plan on having any success in making sense of your medical claims. At this time, it may also be a good idea to consider whether you will need additional help from either in-house or external expertise.

Understanding the concept of MDCs, DRGs, and ICDs is the easy part. Believe it or not, the real challenge begins once you make your requests for additional information from your insurer or TPA. This brings us to the second phase of making sense of your claims data.

Phase II: Requesting the Right Information

While wading through the existing claims information is challenging, the second step—making your request for additional information known (and heard)—can be equally challenging. While this step might seem like a no-brainer, it's not. In fact, obtaining additional information above and beyond the standard reports that your insurer or TPA provides will take political acumen, perseverance, and, in some instances, tenacity (2). If you are fortunate enough to obtain the additional claims information, it's now time to immerse yourself in the data.

Most employers receive their claims reports formatted solely by MDCs. As you will recall, MDCs are generic classifications that do not reveal the specific nature of a person's diagnosis, condition, or disease. By breaking MDC claims data into DRGs or ICDs, you can identify specific conditions, illnesses, or disabilities, such as backache, high blood pressure, and diabetes, and be able to more effectively target health promotion and disease management and be able to demand management efforts around prominent and costly claims. In summary, the second important step in

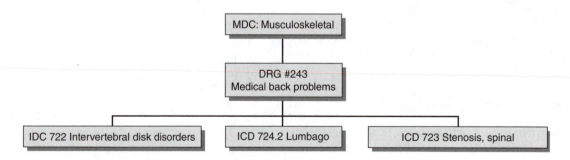

Figure 20.1 A condensed view of a MDC, DRG, and ICD hierarchy.

making sense of your medical claims is a matter of soliciting—in their entirety—the appropriate claims data. Once the requested information is in hand, you can turn your attention to reviewing and prioritizing this data.

Phase III: Thinking Strategically

As you might have guessed, the third step in making sense of your medical data is a detailed analysis of the actual claims themselves. This detailed analysis is conducted for the express purpose of identifying future strategic directions for your company's health promotion programming efforts. If done well, this analysis will serve as a blueprint to improving the health and well-being of your employees. Ultimately, this final step culminates in the formatting of a concise and readable report for key decision makers.

In your quest to make sense of your company's health care claims, you have identified the medical claims data that you currently possess and the additional data that you need. Furthermore, you have formally submitted your request for supplemental information to your insurer or TPA. Once the additional data have been received, you are finally in a position to begin using the data strategically.

As you begin to immerse yourself in the data, it may be helpful to recognize that at this point most health promotion practitioners feel like they have wandered into a strange and confusing land. While there is little guidance to help you make sense of it all, there are some tips and techniques that can make the process a whole lot easier:

- Develop a spirit of inquiry. For most people, making sense of the medical data is a new but very important skill. You'll need to develop an optimistic spirit of inquiry if you expect to learn more and, at the same time, stay energized.

- Look for trends and correlations. Once you get comfortable with the layout and content of the actual reports, begin looking for trends and major cost centers. With concentrated attention, you'll be amazed at what the data will reveal. Focus on conditions that are treatable. There are numerous acute and chronic medical concerns that fall outside of lifestyle-related issues. For example, focusing on congenital birth defects may not be prudent in planning an employee health promotion initiative. However, highly treatable conditions such as musculoskeletal complaints (e.g., low-back pain) make for a fertile area of concentration.

- Monitor reports consistently. While claims data are important to the success of any health promotion initiative, few practitioners use them effectively. If you are to be successful, you'll need to commit to the process and regularly monitor the data.

- Embrace ambiguity. When it comes to obtaining medical claims data, the entire process is riddled with ambiguity. Health plans change and claims administrators come and go. What's more, the way that claims data are stored and reported constantly changes. All of this can spell frustration for practitioners. Still, progressive-minded health promotion professionals wrestle with this ambiguity and make the best of it.

Case Study

A county government on Florida's gulf coast utilized several outsourced vendors to provide claims administration, health risk appraisals, workers' compensation administration, pharmacy benefits management, disease management, absence management, and more. Each vendor provided periodic summary reports, but the employer could not integrate the information to identify health, productivity, and cost trends across the workforce. RiskFlag (from the Outcomes Group)—a Web-based health care solutions support tool that enables health and productivity management professionals to enact workforce intervention strategies based on a total picture of an employee's health conditions, health care system utilization, health risks, productivity, and work injury history—was used to create a list of candidates who were highly likely to incur excess costs due to health-related or functional problems. The Web-based system integrated, queried, and stratified data from distinct health care and human resource data sets, flagging those individuals who meet research and evidenced-based profiles indicative of impending health cost, productivity decrease, or workplace injury. Consequently, a trend toward particular workplace injuries was identified and a targeted intervention was recommended to the client.

Beyond Claims 101—The Opportunities

When the field of prospective medicine was conceived in the early 1960s, there was virtually nothing to guide data analysts in calculating the costs of major risk factors. Eventually, the traditional model of risk-factor influence was born and provided data analysts with a *relative* understanding of how lifestyle, environmental, genetic, and health care factors can influence a person's health status. Yet, in most cases, it was customary to link major risk factors to a *single* influence, such as obesity with lifestyle. Eventually, this one-to-one (unilateral) concept gave way to a more contemporary concept known as *multi–risk factor causation,* which is based on the premise that many illnesses and diseases are caused by *multiple* risk factors across the lifestyle, genetic, environmental, and health care spectrum. Thus, by subjecting group-level claims data to various analyses, program and policy decision makers can better identify and address the root causes of health care demand and associated costs. Figure 20.2 depicts this process.

The Proportionate Risk Factor Cost Appraisal

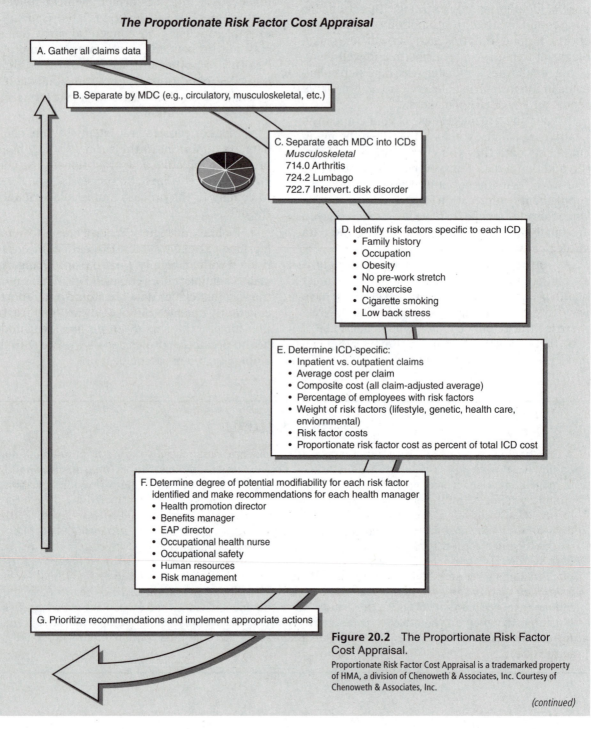

A. Gather all claims data

B. Separate by MDC (e.g., circulatory, musculoskeletal, etc.)

C. Separate each MDC into ICDs
Musculoskeletal
714.0 Arthritis
724.2 Lumbago
722.7 Intervert. disk disorder

D. Identify risk factors specific to each ICD
- Family history
- Occupation
- Obesity
- No pre-work stretch
- No exercise
- Cigarette smoking
- Low back stress

E. Determine ICD-specific:
- Inpatient vs. outpatient claims
- Average cost per claim
- Composite cost (all claim-adjusted average)
- Percentage of employees with risk factors
- Weight of risk factors (lifestyle, genetic, health care, enviornmental)
- Risk factor costs
- Proportionate risk factor cost as percent of total ICD cost

F. Determine degree of potential modifiability for each risk factor identified and make recommendations for each health manager
- Health promotion director
- Benefits manager
- EAP director
- Occupational health nurse
- Occupational safety
- Human resources
- Risk management

G. Prioritize recommendations and implement appropriate actions

Figure 20.2 The Proportionate Risk Factor Cost Appraisal.

Proportionate Risk Factor Cost Appraisal is a trademarked property of HMA, a division of Chenoweth & Associates, Inc. Courtesy of Chenoweth & Associates, Inc.

(continued)

During these same years, health management and human resource professionals have struggled to identify early on the individuals at the highest risk for increased health care utilization, impaired productivity, chronic disease, and workplace injury. It wasn't until the 1990s that research identifying the profiles of employees who populate these high-risk categories became available. As the body of research has grown, the industry of *predictive modeling* has emerged, bringing the capability to stratify populations based on many distinct data attributes. However, the population size necessary for the predictive modeling process remains upward of 50,000, with costs to run the models around the $100,000 U.S. mark.

Consequently, there was not an increase in the application of that research in the employer community, except at the largest employer level. Midsize and small employers, for the most part, found themselves excluded from utilization of the research and predictive modeling tools, unless they received such services as part of health plan strategies under fully insured considerations. Most self-insured small to midsize companies do not have ready access to these types of services and products.

Today, however, this market void has been addressed by products and services that provide sophisticated yet affordable technologies and interpretive functions. Thereby, these products provide support to the small and midsize self-insured employer market. Any size employer can integrate distinct data sets, run queries seeking to identify highest risk employees, and target interventions to the most appropriate subsets of the workplace. Trending of data over time and reporting of outcomes from interventions can also be part of the services provided.

Conclusion

While the idea of using medical claims data to guide corporate wellness programming is often discussed, the reality is that very few practitioners actually do it. We believe that the major reason why so few people rely on this important source of data is that the vast majority simply do not understand how or where to get the reports and what to look for once they have the information in hand. By making the commitment to follow the simple three-phase process outlined in this chapter, you can confidently embrace the challenge of making sense of your company's medical claims data. A case study describing the experience of a Florida county government has been provided to highlight how the claims-based strategy may be used.

Chapter Review Questions

1. Distinguish between basic assessment questions and problem-focused questions.

2. Briefly explain several factors you should consider before choosing to do an in-house analysis.

3. Identify several advantages of obtaining claims data coded by DRGs or ICDs compared with MDCs.

4. Describe 2 or 3 ways you can use claims data analysis to improve employee and organizational health status.

Part

IV

Program Design and Implementation

Part IV presents a series of chapters focused on the main message of this book—specific guidance in designing and implementing evidence-informed worksite health programs. Part I provided important issues and factors to consider that relate to the context of a worksite health program. Part II introduced you to the role of evidence of effectiveness and how to consider such evidence in the application of practice (i.e., real world program implementation). In Part III, the importance of considering evaluation design prior to implementation of the program was delineated and approaches to selecting the right assessment and measurement tools were discussed. Part IV is organized to provide insight into the "what and how" of program design and implementation while keeping the topics of Parts I, II, and III in mind.

Chapter 21 focuses on organizing consumer, employee and employer data to optimize participation, and engagement in interventions. Chapter 22 addresses the role of behavior change theory in program design. Chapter 23 addresses the idea of a culture of health with a focus on the importance of ensuring that healthy workers maintain their health and do not increase their health risks over time. Chapter 24 explores the alignment and connection of the worksite health program and the core business objectives of the company. Chapter 25 addresses diversity in the workplace. Chapter 26 extends the discussion on a culture of health in the worksite setting by presenting a definition and considering how to create and sustain it. The emergence of technological solutions in a web-based or online environment is addressed in Chapters 27 and 29—Chapter 27 introduces you to the use of technologies in creating online communities with a focus on health whereas Chapter 29 places its major focus on how to implement online technologies to optimize health benefit design and provide incentives for employees to participate. Chapter 28 presents an in-depth discussion on incentives and includes a set of principles that help guide program design and implementation. Chapter 30 is heavily focused on the promise of integrating worksite health promotion and occupational safety and health and not only provides compelling arguments for companies to do so, but also presents an in-depth overview of the research to support such an argument. Chapter 31 addresses the role of the built environment in worker health. Medical self care is presented in Chapter 32 and Chapter 33 provides a focus on disease management. This section of the book presents many components across multiple chapters and therefore Chapter 34 is designed to pull all of these topics together in a single overview on how to design, coordinate, implement, evaluate, and report on a comprehensive worksite health promotion program.

The organization of Part IV of this book allows for easy access to a variety of specific topics when you are searching for information on any one of those. However, it also pulls all of these topics together into a single chapter that may be helpful when you are trying to uncover where in the context of a comprehensive program any single topic should be positioned.

21

Organizing Intelligence to Achieve Increased Consumer Engagement, Behavior Change, and Health Improvement

Stephanie Pronk, MEd

Do we know consumers well enough to get them to engage in health improvement programs, change their behavior, and, as a result, improve their health? Case studies tell us that successes are possible, but overall reported participation rates remain low. Why is that? As an industry, worksite health promotion has been very focused on the amount of health care costs consumers incur, health care utilization patterns of consumers, and conditions and risks consumers may have. This information provides good insight on the problems and concerns that underscore the need for solutions; however, it does not necessarily provide the critical data elements or information to support consumers in changing behavior and sustaining that behavior over time. It is fair to conclude that there is an emerging need to expand and organize data and information intelligence differently in order to boost participation rates and truly affect population health.

In the United States, of the trillion dollars spent on health care, 95% goes directly to medical care services for treatment of illness and injury, while only 5% is allocated to disease prevention. Interestingly, 70% of all chronic and acute diseases are caused in part by lifestyle behaviors, such as smoking, overweight and obesity, and physical inactivity (7). Lifestyle choices and patterns exert a major influence on the overall health of the population (3,7).

Understanding individual consumers and working with them to change their health and care-seeking behaviors require different data and methodologies than health care management use today. This chapter introduces new and innovative ideas in how to organize and use a broader set of data to engage consumers, change behaviors, and improve health. Specifically, this chapter addresses four areas. First, we explore a whole new level of consumer insight by leveraging traditional and nontraditional data and turning these data into a multidimensional view of the consumer. Second, we discuss data segmentation strategies for identification and stratification that support identifying unique characteristics of a population, selected target groups, and specific individuals at a higher level of accuracy and connect the consumer to the right intervention. Third, this chapter presents an overview of an engagement approach that uses data to develop deep insights into consumer habits, practices, and attitudes and then uses the information in ways that consumers view as personally relevant and nonintrusive and that prompts consumers to take the right actions to maintain, improve, or manage their health. Finally, the activities related to tracking, measuring, and reporting program effect are discussed. This approach allows for a feedback loop that connects experience to continued database enrichment over time. Figure 21.1 depicts the overall approach (9).

Creating a Multidimensional View of the Consumer

Who really knows consumers? What industries or organizations are good examples of truly understanding their customers and consumers? Without a doubt, the retail and product industries

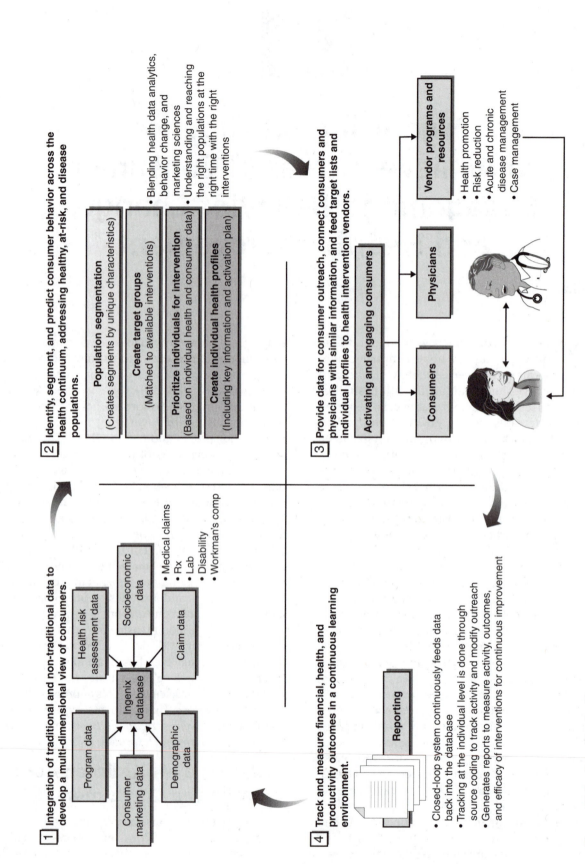

1 Integration of traditional and non-traditional data to develop a multi-dimensional view of consumers.

- Medical claims
- Rx
- Lab
- Disability
- Workman's comp

Program data
Health risk assessment data
Socioeconomic data
Consumer marketing data
Ingenix database
Demographic data
Claim data

2 Identify, segment, and predict consumer behavior across the health continuum, addressing healthy, at-risk, and disease populations.

Population segmentation
(Creates segments by unique characteristics)

Create target groups
(Matched to available interventions)

Prioritize individuals for intervention
(Based on individual health and consumer data)

Create individual health profiles
(Including key information and activation plan)

- Blending health data analytics, behavior change, and marketing sciences
- Understanding and reaching the right populations at the right time with the right interventions

3 Provide data for consumer outreach, connect consumers and physicians with similar information, and feed target lists and individual profiles to health intervention vendors.

Activating and engaging consumers

Consumers
Physicians
Vendor programs and resources

- Health promotion
- Risk reduction
- Acute and chronic disease management
- Case management

4 Track and measure financial, health, and productivity outcomes in a continuous learning environment.

Reporting

- Closed-loop system continuously feeds data back into the database
- Tracking at the individual level is done through source coding to track activity and modify outreach
- Generates reports to measure activity, outcomes, and efficacy of interventions for continuous improvement

Figure 21.1 Organizing intelligence.

demonstrate this understanding. Businesses such as Wal-Mart, Target, Macy's, Nordstrom, Best Buy, Pepsi, Coca-Cola, General Mills, and others (the list could go on and on) not only know their audience but also have developed a combination of art and science in using consumer data through database direct marketing to truly understand and influence consumers' choices, buying behaviors, and purchasing patterns. Thus, the health improvement industry needs to look to and learn from these other industries that truly understand the consumer. The retail and product industries are at the transparency intersection of revolutionizing how consumers engage and buy, how products are sold, and how social and business networks collaborate due to robust data, advanced technologies, and accelerating consumer demands (1).

Let's explore the type of consumer data and information from the retail and product industries needed to create a multidimensional view of consumers that would allow us to drive higher engagement, successful behavior change, and improved population health. Combining traditional health and health care data with nontraditional consumer marketing data allows us to develop deep insights into consumer habits, practices, and attitudes; to use this information to build trust-based relationships with consumers; to improve the health of consumers; and to successfully change and sustain desired health behavior. When we look at consumers from only a clinical perspective (e.g., by using only claims-based data), we merely consider them from a single view and we'll certainly miss the opportunity to understand them as consumers of health promotion products. By leveraging multiple new sources of consumer data, we will gain new dimensions in understanding the target populations that will allow for more accurate population health analyses, targeted outreach, and prioritization of consumer segments for intervention.

There are many publicly available consumer marketing data sources available today. Companies such as Acxiom, Fair Isaac Corporation, PATH Institute Corporation, and many others provide data, supporting technologies, and consulting services to help businesses understand and reach their target audience. Typically, these organizations research, develop, purchase, and combine massive amounts of information on consumers. This information ranges from demographic characteristics (such as occupation, household income, age, gender, home owner versus renter, children, marital status, mortgage amount and date, ethnicity, and so on) to specific consumer behaviors (such as lifestyle characteristics, shopping behaviors, health conditions, commuting distance, mail-order and Internet purchases, charitable contributors, and so on). By combining data we use in health today with the powerful consumer data available from these sources, we will begin to understand the why of consumer behaviors that will allow tailoring of health messages, programs, and approaches in ways never possible before.

As a result of the integration of the multiple data sources, we will move from a one-size-fits-all tactic that has long been the industry standard to a data-driven methodology that provides a multidimensional, individualized, and tailored health approach for every consumer in a personally relevant and meaningful manner. In other words, health messages, programs, and activities will meet consumers where they are at, where they direct their attention, and where they place their preferences.

Segmentation, Identification, and Stratification

In order to move away from a one-size-fits-all intervention approach, segmentation, identification, and stratification approaches need to be rethought and formulated differently. As a result of the integration of multiple data sources and the new ability to understand the consumer at this multidimensional level, the types of analyses performed for population segmentation, target group identification, and individual-level prioritization and stratification are changing. Let's explore how.

The population segmentation analysis is intended to discover what is unique about and distinguishes a particular subpopulation. Typically, health care claims and risk data are used to understand a population, but this approach produces very similar results from one population to another; while rank order may differ, typically population analyses find relatively similar risks and conditions. Combining traditional and nontraditional data sources creates the opportunity to find very unique and distinguishing characteristics of a population or various subpopulations. Statistical techniques that identify and single out the most powerful variables in one consumer cluster versus another cluster in a given population reveal the structures and variables in the data that are unique. This approach provides the data and information to review the characteristics of unique population clusters across the health continuum by providing a deeper understanding of the health drivers, health needs, and distinctly relevant health and consumer characteristics.

In the context of health interventions, the segmentation approach provides the data intelligence to perform gap analyses on the types of programs, delivery modes, language needs, and so on needed to support a given population. The data may reveal that a specific consumer cluster needing smoking cessation services is much more likely to respond favorably to a Web-based intervention than to a group-based program. By providing these types of population analyses, an organization is able to not only understand its unique population clusters but also provide evidence-based information that helps select the most appropriate interventions, activities, and approaches for the overall population or the subpopulations.

The target group analysis is intended to identify specific targets within a population. Unlike the population segmentation analysis, target group analysis requires health, clinical, and specific business logic to be developed in order to identify target groups and match them to available health and care interventions. In addition, budget requirements are introduced into the rule set to determine appropriate investment tactics.

Once target groups have been identified, the next analysis applies stratification rules in order to prioritize individuals for outreach within a given target group. By using this multidimensional data-driven approach, stratification takes on a completely new meaning. Stratification not only assesses severity of risks, conditions, readiness to change, and motivation to engage but also takes into account consumers' priorities, attitudes, and values. Moreover, it considers the way a consumer thinks, responds, and behaves. All this is consolidated not only through the prioritization of interventions but also through the creation of individual profiles of consumers within each cluster. These profiles are subsequently linked to personally relevant and meaningful communications created to support tailored health and care interventions.

Outreach and Engagement Techniques

For consumers to engage and participate in health and care programs or to make appropriate health and care decisions, they must have easy access to accurate, timely, and personally relevant information. Additionally, they must be prepared and ready to turn that information into action. How information is presented may be as important as what information is presented (2).

Besides considering the data relevancy strategies that retail and product industries use in engaging consumers, the health and care management industry needs to consider its marketing techniques. The health and health care industry typically has used mass marketing to build awareness and educate consumers. Mass marketing is a low-involvement marketing technique. It sends the same message to everyone and is largely a one-way communication that doesn't support building a long-term relationship that is directly relevant to adopting and sustaining new behaviors. The industry has also used targeted marketing to engage narrowly defined consumer segments with specific messages (6).

Recently, tailored health messaging has been introduced, and it has become clear that tailored messaging holds great promise for engaging, changing, and sustaining behaviors and improving health (4). The theory and science behind tailored health messages and materials are that consumers are more likely to actively and thoughtfully process information if they perceive it to be personally relevant. Compared with nontailored messages, tailored messages are more likely to be read, remembered, saved, discussed, and perceived by readers as interesting, relevant, and having been written especially for them (5). Tailored materials have been found to affect behavior change more than nontailored materials affect such change.

In the marketing space, one-to-one marketing creates different and highly personalized messages for every consumer and allows for a deeper, more trusting relationship to develop (8). Relatively new to the marketing horizon is consumer-centric marketing. The goal of this type of marketing is to develop deep insights into consumer habits, practices, and attitudes and then use the information to build trust and change behavior (6). Just think of the strength and potential effects of incorporating consumer data intelligence (outside of traditional health risks, costs, and condition information used today) with consumer-centric marketing that uses the tailoring science to produce the gold standard of individually effective behavior change and health improvement messages, materials, and programs.

Integrated Tracking and Reporting Using a Closed-Loop System

The health and care management industry grew up in silos (3). Every vendor had its niche of expertise (worksite wellness, health risk assessment, lifestyle behavior change, decision support, nurse line, disease management, case management, and so on) that was respected and admired by others, and by and large, everyone stayed in their own space. The motto driving the industry was, "We specialize in . . . !" This setup tended to bring many best-in-class companies together at the level of the customer. Today, the industry is increasingly being consolidated, and the resulting companies consider themselves (or at least market themselves) as being a comprehensive solution to market needs and demands. In effect, the motto has turned into, "We are a single solution!" This setup brings integration to the level of the vendor. Unfortunately, all too often the integration is not delivered at the level of the company, mainly due to the limitations of technologies needed to truly integrate the data. Given how the industry grew up, the data, systems, and technologies vary greatly, and consolidation has created very real and expensive challenges. Many organizations discover that the data, the data systems, and the technology platforms are not designed to work together—let alone integrate. The fact is that the industry is not well connected and integrated, especially as it relates to a comprehensive health improvement program that focuses on healthy, at-risk, and disease populations.

Unfortunately, this situation impedes implementations and limits the effectiveness of the health programs for consumers and the organizations that invest in them. Developing an approach that creates the foundation for programs to work together and simultaneously eliminates redundancies would add significant value to the industry. Clearly, creating a tracking and reporting system that learns while it operates, grows, evolves, improves its ability to understand and influence consumer behaviors, and documents improvements in health, short- and long-term behavior change, and bottom-line return on health would bring a much-needed innovation to the industry.

Creating this type of reporting incorporates data collection, data processing, identification, stratification, prioritization, delivery, and reporting into a closed-looped system. Figure 21.2 shows the configuration of a comprehensive closed-loop system of this kind (9). This system enables continuous improvements in population identification and outreach, driving increased ROI and health outcomes. Developing a comprehensive system that allows tracking and reporting of intervention activity, messaging and outreach effectiveness, integrated health and financial outcomes, and effectiveness of specific intervention program components at the population, target group, and individual levels would propel the industry to higher standards of performance.

Conclusion

The combination of traditional and nontraditional data intelligence creates an opportunity for a continuous learning environment. Organizing intelligence to create a multidimensional view of the consumer allows us to understand and influence health behavior and optimizes the process for population, target group, and individual behavior change across the entire health continuum. It will also provide insights on health needs and gaps for specific populations, target groups, and individual consumers. This organization of data and information intelligence should be used to identify, match, and prioritize individuals for health interventions and to create individually tailored messages, health profiles, and programs that allow more successful health behavior change. In addition, by organizing, integrating, and centralizing the data intelligence, more comprehensive measurement approaches can be created in order to measure intervention activity, health and financial outcomes, and effectiveness of specific components and characteristics of behavior change interventions.

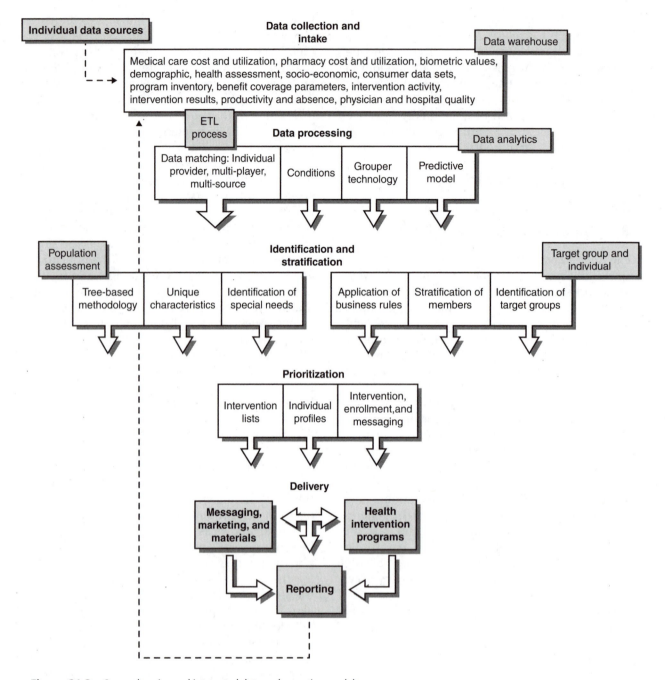

Figure 21.2 Comprehensive and integrated data and reporting model.

Chapter Review Questions

1. What factors contribute to the health and care management industry's inability to know consumers at the level needed to change behaviors?

2. What is the typical marketing approach used today in the health and care management industry?

3. How does the new approach to population segmentation help find the unique and interesting characteristics of a specific population?

4. What challenges exist today impede the industry's ability to influence and change consumer behavior?

5. How can we use integrated traditional and nontraditional data sources to make programs, activities, messaging, and materials personally relevant to the individual consumer?

22

The Application of Behavior Change Theory in the Worksite Setting

Karen Glanz, PhD, MPH

Worksite health promotion programs provide important opportunities to provide employees and their families with information, motivation, skills, and supportive environments to enhance their health. Worksites have several advantages as settings for health promotion interventions: They are convenient for workers, they can harness social support and social influence among coworkers and management, and they enable follow-up, monitoring, and reinforcement (10). For employers, a healthier workforce is more productive and satisfied and may incur lower health care expenditures. Nonclinical community settings such as worksites are now widely recognized as being important settings for health promotion, especially with the growing and widespread concerns of obesity and diabetes (16).

Successful programs are most often based on a solid understanding of the workforce and the influences on employee health behaviors, and this understanding is often acquired most efficiently by applying health behavior theories. This chapter introduces contemporary theoretical bases for health behavior change programs in worksite settings and discusses their applications in practice. More specifically, this chapter (a) introduces key concepts related to the application of behavior change theory in understanding and improving health behavior in worksites, (b) describes several current theoretical models that can be helpful in planning and conducting worksite health programs, and (c) highlights important issues and constructs that cut across theories.

The Importance of Understanding Influences on Health Behavior

Interventions to improve health behavior can be best designed when the designer has an understanding of relevant theories of health behavior change and the ability to use them skillfully (12). Emerging evidence suggests that interventions developed with an explicit theoretical foundation are more effective than those lacking a theoretical base (2) and that some studies combine multiple theories (18).

Four theoretical models are identified that are currently in use and are particularly useful for understanding the processes of changing health behavior in worksite settings: the social cognitive theory, the stages of change construct from the transtheoretical model, the theory of planned behavior, and the social ecological model (12,21). The central elements of each theory and the ways in which these theories can be used to help formulate worksite health promotion interventions are described in this chapter.

Multiple Determinants of Health Behavior

Many social, cultural, and economic factors contribute to the development, maintenance, and change of health behavior patterns. No single factor or set of factors has been found to adequately account for why people eat healthily or do not eat healthily, smoke or do not smoke, and exercise or do not exercise. Knowledge, attitudes, reactions to stress, and motivation are important individual determinants of health behavior. Families, social relationships, socioeconomic status, culture, and geography are other important influences. A broad review of key factors and models for understanding behavior and behavior change can provide a foundation for well-informed worksite health program, help identify the most influential factors for a particular employee or type of worker, and enable employers to focus on the most salient issues.

Multiple Levels of Influence

It is now generally recognized that health promotion interventions are more likely to be effective if they embrace an ecological perspective (21,27). That is, they should not only target individuals but also affect interpersonal, organizational, and environmental factors influencing health behavior. This is clearly illustrated in the context of employees purchasing food and eating during the workday. Employees may bring their food with them from home or buy food from workplace cafeterias and vending machines. Their choices are influenced by personal preferences, habits, nutrition information, availability, cost, and placement, among other things. The process is complex and determined not only by multiple factors but also by factors at multiple levels.

Traditionally, health promoters focused on intraindividual factors such as a person's beliefs, knowledge, and skills. Contemporary thinking suggests that looking beyond the individual to the social milieu and environment can enhance the chance of successful health promotion (27) and that such an approach fits particularly well in worksite settings. Program planners can and should work toward understanding the various levels of influence that affect employees' behaviors and health status. This will be discussed further later in this chapter.

What Is Theory?

A theory is a set of interrelated concepts, definitions, and propositions that presents a systematic view of events or situations by specifying relationships among variables in order to explain and predict the events or situations. The notion of generality, or broad application, is important (12). Even though various theoretical models of health behavior may reflect the same general ideas, each theory employs a unique vocabulary to articulate

the specific factors considered to be important. Theories vary in the extent to which they have been conceptually developed and empirically tested.

Theory can be helpful when planning, implementing, and evaluating interventions. Theories can be used to guide the search for reasons why people are or are not being physically active, smoking, or obtaining routine recommended health screenings. They can help pinpoint what you need to know before working effectively with an employee or a group of workers. They also help to identify what should be monitored, measured, or compared in evaluating the efficacy of interventions.

Explanatory and Change Theories

Theories can guide the search to understand *why* people do or do not practice healthy behaviors, help identify *what* information is needed to design an effective intervention strategy, and provide insight into *how* to design a program so it is successful (12). Theories and models help *explain* behavior as well as suggest how to develop more effective ways to influence and *change* behavior. These types of theory often have different emphases but are quite complementary. For example, understanding why an employee smokes is one step toward a successful cessation effort, but even the best explanations aren't enough by themselves to fully guide change to improve health. Some type of change model will also be needed. All of the theories and models described in this chapter have potential as both explanatory models and change models, though a given theory might be better for one or the other purpose. For example, the theory of planned behavior was originally developed as an explanatory model, whereas the stages of change construct was conceived to help guide planned change efforts.

Important Theories and Their Key Constructs

There are several available and widely used models and theories of behavior change that are applicable to workplace intervention. This section describes four theoretical models that are currently in use and make unique contributions to the interventionist's tool kit. As mentioned earlier, they are the social cognitive theory, the stages of change construct from the transtheoretical model,

Table 22.1 Statements Representing Theoretical Approaches to Health Behavior Change

Theory	Statements
Social cognitive theory	If the company provides a fitness facility or arranges for reduced-cost fees at a nearby gym, employees may find it easier to keep a regular exercise regimen. The use of incentives or point systems for reaching specific fitness milestones—especially if they involve team cooperation—can provide additional reinforcement.
Stages of change	If smokers feel that the time is right and are ready to change, they will probably be more successful at quitting.
Theory of planned behavior	If an individual who plans to get a mammogram at the company health clinic or screening van specifies what, when, how, and where she will be screened by making an appointment, she is more likely than a woman with a more general plan to follow through on the mammogram. Furthermore, if she thinks that her supervisor will be supportive of her getting screened during the workday, her motivation will be higher.
Social ecological model	If healthful food is easily available and low in cost, and the company provides good cooking and food preparation facilities, workers will be more likely to follow healthy eating patterns.

Adapted from K. Glanz, B.K. Rimer, F.M. and Lewis, (eds.), 2002, *Health behavior and health education: Theory, research and practice,* 3rd ed. (San Francisco: Jossey-Bass), 583.

the theory of planned behavior, and the social ecological model. Table 22.1 provides illustrative statements of the application of each theory.

Social Cognitive Theory

Social cognitive theory (SCT), the cognitive formulation of social learning theory that has been best articulated by Bandura (5), explains human behavior in terms of a three-way, dynamic, reciprocal model in which personal factors, environmental influences, and behavior continually interact. SCT synthesizes concepts and processes from cognitive, behavioristic, and emotional models of behavior change, and so it can be readily applied to nutritional intervention for disease prevention and management. A basic premise of SCT is that people learn not only through their own experiences but also by observing the actions of others and the results of those actions. Key constructs of SCT that are relevant to worksite health programs include observational learning, reinforcement, self-control, and self-efficacy (12).

Principles of behavior modification, which have often been used to promote health behavior change, are derived from SCT. Elements of behavioral interventions that are based on SCT constructs of self-control, reinforcement, and self-efficacy include goal setting, self-monitoring, and behavioral contracting (4). Goal setting and self-monitoring seem to be particularly useful components of effective interventions.

Self-efficacy, or a person's confidence in his or her ability to take action and to persist in that action despite obstacles or challenges, seems to be especially important for influencing efforts toward health behavior change (4). Worksite programs can incorporate deliberate efforts to increase patients' self-efficacy by using three types of strategies: (1) setting small, incremental, and achievable goals; (2) using formalized behavioral contracting to establish goals and specify rewards; and (3) providing for monitoring and reinforcement, including incentives and patient self-monitoring by keeping records. The use of financial incentives for smoking cessation has been found successful at increasing participation as well as quitting success in worksite programs (13,29).

The key SCT construct of reciprocal determinism means that a person can be both an agent for change and a responder to change. Thus, changes in the environment, examples of role models, and reinforcements can be used to promote healthier behavior. This core construct is also central to social ecological models and is more important today than ever before.

Stages of Change

Long-term changes in health behavior involve multiple actions and adaptations over time. Some people may not be ready to attempt changes, while others may have already begun implementing changes in their smoking, diet, physical activity, and so on. The construct of stages of change is a key element of the transtheoretical model of behavior change and proposes that people are at different stages of readiness to adopt healthful behaviors (25). The notion of readiness to change, or stages of change, has been examined in health behavior research and found useful in explaining and predicting changes in smoking, physical activity, and eating habits (11,14,26).

Stages of change is a heuristic model that describes a sequence of steps in successful behavior change (25): precontemplation (no recognition of need for or interest in change); contemplation (thinking about changing); preparation (planning for change); action (adopting new habits); and maintenance (ongoing practice of new, healthier behavior). People do not always move through the stages of change in a linear manner—they often recycle and repeat certain stages. For example, individuals may relapse and go back to an earlier stage depending on their level of motivation and self-efficacy.

The stages of change model can be used both to understand why employees might not be ready to attempt behavioral change and to improve the success of health promotion. Patients can be classified according to their stage of change by their responses to a few simple questions. For example, a health counselor examining readiness for dietary change might ask patients if they are interested in trying to change their eating patterns, thinking about changing their diet, ready to begin a new eating plan, already making dietary changes, or trying to sustain changes they have been following for some time. By knowing their current stages, the counselor can determine how much time to spend with each employee, whether to wait until he or she is more ready to attempt active changes, whether to make a referral for a group program or in-depth nutritional counseling, and so on.

Another application of the stages of change model in worksites involves conceptualizing entire organizations along the continuum of stages according to their leaders' and members' (i.e., employees') readiness for change (24). A recent study applied the organizational stages of change construct to provincial health authorities in Canada. The authors found substantial variance among individual managers within the same organizations and observed that organizational readiness did not predict how well health promotion was addressed (6). These authors concluded that assessing individuals' stages of change might be more useful. More studies of this issue may further inform program planners on which way to go.

Theory of Planned Behavior

Often people's health behavior choices are influenced by how they view the actions they are considering and whether they believe important others such as family members or peers would approve

or disapprove of their behavior. The theory of planned behavior (TPB), which evolved from its predecessor, the theory of reasoned action (TRA), focuses on the relationships between behavior and beliefs, attitudes, subjective norms, and intentions (23). The concept of perceived behavioral control involves people's beliefs about whether they can control their performance of a behavior (23)—that is, people may feel motivated if they feel that they can do it. A central assumption of TPB is that behavioral intentions are the most important determinants of behavior (1).

TPB has been applied widely to help understand and explain many types of behavior. The theoretical constructs of attitudes, behavioral beliefs, and behavioral beliefs about certain behaviors such as eating have also been examined within community interventions (8) and found to mediate outcomes of the interventions. The constructs help explain why some people change and others do not after a health communication campaign.

Although the idea that behavioral intentions are important is central to TPB, there has been some concern that they are too far removed to be good predictors of actual behavior. The concept of implementation intentions involves encouraging patients or people receiving an intervention to be very specific about how they would change. One recent worksite smoking cessation study found that providing implementation intention prompts worked best for people who were motivated to quit at baseline (3).

Social Ecological Model

The last conceptual model is the social ecological model, which helps to explain factors affecting behavior and also provides guidance for developing successful programs through social environments. Social ecological models emphasize multiple levels of influence (such as individual, interpersonal, organizational, community, and public policy) and the idea that behaviors both shape and are shaped by the social environment (21,27).

The principles of social ecological models are consistent with social cognitive theory concepts that suggest that creating an environment conducive to change is important to making it easier to adopt healthy behaviors (5). Given the potential effect of worksite environments on employees' health behaviors, a focus on social and physical environmental contexts has received increasing attention (7,9,28).

Selecting Appropriate Theoretical Models

Effective health promotion depends on marshaling the most appropriate theory and practice strategies for a given situation (12). Different theories are best suited to different individuals and situations. For example, when attempting to overcome an employee's personal barriers to increasing physical activity, the theory of planned behavior may be useful. The stages of change model may be especially useful in smoking cessation interventions. The choice of the most fitting theory or theories should begin with identifying the problem, goal, and units of practice—it should *not* begin with simply selecting a theoretical framework because it is intriguing or familiar. The use of a systematic planning process such as intervention mapping can be helpful in developing and evaluating theory-based worksite health programs (17).

When it comes to practical application, theories are often judged in the context of activities of fellow practitioners. To apply the criterion of usefulness to a theory, most providers are concerned with whether it is consistent with everyday observations (12). In contrast, researchers usually make scientific judgments of how well a theory conforms to observable reality *when empirically tested*. Health promotion planners should review the research literature periodically to supplement their firsthand experience and colleagues' advice.

A central premise in applying an understanding of the influences on health behavior to behavior change programs at worksites is that you can gain an understanding of an individual through an interview or a written assessment, and then you can better focus on that individual's readiness, self-efficacy, knowledge level, and so on. Clearly, it is necessary to select a short list of factors to evaluate, and this list may differ depending on the program focus, worksite context and policy, or the person's clinical risk factors. Once there is a good understanding of the person's cognitive and behavioral situation, an individual-level intervention can be personalized, or tailored. The challenge of successfully applying theoretical frameworks in worksite health programs involves evaluating the frameworks and their key concepts in terms of both conceptual relevance and practical value. The integration of multiple theories into a comprehensive model tailored for a given individual or community group requires careful analysis of the audience and frequent reexamination during program design and implementation.

Constructs and Issues Across Theories

The various theories that can be used for health promotion intervention are not mutually exclusive. Not surprisingly, they share several constructs and common issues. It is often challenging to sort out the key issues in various models. This section focuses on important issues and constructs across models. The first of these is that successful behavior change depends on a sound understanding of the employee's, or consumer's, view of the world.

The Individual's View of the World: Perceptions, Cognitions, Emotions, and Habits

Unhealthy behaviors often arise because people do not have the necessary behavioral skills to make changes. Following a heart attack, for example, an employee might understand the importance of quitting smoking or adopting dietary changes but be unable to make those changes. There will be other circumstances where employees might not understand the importance of such changes and may even believe that such changes pose an additional risk to their health. In other circumstances still, a person might be experiencing depression, a major barrier to compliance.

Traditionally, it has been assumed that the relationship among knowledge, attitudes, and behavior is a simple and direct one. Indeed, over the years many prevention programs have been based on the premise that if people understand the health consequences of a particular behavior, they will modify it accordingly. Moreover, the argument goes that if people have a negative attitude toward an existing lifestyle practice and a positive attitude toward change, they will make healthful changes. However, we now know from research conducted over the past 30 y that the relationships among knowledge, awareness of the need to change, intention to change, and an actual change in behavior are very complex.

Ideally, each person should be treated as an individual with unique circumstances and a unique health history. Still, epidemiological research indicates that certain demographic subgroups differ in terms of risk factors and health behaviors. Understanding social disparities is important in today's diverse workplaces (28). It is important to be sensitive to group patterns and yet avoid stereotyping in the absence of firsthand evidence about an individual. Within this general context, various theories and models can guide the search for effective ways to reach and positively motivate workers.

Behavior Change as a Process

Sustained health behavior change involves multiple actions and adaptations over time. Some people may not be ready to attempt changes, some may be thinking about attempting change, and others may have already begun implementing behavioral modifications. One central issue that has gained wide acceptance in recent years is the simple notion that *behavior change is a process, not an event*. It is not a question of someone deciding one day to quit smoking and the next day becoming a nonsmoker for life! The idea that behavior change occurs in a number of steps is not particularly new, but it has gained wider recognition in the past few years. Various multistage theories of behavior change date back more than 50 y (12).

While the stages of change construct cuts across various circumstances of individuals who need to change or want to change, other theories also address these processes. In the following sections we look across various models to illustrate three key concerns in understanding the process of behavior change: (1) motivation versus intention, (2) intention versus action, and (3) changing behavior versus maintaining behavior change.

Motivation Versus Intention

Behavior change is challenging for most people even if they are highly motivated to change. According to the transtheoretical model, people in precontemplation are neither motivated nor planning to change, people in contemplation intend to change, and people in preparation are acting on their intentions by taking specific steps toward the action of change (26).

Intention Versus Action

The transtheoretical model makes clear distinctions among the stage of contemplation, the stage of preparation, and the stage of overt action (25,26). A further application of this distinction comes from the TPB (1,23), which proposes that intentions are the best predictor of behavior. Implementation intentions are even more proximal and may be even better predictors of behavior and behavior change (3).

Changing Behavior Versus Maintaining Behavior Change

Even when there is good initial compliance to a lifestyle change program, such as quitting smoking or adopting an exercise routine, relapse is very common. It is widely recognized that many smokers quit only to begin smoking again within a year. Thus, it has become clear to researchers and clinicians that undertaking initial behavior change and maintaining behavior change require different types of strategies. The Transtheoretical Model (TTM) distinction between action and maintenance stages implicitly addresses this phenomenon (25,26). Relapse prevention specifically focuses on strategies for dealing with maintenance of a recently changed behavior (20). It involves developing self-management and coping strategies and establishing new behavior patterns that emphasize perceived control, environmental management, and improved self-efficacy. These strategies are an eclectic mix drawn from social cognitive theory (5), the TPB (23), applied behavioral analysis, and the forerunners of the stages of change model.

Barriers to Actions, Pros and Cons, and Decisional Balance

According to social cognitive theory (5), a central determinant of behavior involves the interaction between individuals and their environments. Behavior and environment are said to continuously interact and influence one another, which is known as the principle of *reciprocal determinism*. The concept of barriers to action, or perceived barriers, can be found in several theories of health behavior, either explicitly or as an application. It is part of social cognitive theory (5) and the TPB (23). In the transtheoretical model, there are parallel constructs labeled as the *pros* (the benefits of change) and *cons* (the costs of change; 25,26). Taken together, these constructs are known as *decisional balance*.

The idea that individuals engage in relative weighing of the pros and cons has its origins in Janis and Mann's model of decision making, published in their seminal book more than 20 y ago (15), although the idea had emerged much earlier in social psychological discourse. Lewin's idea of force field analysis (19) and other work on persuasion and decision counseling by Janis and Mann predated that important work. Indeed, this notion is basic to models of rational decision making, in which people intellectually think about the advantages and disadvantages, obstacles and facilitators, barriers and benefits, or pros and cons of engaging in a particular action.

Implications and Opportunities

Theory and research suggest that the most effective health behavior change interventions are those that use multiple strategies and aim to achieve multiple goals of awareness, information transmission, skill development, and supportive environments and policies (2). The range of possible intervention tools and techniques is extensive and varied. Programs will differ based on their goals and objectives, the needs of employees, and the available resources, staff, and expertise. Behavior-specific programs can stand alone or can be part of broader multicomponent and multiple-focus health promotion programs (28).

What can be expected? Program design relates closely to what can be expected in terms of results. Generally speaking, minimally intensive intervention efforts such as one-time group education sessions can reach large audiences, but they seldom lead to behavior changes. More intensive programs typically appeal to at-risk or motivated groups, cost more to offer, and can achieve relatively greater changes in knowledge, attitudes, and eating patterns (22).

Behavior change interventions must be sensitive to audience and contextual factors. Behavioral patterns exist for many reasons other than health, and health promotion strategies must take these issues into consideration. The health promotion motto "Know your audience" has a true and valuable meaning. Planning processes can consider multiple theories in a systematic way through approaches such as intervention mapping (17).

Furthermore, change is incremental. It is unreasonable to expect that significant and lasting changes will occur during the course of a program that lasts only a few months. Programs need to pull participants along the continuum of change, being sure to be just in front of those most ready to change with attractive, innovative offerings.

In population-focused programs, it appears to be of limited value to orient a program solely toward modifying individual choice (e.g., providing intensive counseling and nicotine replacement therapy). A more productive strategy also includes environmental change efforts, (e.g., smoking bans that are routinely enforced and benefits coverage of cessation adjuncts; 22). When such efforts are combined with individual counseling and support, long-lasting and meaningful changes can be achieved.

Finally, when planning interventions we should strive to be creative. Health promotion interventions should be as entertaining and engaging as the other activities they are competing with. People will want to participate if they can have fun with these programs. Communication technologies are opening up many different channels for engaging people's interest in better health. The communication of health information, no matter how important, is secondary to attracting and retaining the interest and enthusiasm of the audience.

Conclusion

This chapter has introduced contemporary theoretical bases for health behavior change programs as applied to the worksite setting. The major theories identified and discussed include social cognitive theory, the stages of change construct from the TTM, the Theory of Planned Behavior, and social ecological models. Important issues related to the use of the theories have been discussed and cross-cutting issues have been considered.

Chapter Review Questions

1. Describe three advantages of conducting health promotion programs in worksites and their implications for applying theories of behavior change in designing these programs.

2. Explain the multiple levels of influence that affect employees' health-related behaviors and the implications for using an ecological perspective in developing health promotion programs in worksite settings.

3. What are the major differences between *explanatory* theories and *change* theories?

4. The idea of health behavior change as a *process*—not an event—cuts across several behavior change theories. Explain how this idea can be put into action for either healthy eating or smoking cessation, using constructs from either the stages of change model or the theory of planned behavior.

23

Keeping Healthy Workers Healthy
Creating a Culture of Health

Shirley Musich, PhD; Howard Schubiner, MD; and Timothy J. McDonald, MHSA

A healthy workplace has been defined as any organization that maximizes the integration of worker goals for well-being and company objectives for profitability and productivity (44). Implied in this definition of a healthy workplace are two components: the performance of the organization and the health of the workers. A key premise characterizing a healthy organization is that human capital is maximized by optimizing the quality of the work life within the organization (12). Included in the definition of organizational health are the actual structural and organizational characteristics of the organization, including job demands, work scheduling, interpersonal aspects, and management style as well as organizational practices and policies (12). As we explore strategies for maximizing the health of employee populations, we need to recognize the joint responsibility of the organization and of the employee in managing the health and well-being of the individual and the performance of the organization—in other words, in creating and maintaining a culture of health within the corporation.

In the United States, the responsibility for health largely has been considered to be an individual responsibility. Health promotion activities have typically targeted the improvement or maintenance of individual health behaviors with expected outcomes of improved health status (22), medical cost savings (38), and increased productivity (42). More recently, health management programming has been expanded to include disease management and case management programs that provide resources to the individual along the entire continuum of health (34; see figure 23.1).

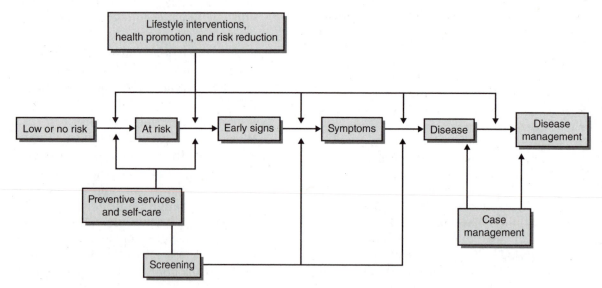

Figure 23.1 Opportunities for population health management. Population health management strategies involve stratification of the population to categorize individuals along a continuum of health from low-risk to diagnosed disease.

Reprinted, by permission, from S.A. Musich, W.N. Burton, and D.W. Edington, 1999, "Costs and benefits of prevention and disease management," *Disease Management and Health Outcomes* 4(3): 153-166.

Despite attempts at population health management, most health management programming typically targets individuals with multiple health risks or diagnosed medical conditions. Fewer health promotion resources are available to currently healthy individuals, as cost-containment strategies consistently target higher-cost subgroups. Thus strategies involving the integration of lower-cost options, including synergies between corporate practices and policies, work environment, and partnerships with medical services, are of critical importance in managing the health of a given population. Effective population management strategies with stated goals of maximizing the health of the entire population should include risk reduction and disease management but also must include programs and defined strategies targeting maintenance of low-risk status—that is, programs designed to assist currently healthy individuals in maintaining health status over time with the stated purpose of maximizing their well-being and vitality, of minimizing injuries, and of preventing disease morbidity often associated with aging.

In focusing on health maintenance strategies—keeping healthy people healthy—there is a recognition that a healthy worker must operate within the context of a healthy work environment, including both physical and psychosocial dimensions. Table 23.1 presents an overview of physical and mental health dimensions in the context of both organizational and individual perspectives. In fact, there is increasing evidence that organizational aspects of work life, including job design (26), job efforts and rewards (45), organizational change and job security (28), and work–life imbalance (53), mediated through worker stress, can have major effects on the health status of employees and their ability to do their work. High stress has been directly linked to the productivity metrics of increased absenteeism (3,39,50,53) and disability (7,23,41). Recommended strategies for maximizing the health of workers thus involve a multidimensional approach that includes four components contributing independently to creating a comprehensive corporate culture of health (see figure 23.2):

- Organizational practices and policies
- Corporate environment
- Health management programming
- Medical services

In this chapter, we explore each of the four components and include recommendations that address dimensions of both physical and mental health (i.e., stress) in the creation of a healthy workplace. Our perspective for each component will be from the assumption of a current healthy state, and for each dimension we will explore strategies and recommendations for maintaining and improving employee health and well-being.

Organizational Practices and Policies

Efforts to maximize the health and well-being of a workforce should begin with considerations of the organization itself (figure 23.2). Expanding the concept of health promotion to the organization implies an internal review of how the workplace is organized and how corporate practices and policies affect the individual worker's ability to do work as well as how these practices and policies are detrimental or beneficial to employee health.

Building a healthy organizational culture involves both the physical work structure and the employees' perception of that work environment. Organizational research has shown positive effects on employee health and well-being, reduced absenteeism, and improved organizational commitment associated with corporate practices that increase job control with flexible work schedules (20), offer opportunities for employee input (33,49), provide worker evaluations with constructive feedback (33,49), and implement family friendly policies (20,53). Other practices might include building a cooperative work environment that emphasizes teamwork with nonharassment and equal opportunity policies.

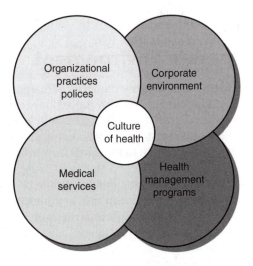

Figure 23.2 Healthy workplace culture model. Recommended strategies for maximizing the health of workers involve a multidimensional approach including these four components contributing independently to creating a comprehensive corporate culture of health.

While these organizational issues address the physical structure of the workplace, there is increasing awareness of the detrimental effects of long-term work stress. Work stress has been linked to job characteristics in two alternative job stress models: (1) the job strain model with dimensions of psychological job demands, job control, and social support (26) and (2) the effort-reward imbalance model assessing the balance of extrinsic and intrinsic efforts at work and subsequent rewards such as money, esteem, or status control (45). Health consequences of long-term stress include hypertension (39), depression (40), myocardial infarctions (6), medical symptoms (e.g., headaches, heartburn, tiredness, stomach pain, and so on; 30), musculoskeletal disorders (3,23,41), and decreased self-reported health status (29). These consequences result in increased illness absenteeism and disability among employee populations in several countries, including the United States (3,7,13,23,39,50,53).

Companies should develop an awareness of how dramatic changes and uncertainty within the corporate organization can affect worker stress. One of the strongest predictors of positive corporate health is maintaining strong communication practices that promote both top-down and bottom-up discussions (33). Organizational changes such as downsizing, acquisition, new patterns of work, and job insecurity have been directly associated with increased worker stress (28,50). Continued up-front communications, stress management, awareness of behavioral health resources, management support, and coworker support mitigate detrimental consequences of rapidly changing business structures and circumstances (23,33,50).

Corporate Environment

While in the United States the focus of maintaining healthy lifestyle has been on individual choices, increasingly attention has shifted to include corporate policies and corporate environment as options that have the potential to influence the entire population (see figure 23.2). At the most basic level, work environment can be defined as the physical characteristics of the workplace, including safety policies, noise levels, lighting, air quality, and ergonomically adapted equipment and furniture. More recently the concept of the work environment has been extended to include healthy eating options and updated cafeteria menus, smoke-free policies, and opportunities for physical activity. The positive effects of environmental changes are strongly supported for improving nutrition and healthy eating and decreasing smoke exposure due to secondhand smoke (8,15). Modifications that stimulated changes in dietary intake used food labeling (point of purchase), expanded availability of healthy products, enhanced visibility of available healthy foods in company cafeterias, and healthy food offerings in vending machines with changes supported by the distribution of posters and bulletins (15).

In 2006, a CDC analysis of the 2005 Behavioral Risk Factor Surveillance System (BRFSS; a representative national telephone health survey) reported that the median percentage of persons who worked mostly indoors and reported that smoking was not allowed in any work areas within their workplace (i.e., complete smoke-free workplace policy) was 73% (8). Secondhand smoke exposure has declined substantially within the past 20 y, a result of employers, communities, and some states implementing smoke-free policies and laws. The 2010 goal established by *Healthy People 2010* is to increase the proportion of workplaces and workers that are covered by smoke-free policies to 100% (8).

The effects of providing walking paths or other opportunities for physical activity (i.e., use of stairs) are less conclusive and generally involve examining work schedules to increase availability, ensuring safety of outdoor options, and mounting awareness campaigns in order to be effective (15). Promoting referrals to community services and programs that may serve as effective resources for workers and their families can be effective as well.

Building a culture of health within a company also requires an awareness of worker perceptions of the work environment. Perceptions of a healthy work environment have been related to job satisfaction, commitment to the organization, morale, number of self-reported absence days, and attempts to look for another job (33). Again the strongest correlates of a healthy work environment were measures of good communication and maintenance of managerial and coworker support. The advantage of environmental policies and practices is that most are relatively low cost and have the potential to affect general populations of individuals. While it is not sufficient by itself to promote rapid health behavior change, a healthy work environment can be synergistic in maximizing the effect of individual health promotion programs—that is, a healthy work environment can make healthy choices at the workplace easier (38).

Health Management Programming

Traditionally most of the emphasis in promoting health within an organization has been associated with designated health promotion programming (see figures 23.1 and 23.2). Focus for programming has included health awareness and education as well as interventions—on-site and, more recently, online. As health promotion developed as a field, most programs focused on activities reducing health risks such as overweight, physical inactivity, high blood pressure, high cholesterol, and smoking. While mental health has been recognized as being influential on overall health, less programming has been directed toward maintenance of mental health, such as programs addressing stress, life and job satisfaction, coping skills, work–life balance, and job demands.

Modern approaches to health management generally involve stratification of the population, often using some version of health risk appraisal (HRA) to broadly categorize individuals along a continuum of health as low risk, high risk, having medical symptoms but undiagnosed disease, and having diagnosed disease (figure 23.1). A suite of programs can then be targeted to serve the health needs of each respective population. In practice, however, most resources are typically directed toward individuals with multiple risks and diagnosed disease—often restricting program eligibility to as little as 20% to 40% of the population (e.g., highest risk and cost subgroups). For effective population management, the needs of the entire population should be addressed—in other words, the remaining 60% to 80% of the population also require defined health management strategies. Providing health tools designed to manage health risks for currently low-risk individuals maximizes health over time by promoting healthy aging (52,56), preventing physical and mental disability (24,48,49), and delaying or reducing disease development (1,25,52,56).

Promoting Healthy Workers: Risk Management

To manage health risks within a population, we must not only understand the prevalence of health risks within the targeted population but also have effective tools to track the baseline prevalence of health risks as well as monitor changes in health risks over time and measure the effectiveness of any programming that should be implemented. For

this, the HRA is generally recommended. While use of HRAs has a long history, most HRAs have been used as voluntary programs with typical annual participation rates of about 10% to 30% (22,38). Use of the HRA as a tool for population risk management implies that a majority (greater than 50%) of the population is measured on an annual basis. Generally, reaching these higher engagement rates within a population requires a defined incentive structure. Ongoing involvement in health management has been recognized as necessary for effective maintenance of health behaviors over time. Nevertheless, risk-management strategies have been shown to be instrumental in healthy aging (24,48,49,52,56), primary and secondary injury prevention (7,17,23,31,51), and primary and secondary disease prevention (1,5,9,25,34,36,40,52,56).

Healthy Aging: Risk Management

An important conclusion of research into healthy aging is that programs should shift their focus from protection against illness to promotion of health and functionality (48). Maximizing health within an aging workforce has increased the urgency to not only understand what predicts healthy aging but also devise interventions that enable workers to continue to function effectively in whatever job they have chosen for however long they should choose to work. Research studies on healthy aging of the workforce indicate that promoting work ability (24,48,49) within a workforce requires (1) adjustments in the physical work environment, (2) adjustments in the psychosocial work environment, (3) health and lifestyle promotion, and (4) updating of professional skills (24). The first two requirements are focused on work content and work environment, while the latter two focus on individuals. While all ages might benefit from these adjustments, older workers (45+ y) benefit the most from these four actions. Adjustments in work content and physical work environment involve ergonomics along with decreases in physical workload, increases in recovery time, and decreases in repetitive work. Psychosocial adjustments might include flexible work schedules, team building, positive attitudes toward aging (both that of self and of others), and open communication as work conditions change. Research studies also indicate that increased job satisfaction and general happiness are positively related and that older workers (65+ y) are more likely to be satisfied with their jobs (46). In addition to being a source of income, working has been shown to be an important source of social standing, self-definition, and good health both physically and mentally (24,46,48). Thus working beyond retirement age may present a positive alternative to retirement for older workers (46,48).

Lifestyle and health promotion studies indicate that physical activity programs to support healthy aging are more important than programs addressing other lifestyle behaviors. In fact, Blair and colleagues (5) have shown that low physical fitness is the strongest predictor of mortality, exceeding the risks of smoking, high blood pressure, high cholesterol, and obesity. In another study, the benefits of increased physical activity in promoting physical health were associated with improved mental abilities while on the job (24). Updating skills and knowledge have become increasingly important in today's work environment but are especially important among older workers to help them remain competent with continued changes in job responsibilities, characteristics, and technology.

In other longitudinal studies conducted in the United States, smoking status, weight, and exercise patterns in midlife and late adulthood were health risk predictors of subsequent disability. People maintaining low-risk activities over time were able to delay morbidity (minimal disability) by 5 to 7 y (52). Furthermore, men with high grip strength and men who avoided conditions of overweight, hyperglycemia, hypertension, smoking, and excessive alcohol consumption (thus maintaining low-risk status) were associated with high survival rates from heart disease—as high as 60% for men with no risk factors and as low as 22% for men with 6 or more risk factors (56).

Primary Injury Prevention: Risk Management

Musculoskeletal symptoms, of which low-back pain makes up a large portion, are a leading cause of work disability and productivity losses among working populations (19). Direct medical costs for low-back pain account for 41% of musculoskeletal costs, and indirect costs associated with morbidity and mortality account for 59% (4). Considering its lifetime prevalence of 60% to 85%, low-back pain will eventually affect almost everyone (19). Programs at the workplace primarily have focused on prevention through ergonomic changes in equipment and furniture and on disability management programs promoting earlier return to work,

alternative job options, and medical interventions to facilitate pain management and rehabilitation (2). Less attention has been given to primary prevention of injury through risk management. Health risks associated with increased prevalence of injuries (especially low-back pain) include smoking (17,31), physical inactivity (51), high blood pressure (31), obesity (31), and high triglyceride levels (31). In addition, increased worker stress mediated through psychosocial factors including high job strain (high demands and low control) and low social support was associated with increased occurrence of low-back (23,41), neck, and upper-limb pain (3,23).

While physical inactivity is not always an independent predictor of musculoskeletal injuries per se (31), there is strong evidence that increases in physical activity are protective and associated with decreased risk of future musculoskeletal disorders (51). Job satisfaction is a strong predictor of return to work after back surgery and is also a strong predictor of disability. Efforts to enhance and maintain job satisfaction are critical in any company. Methods of improving job satisfaction include the following: (1) providing consistent reminders about the reasons why workers do their work (such as reminders of both monetary and nonmonetary benefits to society, the local community, families of workers, and the workers themselves), (2) asking workers how to improve their jobs on a regular basis, (3) providing feedback to workers on the job they are doing with an emphasis on positive feedback, (4) promoting flexibility in working arrangements, and (5) developing a culture of excellence within the workplace so that workers feel that they are part of an organization that provides quality products and an excellent workplace environment.

Primary Disease Prevention: Risk Management

The relationship between unhealthy behaviors (e.g., smoking, sedentariness, obesity, and excessive alcohol use) and increased morbidity and mortality has been well established (1,52,56). These risk factors have been associated with increased risk of developing cardiovascular disease, a variety of cancers, and type 2 diabetes. Furthermore, the co-occurrence of health risk factors substantially increases the risk of disease (e.g., the Framingham risk score for probabilities of cardiac mortality and metabolic syndrome predicting likelihood of developing diabetes or cardiovascular disease is considered in the context of risk clusters, not single risks; 9,32,43). In general, the risk of most chronic diseases increases with an increasing number of health risks (43); consequently, individuals with multiple health risks account for substantial excess spending in medical and pharmaceutical costs (36). Multiple studies performed within the context of health promotion programs have demonstrated that health risks are prevalent and often cluster and that changes in one risk factor can stimulate changes in other risk factors. These findings give credence to risk-management strategies (e.g., increased physical activity is associated with decreased obesity, smoking, and stress; 43). From the contrasting viewpoint, minimizing the number of health risks within a given population over time using strategies for health maintenance rather than risk reduction is a complementary strategy. This strategy offers the potential to help a substantial portion of the population reduce the probabilities of developing chronic disease typically associated with aging and hence maximize health status, decrease morbidity and mortality, and, consequently, increase quality of life over a longer portion of life (52).

Secondary Disease Prevention: Risk Management

Disease management programs have been associated with improvements in the compliance of selected clinical metrics and quality of life as well as cost savings in the number of hospitalizations and emergency room visits for a number of chronic conditions, including congestive heart failure, asthma, and diabetes (16). Less attention has been given to the importance of health behaviors within the context of diagnosed disease. However, several studies have shown the benefits in decreased morbidity (lower medical costs) associated with maintaining low-risk status even among employees with diagnosed disease (36).

Risk Management Programs: Physical Versus Mental Health

Maximizing the health of a population, as discussed previously, requires strategies and programs not only to help individuals who have health risks improve their health status but also to help currently healthy individuals maintain their healthy behaviors over time as they age. Strate-

gies should include programming to maximize risk management that addresses both physical and mental health within the target population.

Physical Health

Health promotion programs typically have focused on physical health risks known to be predictors of heart disease and diabetes: overweight and obesity, physical inactivity, high blood pressure, high cholesterol, and smoking. Numerous studies have documented the results of targeted health promotion programs in improving individual health behaviors and reducing the risk of developing disease (22,38). Fewer strategies have been implemented that address dangerous risk combinations that predict disease, such as metabolic syndrome and Framingham risk components. One example of a 2 y program addressing cardiovascular risks included exercise training, dietary counseling, stress management, and therapeutic education (25). Strategies focused on maintaining health (maintaining a risk status of 0 to 2 health risks) require a selection of prevention programs not unlike the suite of typical programs used to address risk reduction: an HRA that facilitates the overall awareness of current health status as well as changes in health risks from year to year, biometric screening (through on-site vendors or on-site clinics) to monitor currently normal biometric values for early detection of adverse changes over time, weight management programs that focus on healthy eating and avoiding weight gain with age (typical weight gain is 25 lb, or 11.3 kg, between 35 and 60 y of age), and physical activity opportunities that facilitate maintaining already active lifestyles with interesting and challenging programming. Healthy aging studies have indicated that weight management (maintaining normal weight; 1), physical activity (vigorous leisure-time physical activity; 49), and not smoking (49) are the most important health risks associated with improved health status, decreased disability, and decreased morbidity and mortality over time.

Most health promotion programs limit health coaching to those individuals who have multiple health risks. Serious consideration should be given to providing lower-intensity coaching programs that focus on helping individuals maximize their health potential over time rather than focus exclusively on risk reduction. Additionally, program strategies should increase their focus on relapse prevention for those who have made improvements in their lifestyles. Too often programs are short term and, while initially successful in promoting lifestyle changes, have no strategies to assist individuals during the maintenance phase. One example of a successful weight loss program found that initially it was most effective to focus on weigh-loss strategies (calorie counting, nutrition, and so on) to facilitate weight loss but, after 6 mo, participants who continued to lose weight had changed their focus to increased physical activity and self-efficacy training (47).

For people with diagnosed disease, even given the specific disease, minimizing the number of health risks carried by the individual maximizes the health status of that individual. For example, it is well known that among people with diabetes or cardiovascular disease, weight management, physical activity, and medical management of blood pressure and cholesterol can minimize morbidity as measured by medical costs (36). Hence, disease management programs should increase their focus to include lifestyle behaviors in addition to critical clinical metrics.

Certainly not to be minimized is the physical work environment of the corporation. This environment involves safety programming, ergonomics assessments of equipment and furniture, and physical attributes of the workplace such as cleanliness, noise, air quality, and smoke-free work areas.

Mental Health

Maintaining a healthy lifestyle implies a component of mental well-being. In the work environment, the detrimental effects of worker stress have been well documented. People who experience work stress are known to engage in greater numbers of risky lifestyle behaviors (29) and to be at greater risk for developing metabolic syndrome (9). Both job strain and effort-reward imbalance models predict adverse effects on employee well-being that are operationalized as emotional exhaustion, psychosomatic health complaints, physical health symptoms, and decreased job satisfaction (11). Typically, fewer interventions are available that target stress management and improved psychosocial factors. Furthermore, those programs that are available typically target the individual's ability to cope rather than address the possibility of reviewing job characteristics. The Web site of the American Psychological Association (in collaboration with NIOSH) promotes psychologically healthy work environments (see www.phwa.org/resources/creating_a_healthy_workplace.php). Key components targeted include work–life balance, employee growth and development, recognition, and employee involvement (18). The site has been designed to provide resources to

corporations and to highlight organizations that are currently functioning as centers of excellence in the United States.

A Canadian healthy workplace resource (www.nqi.ca) provides seminars, written resources and guidelines, and recognition for excellence in the implementation of healthy workplaces within Canada. Longitudinal aging studies (49) have indicated that the significant factors associated with an improved ability to continue working and to avoid physical or mental disability over time include physical components (decreased muscular work, decreased difficult work postures, and physical work climate), psychosocial components (possibilities for development and influence at work, clarity of work roles, inspiring work), and lifestyle components (increased vigorous exercise in leisure time).

Medical Services

Too often health promotion programming has existed in silos within corporate wellness, benefits, or human resource departments with little or no coordination with physicians providing medical services. Optimal use of medical resources available through benefits structures via covered benefits has the potential to promote an integrated strategy of preventive medicine (figure 23.2). Integral to prevention and early detection of medical conditions is access to care through the primary care physician. One of the most powerful predictors not only of access to care but also of continuity of quality care is having a primary care physician (55). From the corporate perspective, this means promoting an awareness of benefits structures, the importance of regular physical examinations, and compliance with preventive services.

From the provider perspective, the physician or midlevel provider can play a critical role in promoting healthy lifestyle behaviors such as smoking cessation, weight management, physical activity, and management of blood pressure and cholesterol. The provider can promote early detection for acute and chronic conditions through clinical preventive screening, including blood pressure and cholesterol, obesity, cancer, osteoporosis, vision, and hearing screening, with awareness, education, and follow-up reminders to facilitate regular compliance. The provider can also promote awareness and compliance with immunizations and provide counseling for improvement or monitor maintenance for weight control, smoking status, nutrition, sun exposure, injury prevention, and polypharmacy (37).

When pharmaceutical management is recommended for given conditions, the physician can assist in promoting adherence by taking an active role in patient education and follow-up. Identifying barriers to medication adherence and actively engaging patients in shared decision making regarding their treatments have been shown to facilitate adherence for hypertensive medications (21). In the management of chronic conditions, continuity of care with a primary care physician and medical management teams including nurse managers and integrated databases with electronic medical records, laboratory values, and prescription renewal monitoring have been associated with improved outcomes among patients in the primary care setting (14).

Avoiding disease and disability and maintaining physical function imply an awareness of mental functioning of patients. Screening for stress and depression as comorbidities with other chronic conditions is especially important. Challenging patients in order to encourage self-management of medical conditions necessitates education and training and continued support through care coordination and continuity of care strategies for continued success (14).

There is increasing awareness of the prevalence of pain within populations. The lifetime estimates for the incidence of back pain are as high as 85% (23). Given that few individuals will never experience pain, pain management strategies emphasizing self-management approaches to chronic pain should be integrated into injury prevention and recovery programs (27). Research studies focused on causes of pain disability and remission have confirmed that psychosocial variables rather than physical characteristics or severity per se are more likely to predict remission. This finding suggests that more attention should be given to indicators of psychological distress, including depression, perceptions of pain severity, and fear-avoidance beliefs related to pain, physical activity, and work (7).

Stressors produced by factors outside of the workplace (i.e., family situations, financial worries, and so on) affect work performance (20,53). Workers should be made aware of how long-term stress can affect health and put them at risk for physical or mental symptoms (53). The link between emotional stress and both psychological and physical disorders thus becomes explicit, and interventions can be implemented to deal with specific situations. Information about the mind–body link should be disseminated on a regular basis to workers, EAP staff members, company medical providers, and local primary care physicians. When more people are aware of the role of stress in the development of seemingly purely physical symptoms such as back pain, neck pain, carpal tunnel syndrome, headaches, and other syndromes, the rates of these disorders may diminish with earlier detection and targeted interventions. If workers are asked to become aware of stressors in their lives, they can then take actions using occupational mental health resources to improve their coping skills and decrease the need for time away from work. Programs that may improve the ability of workers to cope with stressors in their lives can include exercise programs, yoga classes, meditation classes, and stress management classes. EAPs should have providers who are trained in the relationship between emotional stress and both psychological and physical symptoms. Efforts to increase the use of EAPs by workers should be undertaken. Counselors in these programs should give brief presentations on a regular basis to all units within a company. EAP counselors should be visible and make themselves available for brief curbside consults.

Company physicians and local primary care physicians can play a role in keeping healthy workers healthy. Screening for stressors using instruments such as the Weiss Stress Response Rating Scale (54) could become a standard of care. If workers report high levels of stressful events, they should be assessed for psychological disorders and physical symptoms that may result from these events and be considered for temporary adjustments in workloads. Physicians can lend credibility to the need for coping with stressors by emphasizing the importance of mental well-being and the effectiveness of stress management programs that are available for the worker. Physicians can emphasize the importance of leisure-time physical activity along with weight management and nonsmoking as key to successful physical aging (5,24,37,52,56). They can also emphasize the value of managing stress levels and mental health in maintaining personal well-being (11).

Measuring the Value of Low-Risk Maintenance

As with the implementation of any health promotion strategy or programming, it is of utmost importance to track the effects, including several levels of potential success: participation, health status change, and medical and productivity cost outcomes (ROI).

As an early indicator of success, participation levels for all programming should be monitored and program content and selections should be adjusted over time as needed. It is critical to evaluate the demographics of participants to determine not only who shows up but also who is being missed. Engagement in health is a lifelong process; hence, program strategies must be long term with sustainable efforts. Initial participation, whether intrinsically or extrinsically motivated, must be sustained over the long term for participants to continue to benefit from program effects. The effects of program participation typically last 1 to 2 y depending on the intensity of the program, with participants returning to nonparticipant trends when they drop out or when programs are discontinued.

The second level of success for health maintenance programming should be monitored with the HRA. The goal of any health promotion programming or population management strategy should be to increase the number of individuals at low risk over time. Again, baseline participation is important, but continued health assessments (preferably annual assessments) assist the individual in

ongoing health awareness and early detection of adverse health changes.

One method to monitor changes in health status over time is by tracking the risk transitions occurring between assessments. Tracking should include not only net changes in the number of individuals in low-, medium-, and high-risk categories but also each of the nine possible risk transitions: low risk to low risk, low risk to medium risk, low risk to high risk, medium risk to low risk, medium risk to medium risk, medium risk to high risk, high risk to low risk, high risk to medium risk, and high risk to high risk (35; see figure 23.3). The net gain or loss in percentage points for each respective category of health status—low, medium, or high—is the result of some individuals improving their health status (dashed arrows) with risk reduction, some people gaining health risks (dotted arrows), and some people remaining within the same category over time (solid arrows). The key metric for low-risk maintenance is the number of individuals remaining low risk over time (see percentage next to the solid arrows in figure 23.3). In a steady state, about 80% of individuals will remain low risk; however, with a comprehensive program, this percentage

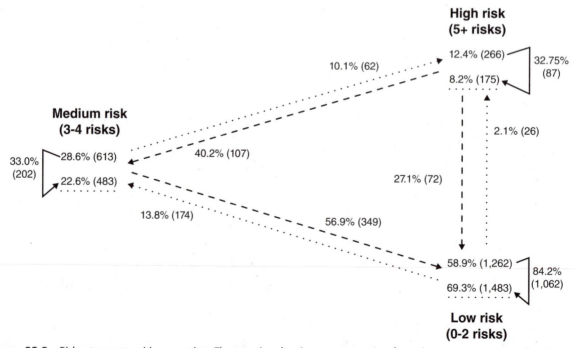

Figure 23.3 Risk category transitions over time. The net gain or loss in percentage points for each respective category of health status, low, medium or high, from Year 1 to Year 5 was the result of some individuals who improved their health status (dashed arrows) with risk reduction, others who gained health risks (dotted arrows) and some who remained within the same category (solid arrows). The numbers of risk factors associated with the low, medium, or high risk status are presented in parentheses below the Risk Status indicators.

can be increased to 85% to 90% (35). Maintaining a currently healthy behavior is always easier than motivating change in individual lifestyle behaviors and then preventing relapse.

The third level of success for health programming is found in the medical and productivity gains associated with a healthy workforce. The lowest medical cost group with the lowest levels of productivity losses (absence, disability, workers' compensation, and presenteeism) is the subgroup of low-risk employees who remain low risk over time. Maximizing the population of individuals at low risk (remaining at low risk) while minimizing the population with multiple risks, promoting management of disease, and providing a healthy workplace environment for all assures the organization of the lowest possible medical costs and the highest gains in productivity with subsequent increases in job satisfaction and commitment to the organization. In general, comprehensive health promotion programming effects on medical cost metrics have been quite consistent with a balance of risk reduction and health maintenance programming in achieving 3:1 ROIs over 3 y (10).

Conclusion

Building a culture of health within an organization requires an integrated, comprehensive approach involving organizational practices and policies, corporate environment, health management strategies and programming, and integration with medical services (figure 23.2). Maximizing the health and well-being of a population over time implies awareness and attention to dimensions of both physical and mental health from both the organizational and the individual perspective (see table 23.1 as well). Healthy workers functioning within a healthy work environment have the potential to work to the best of their abilities, to minimize morbidity and disability over time, and to maximize health, well-being, and quality of

Table 23.1 Keeping Healthy Workers Healthy: Addressing Physical and Mental Health Dimensions at Work

Dimension of health	Physical health	Mental health
Organizational practices and policies	Flexible work schedules Benefits design, including co-payment structures and incentives Worker evaluations and worker feedback Teamwork Nonharassment and equal opportunity	Culture of excellence Continuing education and career opportunities Opportunities for employee input Management support Management communication Effort-reward balance Job strain and job stress Job security
Corporate environment	Physical work environment (noise, safety, lighting, air quality, cleanliness, ergonomics) Cafeteria menus Smoke-free environment Physical activity opportunities	Work–life balance Job satisfaction Corporate communication Coworker support
Health management programming	HRA and biometric screening Weight management Physical activity programs Health risk coaching Disease management Ergonomics	Stress management Coping skill building EAP (awareness and promotion) Relationship building and social ties Meditation and relaxation programs Team-building programs
Medical services	Annual physical examinations Preventive service compliance Drug adherence management Health advocates and care coordination On-site clinics	Screening for stress (Impact of Events Scale by Weiss and Marmer, 1997) Pain management EAP programming Self-management

life. Risk-management strategies assure healthy aging, prevent injuries, and delay early onset of chronic disease. Our medical system has been designed to diagnose and treat disease. Going forward, the paradigm shift should be to build an integrated system focused on prevention, a system that promotes health and well-being from multiple perspectives, assuring a balance in physical and mental dimensions.

Chapter Review Questions

1. A healthy workplace requires a multi-dimensional approach that includes strategies addressing what four components necessary in creating a corporate culture of health?

2. Provide four examples of organizational practices that have been shown to have positive effects on employee health and well-being.

3. What are the key advantages of including environmental policies and practices in corporate health management strategies?

4. Risk management (maintaining low-risk status) over time has been associated with what aspects of individual health, well-being, and quality of life?

5. What role can the primary care physician play in keeping healthy workers healthy?

24

Connecting the Program to Core Business Objectives

Steven P. Noeldner, PhD

Good health is good for everyone. But while businesses and business leaders may agree that good health is important, they may not readily agree that it is a company's responsibility to promote good health among its employees. After all, they might argue, companies are in business not for their employees but to make products or to provide services, which in turn produces profits for their owners or shareholders.

If health promotion is to be embraced and supported by business leaders, a clear and compelling connection between the improved health of the workforce and the company's core business objectives needs to be established. Employees need to be seen as essential human capital, able to produce products or services at lower cost and more profit for the company if they attain and sustain optimal health.

How Business Executives Think

To make an effective business case for health management, it is important to understand how business executives think. First and foremost, business leaders know that to ensure the fiscal health of their companies, they must generate enough revenue to cover all business expenses and maintain a reasonable profit margin. Business owners or shareholders expect this.

Businesses exist in a competitive environment. Innovation and expansion are constant themes for businesses wanting to maintain a competitive edge. These require financing, which often comes directly or indirectly (via debt service on borrowed money) from business revenues. This demonstrates one of the core considerations for business executives: In which of the many competing internal and external initiatives should the company invest?

Consider the variety of ways corporate executives could spend their company's money. Large amounts of capital are often needed to research and develop new or improved products and services. Expansion of manufacturing and production capabilities requires substantial spending for some companies. Sales and marketing expenses can be considerable. Corporate infrastructure (e.g., technology, corporate real estate, and so on) and staffing also require funding. With all of these competing needs, business executives must have a compelling reason to consider health management a core business objective.

Business Objectives

Successful businesses typically have clear goals and objectives to guide their decision making and actions. One obvious business objective is to produce desirable products and services that customers will buy. Other objectives may include obtaining dominant market share, becoming a household brand name, or being the first to develop new technologies. There are also companies committed to making positive contributions to the community, the nation, the world, or mankind. Of these various business objectives, however, profit is typically one of the most important.

Indeed, for many businesses, success is equated with profit. This is especially true for publicly traded companies that are beholden to quarterly earnings reports, equity analysts, and shareholders. Owners of privately held businesses also see profit as a measure of success.

Almost all businesses recognize that they need profits to fund innovation and growth and even to remain solvent during business downturns. One of the ways to ensure recognition and value for worksite health, then, is to link it to corporate profitability. If business leaders recognize that healthy workers are linked to improved corporate revenue and profit, they are more likely to invest in programs that manage and promote health among their employees.

People Produce Profit

Even in today's world of high technology and advanced automation, people remain essential to corporate success. People innovate. People produce and deliver products and services. People create intellectual capital. People establish and sustain company cultures that encourage productivity. Business leaders understand this. What many corporate executives have only recently begun to realize, however, is that the health of the workforce can have a direct effect on the company's bottom line in a number of ways. Consider, for example, how employee health can affect the cost of health insurance—which is a common benefit in the United States—and thus affect corporate financial performance.

Health Insurance for Employees

Until the 1940s, corporations in the United States did not offer or fund health insurance for their employees. Facing a post–World War II wage freeze across the nation, companies began to offer health insurance as a differentiator to attract employees (16). Over the next half century, health insurance became an inextricable benefit that employees expected to receive and that most moderate- and large-sized companies continued to at least partially fund. Since the late 1990s, when health care costs resumed trending at nearly double-digit annual rates, more and more corporate revenue has been required to fund health care expenses. For example, Safeway, a large U.S. grocery chain, reported spending $1 billion U.S. on health care in 2005, which represented 119% of its corporate net profit (4). Another practical example of the effect of health care costs on business is General Motors' estimate that in 2004, employee and dependent health care expenses added approximately $1,500 U.S. to the cost of each automobile it manufactured (2).

While many companies have accepted health care spending as a cost of doing business, some have shifted more of the cost to employees. Much of this cost shifting has been accomplished by raising insurance premiums, co-payments, and deductibles. Mercer's 2006 National Survey of Employer-Sponsored Health Plans reported that when employers were asked to rate the importance of six cost management strategies to their organizations over the next 5 y, implementing health management programs was ranked highest by employers (43%). Only 31% of employers said that shifting cost to employees or scaling back benefits would play an important role in controlling cost (11). Clearly, businesses are recognizing that they cannot rely solely on cost sharing, as they have in the recent past, to manage their total health care spending. Business leaders now recognize that there is value in reducing the demand for health care by focusing on improving and maintaining employee health.

Health Care Costs Directly Relate to Employee Health Status

In the 1970s and 1980s, when worksite health promotion was in its infancy, there was limited published evidence that these programs would produce a positive financial effect. The companies that pioneered worksite health promotion and disease management programs launched their efforts based on the belief that it was the right thing to do for their employees or that health care costs might be saved. In recent years, business leaders have increasingly demanded evidence that funding health management programs is a good business investment (13).

Some business executives will find the direct relationship between employee health status and health care costs to be persuasive when they consider the evidence from a number of studies (5,12). Edington analyzed health care costs and health risk data for more than 2,000,000 individuals and reported that employees who had multiple health risk factors (high risk) had annual health care costs that were higher than those of employees who had few or no health risks (low risk) and that additional health risks added more cost (5).

Health and Productivity

Employee health can also influence corporate revenue and profit whenever poor health has a negative effect on productivity. It has been estimated that the indirect costs of lost productivity can be 2 to 3 times the value of direct medical costs (3). The exact cost of lost productivity can be difficult to measure because most companies do not maintain precise metrics on worker productivity. Measures that have been used in health-related productivity studies are absenteeism, presenteeism (defined as reduced effectiveness on the job due to health-related issues), and employee turnover and replacement costs (10). In addition, self-report instruments such as the Health and Work Performance Questionnaire (HPQ; 8), the Work Limitations Questionnaire (WLQ; 9), and the Work Productivity and Activity Impairment questionnaire (WPAI; 17) have been designed to estimate the cost of the effects of health problems on productivity in terms of reduced job performance, sickness absence, and work-related accidents and injuries.

Total Health Management

The business case for considering health management as an essential core business objective becomes even more compelling when the interrelationship of various employee health and work-life factors are considered. Beyond direct health care costs and measurable losses in productivity, there are other factors that contribute to the overall effect of employee health on corporate spending. Factors such as worksite environment, company culture, health plan design, corporate policies, and access to health management programs all contribute to a company's health-related cost burden. Serxner, Noeldner, and Gold (15) have described how an integrated approach to addressing these factors and to delivering health management programs is likely to produce the largest positive effect on health-related spending.

The emerging concept of *total health management (THM)* expands the health-related cost equation to include the overall work-life experience throughout an employee's tenure with an organization. THM attempts to account for and address the variety of physical, mental, social, and spiritual factors that may affect employee health and productivity. For example, a comprehensive THM program may begin with a health assessment and establishing a personal health record at the time of employment. The company's policies and benefits plan designs will then encourage employee participation in healthy activities and in making efficient (low-cost, high-quality) health care choices through the use of incentives. Decision support services, such as health advocacy programs, online tools, and provider scorecards, may be provided to assist employees in making appropriate choices among high-performing health care providers.

An effective THM program also coordinates care for behavioral health, medical, and disability needs. In addition, it provides functional, emotional, and social support for employees to return to work.

The successful THM program is grounded in a culture that champions healthful activities as well as the employees who practice them. A healthy corporate culture is characterized by nutritious food choices in cafeterias and vending machines and by the food that is provided for meetings and celebrations.

A culture of health also provides accurate depictions of the challenges people face when they attempt to make healthy lifestyle changes. For example, instead of telling only the stories of those who turned their lives around with relative ease, it relates more typical experiences of those who struggle to get started, fall back, and restart again—often multiple times and against multiple obstacles—to finally establish a healthy habit.

Furthermore, organizations that embrace THM seek to eliminate the stigma often associated with behavioral health issues. They provide easy access to behavioral health services at the worksite and from home and encourage the understanding and acceptance of people who experience behavioral health issues. Figure 24.1 demonstrates a framework for an integrated THM program.

To date, there are few studies that have quantified total costs associated with the various components included in the THM model, largely because of the difficulty in obtaining all pertinent information, on an individual employee level, in a single database. Goetzel and colleagues conducted one of the first studies that attempted to quantify the costs associated with health, absence, disability, and presenteeism on specific health conditions. The average combined cost of direct medical expenses (medical and pharmacy), absenteeism (absence and short-term disability), and presenteeism (using several survey tools) ranged from $353.50 to $218.55 U.S. per employee per year when using average (61%) and low (18%) estimates of presenteeism costs as a percentage of total expenditures for 10 specific health conditions (7). These results underscore the importance of including all health-related factors that contribute to corporate spending when considering the potential savings or measuring the actual outcomes of health management programs.

Return on Investment

ROI, or how many dollars are earned or saved for every dollar that is invested, is another important consideration for connecting health management

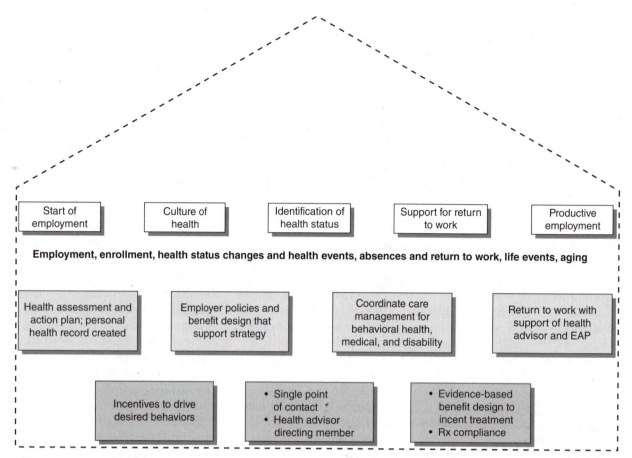

Figure 24.1 Total health management.

programs to core business objectives. In fact, few businesses consider investing discretionary capital on programs or services without the expectation of receiving a meaningful ROI. One way to quantify health management program outcomes is in terms of health care cost avoidance, or savings. A thorough review of recently published literature reported that average annual cost avoidance (or savings) for health promotion and risk reduction programs ranged from 2% to 4% of total health care claims and for disease management programs ranged from 2% to 4.5% for programs that were in place an average of 2.5 y and available to employees and dependents. The ROI or cost-benefit ratios for the same programs ranged from 1:1.5 to 1:3.0 for health promotion and risk reduction programs and 1:1.2 to 1:1.8 for disease management programs (14). It should be noted that, in addition to having cost-effective programs in place, a variety of other factors can influence the success and financial outcomes of health management programs, such as evidence-based program design, robust communication and promotion campaigns, meaningful participation incentives, high participation rates, targeting and tailoring of services, integration of vendors, support from key stakeholders, and a well-established culture of health.

Value of Investment

While published reports of positive health care cost avoidance or savings and ROI results are sufficient for many businesses to invest in health management, enlightened organizations take an even broader view of savings and ROI. Progressive organizations realize that beyond the direct financial benefits of improved employee health, effective health management programs can have a positive effect on other value factors such as employee attraction and retention, improved morale, reduced absence, and enhanced company loyalty. Thus, when considered in terms of their total value to an organization, health management programs have the ability and potential to connect with core business objectives in very meaningful ways.

Fully Insured Versus Self-Funded Health Care

To this point, no distinction has been made between organizations that are fully insured through a group health insurance plan and organizations that self-fund their health care claims costs. Many smaller companies elect to purchase health plans directly from an insurance carrier. Some larger companies, alternatively, elect to accept the risk of self-funding their employees' and dependents' health care costs.

Health management programs have the potential to provide value for all organizations regardless of their size and health care funding mechanisms; however, some fully insured businesses may ask why they should consider paying for health management programs when their companies may not see lower health care costs in reduced health care claims. One response to this question is that most fully insured health plans are experience rated. When a health plan is experience rated, future premiums may be adjusted downward by the health insurance carrier when the plan's covered lives (employees and dependents) spend less on health care. Another argument for fully insured companies is the experience of businesses in countries with socialized medicine models, such as England. In these countries, the value proposition for investment in health management is not focused on health care claims savings but on productivity gains alone.

For businesses that self-fund their health care expenses, the case for investing in health management programs is even stronger. As indicated previously, comprehensive and integrated health management programs can deliver substantial health care cost avoidance or savings and ROI, which can directly affect organizational finances and ultimately corporate profitability.

Building a Business Case

By using the information provided in this chapter and other references, it is possible to build a business case to persuade senior executives to support and invest in health management. The most sophisticated approach to building a business case begins with a thorough analysis of health care claims to (1) identify the diseases and conditions that are the top drivers of health care costs, (2) determine the prevalence of the top conditions, (3) quantify the costs of the top conditions, and (4) quantify potential cost savings if effective health management interventions are employed. Because health care claims data contain personal health information that is protected by HIPAA, individual-level claims analysis must be conducted by a third party (for most organizations). As well, to understand the actual prevalence and cost of diseases and conditions, both medical and prescription medication claims should be combined at the individual level to capture the total cost of care related to specific conditions. While this may seem daunting, there are a number of consulting and health management organizations that provide this type of analysis on a fee-for-service basis.

An alternative method to building a business case, though much less precise, uses aggregate reports that most health insurance or managed care organizations are able to provide. Aggregate reports do not typically include merged health care and prescription claims at the individual level and therefore may underestimate some diseases or chronic conditions. For example, individuals with asthma may have relatively higher prescription drug costs, with minimal or no medical claims, when their condition is well controlled. When using either an individual-level claims analysis or an aggregate claims report to estimate the costs of actionable diseases and conditions, it is possible to estimate the potential effect of health management programs in terms of cost avoidance or savings or ROI. While it is beyond the scope of this chapter to provide a detailed discussion on the subject, several methods for estimating health care cost avoidance or savings and ROI are provided in table 24.1. Please be aware that these methods provide only order-of-magnitude estimates and are predicated on a number of assumptions (which are noted within the table).

Another approach to quantifying the potential financial effect of a worksite health program utilizes estimates of costs associated with health risk factors. HERO published two landmark studies that quantified health care costs associated with various risk factors such as stress, elevated cholesterol, high blood pressure, high BMI, lack of exercise, poor nutrition, depression, and smoking (1,6). Using information from the HERO studies, it is possible to estimate the prevalence of health risks in an employee population and the excess health care costs associated with those risks. It would be reasonable to set a goal to reduce excess health care costs by 10% annually after risk reduction programs have been in place for at least 2 to 3 y.

Table 24.1 Estimating Cost Avoidance or Savings and ROI Associated With Health Risk Management Programs (Example based on a company with 5,000 employees [EE's])

Method 1: Annual cost avoidance/savings as a percentage of healthcare claims			
	Total Annual Medical and Rx Costs	% Medical costs	Projected Costs Avoided
Health Promotion-Risk Reduction Programs*	$40,000,000	2%	$800,000
Estimated Productivity Savings/Gains (as a multiple of healthcare cost avoidance/savings)		2 × $800,000 =	$1,600,000
Method 2: Annual cost avoidance/savings as a percentage of payroll			
	Average Salary	# EE's	Total Payroll
Annual company payroll	$40,000	5,000	$200,000,000
Health Promotion-Risk Reduction Programs (as percentage of payroll**)	0.5%		$1,000,000
Estimating ROI			
Health Promotion-Risk Reduction Programs	**Cost PEPY**	**# EE's**	
Estimated annual healthcare cost avoidance/savings			$800,000
Estimated annual program costs	$100	5,000	$500,000
Estimated annual ROI (savings/costs = ROI)			$1.6:$1.0

Assumptions

Evidence-based program design

Cost-effective programs

Effective communication/promotion strategy and execution

Meaningful incentives provided to all participants

High participation rates (e.g., > 60%)

Integration of vendors where possible

Key stakeholder and cultural support

Program in place 2+ years

*Mercer, MedForecast™, 2007

**Mercer, Total Health Management, 2007

Connecting the Health Management Program to Core Business Objectives

Using the information and references provided in this chapter, it is possible to build a credible argument to connect a health management program to core business objectives. The following list of action steps can be used to develop a compelling case:

1. List the company's or organization's stated business objectives.

2. Identify expected health management outcomes that may be related to existing business objectives.

3. Estimate the potential value of health care cost avoidance or savings and productivity improvements.

4. Relate potential financial outcomes to corporate finances (profit).

5. Estimate program costs including services, incentives, and communication.

6. Develop a proposal that clearly articulates the total value proposition of a health management program (including both financial and nonfinancial factors).

7. Present the proposal to key stakeholders in the organization (consider multiple audiences reached with a variety of messages).

To begin, list the company's existing core business objectives. Next, look for associations between and among the company's business objectives that could be affected by positive health management outcomes. For example, if one business objective is to reduce total health and welfare costs, provide examples of other companies that have reported health care cost reductions (or avoidance) attributed to health management programs.

One of the various methods referenced in this chapter may be used to quantify the expected financial benefits of health management programs. Depending upon the magnitude of estimated cost avoidance or savings, it may be effective to state the financial benefits of health management in terms of the potential effect on corporate profit or on earnings per share for publicly traded companies. In other cases, showing the projected financial benefits of health management alone can be effective.

Most organizations will want to know how much they will have to invest in programs and services. Program and service cost estimates can be obtained from health management vendors.

Finally, it is important to develop one or more focused presentations that are directed to the intended audiences who will support or invest in the health management program. For example, a presentation intended for senior executives will emphasize the total value proposition (financial, productivity, attraction and retention, and so on) of a health management program. A presentation to middle managers, on the other hand, will emphasize how a health management program can affect employee morale, absenteeism, presenteeism, and work–life balance. Regardless of the audience, be prepared for skeptical responses and numerous questions. Thorough research and adequate preparation will assure that a compelling case can be made to connect health management to the company's core business objectives. If the first attempt is unsuccessful, consider revising and repackaging the presentation based on the feedback received from the initial presentation.

Conclusion

This chapter has focused on the methods and strategies that could be deployed to create a clear and compelling connection between the health of workforce and company's core business objectives. To consider health management a core business objective, executive leaders need to be able to connect employee health to the profitability of the company. As a result, health management programs should find ways to clearly document that the people in the company are the strongest assets in producing the company profits. Using a total health management strategy that recognizes the impact of the program on both direct (medical) and indirect (productivity) costs is likely to be the most effective approach.

Chapter Review Questions

1. Why would or should a business executive consider investing in health management programs for employees?

2. How can employee health status be tied to corporate health care costs?

3. What areas other than health care costs can be affected by effective health management programs?

4. When building a case to connect health management to core business objectives, what are the various factors that should be considered?

5. Why may it be valuable to prepare different presentations or proposals for connecting worksite health management programs to core business objectives?

25

Addressing Diversity and Health Literacy at the Worksite

Antronette K. (Toni) Yancey, MD, MPH; A. Janet Tomiyama, MA; and Nicole R. Keith, PhD

The U.S. workforce is becoming increasingly diverse, primarily as a result of immigration and aging, particularly of ethnic minority populations. Ethnic minorities are projected to make up more than half of the U.S. population by the middle of this century; the largest growth is expected to occur among Latinos and Asians. Currently Whites make up the largest plurality but are no longer the majority of Californians. When developing or assessing health promotion policies and programs, it is important to consider the many definitions, connotations, and interpretations of diversity and to recognize that many distinct groups exist within each worksite. Thus, cultural proficiency and inclusiveness are critical components of worksite health promotion programs and policies.

In general, public health researchers and practitioners have focused on four types of diversity. First, *gender* diversity addresses the relative representations of women and men within the power structure of an organization and across organizations, industries, and sectors. Gender diversity is important to consider in workplace health promotion because research shows that work requirements can affect women and men differently in terms of physical and mental health. For example, working overtime is associated with increased risk for cardiovascular disease in women but not in men. *Racial and ethnic* diversity addresses the relative representations of Whites and individuals of minority status based on race, ethnicity, religion, or nationality. *Socioeconomic* diversity addresses the representations of persons from all economic and sociodemographic backgrounds, particularly marginalized groups, including social class. *Underserved populations* are minority groups that are or have been systematically denied full access to equality of opportunity because of discrimination, marginalization, or exclusion. *Underrepresented populations* are a subset of underserved populations in which a small fraction of their representation in the general population is found among physicians, health administration executives, university professors, research investigators, and other positions with power in the public health establishment. These are generally African Americans, American Indians and Alaska Natives, Latinos and Hispanics, and Pacific Islanders.

Effectively addressing issues surrounding diversity in worksite health promotion is critically important for a number of reasons. First, major health disparities currently exist in the United States, particularly in underserved populations. Members of underrepresented ethnic groups have substantially higher rates of morbidity, disability, and mortality. During the 20th century, life expectancy increased by 30 y overall, but (as an example) African American men still live 15 y less, on average, than Asian American women live (www.lapublichealth.org). Race and ethnicity and socioeconomic status, however, are highly confounded, with lower socioeconomic status explaining most but not all health disparities. In fact, poverty is the single most powerful determinant of health status.

Second, many studies have found that health promotion efforts are less successful in underserved populations. However, it is frequently not clear whether the intervention strategy itself is ineffective or whether the marketing or communications and messaging within the intervention are insufficiently culturally targeted. Therefore attention to implementation is particularly important in studies of these populations. For example, in a community intervention using stair prompts to promote taking the stairs, Whites significantly increased their stair usage, whereas Blacks did not significantly increase their stair usage (2). However, in a subsequent study by the same investigators, signs that were culturally targeted to African Americans were effective in both ethnic groups (3).

Third, *health literacy,* or the ability to understand and act appropriately on health information, depends on multiple competencies, including language fluency in standard English, rudimentary scientific comprehension (e.g., anatomy, physiology), basic math skills, reading ability, manual dexterity, visual and auditory acuity, and familiarity and comfort with mainstream American culture. Health literacy is generally lower in underserved populations, and this poses potential problems for successful health promotion in the worksite. Health promotion materials provided to employees may be understood incorrectly or incompletely among employees with lower levels of health literacy, leading to poorer intervention outcomes.

Health literacy may also be an issue for a fourth type of diversity, *cultural* diversity, or the representation of persons who are from cultures other than the dominant or mainstream American culture. People who have language barriers, people who are in an ethnic or sexual minority (lesbian, gay, bisexual, or transgendered individuals), people with disability, or immigrants who are less acculturated may also have different cultural norms and values regarding health and health promotion. Even the simple definition of health and illness may differ across cultures. For example, some cultures do not view obesity as unhealthy, and so worksite health promotion programs that promote healthy nutrition and physical activity as strategies for weight loss may be less successful. Culturally salient interventions increase program recruitment and retention as well as adherence to programmatic goals.

This chapter examines issues pertinent to diversity in the workplace, in the context of efforts to improve the health of all workers. Health literacy is an important topic and is discussed in greater detail in the following section. The chapter then examines health disparities, focusing on obesity and physical activity. The economic, environmental, and sociocultural challenges associated with diverse and underserved populations with relevance to worksite health promotion are summarized, and the chapter concludes with an overview of potential solutions and case studies of physical activity and healthy eating interventions in the workplace.

Health Literacy

Health literacy is more formally defined as "the degree to which individuals have the capacity to obtain, process, and understand basic health information and services needed to make appropriate health decisions" (18; p. 32). Health literacy is important because it strongly predicts the health status of an individual—the higher a person's health literacy, the better the person's health. While the majority of American adults have intermediate health literacy, there are disparities in health literacy that mirror health disparities in general. African Americans, Latinos, American Indians, Alaska Natives, and people identifying as multiracial on average have a lower health literacy than Whites, Asians, and Pacific Islanders have, and adults living below the poverty line have a lower health literacy than more affluent individuals have.

Health literacy may be conceptualized as a potential *barrier* to successful worksite health promotion or as a *goal* of worksite health promotion. As underserved populations begin with a smaller foundation of health literacy, programs can be less effective for them. Therefore, a useful main goal of a worksite health promotion program might be to increase health literacy. If, however, a program has identified other primary goals, health literacy is an important secondary factor to consider when implementing and evaluating such a program.

Health literacy usually is discussed in the context of health care, involving issues such as medication compliance, inappropriate use of emergency services, or inability to interpret test results. However, it certainly has applications to prevention, as the behaviors promoted generally require more frequent and sustained adherence. It is important to clarify that simple *knowledge* of health information generally does not translate into actual health improvement. For example, researchers have conducted smoking interventions that are designed to explain the adverse health effects of smoking in order to encourage quitting. While these types of interventions may have increased health literacy with respect to the unhealthy consequences of smoking, they did little to change actual smoking behavior. What was needed instead was a different kind of health literacy—knowledge of *how* to make and maintain changes in lifestyle and environment. In the case of smoking, such knowledge includes learning how to set a quit date and to ask for the support of coworkers, family, and friends.

Diverse worksites include employees with varying levels of health literacy—while all employees might understand that smoking is bad for health, they may differ in their knowledge on how to make effective behavioral changes resulting in staying quit. Furthermore, members of different types of worksites likely pose an equally varied set of challenges. For example, smoking rates are higher among certain ethnic minority groups, people living in poverty, and people with low levels of formal education. Turning to friends and family (a common source of health information) for support may not be as effective a strategy when the family and friends also smoke. Similarly, reliance on friends and family for advice on weight management may only reinforce less healthful norms, values, and practices, interfering with behavior change.

Health Disparities

The general health of Americans is improving, yet for cultural, behavioral, socioeconomic, biological, or historical reasons, most ethnic minority populations are not following this trend. Additionally, there is evidence that health disparities associated with socioeconomic status are increasing in the United States.

Overweight (BMI = 25-29.9 kg/m^2) and obesity (BMI $\geq$ 30 kg/m^2) are among the most significant risk factors for diabetes, cardiovascular disease, and other chronic disease morbidity and disability. Two-thirds of all U.S. adults are overweight or obese, with non-Hispanic Black women and Hispanics having the highest rates of overweight and obesity. These risk factors and conditions contribute substantially to health disparities, and the costs to society are staggering.

Worksite health promotion is often informed by population-based intervention in the broader community. For example, the CDC initiative to promote stair-climbing and others in the first large wave of such studies likely grew out of two earlier stair prompt studies set in shopping malls and mass transit stations (2,5,17). This intervention was one of the early environmental change approaches, resulting in its identification as a best practice. As is true for most such interventions, however, testing on ethnic minority samples was severely limited. The only stair prompt study available to the CDC at that time that analyzed subgroups by ethnicity found that the stair prompt did not work in African Americans (2). Not surprisingly, few of these worksite policy and environmental change interventions have included substantive ethnic minority samples, a clear opportunity for future research.

In a review of healthy eating and physical activity interventions that targeted or had sufficient representation of ethnic minorities for subgroup analyses, Yancey and colleagues identified just 23 studies from 1972 to 2003 (44). Fewer than one-half of the 23 studies presented outcomes, and 15 of the 23 used convenience samples. The authors noted that of the more than 100 million people from ethnic minorities living in the United States, less than 0.02% have been included in population-based studies to promote physical activity, improve diet, or reduce obesity.

Strategies common to the 23 studies included involving communities and coalitions from study inception, mobilizing social networks, and utilizing social marketing principles such as integrating culturally salient messages and messengers. Cultural targeting is nearly always reported, but it is also necessary to strike a balance between being responsive to the culture of a particular group and accommodating the tremendous individual heterogeneity within the group. The Resource Centers for Minority Aging Research similarly noted the need to engage trusted sources and build trusting relationships when developing and evaluating ethnically and socioeconomically inclusive health promotion programs and policies (4). The following section examines the contributors to obesity-related health disparities and highlights attributes of inclusive interventions with relevance to worksite health promotion.

Addressing Underserved Populations in Workplace Health Promotion: Obesity Prevention and Control

Obesity represents a major public health threat. Addressing obesity as a health concern for underserved populations in the worksite setting is a challenging objective. A discussion on this issue is presented here.

Challenges

American society, as is true of most developed nations, is obesogenic, or obesity producing, and substantial effort and resources are necessary to achieve and maintain a healthy lifestyle when living in the United States. However, obstacles to healthy eating and active living are concentrated in underserved communities. Ethnic minority or lower-income populations experience monumental economic and cultural challenges to healthy eating, physical activity participation, and many other health protective behaviors. Such barriers are inherent in the physical, social, organizational, and political environments of underserved communities. These barriers are detailed in the following discussion.

Economic factors pose enormous challenges to engaging in healthy behaviors (table 25.1). Geographic proximity to healthy foods and physical activity opportunities is strikingly limited for poorer communities. For example, park space in Los Angeles African American, Asian, and Latino communities is less than 1/100 of that in White communities in the same city (39). Similarly, fewer stores stock fresh or frozen produce, and the selection and quality of produce are much poorer. Conversely, fast-food restaurants are more plentiful in low-income and ethnic minority communities. From the higher proportions of inexpensive refined carbohydrate and fat in the food supply to the ubiquitous availability of brand-name sodas and coffee drinks available from vendors and vending machines, dietary quality reflects the nutrition environment of low-income and ethnic minority communities.

Hazardous neighborhood conditions are common. For example, people in low-income neighborhoods are more likely to be located near pollutants (environmental justice issues), face higher levels of exposure to environmental tobacco smoke, and experience higher rates of both intentional injury (due to gunplay or gang infestation) and unintentional injury (due to fewer pedestrian accommodations such as bridges over streets with high traffic volume, speed bumps, sidewalks, and street lamps in good repair). In addition, commercial marketing (including advertising and promotion) undoubtedly influences consumption preferences and purchasing behaviors. Marketing of health-compromising goods and services is pervasive in the United States, but increased exposure to commercial advertising for tobacco, unhealthy foods and beverages, and sedentary entertainment and transportation—as well as decreased exposure to health-promoting goods and services—has been documented in ethnic minority and neighborhoods, ethnically

Table 25.1 Staying Healthy Is Easier for Some Than for Others

	Upper socioeconomic status	Lower socioeconomic status
Education	College+	GED or high school
Housing	Own, safe	Rent, questionably safe
Physical activity	Many gyms and parks, good physical education	Few gyms and parks, poor physical education
Commercial marketing	Little	Pervasive
Neighborhood stores	Fruits and vegetables, food secure	Drugs and alcohol, food insecure
Police	Helpful	Abusive
Health care	Private doctors	Emergency room, Veterans Administration, public clinic
Sick leave	Accrued	None
Leisure priority	Exercise	Rest
Work conditions	Safe, high decisional latitude, flex time	Hazardous, low decisional latitude, no flex time
Child care	Nanny, high-quality facility	Family or neighbor, low-quality facility
Elder or disabled care	Home health workers, high-quality facility	Family or neighbor, low-quality facility
Criminal justice system	Little contact	Much contact
Premature morbidity and mortality	Low	High

Adapted from M. Stolley, 2006, Integrating contextual factors into health disparity research: Examples from obesity, asthma and cancer. In *Society of behavioral medicine* (San Francisco, CA).

targeted publications, and Black audience prime-time television. However, attacks on this predatory marketing are not always politically feasible. Minority media, long ignored by most industries, have literally survived financially on culturally targeted fast-food, soda, alcohol, tobacco, film, and automobile ads that present sociodemographically marginalized groups in a very positive light.

Employment characteristics of lower-income workers present obstacles as well. Those who are lower in the work hierarchy have little flexibility to integrate physical activity into their lifestyles. They have little decisional latitude, rigid schedules (time clocks), and highly structured and supervised (assembly line) work processes. Sites employing a majority of low-income workers, such as low-income residential areas, have fewer healthy food options in close proximity and short lunchtimes. Long commuting times and multiple jobs further constrain leisure, despite higher rates of mass transit use and active transportation.

Leisure-time physical activity and foods with high nutrient value and low energy density are costly for individuals from low-income and ethnic minority backgrounds, both in time and money. Home meal preparation may assume a lower priority than meeting basic needs such as earning sufficient income for household expenses, caring for children and elders, religious observance, and relaxing at home. Federal farm subsidies for corn, used in cattle feed and high-fructose corn syrup, depress the cost of burgers and sodas relative to healthier offerings; the latter are already more expensive because of their more perishable nature, shorter shelf lives, and lower sales volumes (also due, in part, to less aggressive marketing). Low levels of enjoyment of physical activity and suboptimal motor skills may result from exposure to poor-quality physical education as youths.

Sociocultural obstacles to healthy lifestyle adherence are no less—and perhaps even more—influential than economic barriers. Culturally grounded norms, perceptions, and values surrounding physical activity and eating, including gender roles and role modeling, govern the ease or difficulty of participating in healthy behaviors. Many negative perceptions of physical activity have cultural origins with historical underpinnings. Commercially or socially marketed exercise fads and trends have traditionally emphasized sports, structured aerobics, or calisthenics that are consistent with the values of affluent Whites, especially males. Consequently, these exercise traditions have often been dismissed as incongruous by nonmainstream cultures. Sometimes these exercise traditions are even ridiculed—for example, jogging is perceived as a bourgeois waste of time and energy in less affluent or ethnic minority communities. In part, this may be attributed to the traditionally arduous lives of people from socioeconomically marginalized groups. The manual labor of the past has perhaps historically programmed an overestimation of daily work-related exertion and ingrained the need for rest after work to manage stress. A corollary misperception is that sweating reflects moderate to vigorous physical activity (when in fact sweating can accompany minimal exertion depending upon fitness level and ambient temperature).

Similarly, perceptions of healthful foods and healthy eating are culturally rooted. Certain foods, recipes, and food preparation techniques have been associated with particular ethnic identities. One example is the popularity of soul food, typified by fried catfish, fatback-seasoned collard greens, and corn bread, among African Americans. These tastes and smells produce positive affective responses summoning connection to family and nationality or culture of origin. The stressful lives of many individuals from socioeconomically marginalized groups also precipitate the use of nutrient-poor foods (comfort foods) as stress management. Job and residential segregation by income and ethnicity, magnified by the concentration of fast-food restaurants and paucity of dining options with a broader range of cuisines, preclude the usual sampling of a variety of foods as youths become more independent. Since most learning optimally incorporates an experiential component, there is little opportunity for multiple exposures associated with developing preferences for certain foods such as fruits and vegetables, whole grains, and low-fat dairy products (8). This may be compounded by the lack of vigorous exercise, which increases consumption of water and water-bearing foods and decreases preferences for highly sweetened beverages. Even the definition of what constitutes healthy foods varies among groups.

Social roles are key elements of identity influenced by culture of origin. Gender roles reflect culturally grounded notions of femininity and appropriate role behaviors. For example, concerns about maintaining a professional appearance (hair and makeup, skirts, high-heeled shoes) may deter women from exercising during the workday. In very traditional societies, vigorous exercise may even be seen as compromising a girl's virginity and negatively affecting her marriageability. Women are less frequently in positions of authority, and even when they are, expectations of acquiescence may decrease their influence on corporate policy. For women and people from ethnic minority groups, few culturally relevant role models may be available. At the same time, substantial social distance between line staff (who are more likely to be overweight or unfit) and management (who are more likely to be active) may persuade the former to reject healthier behaviors as pretentious or irrelevant.

Potential Solutions

Worksites are captive audiences of adults representing the entire demographic spectrum of a society. They present unparalleled opportunities to leverage organizational policy and practice change to improve the overall health of the workforce and, perhaps, to spur widespread social norm change. However, the promise of worksite health promotion beyond tobacco control has largely been squandered by the differential engagement of younger employees of higher socioeconomic status. The voluntary nature of these interventions, targeted at the individual level, engages primarily the motivated and fit—often fewer than 1 in 20 workers.

Workplace environmental change approaches may be designed to preferentially target ethnic minority and lower-income employees. Particularly, these approaches include *push* strategies that make physical activity and healthy food choices hard to avoid (23). These approaches tend to reduce health disparities, increasing the likelihood of delivering substantial ROI to employers (and to local governments that bear many of the costs of sedentariness) by engaging the more sedentary and overweight population segments less successfully reached by traditional worksite programs. Push strategies include exercise breaks on nondiscretionary time, healthy food services and procurement, walking meetings, vending and vendor restrictions, nearby parking restrictions, and substantive fiscal incentives for mass transit use. They are potentially more sustainable, as they rely less on individual motivation and initiation—the daunting myriad daily decisions and actions that must be undertaken to acquire and prepare healthy foods, to resist the temptations of highly palatable, widely marketed, and nutrient-poor foods and of sedentary entertainment, and to seek out and take advantage of ways to expend energy.

Changing the workplace-driven sociocultural and organizational environment is much more feasible than changing the built environment in these communities. The former changes obviate barriers such as unsafe or unappealing outdoor surroundings, lack of residential access to high-quality produce and recreational facilities, and copious perspiration and lack of enjoyment associated with longer bouts of strenuous exercise. Innovative indoor architectural design (e.g., skip-stop elevators, nested well-lit stairwells, standing workstations), private development of mixed-use neighborhoods, public construction of walking trails, and commercial location of fitness facilities are unlikely to garner a high priority in areas that cannot even regularly secure such basic services as streetlight maintenance, foliage trimming, and sidewalk repair.

Successful health promotion innovations in diverse work settings may share certain fundamental principles, or ingredients. Many, for example, build on cultural assets such as the normative nature of structural integration of group physical activity, in the form of dance or movement to music in social gatherings throughout the life span; the cultural salience of many plant-based foods; and the collectivist versus individualist values. Key ingredients of culturally proficient approaches are outlined in table 25.2.

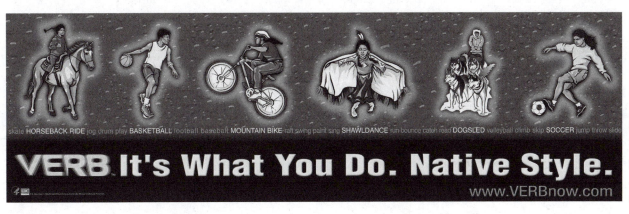

Table 25.2 Key Ingredients of Culturally Proficient and Inclusive Health Promotion Approaches

Ingredient	Sample citations
Building on cultural assets and de-emphasizing cultural deficits and stereotypes	32, 38, 48
Linking to the organization's mission, to outcomes important to regulatory oversight (e.g., occupational safety or injury prevention), or to the bottom line (e.g., employee productivity, to aid in sustainability and institutionalization)	6, 30, 31, 33, 35
Striking a balance between cultural adaptation of a health promotion program or policy to a particular work setting and close adherence or fidelity to program implementation protocols often developed in research settings with affluent White volunteers	9, 22, 48
Compromising on nonessential issues and horse-trading to dodge political minefields and to exercise diplomacy and political savvy	11, 16, 34, 41, 43
Cultivating a participatory process involving employees at all levels of the organizational hierarchy from the outset (cultural insiders), akin to community-based participatory research, in order to build ownership, trust, investment, and visibility	4, 7, 30, 40, 42
Soliciting and utilizing multidisciplinary expertise to assist in innovation development or selection and in implementation (e.g., soliciting help from marketing, human resources, and communications or public relations)	15, 25, 32, 43, 47
Attending to critical intervention targeting elements: *peripheral elements,* such as packaging colors, graphics, and images; *evidential elements,* such as statistics relevant to the target group; *linguistic elements,* such as language, dialect, and reading level; *constituent-involving elements,* such as direct experience or decision making; and *sociocultural elements,* such as integrating group norms, values, and practices into messages and strategies	1, 3, 12, 14, 21, 37
Recognizing that resources are generally insufficient to address the greater challenges of health promotion in diverse settings and that this reality necessitates creativity and flexibility for success	10, 19, 38
Continuously garnering process input from stakeholders and making midcourse corrections to optimize implementation and evaluation	26, 28, 30, 45
Responding rapidly and decisively to difficulties that arise, because information reflecting negatively on the program or policy travels quickly through word-of-mouth dissemination	13, 20, 22, 41

Case Study 1: Integrating Group Exercise Breaks Into Organizational Routine

Incorporating brief, structured exercise bouts into organizational routine in public agency worksites, community-based organizations, private social services agencies (29), corporate worksites, and elementary schools provides a case study of a strategy emerging from predominantly ethnic minority and low-resource practice settings rather than a strategy adapted from research trials with affluent White samples. Yancey and colleagues (45,46) have demonstrated organizational and individual receptivity to integrating 10 min group exercise breaks into daily routines (of staff and clients or members) in health and social services agencies serving Latinos and African Americans in Los Angeles.

The Los Angeles strategy (www.ph.ucla.edu/cehd/activity_breaks.htm [Accessed September 28, 2008]) has been readily disseminated in other settings, providing further evidence of its feasibility and cultural salience (48). These settings include churches, public social services agencies (9), and elementary schools (www.athletescouncil.com). Qualitative data from teachers and administrators implementing the latter adaptation of this strategy, Instant Recess (www.cachampionsforchange.net), underscore the importance of a newly adopted innovation furthering the organizational mission (35).

(continued) ▶

They report that students' enthusiastic embrace of the opportunity to dance to hip-hop music during the school day carries over to their class work and energizes them as well as decreases fidgeting and inattention, outcomes which are similar to those of Take 10! and other comparable interventions (24). Improved self-efficacy or confidence in movement has also been noted during physical education classes, particularly in girls.

While most interventions operate psychologically to motivate behavior change, exercise participation instigated by desire for social conformity adds physiological synergy to the psychological inclination. Enjoyment and enhanced feelings of well-being accompany participation in short bouts of physical activity in a social setting with peers. This positive effect is complemented by a reminder of being a bit out of shape among sedentary, overweight individuals who are surprised by their higher-than-expected perceived levels of exertion at such modest exercise intensity. Evidence also suggests that physical activity initiated in the workplace may generalize from one setting to another and from one type of activity to another.

Case Study 2: Web-Based Promotion of Culturally Salient Healthy Food Choices

Another case study of a worksite health promotion intervention building on cultural assets is provided by the Medical University of South Carolina's and the University of South Carolina's Health-e-AME interactive Web site (22). This intervention was developed from the outset as a community-based participatory research (CPBR) project in collaboration with ministers and the church establishment. It was built on extensive formative research to embed its components in the culture of the Black church and community. Mobilizing mainly church health ministers (usually registered nurses who were members of the congregations) to serve as program champions (www.health-e-ame.com), the Health-e-AME Web site is aimed at providing practical and culturally salient nutrition education and stimulating organizational and sociocultural environmental changes in African American churches, targeting staff and members at high risk for cardiovascular disease.

The central intervention strategy is improving the nutrient value of commonly consumed foods through submission and posting of favorite recipes that the project nutritionists then adapt to lower the fat and increase the fruit, vegetable, and fiber content. These are Web-based recipe upgrades emphasizing soul foods such as collard and turnip greens, cabbage, yams, and black-eyed peas. These healthier food preparations are then integrated into church organizational routine through their inclusion in the food catered at regional church conferences and administrative meetings, meals served after church, potlucks, and refreshments served during church functions. All of these events provide tasting opportunities. Exchange of information across church sites facilitates diffusion of innovative practices.

Other elements of the Web site include a library of downloadable resource materials (e.g., promotional flyers, coupons for healthy food choices at cooperating restaurants and groceries, exercise CDs and DVDs), a technical assistance request function, and a testimonials column. The home page highlights new content, promotes contests and competitions, and invites users to revisit the site. Project staff track usage of the site, solicit enrollment of sites in contests and competitions, and provide feedback. In particular, the home page showcases church activities, success testimonials, digital photos of tasty foods, and active church staff and members.

The Web site has achieved widespread usage, averaging 61,127 successful requests a month and 2,109 requests a day after 3 y. These numbers represent a gradual increase in volume from ≤ 100 requests a day during the first 3 mo. The success of this intervention mirrors a growing body of evidence that Web-based programming is accessible by minority populations and can assist in addressing the particular challenges presented by transportation issues and travel times in low-population density and rural settings.

Conclusion

Embracing diversity in the context of worksite health promotion may be challenging. Diversity is a multifaceted construct that encompasses cultural differences arising from race and ethnicity, nationality, religious affiliation, gender, socioeconomic status, sexual orientation, and many other attributes. The existence of striking health disparities between groups is a major driver of the recent focus on diversity.

In the workplace, the long-term viability and sustainability of health and wellness interventions may depend on the abilities of those implementing the programs or policies to engage the least-empowered segments of the workforce, usually individuals of ethnic minority, women, older people, people who are overweight and sedentary, and people with disabilities. In fact, interventions incorporating policy and environmental changes that rely less on individual motivation and initiative are the current and future direction of health promotion across many content areas.

Tobacco control is an excellent example of this shift. When public health messages emphasized quitting in adults and not starting in adolescents, little change occurred. The advent of better framing of tobacco control as protecting nonsmokers (especially children) from secondhand smoke, taxes on tobacco products, and smoking bans in a range of venues precipitated today's erosion of the social acceptability of smoking, smoking rates, and tobacco-related morbidity and mortality. Organizational practice and policy change, primarily smoking bans in the workplace, drove the legislative policy change that acted in concert to produce current successes.

In order for employers to derive the full benefits from worksite wellness efforts, some may change a lot, but all must change some. Cherry picking healthy and fit volunteers will not generate a substantial ROI. Instead, modest changes to organizational routine that influence the behavior of most, if not all, workers can in turn produce modest but significant outcomes. For example, Lara and colleagues demonstrated an overall 0.32 kg/m² or 1 kg decrease in BMI (p = .05) and a 0.6 in. (1.6 cm) decrease in waist circumference (p = .0009) as a result of implementing a single daily 10 min group exercise break for all staff working in the central administrative building of the Mexican Ministry of Health in Mexico City (23). Had this demonstration project employed a control group, the results likely would have been even more significant, as the secular trends in Mexico, as in the United States, are for annual *increments* in weight and waistlines of similar magnitude. And recent evidence suggests that the accrual of at least some health benefits is the same for 10 3 min bouts of exercise as that conferred by one continuous 30 min bout (27).

Arresting the societal epidemic of obesity-related chronic disease may also be spurred by workplace policy and environmental change innovation. Certain types of worksites may serve as catalysts for social change and elimination of health disparities. In particular, these include organizations serving patients, clients, members, or students that are charged with protecting and improving community health and well-being, including government agencies, health and social services organizations (including health care providers), schools and child care facilities, and religious institutions. Mobilizing these staff members to address their own food and physical activity environments may be a critical step in driving broader social norm change (9). This may also influence client behavior through changes in priorities in their providers' (agency staff's) decision making and through physical (e.g., vending machine selections) and social (conformity with norms, such as others taking the stairs) environmental changes that make healthy choices more available, affordable, and accessible—that in fact make such choices nearly *unavoidable*.

However, the power of commercial enterprise in making health-promoting products highly coveted and widely available should not be underestimated. Pedometers could become as commonly worn as watches, from Timex to Rolex, if corporations became convinced of their marketability and a few early adopter and highly visible icons of popular culture embraced them. These icons, including athletes, entertainers, writers, and politicians, are disproportionately likely to be African American or multiracial and also disproportionately likely to be selected as role models for youths, compared with their population representation (49).

Health promotion in diverse worksites holds much promise for advancing health of the entire country. Prolonged sitting could become as socially distasteful as smoking or drinking and driving, and soda vending machines could become as scarce as those for cigarettes. Workers' sense of entitlement to exercise breaks could rival that for coffee breaks. The extent to which health promotion interventions in the workplace truly embrace and celebrate diversity is a major factor in the fulfillment of that promise.

Chapter Review Questions

1. Name and discuss four types of diversity.
2. Define health literacy and discuss how it applies to worksite health management.
3. Identify and discuss five challenges in addressing underserved populations at the workplace in the context of overweight and obesity. Include potential solutions for each.
4. In a short essay, present a profile of a culturally proficient and inclusive workplace health management program.

26

A Culture of Health
Creating and Sustaining Supportive Organizational Environments for Health

Nicolaas P. Pronk, PhD, FACSM, and Calvin U. Allen, MBA, CHIE

Best-practice and benchmarking studies in the area of worksite health promotion have identified characteristics associated with those organizations that are recognized for their exemplary efforts in supporting health among their workforce. However, not many of these benchmarking projects are sufficiently comprehensive in scope to allow firm conclusions to be drawn. Following a review of the literature, three studies (2,3,11) were identified that met criteria for an inclusive and comprehensive effort and were summarized in a recent article (12). All three of these studies identified best-practice components, many of which overlapped across studies. One component that repeatedly emerged may be described as *corporate culture, organizational values,* or *supportive environment*—in short, whether or not the organization has a culture of health. It is the purpose of this chapter to discuss what a culture of health is, what components may be associated with it, and how it can be shaped or changed.

A Culture of Health Defined

So how does an organization define a culture of health? It seems obvious to consider that a culture of health is conducive to generating good health and healthful practices among workers. However, is there more? What about the norms and values that shape moral awareness of both managers and workers? How are those norms hardwired to support a culture of health? What about the role of work in achieving life goals and purpose? Is a culture of health a static situation that, once achieved, maintains its equilibrium by following

a set agenda? Or, is it more like a dynamic, ever-evolving process that helps guide individuals within the organization toward achieving their best self—achieving self-actualization according to Maslow's hierarchy of needs (9)?

In addition, what are some of the reasons why a company should be interested in creating a culture of health? Clearly, it has something to do with business performance. This does not mean that the company management team is *only* concerned about ensuring that all employees do their work efficiently. Rather, it recognizes that the talents and expertise of workers (the reasons why they were hired in the first place) flourish in a supportive environment, and this has a direct effect on production and the company's competitive edge. As a result, the challenges of balancing work and family are positively addressed with a reciprocal effect on productivity (14). A culture of health will address the worker's expectations of job fulfillment and at the same time address the company's need for business performance. Put another way, healthy employees are likely to have less unexpected sick time and therefore can be more focused on their job, thereby increasing productivity. Companies that pursue a culture of health do so to achieve excellence, not mediocrity, in business performance.

In this regard, a culture of health is defined here as *a workplace ecology in which the dynamic relationship between human beings and their work environment nurtures personal and organizational values that support the achievement of a person's best self while generating exceptional business performance.* Figure 26.1 depicts the interplay of the components expressed in this definition.

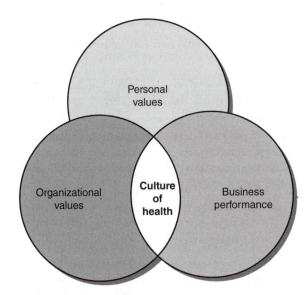

Figure 26.1 A culture of health defined.

Culture of Health Components

As depicted in figure 26.1, the organizational culture may be viewed as the result of the interaction of personal and organizational values and overall business performance. This dynamic interaction is couched in the context of a series of variables that play an important role in generating the desired outcomes. First, there is the organizational paradigm. Next, there is the issue of leadership and the roles that leaders play in the company. Finally, there are the values that the company aspires to that may support and nurture the organizational culture of health. If any of these components conflicts with another, then there will be conflict in the workplace.

Organizational Paradigm

Paradigms, or mental models, are a set of ideas that commit people to shared rules and standards around how they act, work, or practice their trade (8). Information that comes at us is filtered through this set of paradigms under which we operate and hence determines in large part what we believe, conclude, or hold opinions about. In turn, those opinions, conclusions, and beliefs strongly guide our actions.

In order to facilitate changes in organizational behavior that support cooperation and competitive business performance, integrative, inclusive, and overarching types of paradigms are necessary. A narrow view of issues does not lend itself to effec-

tive decision making and cooperation among workers. Rather, it is more likely to lead to fragmented operational behavior and organizational rigidity. When people see the broader implications of their decisions, they see how their actions relate to the overall operations of the company as a whole. In this regard, a direct line of sight to the company mission and vision makes inclusive paradigms very powerful and influential. In a sense, it is a key ingredient to organizational learning (16).

Inclusive paradigms are likely to give rise to organizational practices that are consistent with the best-practice components quantified by benchmarking studies (2,3,11). Examples of inclusive paradigms include the following:

- Alignment of worksite health promotion program objectives with the core business goals
- Strong leadership across the organization
- Creation of a sense of program ownership for employees
- A focus on interdisciplinary and multidepartmental teams
- Multilevel program development

Leadership

The challenge in maintaining consistent organizational values is that individual leaders may hold individual values that conflict with the desired corporate culture. Strong leadership is a key ingredient in shaping and maintaining a healthy organizational culture. Leadership in this context is not defined by a person's position in the organization; rather, it is defined in the context of the behavior of the employee regardless of position in the company. In this way, it is not so much about needing to do things *to* people—to drive them or control them—in order to change a culture. It is much more about combining perspectives and seeing how to learn together. This difference in approach brings to light the notion that leaders can lead by serving others, a concept introduced by renowned sage Lao-tzu in ancient China (circa 600 BC). Lao-tzu said that *the bad leader is he who the people despise, the good leader is he who the people praise, and the great leader is he who the people say, "we did it ourselves"* (paraphrased) (16). The concept was later described in more detail by philosophers such as Hermann Hesse (5,6) and Joseph Campbell (1), among others. More recently, this concept has been elegantly described in the context of organizational behavior by Robert E. Greenleaf in his book *Servant Leadership* (4).

Best-practice components for leadership in worksite health promotion include strong executive management support and identification of champions for the program (2,3,11,12). It follows, then, that leaders should be identified at multiple levels of the organization. Senge (16) identifies that among truly innovative and adaptive companies, a healthy leadership ecology requires three kinds of leaders: local (line) leaders (branch managers, project team leaders, and so on), internal networkers (frontline workers, in-house consultants, and other professional staff who spread ideas throughout the organization), and executive leaders. Without the local (line) leaders, no change or sustaining efforts will go very far into the organization. Without the internal networkers, spread of change initiatives will be limited. Without executive leadership, the overall corporate culture will be like a ship without a rudder, continually in search for innovation but not executing on any opportunity.

The leadership roles that will support the adoption and maintenance of a culture of health vary widely among organizations and may even be unique to specific settings or contexts. However, there is a need for continuity of leadership presence, and as a result several roles have been identified (13). These roles for leaders include the following:

- Visibility across the organization
- Active involvement in (aspects of) the program
- Concern about the program's effect
- Sharing of the vision for a healthy company
- Referral to the program in appropriate manner
- Willingness to support appropriate resourcing of the program
- Active support for program integration into the core business goals and objectives for the company

When combined, these roles lead you down the path of hardwiring the desired culture. It is important for messaging to be consistent, expectations to be clear, and other organizational activities to align with the goals (17). These roles need to be turned into specific tasks that reflect action in order to make such advice real. Clearly, important tasks include the continuous search for optimal organizational paradigms and supporting and aspiring to the highest morals and values for other employees as well as oneself. Table 26.1 outlines several tasks that are directly applicable to leadership roles.

Table 26.1 Examples of Leadership Tasks

Tasks	Comment
Design	Design the governing ideas of purpose and vision and design the core values for the program. Few acts of leadership have more enduring effect on an organization than building a foundation of purpose and core values.
Teach and mentor	Help everyone in the organization, self included, to gain more insightful views of the vision of a healthy company.
Be a good steward	Let your sense of stewardship operate at two levels: stewardship for the people being led and stewardship for the larger purpose or mission that underlies the enterprise. Stewardship interacts directly with the teacher and mentor tasks, the responsible use of allocated resources, the design of the program's vision, and the communication of this vision on a daily basis.
Lead by example	Don't delegate being an example of an active participant. There is no message as strong as actually demonstrating the point.
Be visible	Use every opportunity to reinforce healthy messaging by connecting the message with the leader—in person, on the Intranet, in the newsletter, and so on.
Communicate	Make sure to talk in a variety of ways to all employees. Use written, verbal, and visual methods to communicate, and do it often. Communicate, communicate, communicate!
Report	Let employees and specific stakeholder groups know how the program is doing. When reports become available, use them to identify messages appropriate for such audiences, and remember to put them in a positive light.
Celebrate	Celebrate at any chance you get. Celebrations are great opportunities to relate fun and a sense of accomplishment to the program's experiences. People want to be associated with such feelings.

Cultural Values

Paradigms and values are closely connected—values shape our paradigms and, in turn, paradigms help us understand our values. A paradigm is a set of assumptions about the world around us that helps guide our actions—a theoretical framework of sorts that provides a meaningful context for our behaviors. Values, on the other hand, are core truths by which individuals decide to live their life. Personal values are implicitly related to thoughts that guide us in making decisions. Both paradigms and values guide us toward our beliefs and observable behaviors or actions. Whereas paradigms reflect much about the external world around us, values are inherently within us.

Cultural values are conditions or characteristics that are shared by the members of a group, such as the employees of a worksite. These conditions and characteristics are considered of value to the group and thus tell members of the group how people *should* be or how the group *should* be. As a result, organizational or cultural values are immensely important in shaping strategies around human behavior. Furthermore, values are related to norms of a culture, but they are more general and broad than norms. Norms relate to the rules that guide an acceptable behavior in specific situations whereas values reflect the judgment of such behavior as being appropriate or inappropriate. For example, saying *thank you* after someone helps you out with a particular problem is a norm, but it reflects the value of respect. The interrelationships among paradigms, cultural values, thoughts, beliefs, and behaviors or actions may be depicted as in figure 26.2. The key is how to select the right values for an organization that allow for the creation and maintenance of a culture of health.

Whereas several options may be available, a set of organizational values proposed by the former CEO of Hanover Insurance, William J. O'Brien, stems from several decades of experience and demonstrated results (10). His approach to a values-centered governance calls for four values that nurture the workplace ecology: Localness, merit, openness, and leanness. These values respect and appreciate both organizational and individual capacities and therefore provide positive effect on the health of the organization as well as the employees associated with it. These values serve as the roots of a corporate ecology in which the individuals inside the corporation can find fulfillment through their work.

Localness relates to the notion that the best decisions are made as close to the scene of the action as possible or practical. In this type of situation, individual employees become highly motivated, as they feel more accountability and responsibility for their own actions and results. Localness reflects on the intent to design an organization that allows each person to use the job for both personal *and* organizational development. It involves a set of attitudes, ideas, and actions that leads to effective decision making, guides relationships between people at various levels of the company, and maintains a balance between order and freedom. Localness is not associated with an absence of discipline. In fact, discipline takes on a much more personal role as the values and shared aspirations result in enhanced *self*-discipline instead of *imposed* discipline. Localness is another way to strengthen the line of sight between an employee's performance and the organization's results. This value is closely aligned with the research in organizational development that connects the organization of work with employee health through the dynamic association between job-related decision latitude and psychological demand (7).

Merit refers to the judging of work-related ideas based on their inherent merit rather than their degree of political connivance. In a merit-based company, people are supported in individual initiatives and encouraged to generate open discussion

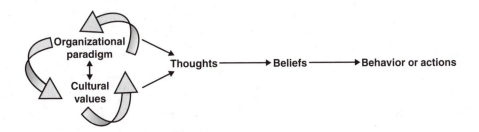

Figure 26.2 Interaction of organizational paradigms and cultural values leading to observable behavior.

and to search for solutions that benefit the larger organization's vision and purpose. For merit to be practiced effectively, company leadership needs to instill among employees a strong sense of responsibility and willingness to speak openly as opposed to blindly following instructions. This willingness to speak out and judge ideas and work based on merit needs to be couched in the context of focus on achieving the organization's goals while adhering to its values.

Openness refers to the unfettered flow of information and ideas throughout an organization. Clearly, openness is an essential ingredient for the merit value, as it provides the inputs and data to evaluate the worth of ideas. Openness is organized according to three dimensions: conversation skill, information flow, and credibility.

- Conversation skill is directed toward an environment in which staff members express their ideas and open themselves up to responses of others—a skill that takes courage and a readiness to accept criticism. However, this skill is essential to both individual and organizational growth.

- Information flow refers to the indicators and data relative to the company's performance in terms of its goals, competitors, and other critical issues. In essence, all those who are part of the discussion should have access to all relevant and important information.

- Credibility addresses the issue of closing the gap between official business statements and reality—it reinforces truthfulness and thereby establishes trust. Credibility is the result of free information flow in an open environment that is observed when everyone gets the same information regardless of what level of the company they work at or which business unit they reside in.

Leanness refers to the wise stewardship of company resources. Whereas localness, merit, and openness are directly related to personal (human) growth and development (health), leanness is directly related to business performance. Leanness is the antidote to excess and addresses the ever-increasing appetite of companies to expand and increase comfort. As it is in human physiology, so it is in organizational health—leanness stimulates appropriate use of resources and generates a healthy company while organizational obesity reflects an unhealthy resource stewardship that may threaten organizational health in times of economic downturn.

Shaping a Culture of Health

Actually changing an organizational culture is easier said than done. Whereas we can identify important corporate paradigms and values to pursue, actually implementing them is a different story. What kind of strategies, tactics, and processes does it take to do this work?

First, taking a simple approach that is easily communicated is a good idea. The approach may be simple; however, the work will be difficult. Gordon Wayne, former CEO of Richmond Wayne, United Kingdom, implemented a culture of health into a large banking system over several years. He notes that "this process is difficult because it allows our vulnerabilities to show, but it can and does work if the willingness and desire to create a healthy workplace are present, especially in those employees who are ready to emerge as leaders in their areas" (18; p. 5). The simplicity of the process used by Wayne is reflected in three key steps that allow the four values of localness, merit, openness, and leanness to be implemented: surfacing, communicating, and aligning.

- *Surfacing* refers to implementing a series of conversations throughout the company—at all levels—and determining what the most important human and operating values are that reflect what matters most to those in the organization and the achievement of the organizational mission. Structured dialogue may be an effective means to facilitate such conversations, as they have shown to work well not only for organizational development goals (16) but also for projects that bring multiple stakeholders together around health-related objectives (15).

- *Communicating* is about connecting the values identified with the processes and stakeholders involved in making the change happen. Providing a forum for open dialogue throughout the organization is a good strategy to ensure that all staff members have a chance to express themselves. For example, a regular e-mail update that is distributed to all staff can include a questions and answers section open to everyone in the organization. Obviously, appropriate management of this activity needs to be in place so that the communications can be implemented orderly, respectfully, and in a timely manner.

- *Aligning* refers to the process by which organizational policies and practices are connected to the identified values, beliefs, and attitudes. The challenge is in the process of providing everyone an opportunity to help shape this culture of health. This change process takes strong leadership to ensure that staff members are engaged and have an opportunity to provide input and feel heard and respected.

Putting the Pieces Together

Based on the discussion in this chapter, the graphical representation in figure 26.3 has been constructed to provide an overview of the process and the results related to creating a culture of health. The process of doing the work is the axle of the change initiative. Around this axle cycles a wheel representative of the results and effects of the process that starts with an open organizational environment and leads to exceptional business performance, which drives additional openness into the organization. The process of surfacing, communicating, and aligning creates an increased free flow of information throughout the organization. This open environment gives

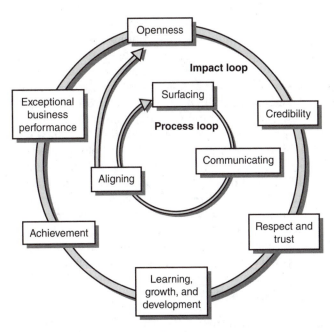

Figure 26.3 Process and effect model for creating a culture of health.

A "Respect Aim" Initiative as a Component of Creating a Healthy Culture at the Workplace

At HealthPartners, a Minnesota-based integrated health care organization, a group of unionized employees asked senior management whether the organization could truly be considered a healthy workplace. There were broad questions regarding employees feeling valued for their contributions to the organization or having an understanding of how their work fit in with the goals of the organization. However, there were also fundamental questions on how to address specific behaviors that many considered offensive and that occurred during the course of the workday. One of HealthPartners' organizational values is *respect*, and, to the credit of the management team, the company listened to the employees and jointly created a rigorous program to address the concerns. By engaging with employees across the organization, leadership was able to identify healthy and harmful behaviors and put them together in a manner that made the program highly visible to all 10,000 employees. The resulting *Respect Aim* initiative addressed the following values and behaviors:

- *R*eliable: I will be dependable and follow through on my responsibilities.
- *E*xcellence: I will go above and beyond to make a positive difference each day.
- *S*how appreciation: I will value and acknowledge your contributions.
- *P*ositive attitude: I will be friendly, optimistic, and helpful.
- *E*mbrace difference: I will honor and learn from your uniqueness and experiences.
- *C*ommunicate: I will listen, seek to understand, and share information.
- *T*eamwork: I will support you, and together we will succeed.

The initiative was implemented across the entire enterprise and connected to annual goals related to staff growth and development. Using an annual measurement approach, the activities designed to address the healthy workplace concerns were tracked over the next 3 y. Employee engagement and satisfaction scores across business units have increased, on average, by 14% over the 3 y.

rise to credibility and generates an increased level of respect and trust among staff members at the company. Being and feeling respected in an environment where trust levels are high leads to personal and organizational growth and development, hallmark features of an organization that allows learning to occur. Learning, growth, and development do not occur in the absence of achievement, and while this is both personal and organizational achievement, since it is pursued in the context of worthwhile pursuits (i.e., the *merit* value), it drives toward improved or exceptional business performance. This strong performance as a business allows for enhanced and continued openness across the organization, so that the process is in essence a loop that feeds on itself.

Conclusion

Creating a culture of health can follow different paths for different organizations. However, a set of principles guiding such efforts appears to be recurring when considering companies that have successfully implemented such change initiatives. Based on experiences reported in the literature, an overview has been presented that provides insights into a change process resulting in an effect or result loop that generates the values and organizational paradigms related to successful efforts. These efforts tend to bring together enhanced personal and organizational values and

business performance in a dynamic and interactive process. The creation and maintenance of a supportive culture for health at the worksite support workers in optimizing their potential—both personally and professionally. As each of us matures from childhood into adulthood, we balance the dynamics of our genetic predispositions, behavioral choices, socioeconomic circumstances, and environmental realities. Companies that pursue an organizational culture that is respectful, trustworthy, supportive of personal growth and development, and appreciative of the relationship between work and health cannot help but succeed at generating a healthy workforce.

Chapter Review Questions

1. Define a culture of health.
2. How would you describe the differences between an organizational paradigm and organizational values?
3. Provide five different leadership roles that support a healthy corporate culture.
4. Briefly discuss what is meant by localness, merit, openness, and leanness.
5. Describe a process to create a healthy culture at a company with multiple locations across the United States and at least 100 employees at each location.

27

Online Communities and Worksite Health Management

Neal S. Sofian, MSPH, and Daniel Newton, PhD

The ever-increasing roles of social networks and online communities affect the way we spend our time in work and out of work. Online communities and social networks have become an important medium for influencing our behavior, particularly as networks are organized around what we call *microcultures of meaning (MoM;* 14) This chapter provides insights into the emergence of collaborative technologies, a rationale for this growth, and an overview of implications of this trend in terms of influencing the future of worksite health.

What Is an Online Community?

Jenny Preece defines an online community as "a group of people who interact in a virtual environment" (10, p. 349). As a group, the community has purpose, is supported by technology, and behaves in accordance with rules and practices defined by the group (11). From a health perspective, this definition could easily apply to an educational classroom, to a project team, or to a support group, with the main difference being that this group interacts in a virtual community. This implies a certain amount of formality or directed purpose, but given the proliferation of technology in how we live our lives, the concept of virtual extends beyond the Web to cell phones, text messages, iPods, and more traditional media such as television. Groups are formed spontaneously for all types of reasons, including sharing photos, recipes, and exercise tips or dispensing advice about living with a disease or condition.

As we explore the growth of these technologies and their influence on our lives, it is important to focus on how we live our lives instead of focusing on the technology itself. Too often, health behavior change programs focus on delivering the same information or program using various technologies and view technology as simply the device of delivery. Each technology influences how we live our lives differently and therefore needs to be understood as a specific tool that may create value in the process of influencing behavior. Influencing health behavior is one of the core objectives of all worksite health management efforts. Figuring out how to deliver messages and programs into individual domains of influence that are meaningful to the user is the real reason to pay attention to online communities and social networks. Research in the *Journal of Science and Medicine in Sport* recently concluded that there is growing evidence that supports the importance of addressing multiple domains of influence to effect the promotion of active lifestyles (1). In the business world, this concept is referred to as an *integrated marketing campaign.* Consumer product companies concluded a long time ago that they can influence consumer buying by creating trust and value in a brand that suggests personal identification or relevance and by communicating these messages in multiple channels (TV, print and Web ads, coupons, direct mail, and so on). In the case of worksite health management, the product can range from participating in health promotion and disease management programs to changing a health behavior to following self-care management guidelines to using the most effective on-site medical care. *The main point to consider as we move forward in this chapter is our understanding of where and how people are communicating and how these environments can be leveraged to influence health.*

The Expansion of Collaborative Technologies: MySpace for Health

From a communications perspective, it is hard to believe how quickly we have advanced and how technology has become ubiquitous in almost all aspects of our lives. Over a 10 y span, cell phone penetration has gone from 34 million to more than 203 million Americans (6). According to Pew Internet statistics, Internet penetration has reached approximately 73% of adults, and broadband adoption was near 43% in early 2006 (8).

The focus on health communication technology in the 90s was about delivering accurate health information and empowering consumers by enhancing access. This led to the establishment and growth of companies such as WebMD Health Services, Healthwise, and other consumer health content providers that offer new venues for medical self-care and self-management. While a significant advancement for consumers, it hasn't been sufficient to merely present static information. As a result, more recent innovations center on what are called *Web 2.0* technologies representing the transformation from static content to collaborative environments in which other members are the main source of content. A Pew Internet study considered the types of activities that are representative of Web.2.0 technologies (9). Table 27.1 presents the findings of this study.

The tremendous success and popularity of Web sites such as MySpace, Facebook, and YouTube provide a glimpse of what the future may hold. Sharing personal information, commenting on everything from hotels to recipes, and rating content and resources are becoming the mainstream in terms of online behavior. MySpace or Yahoo groups have generated hundreds of health communities with tens of thousands of users. Insurers and some integrated delivery systems now offer discussion boards and private messaging with physicians. Employers use e-mail, instant messaging, synchronized calendaring, Web portals, and message boards to promote collaboration. Combine these trends with the recent consumer focus of organizations such as Revolution Health, a Web site that allows users to contribute their own medical treatments and rate those of others, and the paradigm shift from an information-centric approach to intervention to a collaborative approach is clearly underway.

One important dimension that Web.2.0 technologies bring to social networks and online communities *is the movement from a focus on information from an authoritative source to a focus on what many people, including authorities, are saying about*

Table 27.1 Contenders for Web 2.0 Activities

Activity	% Internet users who have done this	Survey date
Used the Internet to get photos developed or to display photos	34	September 2005
Rated a product, service, or person using an online rating system	30	September 2005
Shared files from personal computer with others online	27	May-June 2005
Shared something online that you created yourself, such as your own artwork, photos, stories, or videos	25	December 2005
Took material found online—such as songs, text, or images—and remixed it into your own artistic creation	18	January 2005
Created or worked on your own Web page	14	December 2005
Created or worked on Web pages or blogs for others, including friends or groups you belong to, or for work	13	December 2005
Used online social or professional networking sites such as Friendster or LinkedIn	11	September 2005
Created or worked on your own online journal or blog	8	February-April 2006

Margin of error ranges from ±2% to 4% for each sample.

Adapted from Pew Internet and American Life Project Surveys.

a piece of information, who is saying it, and what credibility they have in saying it. Think about how a person's purchasing decisions or health care decisions are affected by the experiences of a friend, colleague, or close relative. This phenomenon of how people can influence each other led us to focus on the power of online communities, social networks, and MoM.

Not All Information Is Equal

The idea of a heart transplant isn't too hard to grasp. At the risk of oversimplifying a complex surgery, let's explain it as taking out a diseased heart and putting in a new healthy one. But one of the difficulties associated with transplants is often related to rejection. We've discovered that it isn't good enough to just put in a healthy heart. The donor has to be a match. The donor and receiver not only need to have the same blood type but also need for many other markers with regard to organ, donor, and recipient to be as precisely the same as possible. The closer we can match the donor to the recipient, the greater the likelihood that the patient's body will accept the new heart. This heart transplant scenario may be an apt metaphor for thinking about using information to change health behavior.

Information is not simply accurate or inaccurate; its value is often left to how the recipient interprets and perceives it as to whether it is accepted or rejected. Online communities and social networks are important mediums for how we interpret and perceive information. For much too long within the health care world, we have assumed that if we could simply get *all* the right information to people, they would make good decisions about their health. But this is clearly not true. The broad dissemination of health information alone hasn't been sufficient to stem the public health issues we are facing today.

We start from a simple mantra when thinking about the role of information in behavior change, health promotion, and disease management: "It ain't dog food if the dog don't eat it." It is not sufficient to say, "We told him everything he needed to know. He just didn't do it." It may make us feel less responsible but it doesn't solve the problem of improving anyone's health or lowering health care costs.

This same mantra applies to the world of health management and health promotion. It doesn't matter how great your programs or information are or how sound their theoretical underpinnings—if your work is delivered in a way that doesn't match each participant, it won't be widely adopted or generate much effect on the population.

A sound theoretical foundation is essential to the development of effective health behavior change interventions. Whether we consider the transtheoretical model, the theory of planned behavior, or the health belief model, we search for ways to structure our interventions to be effective. But structure alone doesn't guarantee efficacy. If we want to increase the effectiveness of health management and promotion interventions, it is imperative that we focus on reach, mode of transmission, source of delivery, and feel of communication just as much as we pay attention to the structure of the interventions themselves. There is no *one* right way to intervene.

The emergence of not only the World Wide Web but also wireless devices, text messaging, blogging, and remote monitoring devices offers a means of extending the reach and richness of interventions in a way that was not plausible in the past. Innovations in multidirectional communication are making a real difference in the way people understand health issues and approach changes in health behaviors. The key is to deliver interventions in ways that can help people see their health issues as personally relevant, important, and integrated into their everyday lives; it must be the right information, in the right context, by the right source at the time of need.

What Are MoMs and How Do MoMs Happen?

A microculture of meaning (MoM) is a place—real or virtual—where people with common background, purpose, passion, and concerns interact. Depending on the community's needs and the originator's goals, a MoM can be designed to help people take action toward a variety of objectives, including problem solving, finding information, changing health behaviors, socially interacting, developing skills, or finding emotional support (14).

The nature of a MoM within health care is to provide a context that can help people learn and change. As Richard Bandler and John Grinder, the codevelopers of neuro-linguistic programming, write, "Every experience in the world, and every behavior, is appropriate given some context, some frame" (2). Without that frame, information remains indigestible to the user, providing no fuel to take action.

This concept appears to be wired into the very core of the human brain. Eleanor Rosch (12) pioneered much of this work. Rosch describes how human cognition is designed to create nested categories through which we can understand the world from larger to more specific examples within these categories or prototypes of understanding. Rosch and others were able to clarify that though these nested categories are innate to the structure of the human brain, the actual structure of these nests of categories (taxonomies) and our understanding of them are transmitted through our culture. And our culture is transmitted through social relationships. Our capacity for categorization, in other words, has a biological basis, in terms of both individual cognition and our large social interactions. Prototype theory also meshes seamlessly with Wilson's theory of gene-culture coevolution. The human brain appears to have evolved in concert with the social transmission of categorical information. As a result, we are all born with a deep-seated need to understand the world in terms of categories and to share that understanding with each other. (15)

The idea that we rely on nested categories has significant implications for how we need to think about creating individual and group change. Words and concepts such as *health, support, care,* and *diet* don't mean or feel the same to everyone, depending on their life experiences, family history, culture, and demographics. Our job, then, is to help create a context or social transmission that will make this information personally relevant and will lead to a greater likelihood of action. Again, this is an area where collaborative technologies play an important role. One way that has become a major phenomenon on the Web is by providing opportunities for individuals to be surrounded and connected with others with needs and life experiences *pertinent to the user as defined by the user.* In essence the goal is to create a community of people who, through the intimate detail of their personal experience, background, demography, or need, can demonstrate success for others in the struggle of changing health behaviors, coping with health issues, or supporting others in care.

Long before the written word, there were folk tales (metaphors for ways to live) that carried messages for us. We learned, and continue to learn, through stories, oral transmissions of wisdom. Sometimes the transmission via our culture is so powerful we no longer even know why we do what we do. It is just our way. This storytelling is now structured within interventions. Weight Watchers, smoking cessation classes, Alcoholics Anonymous, prenatal classes, the company soft-

ball team, and block watch programs are similar examples of the ways in which people come together to create MoMs in support of each other's health. While a nutritionist may tell a diabetic patient's spouse to change their household diet, it's often a friend of that spouse who has faced the same issue who can explain how to get the husband to eat the diet.

The dance of weaving social relationships with information is not new. However, the increasing capability of communication technology that allows us to create MoMs with vastly broader reach and specificity and more relevance is new. The inclusion of stories, incentives, and ratings is allowing for richer content and resources that can be acted upon and continuously updated. Current interactive voice response (IVR) vendors can measure and adjust automated messages based on intonation. Dating Web sites use complex profiles to match people based on all types of personal data, and advertisers are finding new ways to both target and tailor their product messages to consumers based on Web site usage patterns and increasingly relevant personal information gathered in profiles.

Applying social constructs to behavior is one way to look at improving the relevance and therefore effectiveness of health interventions. In the book *Narrative Therapy: The Social Construction of Preferred Realities,* Jill Freedman explains that the beliefs, values, institutions, customs, labels, laws, divisions of labor, and the like that make up our social realities are constructed by members of a culture as they interact with one another. That is, societies (communities) construct the "lenses" through which their members interpret the world. (5)

Our work with cancer survivors led us to focus on this concept through the phrase *finding people like me.* It was clear to us that the closer we could provide information to survivors from others that they deemed as being credible (people like them), the more likely they were to read and act on what was being conveyed. Figure 27.1 illustrates the path of moving information to action using this contextual paradigm (14).

The credibility of a smoking cessation instructor is often not determined by the teaching track record but by how the instructor answers the question, "Did you smoke?" If the instructor answers *yes,* it allows the instructor to be a legitimate source of advice and relevant resources, and, from the recipient's viewpoint, it makes the context of the communication totally different from the context of the same communication provided when the instructor answers *no.*

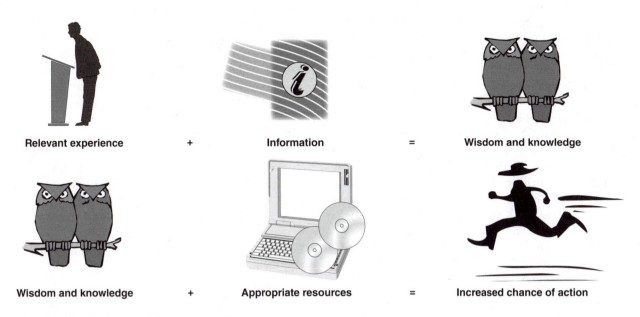

Figure 27.1 Moving from information to action.

Reprinted, by permission, from N. Sofian, D. Newton, and J. DeClaire, 2003, "Strengthen context to enhance health promotion effectiveness," *American Journal of Health Promotions* 7(1): 1-9.

Since each community creates the lens for its members' understanding of reality and how to operate within reality, our interventions should focus on how to leverage this knowledge to create more meaningful communications as well as to build what Robert D. Putnam defines as *social capital.* In his book *Bowling Alone: The Collapse and Revival of American Community* (11), he identifies two types of social capital: bonding and bridging. Bonding social capital allows a group to build identity by creating a sense of exclusivity from others via race, gender, class, membership, and so on. In contrast, bridging social capital allows people to cross lines, building links between disparate groups for the purposes of taking action, accessing resources, and transmitting knowledge. Putnam writes that "bonding social capital constitutes a kind of sociological superglue, whereas bridging social capital provides a sociological WD-40" (11). Support groups demonstrate bridging social capital when they attract people from very diverse backgrounds to rally around a common issue. They demonstrate bonding social capital when subgroups that are alike in some regard find strength in community. For example, while at Alcoholics Anonymous there is a bridge around the common issue of drinking, there is also bonding around members who are in a specific demographic group.

The influence of communities can become sufficiently powerful to overcome even rational objective data. In his book, *The Paradox of Choice,* Barry Schwartz describes how personal relationships bend decision making (13). An example of this, which is based on his concept of the availability heuristic, is the following: One person wants to buy a car that is very safe. His first thought is of a Volvo. Volvo has advertised about safety for decades. But not wanting to be a stooge of Madison Avenue, the buyer decides to do some checking first. After surveying a number of sites he concludes that he really should buy a Kia, which is safe and less expensive. On his way out of the office to start hunting for his car he runs into a good friend. He tells her he is about to buy, but she stops him in his tracks. She tells him a story about how she has seen some graphic stories about terrible crashes that occurred in the very car model he is contemplating buying. But she really likes Volvos. At this moment our buyer is confronted with a dilemma. He has a great deal of vetted information from multiple reliable sources that says he should proceed to buy the Kia. On the other hand he has a personal friend sharing one particularly vivid story from her personal experience. Which car do you think he will purchase? Put your money on the Volvo.

Online Communities and Storytelling

When the major technology of the day was fire, humans transmitted knowledge through oral history. Our stories have been shared as mythology, fairy tales, legends, or oral histories of who we are and how we should operate and act appropriately within our cultures. The accuracy of these stories is almost irrelevant. Their power lies in their deep personal and cultural relevance on the ways we should act in a given circumstance.

This concept is also true for an individual who is ill or faced with a major health issue. Arthur Frank, in *The Wounded Storyteller: Body, Illness, and Ethics* (4), explains that there is a "need of ill people to tell their stories in order to construct new maps and new perceptions of their relationship to the world." The need to tell this story is essentially a social need, suggesting that the story is acknowledged and understood by someone else, even if this acceptance and understanding are not in person. This is a critical understanding that we all too often miss in our delivery of health care information and intervention.

Most health communication today is built with an exclusive focus on accuracy and precision. We have missed the need for story and context. The advent of new media hasn't changed this need; rather, it offers a chance to enhance what was once an oral culture of transmission. In the book *The Cluetrain Manifesto* (7; p. xxxi), Christopher Locke writes, "what if the real attraction of the Internet is not its cutting edge bells and whistles, its jazzy interface or any of the advanced technology that underlies its pipes and wires? What if, instead, the attraction is an atavistic throwback to the prehistoric human fascination with telling tales?"

Walter Ong (16; p. 11) takes this a step further, thinking of how these types of conversations on the Internet show a significant parallel with formerly oral cultures. He refers to this concept as *secondary orality*. From his perspective, "oral traditions are additive rather than subordinative, aggregative rather than analytic, empathetic and participatory rather than objectively distanced, and situational rather than abstract." As we move into a world of managing health, mostly focused on the personal behavior of the consumer, creating the tools and processes that enable these conversations is invaluable. The Internet, text messaging, and other wireless technologies offer significant promise of expanding the reach of such conversations and our ability to convert narrative into action.

Creating Purposeful Social Networks

How can we take advantage of new communication technologies in creating more prolific change while reaching far more people than we ever could have imagined? There is little reason to believe that people with a broken wrist or inflamed tonsils want to become part of a social network of people who share the same transient health issue. To build purposeful and effective social networks, it is important to consider the following factors.

- *Trust:* Participants feel the network is a trusted source of useful knowledge.
- *Relevance:* The knowledge that is shared applies directly to participants on an ongoing basis.
- *Urgency:* The resources shared help members solve a problem quickly and meaningfully. There is often an emotional tie to the issue.
- *Chronicity:* The issue is ongoing and merits getting involved and staying involved.
- *Incentive:* Participation provides a personal benefit. Collaborating helps advance career or job status, personal health, and son on—from the participant's point of view, it's worth it.
- *Serial reciprocity:* Participants believe, "If I help others with my knowledge or experience, they may help someone else, and someone else may help me."

However, in order to build such social networks, we need to know the participant. Criteria that allow us to know the participant are difficult to identify—let alone act upon—given most current uses of new communication technologies. In fact, most of today's computer-mediated or IVR and wireless health interventions tend to offer one-way communication—the producer of the site provides static information about a health topic that goes from the site to the user. It is assumed that accurate information is sufficient to activate a behavior change or at best provide questions with branching logic to deepen the level of detail of the information provided. Even sites that offer bulletin boards are limited. Postings are categorized by topic, and off-topic communication is discouraged. This makes it difficult for people to get to know one another the way they might during the general chitchatting, visiting, and relationship forming that happens in the real world when groups get together regularly around a common topic or cause.

So what are the types of issues that are appropriate for online communities and social networks to address? Here are just a few. On the illness end of the health spectrum, communities can affect diabetes, cancer, obesity, Crohn's disease, Lyme disease, and substance addiction. For caregivers, online communities can help with caring for children with disabilities or for patients with Alzheimer's disease or with end-of-life care. On the health management and health promotion end of the spectrum, areas such as weight loss, smoking cessation, new parent support, and worksite-based team physical activity (cycling, walking, calorie expenditure, and so on) are all suitable targets for online communities.

What are the behaviors we wish to encourage within an online community that will help motivate health behavior change? They are the same behaviors found in other forms of social interactions: receiving support, searching for relevant information and resources when needed, learning how to apply information to personal circumstances, sharing our own stories and resources, and connecting with others regarding our circumstances.

People may share details about their life circumstances or backgrounds that allow them to connect in an infinite variety of unpredictable ways. They may talk about pets, kids, politics, or a local sport team. While such connections may seem inconsequential, over time they allow people to feel a sense of belonging that can build confidence, which is often as significant as the behavior change itself. Without these connections, the participants' bond to the group is only as strong as their interest in the very specific issue that they came for. In the world of social support, such limited interest is rarely enough to sustain the relationship over the long term. The goal is to build as many strands of social capital as possible. You may come to a Web community for one specific reason. You often stay for many additional ones.

So What Does All This Mean for Worksite Health Management?

We are not suggesting that social networks replace existing health management interventions. Quite the opposite! One way for a social network or online community to be used in worksite health promotion is to leverage such tools to increase the participation of employees and their dependents in the many different interventions that are offered by a corporation. The contextually relevant recommendations of others can drive participation through personal stories, ratings, and even incentives tied to using the social network. For example, it is possible to match people with similar fitness interests and goals. The network becomes a place not only to find a cycling buddy but also to create virtual competitions with other employees—regardless of location or department—that can be displayed and shared on the Web. Participants can score points for tracking their times and progress, virtual teams can be formed, stories and pictures can be shared, and people with common interests or capabilities can be matched to encourage ongoing participation.

Not all of this will have to depend on the employee's initiative. Imagine that when you complete a health risk appraisal, it is possible to identify risks you prefer or feel most confident to address. From these data, along with personal profile information, you can be matched to the best programs available from the company. Moreover, you can be provided with an up-to-date search of selected information sources on the Web and then introduced to a support community of people like you. You can read their stories about how they successfully improved their health condition or risk status and then connect with them.

But we can go further yet. By integrating community with coaching, it becomes possible for a telephonic coach to not only intervene with an employee but also facilitate groups of employees receiving similar coaching who can support each other. Instead of a coach making five separate calls to 15 different employees (75 coaching sessions), the coach may only need to complete two calls to each participant, introduce members to each other, and facilitate ongoing sessions. This not only reduces the cost of the coaching intervention but also creates far more opportunities for ongoing support and intervention, taking advantage of employees by making them both recipients and providers of the intervention. In an age of consumer-directed health care, the inclusion of social networks around the existing suite of health promotion interventions creates a more effective and efficient system that actually models the concept of consumer directedness.

Beyond this integration, a community can also provide a means to tie health management to actual health care delivery. There is a growing movement for the use of electronic medical records (EMR) and personal health records (PHR). There is a similar growth in the use of on-site health care clinics. Imagine if we can not only connect phone coaches with employees within the community but also link medical providers to this process, ensuring that there is a closed loop between the employee (consumer) and the whole spectrum of health care and management providers.

To accomplish this sort of integration will require a different set of tools and skills than most programs currently maintain. The expansion of social networking, online communities, and collaborative technologies has several implications for the future of worksite health management. Inherent in these technologies are capabilities that will change the way we communicate and intervene with worksite populations. We will need to collect data not only about risks, diseases, and demographics but also about the preferences of users. We will need to understand that relationships drive behavior as much as information. We will need to understand that knowledge is the domain of the user as well as the provider. Ultimately, our role as professionals will include being facilitators as much as being purveyors of truth.

In return for building these new capabilities, practitioners will be in a position to create a truly integrated approach to delivery of health and medical care within the context of a community of care and caring. The opportunities are exciting and limited only by our imagination. The technology exists to do all this today. The dogs are hungry and ready for us to give them something to eat.

Conclusion

This chapter has provided a focus on the role of online communities in supporting employee health promotion programs in the context of the worksite setting. Online communities and the social networks they represent are an increasingly recognized method to connect with others. Networks can be designed to focus on specific subgroups of the population, such as those who have a chronic illness. On the other hand, they can address risk factors such as low levels of physical activity or obesity. Regardless, they can provide strong motivation to change and be a support mechanism for lasting change among those who use them.

Chapter Review Questions

1. Define *online community* and discuss the concept in the context of a worksite population.

2. Describe microcultures of meaning (MoMs).

3. Identify five factors related to effective social networks and discuss the interactions among those factors and the participant.

28

Rewarding Change
Principles for Implementing Worksite Incentive Programs

Jeffrey J. VanWormer, MS, and Nicolaas P. Pronk, PhD, FACSM

The leading causes of death and disease in the United States are related to lifestyle factors (20). Tobacco use, physical inactivity, and unhealthy eating, for example, rank among the deadliest modifiable behaviors because they account for an estimated 35% of total mortality. As the morbidity burden associated with these lifestyle factors increases in the aging U.S. population, the health care costs associated with these behaviors also increase (25).

Because employers and employees are the primary payers for health care services in the U.S. working adult population, many companies have turned to comprehensive health promotion and disease management programs that aim to improve the health of employees and at least stabilize accelerating health care cost trends. As part of these programs, many companies also include incentives designed to get unhealthy employees engaged in health improvement efforts (16). Indeed, incentives are generally considered a best practice in health promotion (3).

A worksite-based incentive program generally seems like a commonsense and helpful idea. Employees will receive X if they do Y. The prize is received upon completion of the work. The employees are satisfied because they got something valuable, and the employer is satisfied because the employees did something beneficial (usually for both employee and employer). Implementing incentive programs, especially across a large group of people, should not be a casual affair, though. An incentive program can be an exceptionally powerful behavior change strategy, but it is resource intensive and, if applied inappropriately, can eventually have a negative effect on the relationship between the giver and the receiver.

There is a lot at stake with incentive programs, and despite their commonsense appeal, many are delivered in a manner that is either inefficient or ineffective. The purpose of this chapter is to review the core principles of effective incentive programs, highlight how they have performed in the research literature, and discuss how they can be applied to benefits designs. The importance of strong communication strategies associated with incentives is also examined. It is important to emphasize that this chapter does not advocate for an incentives-only approach to worksite health promotion. Incentives are a small component of what should be a comprehensive effort to improve the health of a working population.

Core Principles

Conceptually, incentive programs are simple. An incentive is a contingent relationship whereby an individual does something meaningful to get

A Quick Note on Definitions

Technically, an incentive is an *inducement* to perform work. In other words, it is something received before the work is actually done (to convince a person to do the work). It is commonly used as a synonym for *reward*, so we use it as such here. For the purposes of this chapter, we define *incentive* as a tangible commodity or service given to an individual that is contingent on some predefined action being performed or outcome being realized.

something of value. Most everyone has had at least some experience with incentive programs. For example, parents or grandparents often use them to get children to perform chores around the house.

The picture gets more complicated when trying to implement an incentive program across a large group of people, or population. For example, a worksite-based incentive program must be able to deliver incentives to many employees, individually, all at once. Fortunately, professionals across many disciplines (e.g., education, health, business) have used incentive programs for many years. These collective experiences have enabled behavioral scientists to identify some core principles that optimize incentives; they include value and contingency.

Value

The central tenet of a good incentive program is value (5). The receivers of the incentive must value what they expect to get in order to do the work. For example, a worksite may implement a program in which any smoking employee who quits will be paid $50 U.S. A given employee must feel that the $50 is valuable (relative to the work) for the incentive to be helpful. If not, offering the incentive will do nothing for motivation.

So, what is valuable? There is not a simple solution when dealing with a population because what is a beneficial incentive for one employee may be meaningless for another.* Instead, one type of incentive is usually offered that is believed to be of reasonable value to everyone (or at least most of the group). This requires making some assumptions based on other evidence or past experience.

Incentives for large groups usually involve conditioned items of value, such as cash, discounts, gift cards, or coupons. These are conditioned incentives because people can exchange them for preferred items of value. This also helps make them individualized. Though it will not be the most important factor in sustaining performance (5), some form of money is at least moderately valuable for most people because they can use it to get other things they want. Also, be sure to consider the factors that optimize the value of any given incentive. These factors are discussed in the following sections.

What Is Valuable for Your Workforce?

First, examine any past incentive programs that have been popular. Perhaps the incentives used for them are still applicable. Otherwise, according to Daniels (5), try the following:

1. *Ask:* Poll employees on a list of incentive ideas to see what they like. The literature suggests that about $50 U.S. (at least annually) may be a reasonable minimum (18,23).
2. *Try:* Pilot test the incentive that most people said they would like. Or, just try something novel and unexpected.
3. *Observe:* See how the incentive performs and continue to get feedback on its acceptability. If it's not working, try something else.

Magnitude

Magnitude is a question of how much or how strong. If a gift card is used as an incentive, how much does it need to be worth before people think it is valuable: $10, $50, $200 U.S.? Similarly, if a discounted co-payment for office visits is the incentive, how big should the discount be: $5 U.S. per visit, 25% off, complete waiver? Such considerations require knowledge of the target population. For example, the median salary of a given company may be too high for a $10 U.S. gift card to be valuable. Similarly, the employees may be very young and in relatively good health, making incentives such as reduced office visit co-payments weak. Selecting the appropriate incentive magnitude requires thinking about how deprived the population is of the incentive you are giving. The less the population members have of it, the more valuable it will usually be. Deciding on the appropriate incentive magnitude also involves balancing existing resources. Obviously, there are limits to the costs associated with incentives, depending on the expected ROI. Declines in motivation can also be created by giving so large of an incentive

---

*In the simplest situation, the incentive giver could figure out what is valuable for an individual and basically give individuals the incentive of their choosing. This is often attempted in individual behavior therapy, but at the population level (such as a worksite) such an approach is usually too logistically cumbersome.

that people feel coerced, especially if the incentive is reinforcing weak proxies of actual behaviors (see discussion in 21,22). Generally speaking, the incentive magnitude should be proportional to the work (11).

Frequency

Alongside questions of magnitude, how frequently the incentive is delivered must also be considered. Should incentives be given repeatedly at short intervals or should they be a onetime deal at the end of the year? Again, the driving consideration should be that the incentive frequency is proportional to the work (11). More work should get incentivized more frequently relative to less work. This is because more frequent incentives tend to have higher value. Health promotion programs typically focus on lifestyle changes. By definition, lifestyle changes are long term, so it would seem that incentives should be given frequently over time. For example, weight management involves a combination of behaviors (e.g., eating fewer calories, increasing exercise) that must be sustained acutely over months during the weight loss phase and at least moderately over years during the weight maintenance phase. It makes sense to deliver incentives for such programs at regular intervals, at least in the beginning. As a general rule, it is usually more effective to incentivize early on rather than later (4). The idea is to give people a reason, even if it is an external one, to initiate change and then allow natural contingencies to take over in the long term.

Immediacy

Immediacy is perhaps the simplest component of value, but it is also the most overlooked. It involves the latent period, or lag time, between the target behavior and the delivery of the incentive. This latent period exists on a continuum between immediate and delayed. Incentives are most effective when they are delivered immediately after the target behavior is performed (4,5). The longer the lag time between behavior and incentive, the less certain and weaker the incentive.* In worksite settings, it can be challenging to deliver individual incentives immediately after performance. Part of this is due to the very nature of the incentive.

Gift cards, discounts, and coupons usually require time for people to cash in and get what they want. Also, there are inherent delays due to the logistical problems of gathering information on who has earned the incentive and then actually delivering it. Often, however, too much time is spent trying to pick the perfect kind of incentive and too little time is spent figuring out how that incentive will be delivered. The process of incentive delivery is equally important to ensure that all unnecessary delays are eliminated and that the incentive can be received as quickly as possible after the target behavior has been achieved. A modest, immediate incentive is usually more valued than a large, delayed one (10).

Contingency

The contingency principle is straightforward in that it asserts that the incentive must be earned, or must follow the work. If the behavior of interest is not performed, the incentive is not delivered. When this is done, it creates a true contingent relationship: Do X to get Y. This relationship needs to be understood clearly and delivered with absolute consistency. Individuals need to know exactly what they must do and believe with unqualified certainty that they will get the promised incentive because of doing it (5,24).

Using a Thought Bridge

One way to make delayed incentives feel more immediate (and therefore more effective) is to use a thought bridge. A thought bridge is just something that lets employees know they earned their incentive and when they might expect to get or use it. It can be something as simple as an e-mail message, a printed certificate, or, perhaps most optimally, a face-to-face conversation. The key is to deliver it as quickly as possible after the incentive has been earned. Related to this, be sure to give people frequent progress reports on how close they are to earning their incentive.

*Consider the immediate factors that usually maintain the unhealthy behaviors an incentive program is trying to target. For example, being sedentary after work (e.g., by vegging out or watching television) feels good because it provides a sense of comfort and stress relief. On the other hand, exercising after work may not feel as good, at least not right away, because it involves uncomfortable experiences (e.g., sore muscles and heavy breathing) and its benefits (e.g., improved health and appearance) are more delayed and, by definition, more uncertain.

Among the most challenging parts of setting up an incentive program is figuring out exactly what people should do. At the highest level, it seems obvious. For example, a smoking cessation initiative targets smoking. Individuals who quit smoking get their incentive. Measurement of the target behavior, however, becomes critical at this point. In order to create a true contingent relationship between a behavior (or outcome) and an incentive, the behavior of interest must be verifiable. In this example, it means figuring out how to define and measure smoking cessation. Is it being quit for a day, a week, or half a year? How do you know who has quit? These considerations will, again, have to balance resource, legal, and privacy concerns.

In population-level incentive programs, compromises usually have to be made in terms of what outcome is meaningful, what people can realistically achieve, what is affordable to measure, and what people will accept. It is helpful to start with the ideal and work backward. To use the smoking example, not smoking while being an employee would be the ideal target behavior, but can it be reliably measured? Also, is it feasible to measure over the length of employment? Perhaps proxies for long-term quitting could be used that are balanced against what people are likely to achieve given the resources available for incentives. For example, quitting for 30 d is a relatively good proxy for quitting over the next year. As such, it would probably be a worthwhile behavior to incentivize. Remember, however, that the 30 d quit must be verifiable. Ideally, an objective, reliable lab test such as salivary cotinine could be used. But the nature of such a test must be considered before it can be implemented in the real world. Serum cotinine testing is expensive, time consuming, and invasive and would have to be administered more than once to verify a 30 d quit. Instead of using a serum cotinine, it may be tempting to rely on self-report. For most behaviors, self-report is generally reliable. This changes, however, when an incentive is attached to what is reported. In this case, people *saying* they have quit for 30 d is being incentivized, regardless of whether they have actually quit. It could be argued, then, that for some people being untruthful is reinforced.

If objectively measured smoking cessation is too cost prohibitive and self-reported smoking cessation is not reliable, what could be measured? Perhaps the next best thing is completion of a smoking cessation program. It is not directly incentivizing quitting smoking, but if the program is good (i.e., completion and quit rate are high), completion can serve as a reasonable proxy for smoking cessation. More importantly, the target behavior (i.e., completing the program) is clear and can be objectively measured, and there is no incentive to lie about quitting smoking. In short, such an incentive may not be perfect, but it strikes the best balance because participants complete meaningful work to earn their incentive and do not feel coerced in the process.

Incentives in Context: Smoking and Diet

Incentives are not particularly rare or new intervention strategies (24), but they have been understudied, especially as they relate to worksite health promotion. A handful of systematic literature reviews has been conducted on the general topic of using incentives to improve health (8,9,14,28), mainly in clinical or community populations. Findings from these reviews have generally indicated that incentives work well in the short term, especially for simple, clearly defined, and usually short-term behaviors such as attending clinical appointments, completing screenings or tests, filling out surveys, or adhering to medication. In the long term, and for behaviors and outcomes that are more complex (e.g., diet or weight management), the effects of incentives are weaker or poorly studied.

Of specific interest to worksites are incentives that promote changes in behaviors that are ubiquitous at work but strongly related to increased health care costs and decreased productivity. Behaviors such as smoking cessation and healthy eating are common targets of worksite wellness campaigns (13). Of these behavioral domains, smoking cessation has received the most attention in the scientific literature, with several systematic literature reviews and meta-analyses covering this topic in the last decade (6,12,13,19). Incentive programs for healthy eating have been the subject of one recent literature review (27). Results from these systematic reviews are summarized in table 28.1 and generally parallel what has been found in the more general literature reviews on the topic of incentives for health promotion.

Enhancing the Value of Incentives Through Communication

Incentives are just one factor that explains the outcomes of a program. Few employees will truly be in it just for the money, at least not for very long. Most behavioral scientists agree that a monetary

Table 28.1 Summary of Findings From Recent Systematic Reviews of Incentive-Based Interventions for Smoking Cessation and Healthy Eating

Focus area and study	Studies reviewed	Outcome of interest	Conclusions	Comments
Smoking cessation Janer et al. (13)	5 studies (no design restrictions) Limited to worksite settings	Abstinence from smoking	Incentives were effective for improving short-term (i.e., during the incentive phase) quit rates but were not effective and were potentially negative in the long term.	Broad study selection criteria that included some with weak designs
Smoking cessation Moher et al. (19)	5 controlled trials at the group (versus individual) level Limited to worksite settings and studies with pre- and postintervention follow-up	Abstinence from smoking	Incentives did not improve worksite quit rates at 12 mo follow-up or beyond but did seem to increase participation in smoking cessation programs.	Only review of group-level analyses, but can be difficult to detect individual-level effects
Smoking cessation Hey et al. (12)	15 controlled trials Limited to studies with pre- and postintervention follow-up	Abstinence from smoking (most conservative reported)	Incentives improved quit rates at 6 mo follow-up or less and at least marginally increased participation in smoking cessation programs.	Rigorous study selection criteria that minimized bias
Smoking cessation Donatelle et al. (6)	Several studies (no design or setting restrictions)	Abstinence from smoking	Incentives improved short-term quit rates but not long-term rates (i.e., after 6 mo). Program participation likely increases, especially in community or worksite settings.	Broad study selection criteria that included many with weak designs. Scattered presentation of evidence, but only review of laboratory findings and discussion of theoretical bases of incentives Rigorous study selection criteria that minimized bias
Healthy eating Wall et al. (27)	4 randomized controlled trials	Food consumption, weight change, or food sales	Incentives increased consumption or purchase of healthy foods, as well as weight loss, at 12 mo follow-up or less.	Slightly different incentive strategy, however, that usually involved free or reduced-price healthy foods (versus rewards for consuming healthy foods)

reward, used in a vacuum, is a weak intervention (5). To be optimized, tangible incentives should be paired with positive social interactions (2). This is because monetary incentives and social praise, from a respected social source, have a synergistic interaction. Social reinforcement makes a monetary incentive come alive, enhancing its effectiveness by creating a memory of a positive accomplishment that friends, coworkers, and supervisors value right alongside the individual achieving it. Such experiences long outlast the money spent and help employees understand the bigger picture as to why improving health is

a win–win situation for them and the company. In short, even a modest incentive (e.g., $20 U.S. gift card) can become highly valuable if it is delivered in the context of a larger atmosphere or culture of employers and employees who care about the health of the workforce.

Optimizing an incentive program starts (and ends) with a good communication plan. Previously, we empirically showed that stronger communication strategies make incentives more effective in driving participation (18). In an attempt to confirm these findings, we used similar methodology in an additional analysis that included

78 companies (with 22,838 employees invited to complete a health assessment, HA) and once again constructed interaction categories between the incentives and the communications and marketing approach of the program. Participation was measured as completion of the HA. Quantification of the strength of the incentives was based on the type and magnitude, whereas the strength of the communications approach was based on the frequency of messaging and the overall marketing intensity of the program. Figure 28.1 presents the findings, which corroborated those of our previous analysis (18) and again suggested a strong synergistic relationship between combinations of incentives and communications and employee decisions to complete an HA.

Unfortunately, much of the scientific literature in this area is scattered and must be extrapolated from reviews of clinical trial recruitment efforts and survey participation (7,17). Employees obviously need to know about the incentive program, but promotion cannot stop with a onetime message. Reminders increase participation (1), so they should be delivered frequently and include clear messaging about what the incentive program is, why it is important, and how it works. Because people access information in different ways and at various times, communications should also

be delivered by different mass modalities such as e-mails, posters, pay stub inserts, or designated worksite Intranet sections. In addition, more personal forms of communication, such as invitation letters or departmental meetings, can enhance program participation (15). These types of communication methods likely serve to increase awareness among employees, create word of mouth and conversations on the topic, and enhance opportunities for social reinforcement of lifestyle changes.

Application to Benefits Design

The discussion on incentives would not be complete without addressing health care benefits. The idea of providing an incentive that is linked to benefits design is potentially powerful since employees recognize this as a clear value. Moreover, it is a strategy that can also help offset costs for the employer by shifting higher contributions to employees who are not participating in the health improvement programs, thereby paying, at least in part, for the expenses related to the programs being implemented.

There are a variety of ways in which this incentive can be structured. First, participation in a

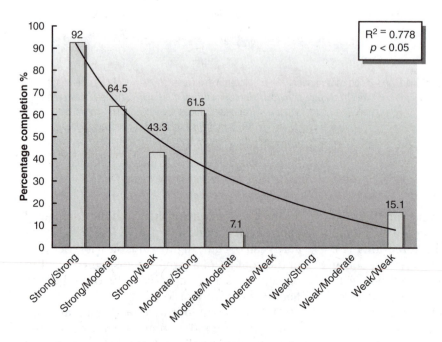

Figure 28.1   Incentives, communications, and HA completion.

program or completion of a health risk appraisal can be linked to benefits as a prerequisite for health insurance eligibility. Next, a reduction in the health insurance premium contribution may be offered. Alternatively, the benefits plan may be adjusted by providing a reduction in the clinic visit co-payments or deductible. For example, a company may decide to structure the incentive such that those who complete a health risk appraisal and a risk reduction program in year one receive a $35 U.S. reduction in their co-payment, a $150 U.S. reduction in their deductible, or a $15 U.S. reduction in their monthly premium (a $180 U.S. annual premium reduction) in year two. One of the first companies to adopt such a strategy was Johnson & Johnson. After the company began offering a $500 U.S. health insurance premium discount for participating in a wellness program (including completion of a health risk appraisal), program participation rapidly increased to 90%.

With the introduction of health reimbursement arrangements (HRAs) and then HSAs as part of consumer-directed health plans (CDHP), many employers began contributing to these spending accounts instead of offering premium differentials or cash bonuses as incentives. There is general agreement that HRAs are more popular than HSAs as funding vehicles for these incentives, because HRAs offer greater flexibility. Table 28.2 outlines several selected characteristics of the HRA and the HSA. Clearly both accounts can be effectively used for the integration of incentives for health promotion activities, although they should be carefully crafted in order to ensure alignment and compliance with federal and state regulations and to ensure appropriate protection of personal privacy. Other chapters in this book provide more detailed overviews of the legal issues associated with incentive designs (for example see Chapter 6).

Important Questions to Ponder

- If you could afford to offer only $10 U.S. worth of incentives per year for each employee, what could you do to enhance the value of that incentive?

- Why might it not be a good idea to incentivize self-reported behavior change?

- What methods of communication would work best for employees where you work? How often do you need to send the message before it is well received?

Table 28.2 Selected Characteristics of HRAs and HSAs

	Health reimbursement arrangement (HRA)	Health savings account (HSA)
Account description	Account funded and owned by employer to reimburse employees' qualified medical expenses	Tax-free account to pay for qualified medical expenses and serve as a retirement savings account
Owner	Employer	Employee
Funders	Employer only	Employee, employer, or both; employee can make tax-free contributions up to an annual maximum defined by the IRS.
Annual contribution limits	No federal limits	Federal limit of $2,850 U.S. (individual) or $5,650 U.S. (family) in 2007
Use	Funds can be used for predetermined medical expenses.	Funds can be used for eligible medical expenses determined by the IRS.
Rollover provisions	The employer determines the annual rollover. Unused funds revert to the employer when the employee leaves or retires from the company—funds are not portable.	Unused funds remain with the employee—funds are portable. Any money left over at the end of the calendar year is rolled over to the next year—interest accrues tax free.
Required companion plan	None required	Must be paired with high-deductible plan (minimum of $1,100 U.S. individual or $2,200 U.S. family in 2007); preventive care expenses are exempt from deductible.

Conclusion

From a population health perspective, worksite-level incentive programs seem to be effective. In the short term, incentive programs can enhance the behavior change effects of health promotion and disease management programs, but they seem to be less effective and not particularly well understood in the long term. Despite this, incentive programs can generate an overall improvement in population-level behavior changes because they tend to garner higher participation in behavior change programs. This point is well demonstrated in table 28.3, which shows results from a small randomized controlled trial by Volpp and colleagues (26). In this trial, the 3 mo quit rate for an incentivized smoking cessation program was higher than the 3 mo quit rate for a nonincentivized smoking cessation program. By 12 mo, the quit rates in each program looked similar, but the incentivized program attracted more smokers to at least try to quit. Therefore the absolute reduction in smoking across the population offered the incentivized program was greater relative to the absolute reduction in the population offered the nonincentivized program.

More recently, the trend for employers has been to initiate incentive plans that are linked to health care benefits design. Such incentives include reductions in deductibles, clinic visit co-payments, or monthly premiums. In addition, incentives have been integrated into specific benefits-related products such as HRAs and HSAs, where contributions are made into those accounts in response to achievement of a prespecified health promotion activity.

Most incentive programs that are delivered in today's workforce are not as optimal as they could be, or, perhaps more aptly described by Daniels (5; p. 151), they are "too little, too few, too late." This is because the incentive structure does not adhere well to the core principles outlined in this chapter. Even in the scientific literature, incentive-based interventions suffer from methodological and design flaws such as small incentive magnitude, delayed delivery, and extremely heterogeneous populations. Given the largely unstudied area of combining incentives with strong communications that can enhance their effectiveness, we might also add *too impersonal* and *too unpublicized* to Daniels' list.

It is important to keep a broad view of behavior change in mind when implementing worksite-level incentives. Even optimally designed programs will probably not be strong enough, if used alone, to maintain the health of a population. Given the current knowledge base in this area, it is best to conceptualize an incentive program as a relatively short-term intervention that gives employees a reason to get excited about healthy lifestyle changes and be rewarded for initiating them. The idea is that the incentive convinces employees to quit smoking, lose weight, improve their diet, or increase their physical activity in the near term so they can be exposed to natural contingencies that maintain such behaviors in the long term. The bottom line is that a $100 U.S. gift card cannot compete (for very long) with feeling stronger, more attractive, and healthier—not to mention the social benefits tied to such outcomes. If an employee does not get at least some of these more elastic benefits from the lifestyle changes that are being encouraged, the dollar amount of the incentive will be irrelevant and cost prohibitive.

Given the wide variety of needs, preferences, and logistical obstacles in any given workforce, implementing a worksite-level incentive program will almost always involve compromises from the ideal. So what is an employer to do? Several design considerations for worksite-level incentive programs are reviewed in the list on p. 247. The overarching theme is to make sure the incentive is paired with something meaningful. Good programs, moderately valuable and valued rewards, and clear rules are a necessary start.

Table 28.3 Smoking Cessation Rates Across Incentivized and Nonincentivized Programs

	Nonincentivized program	Incentivized program
Offered the program	100%	100%
Enrolled in the program	20%	41%
Completed the program	12% (59% of enrollees)	25% (61% of enrollees)
Quit at 12 mo follow-up	5% (24% of enrollees)	7% (16% of enrollees)

Keys for worksite-level incentive programs

- Keep the incentive at a moderate but meaningful magnitude. Earned incentives of about $50 U.S. per year are a reasonable minimum that promotes the initiation of healthy lifestyle changes without fostering feelings of coercion, dependence, or overjustification.

- The best types of incentives are not established but are conditioned items of monetary value such as cash, gift cards, coupons, or discounts. Other, more tangible items such as T-shirts, gadgets, or mugs may be less generalizable across a large group of individuals.

- Enhance the overall value of the incentive as much as possible by
  - delivering it as immediately as possible after the target behavior or outcome is achieved;
  - delivering it frequently, especially early on;
  - pairing it with frequent praise from a meaningful, respected source (e.g., supervisor or department head);
  - using strong communication strategies that keep people aware and informed of expectations, progress, and benefits.

- Make sure the incentive is contingent on the behavior or outcome of interest. If the behavior or outcome of interest cannot be acceptably measured, use the closest possible indirect measure. If the behavior is not at least reasonably verifiable, do not incentivize it.

- Think of incentives as a tool to initiate change. They should be used as a complement to high-quality health promotion programs so the internal benefits of a healthy lifestyle eventually take over. Natural contingencies, not frequent payments, seem best suited to maintain long-term change.

More importantly, employees need to buy into why improving their health is important in the first place. Incentives are a great way to get employees' attention and to get employees focused on making behavior changes they may not have considered otherwise. The success of any worksite incentive program ultimately falls back on the relationship between the giver and the receiver. Frequent, straightforward, and personalized communications regarding what is asked of employees, why it is important, how it benefits all involved, and how things are progressing are essential in keeping employees invested over the long term and in creating a worksite culture that values the health of its employees.

Chapter Review Questions

1. Define the term *incentive*.
2. Which two core principles optimize incentives?
3. Explain the concept of immediacy.
4. Describe a situation in the context of a worksite health management program where a thought bridge is used to manage the incentive component of the overall program.
5. Discuss how incentives may be integrated into an insurance benefits design program.

29

eHealth for Employee Health and Wellness

Optimizing Plan Design and Incentive Management

David K. Ahern, PhD; Lauren Buckel, BA; Edward W. Aberger, PhD; and Michael J. Follick, PhD

A fast-growing area, eHealth is of interest for consumers, health care providers, and employers alike (9). *eHealth* is defined as the use of emerging *interactive* technologies (e.g., Internet, interactive TV, interactive voice response systems, kiosks, or personal digital assistants) to enable health improvement and health care services (6). For the purposes of this chapter, we distinguish among eHealth *platforms* (interactive Web sites and Web portals), eHealth decision-support *tools* (specific, *interactive* applications addressing a particular target behavior or condition such as smoking cessation or diabetes), and eHealth *programs,* which use eHealth platforms and tools to implement a coordinated set of management and evaluation services to achieve overall health improvement as well as to control the increasing trend in health insurance costs.

To guide the reader in understanding the value of eHealth to employers and their employees, this chapter is organized into two major sections: (1) eHealth Platforms and Tools and (2) eHealth Programs to Optimize Plan Design. Useful resources and practical advice are given to enable employers to make informed decisions about using eHealth with their employees.

Growth of eHealth

Across the globe, 80% of Internet users seek health care information online, with increased interest in information regarding doctors and hospitals (14). Increasingly, the Internet is viewed as a primary source of health information, supplementing the information and recommendations received from physicians (12). In addition to static health infor-

mation, increasingly sophisticated interactive and individually tailored applications are accessible through the Internet and Internet-enabled devices for health behavior change and chronic disease management, such as smoking cessation, weight loss, diabetes monitoring and management, and so on. Emerging evidence provides support for the beneficial effects of these types of interactive eHealth applications (1).

Employers and their employees are also benefiting from the burgeoning growth of eHealth. Many employers, especially midsize to large companies, are relying on Web-based platforms and tools to support human resource functions, to help employees manage their health benefits, and to provide links to a range of health-related Web sites and decision-support tools. Increasingly, employers are recognizing the importance of having a healthy workforce not only in terms of controlling the growth of health insurance costs but also in terms of reduced absenteeism and presenteeism and improved productivity. Employers view eHealth as one of a variety of strategies to improve the health of their workforce.

eHealth Strategies for Employers

Table 29.1 presents the various strategies for using eHealth that employers can consider to promote healthy behaviors among their employees. In terms of the most common uses, eHealth tools are being deployed in the employment setting to encourage healthy eating and nutrition, weight loss, smoking cessation, and greater physical activity. In the employer space, eHealth tools are becoming more transactional and tailored to

Table 29.1 Strategies for Using eHealth to Promote Healthy Behaviors

Strategy	Example
Assess health risks of employees.	Provide online, interactive health risk assessment (HRA).
Understand employees' readiness to change and level of activation.	Provide online assessment of state of motivation to change or measure of activation.
Personalize feedback and recommendations for each employee.	Provide individually tailored plan based on baseline health risk behaviors, motivation to change, self-efficacy, and activation level.
Use incentives to encourage employee participation and reinforce target behaviors.	Utilize a Web portal to provide feedback, monitoring, goals achieved, and incentives earned.

personal characteristics, thereby having greater appeal and potential for effect.

eHealth Platforms and Tools

The wide range of available eHealth platforms and tools contributes to the versatility of these interactive technologies. Online health risk assessments (HRAs), e-mail, interactive health promotion and disease management applications, and personal health records are the predominant eHealth platforms and tools that employers have begun to implement as a part of their health and wellness or disease management programs. The following section provides a more in-depth explanation of the uses and benefits of each of these tools as well as discusses factors that act as barriers to their adoption. One common element to all of these eHealth platforms and tools is the tailoring of content and messaging to the individual. Research shows that information that is personalized is more likely to be read and acted upon. Examples of these approaches are given to illustrate the reported effect and value to both employers and employees.

Health Risk Assessments

HRAs are survey instruments designed to assess the health status of employees across a broad range of topics including demographics, health behaviors, risks, and existing conditions. Over the past 20 years, research evidence from the occupational health literature has demonstrated the importance and value of determining employee health status as a first step in identifying patterns of risk factors and prevalence of chronic conditions. Information gained from an HRA can then be used to target intervention programs, and a

postintervention HRA can be used to evaluate the effect of programs. There are many vendors in the HRA marketplace that provide a range of both online and paper versions of HRAs and related services. For employers, the decision to choose one HRA vendor over another is a challenge. Although the actual questionnaires themselves are comparable in terms of their content and questions, there are a number of factors to consider in making an informed choice that meets the needs of the organization. Can the HRA be customized with additional questions? Are biometrics such as blood pressure, BMI, and so on and laboratory information collected? Does it take multiple sessions to complete the HRA? Can the user complete the HRA in multiple sessions? These are just a few of the questions an employer will want to consider. A template to assist employers in evaluating HRA instruments and vendors in terms of the major features and functions of interest is available in table 29.2. Additionally, chapter 16 provides an in-depth overview of health risk assessment tools.

Online HRAs are becoming increasingly popular for obvious reasons relating to their ease of administration, reduced respondent burden, reliability of responses, immediacy of results, and more rapid availability of aggregated information in a database. Providing an online, interactive HRA allows employers to reach a wide geographical range. For example, Chevron Corporation is a self-insured, large employer with facilities and employees spanning the globe. It began its deployment of an HRA with a paper-and-pencil version but from this experience quickly recognized the value of leveraging the Internet in order to scale the application to its more than 50,000 employees and dependents.

Table 29.2   HRA Vendor Selection Template

Questions	Vendor 1	Vendor 2
License Algorithms & Modules		
Level of Customization		
Add/Remove questions		
Interaction with data		
Modification of look and feel		
Modification of flow and output		
Multiple HRA capabilities over time		
Are updates available?		
Host Health Risk Appraisal (Embedded and standalone with link to site)		
Single sign on		
Exchange of data		
Flow interruption		
Modification of look and feel		
Modification of flow and output		
Timeline for data exchanges (real time)		
Can they provide a test platform?		
Is technical support included?		
Multiple HRA capabilities over time		
Are updates available?		
Pricing Options		
Other vendor selection questions		
How many questions?		
Grade level		
Electronic (yes/no)		
Paper (yes/no)		
How long to complete?		
Does it include interest survey questions?		
What is the CVD algorithm used?		
How long is the member report?		
Is there an employer report?		
Can the participant report be customized?		
Can they provide a sample report?		
Can they provide a sample survey?		
Can the participant leave the instrument and finish completing later?		
Can they provide 3 clients using the instrument who have been using it for at least 2 years?		
Contact information		

Chevron Corporation

The Chevron Corporation, headquartered in San Francisco, California, is one of the three largest energy companies in the world. It employs more than 50,000 people in 180 different countries. Five years ago, the company made the switch from a paper-and-pencil HRA that was completed only once every 2 to 3 y to an interactive online HRA that encourages regular use by employees. By instituting a Web-based HRA, the Chevron Corporation has been able to reduce health risks among its employees and dependents. The online tool is available for use by employees and their families and can be taken regularly, providing the company with more accurate information about the health of its employee population. Furthermore, the online assessment allows for a dynamic set of questions that can be tailored to each employee depending on age, gender, health history, and readiness to change. The new design also enables integration of the HRA results and other health promotion programs offered by the company. As of October 2006, 4,158 users had registered. Approximately one-quarter of those users were found to have at least three major risk factors. The company is working to reduce those health risks by integrating the HRA with other programs. In 2001, 87% of participants had either improved or completely eliminated at least one health risk. Overall dropout rates have been very low, which supports the continued use of the program. The Chevron Corporation has had much success with the online HRA and is continuing to work on ways to improve the integration and adoption of the program (8).

E-mail Communications

E-mail is becoming, albeit slowly, a mechanism for communication between providers and patients. Research consistently shows that patients want to e-mail their providers with questions about their health and conditions. Providers are less sanguine about the benefits of e-mail and are concerned about being overwhelmed with questions and increased liability for uncompensated care.

E-mail in the workplace has become ubiquitous and is used as a major channel of communication. Furthermore, it has the potential to serve as a platform for providing health information and tailored health messages to employees as part of an overall health improvement program. One illustration

Promoting Health Through E-Mail

A preliminary study conducted by Patricia Franklin and colleagues (7) that evaluated the use of e-mail for health promotion found this eHealth platform to be an effective method of reaching a broad population and improving participation in health care. Conducted at a large health insurance company in upstate New York, this study involved e-mailing daily health tips from RealAge (www.realage.com) to participants on Mondays through Fridays for 26 wk. Topics addressed in the e-mails included fruit and vegetable intake, physical activity (both aerobic and muscle strengthening), and general healthy living. Over the course of 6 mo, the researchers measured the total number of e-mails participants opened, the number of days participants opened the e-mails, the frequency in which participants opened more than four e-mails per week, and the participants' use of health-related Web links that were embedded in the e-mails. Despite the fact that the modern worker must sort through many e-mails each day, the researchers found that a vast majority of participants (81%) opened the daily e-mails for 23 wk or longer. More than 50% of participants continued to open the e-mails for all 26 wk. Furthermore, the majority of participants opened 4 to 5 e-mails per week throughout the course of the study, and almost all participants (90%) went to the Web links at least once for further information. Another important finding was that the rate of participation did not depend on the employees' baseline health behaviors. The study gives support to the effectiveness of eHealth tools such as e-mail health promotion programs for reaching a wide variety of employees in the workplace and encouraging active participation in health care (7).

of this approach is a study conducted in a large insurance company in upstate New York.

The fact that regular e-mail is not secure, however, limits its widespread use for tailoring health information and content. Moreover, there is increasing concern about the overwhelming amount of e-mail that employees receive, which may preclude its use for reliable and effective messaging.

Interactive Tools for Behavior Change and Disease Management

The eHealth movement has led to a surge in the development of interactive decision-support tools to assist employees in changing their health behaviors (e.g., exercise and weight management, smoking cessation, nutrition, alcohol and other drug use) or managing chronic diseases (e.g., diabetes, asthma, heart disease). These interventions can be delivered via CD-ROMs, wireless networks, the Internet, or stand-alone devices that connect to telephone lines and may include components as vastly different as biometric monitoring, simple questions about health risks, remote transmission of this information to providers, and reminders and prompts such as a reminder to take prescription medication. Current studies on these and other interactive eHealth applications note encouraging trends in behavior change or support the deployment of Web-based tailored interventions. However, they also highlight difficulties, such as lack of generalizability to diverse populations or health and disease states, maintaining participant enrollment in programs, sustaining changes over time, and integrating these systems into office work flow and showing ROI. There is some emerging evidence that indicates that remote disease monitoring is a cost-effective component of disease management programs and that patient-centered care can be enhanced with an electronic shared decision-making system. However, because these interventions are in the nascent stage of evolution, no single standard or approach stands alone as best of breed.

Employers, often through their TPAs or outsource vendors, are benefiting from these interactive applications as part of their health and wellness and disease management programs. As an example, Pfizer implemented a targeted program using a tailored Web portal with multiple functions including an HRA, disease management resources, and health coaching. Incentives were also included in this program to encourage enrollment and participation in screening.

Healthy Pfizer

The Healthy Pfizer initiative began in 2005 as a targeted health and wellness program for the company's 41,223 U.S. employee members and their dependents. As a part of this multifaceted plan, a tailored Web portal is offered to assist members in the management of their health. Through the use of this portal, employees have access to an online health questionnaire (used as a risk assessment tool), health coaching, disease management assistance, online health advisors, and an electronic data warehouse that is used to record progress. As of December 2006, more than 13,000 members had enrolled in the program, which is expected to lower the company's overall health care costs and improve overall population health. In order to encourage employee participation, Pfizer has offered incentives in return for use of the program. In the first year, Pfizer attempted to increase members' engagement with their health care by offering $100 U.S. in gift cards and a 20% discount on insurance premiums to those employees and their dependents who completed the health questionnaire and screening. In the second year of the program, Pfizer encouraged further involvement by requiring participants to retake the questionnaire, receive an annual physical, enroll in the coaching program and participate in at least two sessions, join a walking program, and start putting together a personal health record in order to receive the maximum incentive. Although this is a relatively new eHealth initiative, Pfizer has already seen improvements among the health of its employee members and expects that trend to continue in coming years (4).

Personal Health Records

There is growing interest among employers in the potential value of the personal health record (PHR) as part of a strategy to encourage employees to engage in their own health care and to empower personal responsibility for health. Unlike electronic medical records (EMRs), PHRs allow employees to control the information and the access to data within their PHR. Conceptually, the PHR is not linked to a single provider or health plan, spans an employee's lifetime, and can contain data entered by employees that might not normally be part of a medical record (e.g., nonprescription medications and supplements, alternative and complementary modalities of care). However, there are some concerns about employees' willingness to use a PHR if offered one by their employer. Trust and concern about confidentiality and security appear to be the major factors that contribute to this reluctance. Nevertheless, employers are looking carefully at PHRs as yet another eHealth tool to convey to their employees the importance of personal responsibility for health. At this early stage of development, many PHRs are limited in functionality, and people continue to raise questions about access to them, especially in emergencies. Additionally, most health care providers do not have their medical records stored in an electronic, interoperable format, which limits the transfer of data from that source to an individual's PHR. Nevertheless, results from the Personal Health Working Group, part of the Markle Foundation's Connecting for Health initiative, indicated that more than 70% of respondents (from a national survey of 1,246 U.S. households) would use one or more features of a PHR to e-mail their doctor, track immunizations, note mistakes in the record, transfer information to new providers, and get and track test results (10).

Recently, a coalition of large employers, including Wal-Mart and Pitney Bowes, has formed to develop and implement a PHR for their employees. Also, Microsoft has just announced the availability of a secure PHR called *HealthVault* that is available free to the public with partnerships with health care providers and institutions to enable interoperability of information flow between the PHR and the EMR. Time will tell if these early demonstration projects are successful.

Examples of eHealth Platforms and Tools for Specific Behaviors and Conditions

The variety of available eHealth tools provides ample opportunities for interventions that promote behavior change among employees. The most common target behaviors and conditions on which eHealth interventions have been focused are obesity, sedentary lifestyle, nutrition, chronic disease management, access to and use of medications, and detection of underlying health risks. Table 29.3 provides some possible uses of various eHealth platforms to improve health outcomes in each of these areas. Table 29.3 is meant to provide examples rather than serve an all-inclusive list. While some behaviors have the potential of being

Table 29.3   eHealth Platforms and Tools for Promoting Behavior Change

Condition or behavior	eHealth platform or tool	Example
Obesity	Web site	Interactive Web site that provides online counseling, discussion board, calorie calculators, sample weekly menus, and so on
Sedentary lifestyle	E-mail	Weekly e-mail tips on practical ways to increase physical activity, sample exercises, and health facts about the benefits of physical activity
Nutrition	Computer-tailored magazine	Tailored program that assesses nutritional areas that need improvement and provides individual feedback on healthy eating tips and so on, focused on areas employee needs the most
Chronic disease management	Secure online portal	Portal that allows employee to communicate with the clinic to request refills, follow-up appointments, and so on
Enhanced access to and improved use of medications	Interactive Web-based program	Program that provides access to educational information about appropriate use of medications as well as incentives for cost-effective medication choices, provides access to online medication records, and provides platform to confidentially ask medication-related questions
Undetected health risks or problems	Online HRA	HRA that allows for more frequent monitoring of employee health and behavior and that can be easily integrated into other aspects of a health promotion program

influenced by several different platforms and tools (or a combination of these), others are tied to a more specific mechanism. For example, the high prevalence of obesity can be addressed by using an interactive Web site that encourages accountability for behavior change. This can be done by allowing registered members to track their progress over time, to participate in online counseling sessions with certified counselors or to join discussion board sessions with other members, and to access supplemental tools such as calorie calculators and sample menus for healthy eating. At the same time, the behaviors contributing to obesity can also be influenced through the use of weekly e-mails that provide tailored weight loss tips or advice from a counselor.

On the other hand, the detection of health risks among the employee population is best done through the use of a comprehensive online HRA as discussed previously. As seen with the example of the Chevron Corporation, the online HRA provides many advantages over the traditional pencil-and-paper one, as it has the ability to provide immediate feedback, allows for more regular monitoring of health status, and can be easily integrated into other health promotion programs that may already be established in the company. Additionally, due to the ease of capturing and storing data with online HRAs, employers have the potential to combine various platforms to provide a more comprehensive intervention for their employees. For example, an online HRA can first be used to identify individual risk factors, after which the employee can be directed to a Web-based program intended to influence specific behaviors (obesity, medication compliance, nutrition, and so on) that attempt to reduce the discovered risks.

It is important to note, however, that eHealth platforms and tools in and of themselves are not the solution to improved employee health and wellness. Rather, they are useful components of an overall *eHealth program,* a process that integrates health plan design, strategic use of incentives, and management and evaluation services. The next section describes how eHealth programs can play an important role in making health plans more effective.

eHealth Programs to Optimize Plan Design

Recently, commercial health insurance has been moving toward innovation and change in health plan designs. As costs of health care continue to rise, employers can attempt to control these increases by giving employees and their dependents more responsibility for the costs and self-care of their own health. Two types of plan designs relying on this principle that have become increasingly popular among employers are consumer-directed health plans (CDHP) and value-based health plans (VBHP). The CDHP combines a high-deductible plan with an emphasis on *transparency* in the quality and costs of health care (3). The majority of the financial risk in this design rests with the employee. In order to be successful, the CDHP is dependent on the transparency of information, as it relies on a patient's ability to discriminate between services that are essential and services that are less necessary. The VBHP, or evidence-based health plan, on the other hand, promotes consumerism through support for healthy behaviors and receipt of evidence-based care leading to improved health outcomes. In order to do this, the VBHP relies on structured incentives and a system based on value. One main area of health care in which this is implemented is employee medication benefits. Under this design, the inherent benefit of the medication in terms of its effect on health improvement is held in the same regard as the cost of the medication. A tiered benefits system is still utilized, but instead of being tiered on cost alone, co-payment rates are tiered on the value of the medication (3), with the highest valued medications (generally drugs deemed as lifesaving) set in the lowest tier, regardless of whether they are generic or brand name.

Health Plan Design, eHealth Platforms, and eHealth Tools

The successful utilization of these emerging plan designs illustrates another important role of eHealth platforms, tools, and programs. In this regard, eHealth can be used to assist companies in a variety of ways. At the very least, electronic resources have the ability to facilitate employees' understanding of health plan benefits and how they operate. As health plan designs continue to evolve and become more complicated through the implementation of higher deductibles, differential co-payments for services, and differential out-of-pocket costs for use of different providers, Internet-based tools can be used to offer employees easy access to the various aspects of their health plan. Furthermore, eHealth tools can also provide a mechanism for employees to access and choose networks of providers and other services, which is particularly essential for health plans that follow a consumer-directed approach.

Online tools can also be used to educate employees to become careful consumers of health care. The very nature of eHealth gives it the potential to increase transparency of information regarding both cost and quality of various health care services. Providing online data regarding the cost of various physicians, specialty practices, and services as well as quality data for local hospitals gives patients the ability to evaluate their options as they decide how best to spend their health care dollars.

However, the greatest opportunity and value of eHealth lie not only in educating members about their benefits and the costs of care but also in being synergistically integrated with plan design to help achieve improved health outcomes and ultimately reduced costs. One feature of eHealth that enables this integration is the ability to organize and manage various aspects of the health plan. The successful implementation of these plan designs depends on the organization of data from many different sources. eHealth tools allow for a patient's pertinent clinical information to be incorporated into the benefits design. In this way, a patient's prescription can automatically receive any co-payment waiver or reduction that may be warranted through a value-based design. Additionally, employers can track the progress of employee compliance to determine whether their plan design is having the desired effect.

Even more importantly, there is an opportunity to structure plan designs to incorporate incentives with the use of eHealth. This feature allows for an effective bridge between eHealth tools and health care benefits designs. While many eHealth platforms and tools have been shown to be effective in promoting behavior change, they are limited by low rates of adoption and usage. Through the incentives offered by plan designs, however, use of eHealth tools can be promoted and improved.

Incentives and Incentive Management

Incentives—money and other rewards—are increasingly recognized as an important vehicle for engaging employees and promoting healthy behavior changes. Based on the behavioral principle of reinforcement, incentives can serve as a critically important means for employees to get in the game and take action when they might otherwise stay on the sideline. eHealth platforms and tools can enable and support VBHP or CDHP designs with structured incentives—that is, incentives that are contingent on specific, targeted

health behaviors. Conversely, the health plan designs can help increase participation in various eHealth initiatives, thereby increasing their potential to reach a large population and produce significant behavior changes. Examples include co-payment reductions for employees who take part in an online nutrition program or lower premium contributions for employees who complete an online tailored HRA. Using eHealth technologies to promote health requires fewer resources than those required by traditional health promotion programs offered at worksites, because both the start-up and maintenance costs are relatively low. Even after providing financial incentives to employees who enroll, employers should expect to see significant cost savings from the overall reduction in adverse health outcomes.

In turn, eHealth can promote improved consumerism and self-care as well as reduction of risk factors and other health problems, which can help plan designs achieve the critical goal of optimizing health and health outcomes. The synergy of plan designs that promote health and wellness combined with online tools that make resources for their improvement easily accessible and widely disseminated can help employers move toward a healthier (and therefore more productive) workforce.

One example of a successful integration of an eHealth program with employer benefits design is the *myMedicationAdvisor* program developed by Abacus Health Solutions (Cranston, Rhode Island). This eHealth program is meant to be integrated into a preexisting pharmacy benefits plan and promotes the safe and cost-effective use of prescription medications. Additionally, the program incorporates a transactional Web portal, medication records, and risk profiles for members.

Another illustration of the integration between eHealth and benefits design is the *Good Health Gateway,* also developed by Abacus Health Solutions. This comprehensive eHealth program utilizes the principles of value-based plan design and uses a secure Web platform to promote better health through diabetes management. Members with diabetes can enroll in the program to receive waivers on both co-payments for generic medications and costs for any diabetes durable medical equipment. The use of an eHealth platform is pivotal to the success of the program. By enrolling, employees are given a tangible set of goals to manage their condition that they can view each time they log on. This results in improved health outcomes and cost savings for the employee and employer alike. All necessary information for

Enhanced Access
to Cost-Effective Medication: myMedicationAdvisor

The myMedicationAdvisor program is an interactive Web site that can be used as an add-on to the existing employer-provided pharmacy benefit. Features of the Web site include the following:

- Educational text regarding medication use and safety
- An In the News section with current updates
- A Medication Record for use with prescribers and pharmacists
- An interactive Medication Error Risk Profile with feedback to reduce individual risk
- A Choose the Best Medication section that suggests important considerations to discuss with providers regarding medication options
- An Ask-a-Pharmacist service for confidential responses to medication-related questions
- Interactive Therapeutic Lifestyle Change Web tools to support and enhance medication value through a comprehensive behavioral approach to the treatment of cholesterol, hypertension, and related conditions

myMedicationAdvisor also includes an incentive program that can be customized to the individual employer and allows for the integration of products from outside vendors. Incentives are intended to reward members for working with their health care providers to select treatment options with maximum value, such as generic alternatives to brand-name medications. Members who elect to use these savings programs obtain their prescriptions for free (the co-payment is waived). To date, the myMedicationAdvisor program has been used successfully by 90 municipal entities in New England as well as by a consortium of public schools in California covering an additional 112,000+ lives. On average, the program has resulted in savings of $40 to $60 U.S. per 30 d prescription.

program progress is organized in one location, allowing plan members as well as their employers to track that progress. Furthermore, the Good Health Gateway allows for implementation of feedback, dispersal of incentives and rewards, and aggregation of progress reports for the employer. An additional component to improve overall health that this program provides is access to other valuable health management tools, such as heart age and BMI calculators.

The Good Health Gateway diabetes initiative constitutes a direct investment by the employer in integrating eHealth support and benefits design modifications to enhance pharmacy access to its health plan membership. Good Health Gateway, as the vehicle for incentive administration and delivery, is designed to attract members' interest and encourage frequent, regular use of the eHealth platform and tools, providing ongoing education, support, and direct reinforcement for proactive diabetes self-care. The employer investment is predicated on well-established evidence demonstrating the economic case for application of evidence-based standards to the management

of diabetes. In a review of the literature, Berger (2007) documented the substantial differences in both short- and long-term direct health care costs for those whose diabetes is effectively managed versus those with ineffective management: Annual costs are 32% lower ($1,171 U.S. per person) in the effectively managed population (2,13). Berger reviews the value-based employer initiative by Pitney Bowes, in which reduction of pharmacy co-payments for antidiabetes medications resulted in improved medication adherence, decreased pharmacy costs for individuals with diabetes, decreased emergency room visits, and decreased diabetes-related disability. The latter effect is especially critical, with evidence indicating that the indirect costs of diabetes to employers in the form of lost productivity are 4.5 times the direct health care costs (5).

The value proposition to employers is clear for providing an eHealth program to enhance pharmacy access and adherence to diabetes standards of care. The value proposition to covered health plan members is equally compelling. Employees and covered dependents receive direct and

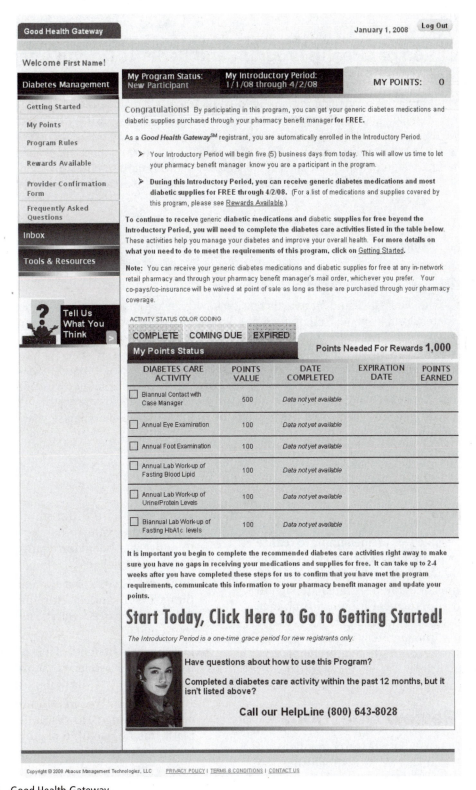

Figure 29.1 Good Health Gateway.
Reprinted, by permission, from Abacus Management Technologies LLC.

immediate value through reduced out-of-pocket costs for antidiabetes medications and supplies. In addition, they are able to access tools and support for understanding and managing their condition as well as obtain intermediate and long-term value in avoidance and reduction of the sequelae and comorbidities associated with unmanaged diabetes.

A screen shot of the Good Health Gateway can be seen in figure 29.1. A more in-depth description of the program is given in the following sidebar.

An Illustration of eHealth Program and Benefits Design Integration: Incentives for Managing Diabetes Among Employees

A large national financial services company is introducing an insurance plan that includes a new initiative for employees and adult dependents with diabetes. The program is designed to improve access and provide rewards for those members who attempt to actively manage their diabetes and work to improve overall health outcomes. Using an eHealth platform called the *Good Health Gateway,* the benefits design provides incentives for employees who maintain certain evidence-based standards of diabetes care. In order to qualify for the incentives, participants must complete the following:

• Annual eye examination

• Annual foot examination

• Annual laboratory workup of fasting blood lipids and urinalysis

• Quarterly laboratory workup of fasting Hb_{A1c} levels

Employees who meet the listed standards qualify for 100% coverage of generic diabetes medications and diabetes durable medical equipment purchased through the company's pharmacy benefits managers. Progress toward these goals can be tracked using the *Good Health Gateway* platform. In addition to receiving financial incentives, participating members also have access to diabetes care management staff, with whom they can discuss the importance of the maintenance guidelines recommended by the program. Encouragement for completing any missing or outdated exams as well as a review of overall diabetes self-care is also provided by the support staff. The program was set to launch January 1, 2008, and will be an important step toward managing diabetes among the employed population.

Conclusion

Employers and employees are beginning to realize the powerful benefits of eHealth platforms and tools, especially when offered as components of eHealth programs integrated with plan design to encourage and support health behavior change and chronic disease management. As eHealth advances there will undoubtedly be more opportunity for innovative programs to support employers and employees in their search for better health and affordable health care.

Chapter Review Questions

1. Define eHealth. What are the components of eHealth initiatives? What distinguishes the types from each other?

2. What are some different eHealth tools? Think of an example use for one such tool to address a behavior change intervention for your employees.

3. Why are eHealth and the emerging health plans discussed in this chapter closely linked? How can eHealth be used to optimize these plans?

4. List the main benefits of using eHealth initiatives in the workplace that are discussed in this chapter.

5. Why are incentives important in promoting behavior change? How can eHealth tools and platforms be useful in deploying incentive-based programs for employees?

30

Effective Programs to Promote Worker Health Within Healthy and Safe Worksites

Glorian Sorensen, PhD, MPH, and Lisa Quintiliani, PhD

Risk-related behaviors contribute to a significant proportion of chronic diseases and have important implications for worker health outcomes. Increasingly within the United States, worksites are providing programming to reduce these risk-related behaviors (71). Worksite health promotion (WHP) programs are designed to promote healthy behaviors such as tobacco cessation, weight control, healthy diet, physical activity, seat belt use, influenza vaccinations, adherence to screening guidelines (e.g., mammography, blood pressure, cholesterol), substance abuse prevention, case management (e.g., diabetes), and sun exposure prevention (87,138,140). The WHO describes the workplace as a priority setting for health promotion regarding a variety of behaviors, including diet and physical activity promotion, as outlined in a technical paper prepared for the WHO and World Economic Forum (WEF) joint event on preventing chronic diseases in the workplace (106). As this book clearly documents, the workplace offers numerous advantages for delivery of WHP programs. Worksites provide an important setting for influencing health behaviors through educational efforts designed to reach large numbers of workers not accessible through other channels. Worksites offer the potential for support of long-term behavior changes, mobilization of peer support, use of environmental supports, and offering comprehensive multilevel interventions repeatedly over time as a means of building and sustaining interest in behavior changes (1,6,12,19,23).

WHP programs share the goal of promoting worker health with occupational safety and health (OSH) efforts, which are designed to minimize workers' exposures to job-related risks, including exposures to physical, biological, chemical, ergonomic, and psychosocial hazards (69). These interventions may include changes in the organization and environment, such as the use of product substitution, engineering controls, and job redesign, as well as through individual efforts, including use of personal protective equipment, generally seen as a supplemental measure.

WHP and OSH provide two parallel pathways for promoting worker health within healthy workplaces. A growing body of research conducted by this research team (8,10,68,121,122,127,128)

This paper has been drawn extensively from a previous paper adapted by permission from the National Institute for Occupational Safety and Health: Sorensen, G., Barbeau, E. Steps to a healthier US workforce: Integrating occupational health and safety and worksite health promotion: State of the science. Commissioned paper for NIOSH Steps to a Healthier US Workforce Symposium; October 26-28, 2004; Washington, DC.

Acknowledgements: Our thinking on this topic has been greatly informed by our collaborators, among them Elizabeth Barbeau, Gary Bennett, Karen Emmons, Elizabeth Harden, Mary Kay Hunt, Anthony LaMontagne, Deborah McLellan, Anne Stoddard, Lorraine Wallace, Gregory Wagner, and Richard Youngstrom, and by the worksites and unions collaborating on our research. We additionally appreciate the support of a grant from Liberty Mutual Insurance Company and funding from the National Cancer Institute (1K05 CA108663 and 2R25 057711). The findings and conclusions of this chapter are those of the authors and do not necessarily represent the views of the funding agency.

and others (74,75,103) demonstrates that these parallel efforts can be strengthened when they are coordinated and integrated rather than separate and independent. Going beyond the simple sum of their parts, integrated interventions are a different way of conceptualizing, studying, and intervening to improve and protect worker health. This approach is now recognized within the core principles of numerous international efforts supporting worker health (31,147,149).

The purpose of this chapter is to describe best-practice programs to reduce health risks and optimize worker health, integrating efforts to promote healthy behaviors with those designed to create and maintain a safe and healthy work environment. We summarize the evidence describing key components of effective WHP programs, describe the rationale and evidence for an integrated approach linking WHP and OSH efforts, and outline the evidence for best-practice approaches to implementing these programs.

The Evidence on Worksite Health Promotion

The 2004 National Worksite Health Promotion Survey of 730 worksites found that many companies provide some type of health promotion programming. For example, of the surveyed companies, 26% provided health education, 30% provided supportive social and physical environments, and 24% provided worksite screening (71). According to the National Health Interview Survey in 1994, 61% of U.S. employees aged 18 y and older took part in employer-sponsored health promotion activities, defined to include one or more elements of a comprehensive workplace health promotion program (18). In addition, according to the National Compensation Survey, percentages of U.S. workers with access to workplace health programs have increased in recent years. In 2005, 40% of workers had access to EAPs, 23% had access to WHP programs, and 13% had access to on-site or subsidized fitness centers (139). However, these programs are not equally available to all workers. These programs are less frequently available to employees of smaller worksites, employees earning $15 U.S. an hour or less, employees in blue-collar occupations, and employees working part time (139). Even when programs are available, participation rates are not equivalent across worksites. Participants are most likely to be salaried, white-collar employees whose general health is better than average (72).

WHP research has documented the efficacy of these programs across a wide array of outcomes, including changes in anthropometric measures, health behaviors, life satisfaction indicators, and measures of morbidity and mortality. In general, results from randomized studies of WHP have found modest yet promising effect sizes (11,27,72,107,133). We examined literature reviews of WHP programs and noted when at least one of the studies reviewed indicated a significant finding; figure 30.1 summarizes these results for programs targeting physical activity, nutrition or cholesterol, weight control, alcohol use, and cancer risk factors as well as for multicomponent programs. The studies included have a range of study designs; although authors of these reviews place the most weight on the results of randomized controlled studies, other study designs were included. Methodological limitations to the studies included in these reviews are inadequate sample sizes; the use of nonrandomized designs; differential attrition across study groups; analysis at the individual level failing to take into account group randomization; and the use of inadequate measures, including relying solely on worker self-reports rather than using additional objective measures, such as biochemical assessments.

One concern sometimes raised in the interpretation of the results of these studies is the magnitude of effect sizes, even when statistically significant changes in behavior are found. Some observers continue to apply the standard of clinical significance in assessing the magnitude of the results of these trials. Yet, as Rose noted (111,112), small changes in behavior observed across entire populations are likely to have large effects on disease risk. For example, Tosteson and colleagues (137) estimated the cost-effectiveness of population-wide strategies to reduce serum cholesterol and found that community-based interventions to reduce serum cholesterol are cost effective if serum cholesterol is reduced by only 2% or more (137). It is important that the standards used for interpretation of the results of worksite intervention studies be based on the public health significance of the effects.

The OSH Approach

OSH programs have traditionally been concerned with reducing hazardous exposures at work that can lead to work-related injury, illness, and disability (134). These interventions are predominantly within the domain of management

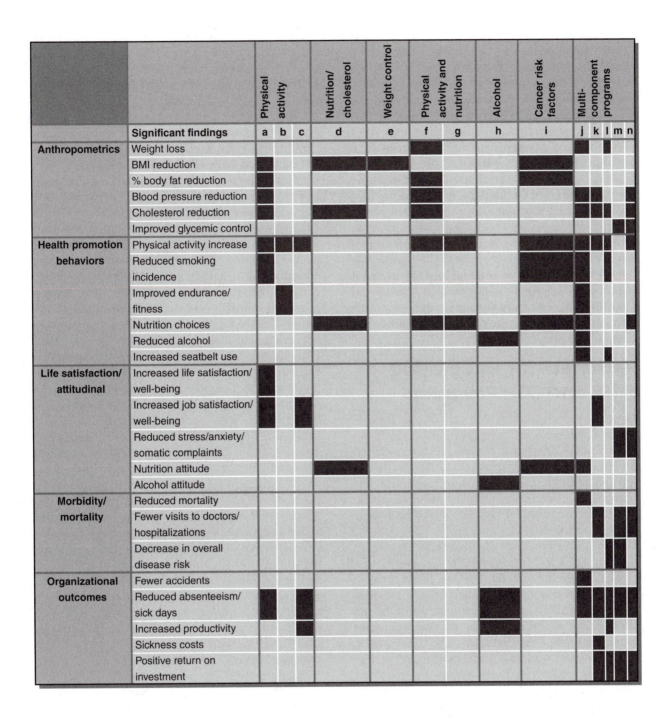

[1] Studies included in each review may overlap.
[2] Literature review, number of studies (years) *(reference)*
a. Shepard 1996, 52 (1972-1994) *(116)*
b. Dishman et al. 1998, 26 (1979-1995) *(26)*
c. Proper et al. 2002, 8 (1981-1999) *(105)*
d. Glanz et al. 1996, Nutr=10, Chol=16 (1980-1995) *(40)*
e. Hennrikus et al. 1996 43, (1968-1994) *(52)*
f. Matson-Koffman et al. 2005 18 (1991-2001) *(78)*
g. Engbers et al. 2005, 13 (1987-2002) *(29)*

h. Roman et al. 1996 24 (1970-1995) *(110)*
i. Janer et al. 2002 45 (1984-2000) *(57)*
j. Heaney et al. 1997, 47 (1978-1996) *(50)*
k. Pelletier 1996, 26 (1992-1995) *(97)*
l. Pelletier 1999, 11 (1998-2000) *(98)*
m. Pelletier 2001, 12 (1998-2000) *(99)*
n. Pelletier 2005 8 (2000-2004) *(100)*

Figure 30.1 Health risk reduction through various WHP methods (by significant findings).

decisions rather than individual worker actions (23,47) and may also be the subject of joint decision making by labor and management through collective bargaining or less formal means. Coordination between OSH and WHP has not been the norm in the United States, and the two fields have generally approached their objectives with differing assumptions, differing priorities, and differing methods. Although, like WHP interventions, OSH interventions operate at multiple levels of influence (individual, organizational, or both), the starting point is more likely to be at the organizational level, depending on the hazards present and the type of workplace. Many occupational health practitioners base their approach to interventions on the well-recognized hierarchy of controls model. As we describe later, this model calls for adherence to a recommended sequence for control of hazards beginning with control as close to the source as possible (90).

Rationale for Integrating WHP and OSH Programs

There have been increasing calls for a comprehensive approach to worker health, based on multidisciplinary, integrated methods aimed at creating health-promoting workplaces (6,12,19,23,109,120,123,143). There are several key reasons that integrating OSH and WHP may have particular benefits for worker health and their work environments.

First, workers' risk of disease is increased by exposures to both occupational hazards and risk-related behaviors (83,86). The effects of these dual risks are not independent of one another (142). Take, as an example, exposure to tobacco (120). Some of the same toxic agents present in tobacco smoke are also hazards in the worksite (e.g., benzene), and thus workers who smoke may be doubly exposed to these agents through their exposures on the job. In addition, tobacco smoke and toxic agents found in the worksite may interact synergistically, increasing the profound effect beyond the simple addition of the two exposures alone (e.g., asbestos).

Second, the workers at highest risk for exposure to hazardous working conditions are also those most likely to engage in risk-related health behaviors. Exposure to both job risks and risk-related behaviors are concentrated among those employed in working-class occupations (38,85,89). Workers in these occupations are more likely to be injured or become ill due to workplace hazards than are professional employees (86). Risk-related behaviors also are concentrated in working-class occupations and workers with lower levels of education. Overweight status is inversely associated with education level (33,36,82,113) and occupation (36,113). There is also evidence that exposure to job hazards and health behaviors are correlated. For example, increased exposure to hazards on the job has been linked with unhealthy dietary habits among blue-collar workers (59,95).

Third, integrating WHP and OSH may increase program participation and effectiveness for high-risk workers. Workers at highest risk for job exposures may be more likely to participate in integrated OSH and WHP programs than in WHP programs alone. There is evidence from the risk communication field that people place highest priority on those risks that are involuntary, outside personal control, undetectable, and seemingly unfair (7,15,35), features that often characterize occupational hazards. Accordingly, workers may perceive management's actions to reduce workers' exposures to occupational hazards as being more important than personal health behavior changes and may feel that the benefits of individual health behavior changes are insignificant in the face of exposures to workplace hazards (120). Skepticism about management's commitment to improve worker health may reduce workers' interest in participating in health promotion programs at work (84,123,144). Conversely, employer efforts to create a safe and healthy work environment may foster a climate of trust and thereby enhance workers' receptivity to messages from their employer regarding health behavior change. In a study of blue-collar workers, we found that workers who reported that their employers had made changes to reduce hazardous exposures on the job were significantly more likely to have participated in smoking cessation and nutrition programs than were workers not reporting management changes (129). Reduction of job risks may be required to both gain credibility and increase the audience's receptivity to health education messages about individual health behaviors (46,127). In addition, programs integrating messages about job risks and risk-related behaviors may increase workers' motivations to make health behavior changes (126).

Finally, integrated OSH and WHP efforts may benefit the broader work organization and environment. A growing literature demonstrates the benefits of WHP programs in terms of both direct costs (e.g., reduction in health care costs; 44,77,94) and indirect costs (e.g., reductions in costs due to lost production as a result of decreased productivity or increased work absence; 3,4,32,43,44,49,92,115). In addition, research also indicates the cost-effectiveness of using OSH interventions to prevent occupational diseases (66,67). Within this growing literature, comprehensive programs integrating employee wellness, disability management, employee assistance, and occupational medicine have been shown to result in long-term savings in medical care utilization and expenditures (94) and reductions in sickness absence (74).

Evidence for the Effectiveness of Integrated OSH and WHP Programs

Evidence is beginning to accumulate documenting the potential benefits of interventions integrating efforts to reduce behavioral risks with OSH initiatives, particularly for worker health behaviors (74,120,121,127). An increasing number of companies and labor unions have reported successful application of integrated approaches, including Johnson & Johnson (56), UAW and GM (28), Chevron Corporation (145), 3M (5), Glaxo Wellcome (GlaxoSmithKline) (131), Citibank (91,93), the Laborers' International Union of North America (122), and the International Association of Bridge, Structural, Ornamental and Reinforcing Iron Workers (8). These initiatives have begun to change the dialogue about approaches to worker health, increasing the focus on integration. This trend is clearly evident in the IOM report *Integrating Employee Health: A Model Program for NASA* (55). This report recommended that forward-looking employers, such as NASA, integrate occupational health, health promotion, and related functions supporting employee health as a means of improving the health and performance of their workforce (55).

Table 30.1 summarizes key studies assessing the effectiveness of integrated OSH and WHP interventions. Included in this table are summaries of a series of studies we have conducted to examine the efficacy of interventions integrating WHP and OSH across multiple levels of influence.

One of these studies, WellWorks-2, was designed specifically to explore the incremental effect of adding OSH to WHP efforts, asking the question, Does the addition of worksite OSH increase the effectiveness of worksite health promotion only (128)? Using a randomized controlled design, 15 midsize to large manufacturing worksites were randomly assigned to receive either WHP only or WHP plus OSH. We hypothesized a priori that the integrated OSH and WHP intervention would have the most relevance to workers in hourly positions, in which exposures to hazards on the job are more common than exposures among salaried jobs. Smoking quit rates among hourly workers in the OSH and WHP condition more than doubled relative to those in the WHP condition (11.8% versus 5.9%; $p = .04$) and were comparable to quit rates of salaried workers. We found no differences in quit rates between groups for salaried workers. We found no significant between-group differences in change in fruit and vegetable consumption, either in the sample overall or by job type. Nonetheless, these findings indicate the potential significant contribution of an integrated OSH and WHP intervention in promoting smoking cessation among blue-collar workers. We also found that worksites in the health promotion and OSH condition made statistically significant improvements in their health and safety programs compared with health promotion only sites (68) and that worker participation in intervention programs was significantly higher in the OSH and WHP condition than in the WHP condition (53). Broad-based dissemination of a program such as this is likely to have significant public health benefits (20).

Characteristics of Best-Practice Programs

An integrated approach to worker health aims to link programs ranging from wellness initiatives to medical benefits design and incentives to short- and long-term disability to workers' compensation to disease management programs to OSH into a single process emphasizing coordination, measurement, and feedback loops from outcomes to further inform ongoing program design (55). In this way, unlike a piecemeal approach, a comprehensive approach to worker health addresses multiple sources of health outcomes, both on and off the job, by offering multiple and coordinated interventions targeting both workers and management (19,23,43,55,119).

In this section, we describe key elements of best-practice programs, following recommendations provided by the IOM (55), the Corporate Health Promotion Consortium Benchmarking Study from the American Productivity and Quality Center (APQC; 14), emerging work from the NIOSH WorkLife Initiative (42,119), and others (124). As described in chapter 22, a key starting point for designing programs to promote worker health is a solid theoretical foundation. Best-practice programs are guided by

Table 30.1 Studies Integrating OSH and Health Promotion

Study	Design	Intervention outcomes	Intervention[‡]	Results	Setting
WellWorks-1 (127)	RCT* worksites	Smoking cessation Dietary habits	● ● ● ●	Significant improvements in smoking cessation and fruit and vegetable consumption for all workers Significant improvements in fiber consumption for laborers	Midsize to large manufacturing worksites (*n* = 24 sites)
WellWorks-2 (128)	RCT* worksites	Smoking cessation Fruit and vegetable consumption OSH exposures	● ● ● ●	Significant improvements in smoking cessation among hourly workers Significant improvements in OSH programs	Midsize to large manufacturing worksites (*n* = 15 sites)
The Brabantia Project (74)	Quasi-experimental pre- and poststudy design	Lifestyle score (smoking, physical activity, hours sleep, BMI, alcohol use, fat intake) Health risk General stress reactions Working conditions Absenteeism	● ● ● ●	Improved cardiovascular health (due to improved serum cholesterol in men) Improved working conditions (due to improved perceived psychological demand and improved ergonomic conditions) Reduced absenteeism (8.1% reduction in experimental group, 4.8% reduction in control group)	Three Dutch Brabantia worksites (*n* = 3 sites)
Healthy Directions– Small Business study (121)	RCT* worksites	Fruit and vegetable consumption Red meat consumption Multivitamin use Physical activity	● ● ● ●	Significant improvements in physical activity and multivitamin use for all workers Larger effects for workers than for managers for fruits and vegetables and physical activity	Small manufacturing worksites (*n* = 24 sites)
MassBuilt (9)	Methods development	Smoking cessation	● ○ ● ●	Meaningful role of unions in daily lives of workers and unions can transmit trustworthy information about health	Construction apprentices in union program
United for a Healthy Future (122)	RCT* worksites	Smoking cessation Fruit and vegetable consumption	● ○ ● ○	Significant improvements in smoking cessation and fruit and vegetable consumption in the intervention group	Unionized construction laborers

*Randomized controlled trial with levels of randomization.
‡ Intervention:

	Individual	**Organization**
OSH	●	●
WHP	●	●

various theoretical frameworks that illustrate the complex web of factors intersecting to influence worker health. These factors involve the individual worker, the immediate work environment, and the larger contexts in which both the individual worker and the worksite are embedded (6,39,55,123). For further information on the application of best practices to programs that target diet and physical activity promotion, please refer to the WHO and WEF technical paper (106). We have organized this discussion to include: (1) program planning and design, (2) implementation of integrated programs, and (3) organizational support.

Program Planning and Design

An effective program relies on careful planning to assure fit with the worksite, workforce, and current policies and practices. Establishing integrated systems across organizational functions facilitates coordination. Worker participation in planning and setting priorities can lay the foundation for broad participation in programs (55).

Needs Assessment

A range of approaches to assessing the needs of the worksite and its workforce can be employed. One commonly used approach is the health risk appraisal (HRA), an instrument that uses personal, medical, and lifestyle indicators to assess the likelihood that an individual will develop a preventable or chronic disease As described in chapter 16, the HRA uses a questionnaire to assess worker risks and health status, thereby providing information to set priorities as part of the program planning process. The HRA has been used effectively as a tool to build awareness of health risks and lay the foundation for health education (28,55). With the overall goal of worker health, it is important to plan for providing the right programs that respond to each worker's needs (114). The needs assessment can help to assure that programs are designed for the specific needs of the worksite and the diverse needs of the workers.

Participatory Approaches

Employee and management participation in program planning and implementation contributes to the design of programs responsive to workers'

needs, readiness for change, cultural backgrounds, and priorities. It also assures that programs are responsive to the overall context and culture of the work organization. This process additionally encourages buy-in to the planning process (55,80). One key strategy for engaging workers and managers in joint planning is through health and safety committees and health and wellness committees or coordination across committees (55). The program support generated by participation in such committees has been shown to influence subsequent worker participation in WHP program activities (136). Focus group interviews or informal conversations with diverse groups of workers are another useful strategy for gaining worker input from the workers not included in these committees. Worker participation may have side benefits as well, including development of skills such as problem identification, problem solving, and communication skills (6,12).

Integrated Systems

Integrated programs address risks arising from occupational hazards and health behaviors, with built-in synergy to promote integration across otherwise parallel efforts. Integrated programs accordingly rely on core best-practice principles guiding interventions for OSH and WHP. Programs may focus on both additive and synergistic effects across risk factors. By finding points of coordination and synergy across points in the organization that have often operated as independent silos, it is possible to improve the effectiveness of occupational health and WHP programs. This model provides a framework for moving beyond the individual as the locus of intervention and responsibility for health in recognition of management's central role in worker health (55,130). Thus, effective programs need to be aimed at and coordinated across multiple levels of influence.

Implementation of Integrated Programs

Best-practice interventions within OSH and WHP are aimed at multiple levels of influence (79,133). At the individual and interpersonal level, interventions aim to educate individual workers and build social norms supportive of health, perhaps through educational classes or one-on-one training programs. At environmental and organizational levels, interventions may promote health through changes in the work environment or organization, such as interventions to improve the work climate and organizational policies, to reduce the potential for hazardous exposures in the physical work environment, to improve the organization of work (such as by reducing work-load), and to increase opportunities at work for healthy behaviors, perhaps through break times promoting physical activity.

Individual and Interpersonal Levels

At this level, interventions aim to educate individual workers and build social norms supportive of health. Educational programs for individual workers include programs to facilitate health behavior changes as well as training and education on workplace safety and health (54). Health education programs include both worksite-wide initiatives and efforts designed to help individual workers make health behavior changes (81,130). Such interventions may include strategies for health education and awareness building ranging from distributing hard copy materials to providing Web-based resources to holding group sessions such as lunch and learn seminars or health fairs. Although these are useful and low-cost ways to build awareness about health issues, these strategies are potentially less effective in promoting health behavior change as isolated activities than when incorporated into comprehensive efforts (50,55). Regardless of whether programs are delivered one on one to individual workers or to groups of employees, it is important that they respond to worker priorities and readiness to make health behavior changes.

These interventions may be offered across a continuum of intensity, with more-intensive programs designed for high-risk workers most ready to focus on health behavior change and less-intensive worksite-wide programs designed to reach a breadth of the workforce. Intensive programs are likely to attract workers most interested in and motivated to make health behavior changes. At the other end of the spectrum, worksite-wide programs generally aim to influence health behaviors among workers at varying stages of readiness for health behavior change. Not surprisingly, these two ends of the continuum differ in their ability to change behaviors. For example, studies on smoking cessation have found that more-intensive programs, with multiple sessions and multiple components, yield higher quit rates than short-term, less-intensive interventions (30,34,81). It is important to keep in mind, however, that because these programs are designed for highly motivated volunteers who are ready to commit to a behavior change program, they may miss important segments of the working population who are not interested in participating in intensive programs. From a public health perspective, the *effect* of an intervention is a product of both its *efficacy* in changing behavior and its *reach,* meaning the proportion of the population reached either directly through participation or indirectly through diffusion of intervention messages throughout the worksite (2,41).

Moving away from the one-size-fits-all approach to interventions, tailoring is one strategy for increasing the intensity of interventions delivered to at-risk populations. Tailored interventions typically are delivered through print communication (61,108,122,141), telephone counseling (21), Web-based approaches (22,60,88), and automated voice messaging (24). Individually tailored interventions are typically algorithm based and utilize expert systems or computer-based programs to match a large library of messages to individuals' varying information needs and levels of motivation to change, combining specific statements and graphics into personalized interventions for specific individuals (63). Tailoring in general decreases the level of distraction caused by information not pertaining to the issue at hand by eliminating extraneous information, thereby increasing the perception of the personal relevance of the message and enhancing the effectiveness (101). Tailoring messages allows researchers and intervention developers to incorporate several best-practice behavioral change elements, such as building self-efficacy, encouraging goal setting, and targeting motivational stages of change (63,73), and has been shown to be effective in improving a range of health behavior outcomes (64,117).

Interventions can also be designed to build social support and social norms supportive of worker health. Social norms can have a powerful influence on how an individual makes decisions (70) and can affect individual health behaviors, program participation, and OSH practices (122). Worksite programs may also facilitate social support, which may take the form of direct assistance, information, advice, and expression of concern (51). For example, in a WHP program conducted with blue-collar women in the southern United States, the intervention planners implemented a natural helpers program in which certain individuals were identified by their fellow colleagues to act as a resource for other workers. This program was part of a larger initiative to improve healthy eating and physical activity (17). The overall intervention reported beneficial changes in fruit and vegetable consumption and strength and flexibility exercises.

Work Environment and Organization Levels

Both social and physical characteristics of the work environment influence worker health outcomes. Reducing the potential for hazardous work exposures within the work environment is the first line of defense for ensuring occupational health and safety (55). A supportive work environment can also facilitate health behavior changes by adding healthier food options to the cafeteria, building physical activity opportunities, and displaying point-of-decision prompts for physical activity (29,78).

OSH interventions generally rely on a hierarchy of controls model, which recommends a sequence for controlling hazards beginning with control as close to the source as possible (90). The ideal choice is substituting safer substances for those that are hazardous, thereby removing the potential hazard. Engineering controls provide a second line of defense for the control of hazards, followed by administrative controls such as job redesign or job rotation. Personal protective equipment used by workers is recommended only as a last line of defense when substitution or engineering controls are not possible. By itself, using personal protective equipment is not an acceptable method of control because its effectiveness is highly variable and not reliable. Thus, in a manufacturing setting a hierarchy of controls model would call first for elimination or substitution of a chemical that gives off toxic fumes, followed by engineering efforts to provide ventilation to reduce workers' exposure to fumes, then by administrative controls such as rotating workers on and off jobs that involve the chemical so as to reduce total exposure to any one worker, and finally by personal protective equipment such as respirators. Another example might be addressing medical errors in a health care setting by focusing at the organizational level to assess whether the staffing plan is adequate to avoid excessive worker overload rather than at the individual level to educate workers how to cope with stress and overwork.

The worksite environment can also be modified to support health behavior changes. Examples of such modifications are instituting tobacco control policies aimed at both protecting nonsmokers from the hazardous effects of environmental tobacco smoke and promoting an environment supportive of non-smoking, increasing the availability of healthy foods in worksite cafeterias, or modifying the built environment to promote physical activity. Worksite policies on tobacco have been shown to decrease worker exposure to environmental tobacco smoke (48,76,132) and to contribute to worker reductions in smoking, including quitting (16,30,58,62,96,102,146). Employer efforts to promote compliance with smoking policies can contribute to an overall climate supportive of nonsmoking (125). Similarly, studies have examined the effects of making healthier food options more frequently available at the workplace (29,78) and have found strong support for the effect of these changes on increased fruit and vegetable intake and decreased fat intake (29).

Organizational Support

The effectiveness of integrated OSH and WHP programs relies on demonstrated support from management and social norms or standards around health (55). Recommendations for best-practice worksite programs have focused particularly on several key indicators of organizational support. These are described in the following sections.

Connecting the Program to Business Objectives

Programs and policies aimed at chronic disease prevention may be strengthened when they support a company's corporate objectives with respect to organizational-wide financial effects as well as individual-level benefits to the health and well-being of employees. Many businesses have recognized the importance of employee health for achieving core objectives; integrated OSH and WHP programs may be seen as strategic initiatives to protect human and financial resources. By promoting wellness and risk factor reduction, businesses may avoid unnecessary health costs, enhance productivity, reduce absenteeism and turnover, and encourage their employees through demonstrated commitment to their well-being. In a survey of 365 large U.S. companies, 80% reported that they believed their wellness program would reduce their health care costs, with the results to be realized over the long term (25).

Management and Labor Support

Substantial managerial support is often essential to generate the human and financial capital required to initiate and maintain successful worksite programs, particularly when the programs are aimed at integrating across traditionally segregated functions such as OSH and WHP (124). Even with respect to primarily employee-driven wellness initiatives, strong and consistent support from company leaders may serve to complement a bottom-up approach, helping to ensure legitimacy and program resources. Programs thrive in organizations that support active worker involvement, input, and participation and rely heavily on leadership commitment to worker health and safety. In organized worksites, union involvement may make it possible to craft programs that are responsive to worker concerns and to provide a voice for workers in program planning.

Incentives

Incentives provide a mechanism to increase participation in worksite programs as well as build and maintain motivation toward health behavior changes (65,135). There are several types of incentives, which can be defined broadly as intrinsic (e.g., participants receive a monthly chart of their progress in increasing their number of steps to 10,000 steps per day) or extrinsic (45). Extrinsic incentives, which are those provided by an outside source, can be built into worksite programs in several ways, ranging from (1) reduced co-payments, lower premiums, and more attractive benefits given by insurance providers for employees performing healthy behaviors; (2) wellness opportunities including sponsored classes such as supermarket tours, health screenings, and walking clubs; and (3) financial incentives to participate in wellness activities (104). In a 2005 survey of 365 large companies based in the United States, nearly half reported offering an incentive to encourage program participation (25). In OSH programs, the use of incentives or safety rewards is under debate; it is important that the use of incentives does not result in reduced reporting (e.g., decreased accident reporting in response to incentives to reduce accidents) and that incentives do not inappropriately shift the burden of responsibility to workers in situations in which employers have responsibility to provide a safe work environment (37).

Program Resources

Successful programs rely on appropriate budgeting, staffing, and resources. An incremental start-up allows programs to begin with modest and achievable goals and to scale up based on initial program experiences. In this way, it is possible to direct resources in focused and strategic direc-tions. An increasing number of vendors are available to assist worksites in program planning and implementation and may be particularly useful in small to midsize worksites that do not have the resources to staff their own programming.

Conclusion

The growing evidence for the contributions of integrated WHP and OSH programs to worker health outcomes provides a stimulus for further dissemination of these programs across a range of work settings. It is imperative that future research document ways in which comprehensive WHP programs may further the mission of the organization through support for healthy and productive workers within healthy worksites (119). Research to develop and test effective intervention strategies integrating OSH and WHP requires an interdisciplinary approach. The belief that worker health begins with individual behavior change sets in motion intervention strategies that differ from interventions of the OSH approach, which starts from the assumption that management bears primary responsibility for worker health and safety on the job (118). Overcoming the segmentation of these fields ultimately will require an inclusive and comprehensive model of work and health that provides for resolution—or at least understanding—of our different assumptions, vocabulary, research methods, and intervention approaches (13). This chapter further underscores the benefits of such coordinated efforts, including the creation of a positive and caring image for the company, improved staff morale, reduced turnover and absenteeism, and improved productivity (150).

Chapter Review Questions

1. Identify four reasons that justify the rationale for implementing integrated programs.

2. Given the evidence provided in support of integrated programs, what are the knowledge gaps in this area that point to the need for further research on the application of integrated programs?

3. List three important components of program planning and design.

4. Identify best-practice approaches for implementing integrated programs by selecting two approaches that correspond to the individual level and two that correspond to the organizational level.

5. What indicators of organizational support are important to program success?

31

Programs Designed to Improve Employee Health Through Changes in the Built Environment

Mireille N. M. van Poppel, PhD, and Luuk H. Engbers, PhD, PT

The increase in the prevalence of obesity in the United States started in the beginning of the 1980s (19), after relative stability. In western Europe the increase in obesity started a few years later but is following the American trend (9,20). However, obesity is a problem not only in Western industrialized countries but also in large areas of Africa, Asia, and Latin America, in which the percentage of the population that is overweight (BMI > 25 kg/m^2) is increasing. In China an alarming increase in the number of overweight and obese people has recently been observed; for instance, 23.9% of the younger population (20-45 y) is obese (BMI > 30 kg/m^2; 3,29,31).

Due to the relatively short time frame during which the increase in prevalence of obesity has occurred, causal factors for obesity are likely to include the environment as much as other factors such as physiology, metabolism, or genetic predisposition. The underlying idea of this assumption is that the human body has evolved for physical activity (37). Throughout most of human history, physical demands were a typical aspect of daily life and an expected part of the everyday world. Nowadays these demands on the human body are no longer present because of the increasing mechanization of society and the increase in televised and computerized entertainment.

The following daily routine is a reality for many employees: Travel to work by car, take the elevator to an office, and sit behind a desk for the majority of the working day. At the end of the day, commute home by car or train and then when at home, continue inactivity with popular computerized and television entertainment. The transition from a physically demanding environment to a predominantly mechanized environment focused on convenience has significantly contributed to the decline in physical activity levels.

Frequently mentioned contributors to the changing and unhealthy dietary habits are the convenience in food availability, the increasing availability of energy-dense but nutrient-poor (ready-to-eat) foods, and the greater amount of meals with large portion sizes consumed away from home (30). This new environment of decreased physical activity and unhealthy foods can be called the *obesogenic* environment, (38) an environment in which the choice to make healthy decisions has become increasingly difficult and—more importantly—less obvious for most individuals. In this perspective, unhealthy behavior has become a normal response to an abnormal environment.

Environmental Interventions in Worksite Health Promotion

In general, (worksite) health promotion strategies can be defined as "the combination of educational and environmental supports for actions and conditions of living beneficial for health" (19; p. 320). The term *environmental supports* or *strategies* in this definition can be interpreted as "all strategies that aim to reduce barriers or increase opportunities for healthy choices, e.g., by providing more healthy options, by making healthy choices more accessible and by establishing policies that require healthy choices, or restrict the number of less healthy options" (18; p. 397). Or, defined more concisely, *environmental supports* or *strategies* are "all strategies that do not require the individual to self-select into a defined educational program (i.e., self-help programs, classes or groups)" (17; p. 398). To address the role of the environment in determining behavior, this chapter includes a description of the theoretical background of environmental strategies in health promotion. In a review by Kahn and colleagues (22), three types of interventions were identified that are specific to physical activity promotion within the community and include environmental and policy approaches. While they may or may not be specific to the work-site setting, all three interventions may be applied in the workplace setting. The three interventions are the following:

1. Informational approaches to change knowledge and attitudes about the benefits of and opportunities for physical activity and a healthy diet within a community (worksite or school)

2. Behavioral and social approaches to teach people the behavioral management skills necessary for successful adaptation and maintenance of behavior change and for social environments that facilitate and enhance behavior change (i.e., physical activity or fitness programs)

3. Environmental policy approaches to change the structure of physical and organizational environments to provide safe, attractive, and convenient places for physical activity (e.g., walking tracks, attractive staircases, and fitness facilities)

In this chapter, only the third type of intervention is discussed.

Theories and Models

One of the earlier models or theories that incorporated the role of the environment into behavior is the social learning theory, or social cognitive theory, from Bandura (4,5) and the related concept of reciprocal determinism. This theory underlines the dynamic relationship between the physical and the social environment and between observable behavior and cognitive personal dimensions. Reciprocal determinism means that "behavior, cognitive and other personal factors, and environmental influences all operate interactively as determinants of each other" (4). Thus, a person can be both the actor of and the respondent to change. Consequently, when changes in the individual and the environment are introduced simultaneously, behavioral changes are more likely to be maintained. However, this model does not specifically describe which environmental factors can be targeted in order to influence behavior.

The ecological model of behavior is more specific about the environmental factors and is often used as a theoretical basis for environmental health promotion strategies. The main principle of the ecological model is that environments restrict the range of behaviors by promoting and sometimes demanding certain actions and by discouraging or prohibiting other behaviors (43; see figure 31.1). A more concrete description of the ecological model is given by Sallis and Owen (33): "Behaviors are influenced by the interaction of interpersonal, social/cultural and physical environment variables and behavior has multiple levels of influence. The environmental

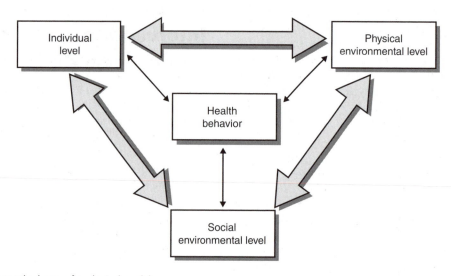

Figure 31.1 General scheme of ecological models.

Reprinted, by permission, from S. Titze, 2003, *Promotion of health-enhancing physical activity. An individual, social and environmental approach* (Aachen, Shaker Verlag GMBH).

approach can influence behavior both indirectly and directly." The human interaction with the environment can be considered as an important explanation in understanding behavior. Consequently, ecological models in health promotion should not be considered as models that predict or explain behavior. Rather, as Titze (39) describes it, "ecological models are conceptual frameworks suggesting that there is much to be gained when intervention goals are moved from the individual to the environmental level." To put it more directly, when the environment is taken into account in addition to intrapersonal factors, a greater effect on behavior change can be expected.

Within the scope of the ecological models, Sallis and Bauman (34) summarize a number of environmental and policy leverage points in the constructed physical environment that can be used in environmental physical activity interventions. Possible leverage points include using radio, TV, Internet, and posters in various settings to provide information and cues to motivate people to be active. At the worksite, shower rooms or (secure) parking spaces for bicycles could be installed, and staircases could be made more attractive. At both the worksite and public buildings, parking lots could be separated from buildings by green space. Besides these changes in the physical environment, policy changes can be considered. Examples of organizational policy changes include subsidized (worksite) health club memberships or stair use competitions. Also, the worksite could give rewards to active commuters. According to Zimring and colleagues (45), the previously mentioned leverage points to promote health in the physical environment can be considered at four separate levels of a spatial scale: (1) urban design, (2) site selection and design, (3) building design, and (4) building element design. These levels can be helpful in designing environmental projects or interventions within a timeline (temporal flow). As Zimring and colleagues (45) described it, "In the case of new construction, most clients choose a site before they design a building, and design a building before they design elements. In building renovation (or an environmental intervention), the order may be reversed, as the assessment of changes to building elements and layouts are considered prior to changes in the building form or the decision to relocate rather than renovate."

Ecological models can be considered to be more pragmatic than many other theoretical models that more specifically attempt to predict behavior. Hence, intrapersonal factors that occur within the individual as a consequence of the social and physical environment are not specified. Models specifying intrapersonal factors are described in detail in chapter 22. An important determinant of behavior that is not usually mentioned in these models is habitual behavior, or habits. Insight into habitual behavior might give additional information in how the environment intervenes on the behavior of the individual. Habits are the result of automated unconscious cognitive processes (1,40). They are formed when a certain behavior is repeated often enough. Thus, (new) habit formation is more likely to occur when the evaluation of a certain behavior is satisfactory to the individual. Habits are also strongly dependent on situational or environmental factors or obstacles (40). Therefore, it is hypothesized that if habits are a strong determinant of a certain behavior, the introduction of new motivational materials or cues in an existing environment will change or momentarily interrupt routine or habitual behavior (e.g., taking the elevator). If this interruption of unwanted unhealthy behavior occurs on several occasions, a new healthy habit can be formed, under the assumption that this new behavior was satisfactory. In addition, information processing is unlikely to occur when behaviors are guided by strong habits. In other words, behaviors that are determined by strong habits are less guided by cognitive or conscious processes (1,7,8,17,18,40,42). For that reason, in many health change interventions there has been a shift from providing information (or counseling) to changing the environment in order to break through unhealthy habits and achieve significant behavioral changes among the target population.

To conclude, lifestyle behaviors at the worksite are determined not only by conscious choices but also by unconscious processes or habits and might be effectively influenced by environmental changes. The next section reviews the literature on the effectiveness of environmental interventions aimed at improving physical activity and diet at work. This overview of the literature is restricted to physical environmental interventions and does not include interventions targeting the social environment at work (see chapter 26) or interventions consisting of changes in policy or legislation (see chapters 6 and 7). Although examples of modifications in the social environment are not mentioned in this chapter, we do acknowledge their importance. Changes in the physical environment affect the social environment and vice versa; the effects of either component will reinforce the other. A recent publication of the WHO (44) mentioned several key elements of successful worksite health promotion programs related to the social environment. These elements include strong management support, effective communication with and involvement of employees at all levels of development and implementation of the intervention, and adapting the program to the social norms within the worksite culture.

Environmental Interventions for Improving Physical Activity at Work

In the available scientific literature, several opportunities and examples for improving physical activity levels among employees in existing worksites are mentioned. These are (1) increasing stair use, (2) stimulating active commuting, (3) stimulating walking at lunchtime or during working hours, and (4) providing opportunities or facilities for fitness and exercise at work (e.g., in company fitness facilities). An overview of each of these examples follows.

Stair Use

A review by Matson-Koffman and colleagues (26) included seven studies (only one at the workplace) in which the effects of environmental interventions on stair use were assessed. The interventions included encouragement to take the stairs that consisted of signs, banners, music, and food in the staircases. Two instances included signs discouraging the use of elevators, such as signs stating, "Elevator for physically challenged and staff use only. Others please use the stairs." Six of these interventions led to increased stair use in at least part of the population. Inconsistent gender differences were observed; with some studies reporting increased stair use only among men and others only among women. In a review by Eves and Webb (15), more emphasis was placed on interventions conducted at the workplace. They concluded that nine interventions conducted at worksites that attempted to increase stair use by reducing elevator use through health promotion point-of-choice signs failed to show compelling results. In a controlled study not included in these reviews, an environmental intervention on stair use resulted in a short-term (3 mo) increase of use, but no long-term (12 mo) effects were observed (12).

The overall lack of effect of interventions aimed at stair use at the workplace is in marked contrast to the uniformly positive results reported in public settings such as shopping malls, airports, and train and bus stations. Eves and Webb (15) state that so far it is unclear whether health promotion initiatives at the workplace have employed suboptimal campaigns or whether the choice of stairs over the elevator at worksites is fundamentally different from the choice between using the stairs or the continuously available escalators in public settings. At worksites, having to wait for an elevator to arrive might be the prompt to take the stairs, because taking the stairs is more efficient. Consequently, health messages are less effective. At public settings, however, health reasons might be the primary prompt to use the stairs, because both options are equally available and accessible.

Another explanation of the difference in the success of interventions implemented in public settings compared with those implemented at work might be that in public settings people are exposed to the intervention infrequently (most people will not visit the intervention site daily) while at work a fixed population is exposed to the intervention the entire day. It could be that after a few days or weeks the worksite population does not consciously notice the intervention materials anymore (the materials become part of the wallpaper), and thus the intervention loses its effectiveness. This might explain the disappearance of the short-term effect observed for the FoodSteps intervention (12) and the lack of effect Marshall and colleagues (25) observed when putting an intervention into place for a second time.

Some critical notes should be made regarding existing studies on stair use. Eves and Webb (15) made some recommendations for the measurement of stair use in worksite settings. They recommend that a clear distinction between ascent and descent has to be made. Climbing the stairs uses three times the energy that descending requires, 8.6 to 9.6 METS as opposed to 2.9 to 3.2 METS (2), respectively. Only when individuals increase their climbing (number of stair ascents per day) are they able to meet the CDC and ACSM physical activity recommendation. This recommendation is equivalent to 40 min of stair *descent* per day, which seems near impossible to achieve in a worksite setting. On the other hand, an increase in weekly stair use (including descent) can certainly contribute toward the accumulation of a sufficient number of minutes of physical activity to meet the CDC and ACSM recommendation.

Furthermore, whereas the design of the staircases themselves is one issue, the design or layout of the building and the placement of the stairs within it are another. Several authors state that these issues are relevant for stair use (12,15,27). In a unique cross-sectional study designed to assess the relationship between stair use and design and location of stairs (27), five themes for potential environmental determinants of stair use were tested. These themes included appeal, comfort, convenience (i.e., proximity, distribution, and accessibility), legibility (i.e., visibility, stair type, and number of turns from entrance or path), and safety. The interventions described previously covered only appeal and legibility (visibility), because these factors can be changed with simple measures such as signs, banners, and music or food in the staircases. Nicoll (27), however, studied whether stair use was related to the physical environmental features of 10 buildings. In contrast to the hypothesis tested in other studies that the attractiveness of the staircase might stimulate the use of the stairs, constructs such as appeal, comfort, or safety were *not* associated with stair use. The only variable from these three constructs that was related to stair use was stair width, an indicator of compatibility of stairs to accommodate travel with social groups (and being able to hold a conversation). Convenience (distribution and accessibility) and legibility (visibility, stair type, number of turns from entrance or most integrated path) were important determinants of stair use. Given these findings, Nicoll stated that "a well-placed stair has more impact on stair use than a well-dressed stair." The buildings included in the study of Nicoll were all three- or four-story academic buildings. Thus the effect of the height of a building on stair use could not be assessed. Other research indicates that when the number of stories in a building increases, stair use decreases, and that four stories is the maximum that subjects are willing to climb (23).

A last point worth mentioning is that data on stair use usually are not collected at the individual level; they provide insight only into the total percentage of people using the stairs. Given the infrared technology applications to head counting used as the measurement of stair use, it is not possible to assess for whom these interventions were (most) effective. In the only controlled study with data at the individual level, the *FoodSteps* study, results indicate that, surprisingly, workers with normal body weight used the stairs more often following implementation of the intervention. Overweight or obese people used the stairs less and consequently did not change their stair use behavior (12).

To advance the field, randomized controlled studies with data on the direction of stair use

(decent or ascent) at the individual level are needed. Preferably these studies will include environmental interventions that are more comprehensive than point-of-decision signs and involve changes in or reconfigurations of the (internal) building layout.

Active Commuting

Regarding active commuting, physical environmental characteristics that can be influenced by the management of a company or organization are the selection of the worksite and its design and certain building elements, such as secure parking places for bikes and showers and changing rooms for employees. Of course, offering discounts or tax reductions for employees who purchase bikes could also stimulate active commuting, but this is a policy, not a physical environmental intervention. Although the effects of environmental interventions would not be difficult to study, almost no controlled studies have been conducted to date.

Vuori and associates (41) studied the effects of a multicomponent intervention aimed at active commuting. Information on the benefits and possibilities for walking or cycling to work was provided. Motivation was increased by lotteries that included chances to win free fitness testing, and arrangements were made to improve facilities for showering and changing. Furthermore, safety of commuting routes was assessed and information on safe routes was provided for employees. These interventions led to a modest increase in walking and cycling to work

Walking at Lunch or During Working Hours

Lunch walking and other walking during working hours can be part of physical activity at work. According to the previously mentioned spatial scales proposed by Zimring and colleagues (45), the spatial scales relevant for this kind of physical activity are the site location and its design. Availability, attractiveness, accessibility, and knowledge of walking routes might be important factors that can influence walking in the vicinity of the worksite. In the study of Pegus and associates (28), the installment of a walking track outside the company was part of a multicomponent health promotion program. Although these authors observed improvements in physical activity and body composition, there were no differences between intervention and control sites at follow-up. Thus no effects could be attributed to the environmental component of the intervention. A team of researchers led by Emmons (11) included exercise space and equipment and a red-lined route for walking during lunch in their multicomponent health promotion program. They observed a significant increase in exercise among employees of the intervention site compared with employees of the control site. Whether or not the walking route was an effective component of the intervention also could not be determined in this study.

Heirich and coworkers (21) compared four worksites that all introduced different interventions to stimulate physical activity levels. Worksite A introduced aerobics classes. Worksite B established a fitness facility with certified trainers. Worksite C introduced aerobics classes in combination with outreach and counseling for employees with cardiovascular disease risk factors. Worksite D introduced outreach, counseling, and organized physical activities for all employees and mapped out walking paths. Sites C and D were most effective in getting employees to exercise. Unfortunately, due to the study design, effectiveness of the walking routes could not be determined.

In a qualitative study at four small manufacturing companies, Gates and associates (16) gathered information on what strategies would aid in reducing barriers for employees to make use of walking paths. At all four companies, walking paths were identified as an appropriate intervention component. In focus groups, employees and managers agreed that the paths should be marked for distance, that safety must be maintained, and that competitions, incentives, and pedometers would increase use. Short lunch breaks and lack of lighting were seen as barriers, and placing exercise stations along the paths and organizing buddy groups were seen as enhancing motivation.

Exercise Facilities at Work

Making fitness facilities available, with or without certified trainers, with or without organized classes, could be considered an environmental intervention, since access and availability are equal for all employees. In the previously described study of Heirich and coworkers (21), participation rates for aerobics classes were low at worksites A and C, and classes were discontinued. A decrease in levels of physical activity was found in worksite B (fitness facilities only, without an outreach program). At worksites C and D improve-

ments in physical activity levels among employees with CVD risk factors were found.

Emmons and associates (11) also combined exercise facilities and equipment, a red-lined walking route, and another intervention component. Similar to Heirich and colleagues (21), they found that physical activity improved. However, as mentioned before, given the design of these two studies, it could not be assessed which intervention components were effective and which were not.

In a review of the effectiveness of worksite physical activity programs, including 26 controlled studies (some randomized), strong evidence was found for an effect on physical activity and musculoskeletal disorders, but limited evidence was found for an effect on fatigue (32). Dishman and coworkers (10) also reviewed worksite fitness programs and concluded that these programs produced a small, nonsignificant effect on physical activity. However, the studies included in these review did not evaluate the effect of merely providing access to facilities or classes; rather, they actively recruited study participants and the effects on various health parameters. An individual who self-selects into a defined fitness program contradicts the definition of environmental interventions given earlier in this chapter. Thus a majority of the interventions described in these two reviews cannot really be considered as environmental interventions.

Moreover, in general only a small percentage of employees make use of exercise or fitness facilities at work, and inactive employees with unhealthy lifestyle habits are usually not reached with this type of intervention (6,24,36). Whether the benefits of these types of facilities outweigh the costs, especially when they are accompanied with certified trainers, is doubtful (36), although no conclusive evidence is available to either prove or disprove the cost-effectiveness. Regardless, although facilities might enhance the image of a company, given the participation rates and costs associated with construction of a fitness facility, on-site fitness centers should not be the only pillar of a company's health policy.

Designing Buildings for Physical Activity

The previously described studies mostly involve interventions in the context of an existing situation. It would, however, be more efficient and probably more effective to design buildings from scratch or to renovate the inside of buildings with physical activity and health in mind. In contrast to the interventions described in the previously mentioned studies, these more fundamental changes might generate lasting effects on the targeted behavior. Considerations would include the placement of elevators, escalators, and stairs and the design and placement of facilities such as meeting rooms, copiers, printers, coffee corners, and workstations. Unfortunately, to date, no data are available on the effectiveness of this type of intervention.

The effect of such an approach might be much greater than that of putting up point-of-decision signs near a staircase that is not optimally designed (e.g., concealed behind an unattractive door and only put in place as a fire exit) or optimally located in the first place. However, the effect is difficult to study with scientifically rigorous designs. Natural experiments, in which employees are relocated from one (type of) building to another, might provide the opportunity to study the effects of different building designs on physical activity, provided that other worksites can be used as control conditions. Also, observational cross-sectional studies are a possibility in which worksite physical activity in various types of buildings is monitored and associated with objective scores of the physical internal and external environment of the building. These studies are common for the built environment (e.g., urban design in relation to physical activity) but to date have been performed only once for worksites (27). This type of study might provide meaningful insights on how the building design interacts with physical activity and how building design can be modified most effectively.

Environmental Interventions for Improving Dietary Habits at Work

Dietary behavior is even more diverse and complex than physical activity behavior; however, it is usually divided into just a few sub-behaviors, such as fruit and vegetable consumption, fat consumption, snack or sweet consumption, and soft drink consumption. In a review conducted by Seymour (35), 10 studies covering worksite-based interventions were identified; 3 studies used information strategies only, 1 study labeled the energy content of food items, and another listed low-fat items on a sign in front of the cafeteria and placed a heart symbol next to each low-fat entrée on the serving line. The author, who limited the review to stud-

ies that considered environmental interventions only (not in combination with other strategies), concluded that most environmental interventions at the worksite resulted in significant changes in the desired direction. This finding was confirmed by the reviews of Engbers and colleagues (14) and Matson-Koffman (26), although both of these reviews included interventions that consisted of environmental components in addition to information or counseling components. They reported positive effects of the interventions on fruit and vegetable consumption and fat intake. The environmental components mostly consisted of labeling food products in a restaurant. These labels provided information on nutritional or caloric content of the products. This labeling of healthier food selections increased the consumption of these products. Furthermore, increasing workers' access to healthier foods (low-fat foods, fruits, and vegetables) in canteens or vending machines might be a successful strategy, resulting in decreased fat consumption and increased fruit and vegetable consumption.

From these three reviews of dietary interventions, the following promising practices for environmental modifications can be identified:

- Increased availability of healthy products in company canteens and vending machines
- Information strategies such as cards or food labeling (i.e., point-of-purchase prompts) displaying caloric content or labels distinguishing between healthy and unhealthy products

Nonphysical environmental (policy) interventions that might be effective are the following:

- Pricing strategies such as reducing the prices of healthy products while increasing the prices of unhealthy products
- Providing incentives so that the number of healthy (labeled) products purchased can result in awards or discounts

However, some limitations and cautions should be mentioned regarding reviews of dietary interventions. As with the physical activity interventions, data were often not available at the individual level—rather, effects of the interventions were assessed using general sales data from the canteen or vending machines. Assigning intervention effectiveness to individuals or subgroups or associating it with other outcomes is therefore not appropriate. Furthermore, not all studies assessed dietary habits outside of work, and the possibility that employees compensated their healthier dietary habits at work with an unhealthier diet at home could not be ruled out.

Conclusion

Overall, no convincing evidence is currently available for the effect of environmental interventions on physical activity. Although some effects were found for point-of-decision prompts on stair use at the worksite, these effects were small and short term. Environmental strategies for the promotion of healthy food seem to have an effect in the desired direction. These strategies consist of healthy food availability and labeling.

With the exception of the studies on stair use, most other studies on physical activity described in this chapter studied the effects of comprehensive multicomponent interventions. Most of these interventions were accompanied by individual counseling strategies. Although a number of these interventions were effective, these effects can not be attributed to the environmental component. More studies are necessary to tease out the added value of the environmental components. Preferably, these studies should be controlled and should gather data at the individual level. This way the results can be associated with individual characteristics of subjects and consequently provide insight on the people (i.e., subgroups) whom the interventions may be more effective.

Perhaps more importantly, studies on the association between physical activity and building design, rather than building elements (e.g., attractiveness), are necessary. The study by Nicoll (27) is a fine and useful example of the type of study that is much needed. Similar to the research on the relationship between urban design and physical activity, the studies on the relationship between building design and worksite-based physical activity could first utilize a cross-sectional design. Cross-sectional studies on urban design cannot rule out that certain people (active or inactive) self-select a certain type of neighborhood, and thus no conclusion on the causal relationship between physical environmental characteristics and lifestyle factors can be drawn. This methodological problem is not likely to occur when studying the relationship between building design and worksite-based physical activity because employees usually have no choice regarding the type of building in which they work. On the other hand, the differences between white-collar and blue-collar employees remain a point of consideration in such studies.

When certain building characteristics are identified as having a relationship with physical activity, natural experiments or controlled intervention studies are the next steps to confirm whether related building modifications will actually change behavior. The studies should be conducted in collaboration with architects and project developers, who may be able to immediately integrate the results of such studies into their work or, at a minimum, take health into consideration when designing new buildings and worksites (see also chapter 11). Regardless of how important the environmental characteristics of the worksite may prove to be for physical activity and diet, the social and political environment should not be forgotten. Optimally, stakeholders in the physical, social, and political environment should work together in the promotion of healthy behavior at work.

Chapter Review Questions:

1. What are essential levels in the ecological model?

2. What is a definition of an environmental intervention?

3. What important differences between a public setting such as a shopping mall and a worksite setting affect the decision to use the stairs?

32

The Design, Implementation, and Evaluation of Medical Self-Care Programs

Don R. Powell, PhD, and Jeanette D. Karwan, RD

Medical self-care is a series of behaviors consumers engage in when experiencing physical or psychological symptoms in order to make an informed decision about when to seek professional medical assistance versus when they can treat themselves at home using self-administered procedures. It usually involves the use of outside resources, such as a self-care book, nurse call line, online content, or family health adviser. It is more often used for decisions about diagnosis and treatment of everyday health problems as opposed to managing already diagnosed chronic conditions. These ongoing conditions need diagnosis and monitoring from a doctor or other health care provider. Medical self-care also includes finding out about and getting appropriate health screenings and immunizations.

Medical self-care is not the same as medical consumerism. The latter is concerned with the usage of the health care system. This includes communicating with doctors and health care providers and choosing and using a health plan. If medical assistance is warranted, however, using a medical self-care resource can prompt a consumer to play a more active role in communicating with doctors and other health care providers. This includes providing accurate information to help with a diagnosis; asking questions about treatment options, risks, and costs; and making a shared decision about what type of treatment to pursue.

Medical self-care is nothing new. In fact, 73% of Americans would rather treat themselves at home than see a doctor (4). Providing a medical self-care program can help people handle common conditions, such as headaches and sore throats, more effectively and knowledgeably.

This chapter presents the need for medical self-care, its goals and benefits, components of a medical self-care program, practical ways to apply medical self-care to employees of a company, and the efficacy of medical self-care programs.

The Need for Medical Self-Care

To understand the need for medical self-care, it is important to know four major sources of demand for health care:

- *Morbidity.* Morbidity is true illness. Illness certainly drives demand for services.

- *Perceived need.* Some people go to the doctor for problems such as a minor skin wound, whereas others walk around with pneumonia. How much people feel the need to be seen by a health care provider will influence their utilization.

- *Patient preference.* After options have been given by a provider regarding such issues as whether to take medication, have a procedure, or undergo surgery, it is up to the patient to make an informed decision.

- *Nonhealth motives.* Demand is also driven by issues unrelated to health, such as wanting to be absent from work or wishing to file a workers' compensation claim when none is warranted.

Major Determinants of Medical Self-Care Utilization

In addition, several factors are important reasons why people decide to use medical self-care programs. The major reasons include endogenous factors, exogenous factors, and physician encouragement. A brief description of each is provided.

Endogenous factors include employees' ages and genders, clinical risk factors, income levels, educational and ethnic backgrounds, personal perceptions, and health behaviors. Also included are employees' attitudes about personal health and health care use, as well as their sense of responsibility to take care of their own health needs.

Exogenous factors include the extent and scope of insurance coverage, geographic access to services, and regional or local practice patterns. Provider incentives affecting diagnosis and treatment decisions also play a role in medical self-care utilization.

Physician encouragement refers to the ability of physicians to empower their patients. They can encourage patients to use a self-care guide, call a nurse line, or go online for self-care content. They should encourage their patients to live healthy lifestyles.

Goals and Benefits of Medical Self-Care

Medical self-care plays a vital role in worker health improvement, including disease prevention, health promotion, and worker productivity. A misconception many people have about medical self-care is that its purpose is to keep people from seeking and receiving care from a health care provider. They believe that medical self-care means taking care of their health needs on their own, without any medical guidance or assistance. In reality, the goal is to get individuals to both choose and use the appropriate level of medical care that addresses their health needs at any given time. In this regard, people applying medical self-care to their symptoms may decide to see a health care provider as readily as deciding it is unnecessary to do so. A medical self-care resource provides information that people can use to gain enough knowledge to evaluate whether to contact a health care provider or to treat a problem on their own. Moreover, a medical self-care resource provides guidelines of specific home care remedies to use for particular health problems.

Goals and Benefits of Medical Self-Care Programs for Employers

There are several reasons why employers may be interested in providing their employees access to a medical self-care program. Such reasons include reductions in health care costs, improved employee health, reduction in medical errors and inappropriate self-care practices, and other benefits.

Reduction in Health Care Costs

The cost increases of health benefits in the United States are more than double the rate of inflation (10) and employee health care costs are expected to continue to rise. According to Towers Perrin, for 2008, the average company health benefits expenditure per employee is expected to be $9,312 U.S. This is an increase of 7% over the average cost in 2007 (19).

"To help curb rising costs, employers and health plans are looking for consumers to take more responsibility for medical costs, lifestyle choices and treatment decisions" (2). Employers can help accomplish this objective by utilizing one or more medical self-care programs. One way a medical self-care program can lower health care costs is reducing unnecessary utilization. By and large, people in the United States are frequent users of the health care system. In 2005, there were approximately 964 million visits to nonfederal office-based physicians, which comes out to about 3.3 visits per person in the United States (22). It has been estimated that about 25% of these visits, or 241 million visits, are deemed to be unnecessary (5). Since the average doctor visit costs about $121 U.S. (21), more than $28 billion U.S. is being spent unnecessarily on them.

In 2005, there were approximately 115 million visits to hospital ERs. This comes out to about 37.8 visits per 100 people (23). It has been estimated that 55% of these visits, or 63 million, are for non-urgent care (5). Because the average emergency visit costs $560 U.S. (21), more than $35 billion U.S. is being spent unnecessarily on emergency visits.

According to Larry Chapman, MPH, senior vice president of WebMD Health Services, "the general findings are that medical self-care books and associated training programs reduce visits to health care providers between 7% and 19%. In addition, there are also studies that show visits for minor health conditions are generally reduced by about 35% as a result of well-designed self-care programs. In general, most self-care programs will show a benefit to cost ratio by between 2:1 and 5:1." (24)

A 3 y study of 1,500 calls to nurse advice lines reported that nurses recommended self-care rather than ER or doctor visit care on nearly 80% of calls (13). According to Christine Tanner, PhD, RN, the lead author of this study, "The evidence shows that it reduces utilization of more expensive services. It significantly saves health system resources." Also, when callers were asked what they would have done without the use of the nurse line, 35% reported that they would have gone to the emergency department; 33% said they would have made a doctor appointment.

Of all areas of wellness, medical self-care has been shown to yield some of the most significant ROI figures. A study conducted by Capital Blue Cross in Harrisburg, Pennsylvania, on a self-care program it implemented for a manufacturing company demonstrated significant reductions in health care utilization. The claims data for 371 employees were analyzed over a 1 y time frame both pre- and postdistribution of a self-care guide. There were no other changes in the company's benefits design during the study. The data showed that employees who received the guide had an 18.4% decrease in the frequency of physician office visits and a 19.8% decrease in the frequency of ER visits. The 12 mo savings was $39.06 U.S. per employee, which amounted to a 24.3% decrease in costs. The ROI was 5:1 (18). The study also demonstrated that the benefits of the self-care program carried over to the dependents of employees as they, too, reduced their utilization. An analysis of all 938 members showed a 12 mo savings of $21.67 U.S. per member. This represented a 17.8% reduction in costs. The frequency of physician and ER visits for members decreased 11%. The ROI was 7:1 (18).

Blue Cross Blue Shield of Massachusetts provided 338,963 members with a self-care guide. The guide was custom designed based on the plan's most frequently used ICD-9 codes. The analysis looked at utilization data for 51,021 members who received the guide and an equal number of members who did not. The two managed care samples were similar with respect to age and gender. Claims data for the group that received the guide were analyzed 9 mo before distribution of the guide and 9 mo after distribution. The results showed a decrease in ER visits of 2.4 per 1,000 members and a decrease in outpatient visits of 8.4 per 1,000 members. During the same time frame, the group that did not receive the guide showed an increase of 2.4 per 1,000 members for ER visits and an increase of 12.0 per 1,000 members for outpatient visits. The experimental group demonstrated a 3.2% reduction in ER visits. The results were statistically significant (9).

The Florida Hospital Medical Center in Orlando gave 4,382 employees a self-care guide. Five months after the guide was distributed, evaluation questionnaires were sent to 1,236 employees and were returned by 365 of them (a 30% response rate). It was determined that these employees had reduced physician office use by 126 visits and ER use by 52 visits. Using the hospital insurance records, it was calculated that the average cost for a physician office visit was $55.00 U.S. and the average cost for an ER visit was $462.00 U.S. This amounted to a savings of $30,954 or $84.81 U.S. per employee in the 5 mo. In addition, employees were absent from work 72 d less. This research was based on self-reported data (17).

In addition to the civilian population, medical self-care research has been conducted in the military. The U.S. Army commissioned the development of a military self-care guide geared toward the issues of basic training. It was researched at General Leonard Wood Army Community Hospital from 1998 to 2000, during which time a total of 77,916 soldiers were enrolled in the self-care program. The research found an avoidance of lost duty time of 33,894 h and an avoidance of provider visits of 17,839. The provider time saved was calculated to be 5,946 h. The U.S. Army's research at five other sites showed similar results leading to the implementation of an army-wide medical self-care program (20).

Improved Employee Health

According to Doing Well Through Wellness: 2006-07 Survey of Wellness Programs at Business Roundtable Member Companies, "healthier employees" was the number one reason for having corporate wellness programs (1). Medical self-care resources can help improve the health of employees as well. They are quick references for treating common health problems so they do not get worse and for information on when to get health screenings that detect problems early when they are easier and less costly to treat. Examples are high blood pressure, dental problems, and cancers of the cervix, breast, prostate, and colon.

Lowered Incidence and Prevention of Medical Errors and Inappropriate Self-Care Practices

In addition to being a quick reference for information on what to do for common health problems, a medical self-care guide provides guidance for addressing emergency situations that occur in the home. For example, in the event that a child swallows a poisonous substance, a self-care guide is a handy resource for providing advice on calling a poison control center, as well as giving a number to call, such as the National Poison Control Center at 800-222-1222. Without having a medical self-care guide to refer to, an individual may resort to giving syrup of ipecac to a child who has swallowed a substance that may or may not be poisonous. However, this over-the-counter remedy for swallowed poisons is no longer recommended by the American Academy of Pediatrics (3).

Additional Benefits for Employers

Getting the appropriate level of care for a health problem can help reduce absenteeism, reduce presenteeism, increase productivity, and improve employee morale. Employees do not need to take time off work for unnecessary doctor office visits. Using appropriate self-care measures for common conditions, such as back pain and the common cold, helps employees function better at work. Following recommendations in a medical self-care resource can help keep problems from getting worse. Examples range from simple recommendations, such as treating a minor wound so it doesn't get infected, to having screening tests that diagnose conditions in their earliest stages when they are easier and less costly to treat.

Goals and Benefits of Medical Self-Care Programs for Employees

There are several goals and benefits associated with medical self-care programs for employees. These include improved employee health, time savings (productivity loss reduction), and increased confidence. These goals and benefits are discussed below.

Improved Health

People's lives have been saved from heeding recommendations from a self-care resource that encouraged them to see a provider or go to the ER when they had life-threatening symptoms they didn't recognize as such. An employee of a large health system in Minneapolis, Minnesota, who received a self-care guide from her employer, credits the guide for helping her get emergency care for severe abdominal pain. She was diagnosed with ovarian cancer that was in an early stage. She received appropriate treatment and was given a clean bill of health. A study done in Australia compared the use of a health self-care program with one that utilized a general practitioner as the advice giver. The health self-care group received self-care information by mail. The second group, ironically called *medical self-care,* saw a general practitioner for health change recommendations. The study concluded that "the analysis of results indicate that variables such as number of days spent in the hospital and total risks scores for the health self-care model were lower than the Medical model" (6).

Time Savings

In the emergency department, the mean waiting time to see a physician is 47.4 min, the mean patient care time is 2.5 h, and the mean duration of an emergency department visit is 3.3 h (22). The mean wait time for a doctor office visit for a patient who has an appointment is 20.4 min (11). Time spent with a physician varies by specialty. Overall, the mean time spent with a physician is 19.7 min (22). These wait times may be unnecessary if a medical self-care resource steers a person to see a doctor versus getting emergency care. Of the some 121 million family households in the United States, 95% have health care expenses. The average out-of-pocket expense is $1,321 U.S. (10). Avoiding unnecessary utilization of emergency department and doctor office visits saves money that consumers would have to pay for deductibles, office visit co-payments, and out-of-pocket costs for services that are not covered.

Increased Confidence in Taking Care of Health Needs

Increased confidence in making health care decisions empowers individuals to be more active health consumers. This can involve teaching people to be more assertive so they are more comfortable communicating with their doctors or health care providers. People are also taught to ask better questions. Empowered consumers demand more information and expect good answers from their health care providers. They seek different opinions or approaches. Then, using all the information they gather, they make an informed decision that may be different than what their health care provider recommends. They write down questions in advance and make sure they get answers during an office visit. They will not allow themselves to be rushed or intimidated by their health care providers.

Components of a Medical Self-Care Program

There are several components of a medical self-care program that should be discussed in more detail. These components include publication materials, the selection of such materials, the distribution of the materials, self-care workshops, nurse call lines and their selection, online content and their selection, and employee engagement and participation processes. These components are discussed below.

Self-Care Publications

A core element of a medical self-care program is providing employees with one or more printed materials. These include medical self-care guides such as books, booklets, and brochures. The guides answer four basic questions that people should consider asking when they are experiencing any physical or psychological symptoms (16):

1. Is this a medical emergency situation?
2. Should I consult a physician or other health care provider, and when should I do this?
3. Can I treat the problem myself?
4. What self-care procedures should I use?

The majority of self-care guides are geared toward common health issues that affect male and female adults of various ages. Self-care guides are also available that address the needs of targeted groups, such as seniors, women, men, children, adolescents, pregnant women, and people experiencing mental health issues.

Selecting a Self-Care Publication

The criteria when selecting a self-care guide include the following:

- *Cost-effectiveness.* Find out if there have been studies conducted on the guide you are interested in and what the results were.
- *Appropriate length.* After considering your target population, determine whether a brochure, booklet, or book is most appropriate for your employees.
- *Appropriate reading level.* After considering the average educational background of your

employees, make sure the self-care publication meets their needs. The Joint Commission estimates that more than 90 million people in the United States have low health literacy; they do not have the means to obtain or understand the health information that they need to make good choices about their health (7). A medical self-care program needs to be given in reading levels appropriate to the individuals using it. Generally, self-care content should be written at a 6th grade reading level in order to appeal to a diverse population.

- *Customization options.* Most self-care guide providers offer a variety of customization options, including a logo on the cover, a totally new cover, an inside cover letter, additions and subtractions, and so on. Organizations can also choose to have a self-care guide custom designed to match their most frequently used ICD-9 codes or to meet the needs of a specific population group, such as pregnant women, women in general, and men. The U.S. Army commissioned a self-care provider to develop a guide based on the issues encountered during basic training. In a number of studies, this guide demonstrated significant reductions in troop medical clinic visits and increased training time, thereby saving the army money while increasing productivity.
- *Common reasons people seek health care services.* Although there are thousands of reasons people go to the doctor or seek medical care, there are 26 prevalent conditions. These conditions account for 90% of physician office visits. Medical self-care programs should address these.
  - Asthma
  - Backache
  - Bronchitis
  - Chest pain
  - Cold
  - Cough
  - Cuts and scrapes
  - Depression
  - Influenza (flu)
  - Diarrhea
  - Earache
  - Eczema
  - Fatigue
  - Fever
  - Hay fever
  - Headache
  - Heartburn
  - Ingrown toenail

- Laryngitis
- Nausea and vomiting
- Premenstrual syndrome
- Sinusitis
- Sore throat
- Sport injuries
- Sprains and strains
- Urinary tract infection

From National Center for Health Statistics 2006.

Medical self-care programs should also address the most common reasons for ER visits. Following are these reasons and the percent of visits they account for.

- Stomach pain, cramps, and spasms—6.8%
- Chest pain and related symptoms—5.4%
- Fever—3.8%
- Headache—2.6%
- Back symptoms—2.6%
- Cough—2.5%
- Shortness of breath—2.3%
- Vomiting—2.3%
- Lacerations and cuts of the upper extremity—1.9%
- Pain (not referred to specific body system)—1.9%
- Throat symptoms—1.8%
- Motor vehicle accident—1.7%
- Earache or ear infection—1.6%
- Accident (not otherwise specified)—1.6%
- Vertigo (dizziness)—1.6%
- Leg symptoms—1.3%
- Injury to head, neck, or face—1.3%
- Labored breathing—1.2%
- Skin rash—1.4%
- Nausea—1.4%
- All other reasons—52.6%

From National Center for Health Statistics 2006.

- *Clinical review team.* Make note of who has contributed and reviewed the guide and their areas of expertise.
- *Publication date.* You need to have a guide or a content that was developed in the last year or two because medical protocols and information change. For instance, over the last few years, guidelines concerning asthma, cardiopulmonary resuscitation (CPR), and the use of over-the-counter cough and cold medicines for children under 6 y have changed.
- *Other languages.* If English is a second language for your employees, you may want a guide written in their native language. Spanish is the most commonly requested self-care guide that is not in English.
- *Cost.* Make sure the guide you select fits within your budget. Price tends to be driven by the length of the publication. Brochures and booklets tend to be less expensive than books, and online content tends to be less expensive than printed materials. A nurse advice line is the most costly of the self-care interventions.

Distribution of Self-Care Guides

Employers can mail a self-care guide to each employee's home address. In this regard, it becomes a resource for the entire family. This is important because women are thought to make 70% to 80% of all health care decisions. Companies that employ mostly males want to be able to make the information accessible to the female dependents. The other advantage of making sure the guide is placed in the home is that dependents of employees are responsible for approximately 70% of a company's health care costs. If a book is sent to the home, it should be accompanied by a cover letter explaining why it is being sent. Communicating ahead of time that the book will be arriving is also beneficial.

Most organizations will distribute the guide to all employees at work to save on mailing costs. Others will give the guide only to people who attend a self-care workshop.

Some organizations use a self-care guide as an incentive for filling out a health assessment or health risk appraisal (HRA), participating in a health screening, and so on. We feel this is a mistake because only 10% to 50% of an employee population will participate in a health screening or HRA and subsequently receive a self-care guide. Because the benefits of self-care are numerous, employers should not limit who receives the guide based upon their participation in another type of wellness activity. We strongly discourage the use of a self-care guide as an incentive. There are many other health books that can be used as an incentive, as well as money, gift cards, paraphernalia, and so on.

Self-Care Workshops

Medical self-care workshops provide instruction on how to use information given in self-care publications. These workshops can be conducted with or without an instructor using a PowerPoint® presentation, a DVD or videotape presentation, or an online presentation. The purpose of the workshop is to explain how to use printed self-care materials, such as a self-care book.

It is generally agreed that providing recipients of a self-care guide with some instruction on how to use it and maximize its benefits is advantageous. Unfortunately, no research to date has compared a medical self-care program that offers a medical self-care guide along with a corresponding workshop with a self-care guide offered without a workshop. It also appears that the more people who receive a self-care guide, the greater the overall savings will be. In this regard, many organizations feel it is better to put a guide into everyone's hands rather than limit it to those who can attend a medical self-care workshop. Also, in many cases, because of a dispersed workforce, conducting workshops is difficult.

Nurse Call Lines

Nurse call lines are a popular type of medical self-care program. They are also referred to as *nurse advice lines* and *telephone triage*. They are staffed by registered nurses who are available to answer calls 24 hours a day, 7 days a week. Services provided include the following:

- A toll-free telephone number.
- Information on health conditions. This can be provided by direct communication with a nurse, as well as through an audio library of prerecorded messages on various health topics. Home mailing of information may also be provided.
- Assessment of the appropriate level of care needed for symptoms reported by the caller.
- The ability to talk to a nurse and ask questions, as well as respond to questions asked by the nurse. This allows the nurse to accrue information that the caller may not think is relevant in assessing the situation.
- The ability to refer a caller to a provider and even access the emergency medical system while on the telephone with the caller, if needed.
- The availability of physician consultation 24 hours a day, 7 days a week, as needed.
- Evaluations and reports. Data collected include total number of callers and what percent of total eligible members this represents, a tracking of nurse recommendations

for appropriate levels of care, and caller preintent and postintent. Other data collected track usage by age, gender, time of call, and reason for the call.

Selecting a Nurse Call Line

Criteria when evaluating a nurse call line include the following:

- Meeting minimum requirements for staff credentialing and experience
- Software and protocols used. Commonly used ones include Barton-Schmidt Pediatric Advisor; Adult Telephone Protocols and Pediatric Telephone Protocols authored by David Thompson, MD; and ones developed by McKesson.
- Accreditation of the nurse call line (e.g., by the URAC [also known as American Accreditation HealthCare Commission])
- The type of telephone and computer technology that is utilized
- The type of backup system for a power outage
- The type and detail of evaluations and reports
- Linkage with other services, such as disease management, prenatal management, case management, and so on
- Cost

A disadvantage of nurse call lines is that, although they provide a valuable service, they tend to be underutilized. On average, only 2% to 10% of an employee member population will call the nurse advice line during a 1 y time frame. This is in contrast to self-care publications, which receive more frequent use.

Online Self-Care Content

Medical self-care information can be provided on a Web site through public eHealth portals, such as WebMD and MayoClinic.com. Although some people prefer to go online for medical self-care content, it is our opinion that most people prefer to utilize a book or call a nurse advice line. Every employee can be issued a printed self-care guide, but not everyone uses the Internet. As of July 2007, about 70% of the American population uses the Internet (8). According to the Pew Internet and American Life Project (14), about 80% of Internet users, or 56% of the total U.S. population, searched for health information online, and 64% percent sought information about a specific disease or medical problem. This means that about 74% of the adult population did not use the Internet for information about a specific condition or medical problem. No survey has looked at the percent of people who search for information on everyday health problems versus chronic conditions.

It was also found that 25% of health Internet users stated they felt overwhelmed by the amount of information they found online. On the other hand, 22% felt frustrated by a lack of information or an inability to find what they were looking for online, and 18% said they felt confused by the information they found online. In addition, 75% of health information seekers do not consistently check the source and the date of the health information they find online (14). Of those who do have Internet access, it may be accessible only at work. They would be unable to access it when at home, which is where most health problems occur. Also, no research has shown that organizations have saved money by putting medical self-care content online. There are many published studies regarding medical self-care publications and some involving nurse advice lines.

Selecting Online Sources

One of the most important criteria in selecting an online resource is choosing one that gives credible health information. Examples are resources that are accredited by Health On the Net (HON) Foundation and URAC.

Methods to Increase Participation in a Medical Self-Care Program

Incentives increase participation in any type of wellness activity. Increasing participation in a medical self-care program benefits the employee and the employer. Some organizations offered employees who receive the guide the opportunity to take a quiz, and those who knew the answers earned a reward. Other organizations called their employees to find out if they could answer questions over the telephone that they would need their self-care guide to answer. Those who answered the questions correctly received a gift certificate to a local restaurant.

A medical self-care program is a process rather than an event. It does not begin and end with the distribution of a self-care guide or providing a refrigerator magnet with the toll-free number of a nurse call line. In this regard, the most successful medical self-care programs are ones that involve ongoing promotion to reinforce utilization of these valuable services. Sample promotional materials include refrigerator magnets, posters, fliers, paycheck stuffers, table tents, postcards, e-mails, and telephone stickers. Also, an employee newsletter can reinforce use of the self-care guide or nurse call line by having an article about medical self-care in each issue and suggesting that people use the medical self-care resources available to them. Employees can receive the best self-care guide in the world, access to the best nurse call line, and access to the best online content, but if it is underutilized, it will not result in the benefits that an organization wishes to receive from its medical self-care program. Distributing a new self-care guide each year is a cost-effective endeavor. It will jump-start the program, remind people that they have a self-care guide, and replace lost copies. In addition, it will have updated information regarding protocols and medical information. A medical self-care question could also be added to an HRA. Doing this would serve as a yearly reminder if an HRA is provided annually.

Legal Implications of Medical Self-Care

Some organizations are initially reluctant to provide a medical self-care program due to concerns about liability. They worry that if an employee has an adverse outcome to the advice given in a self-care program, they will face a lawsuit. It is interesting to note that self-care guides have been in existence for about 30 y and have been distributed to approximately 30 million households. We are not aware of a single lawsuit ever having been brought against a self-care publisher. Even though nurse call lines have been in existence for about 23 y, the authors are aware of only two lawsuits ever having been brought against nurse advice line providers. Even though we live in a rather litigious society, it is quite significant that publications have been litigious free and nurse call lines virtually litigious free (15).

Employee Skepticism of Medical Self-Care

Some employees are resistant to self-care programs because they may perceive such programs as the employer's desire to not have them use health care services. Nothing could be further from the truth, because the goal of these programs is appropriate use of the health care system. In this regard, a self-care program may encourage a person to seek treatment who needs it just as soon as it may recommend self-care as being appropriate. This concept may be illustrated using a brief anecdote that describes how a self-care program prompted appropriate use of medical resources instead of recommending home remedy. This example occurred in a health system in Milwaukee, Wisconsin, that distributed a self-care book to all its employees. An employee of the system said that her husband was having chest discomfort after laying tile in their garage. He sat in a recliner and assumed that it was heartburn. The employee noticed the self-care book sitting on the coffee table, picked it up, and while reading the heart section, realized her husband might be having a heart attack. They immediately went to the closest hospital ER where her suspicions were confirmed. A day later, he had quadruple bypass surgery.

Evaluating a Medical Self-Care Program

Various research designs can be used to evaluate a self-care program. The least rigorous is one that has participants fill out a questionnaire asking them about their use of the self-care guide. Ideally, it should evaluate their use during the 12 mo after receiving the guide. Questions should include whether they avoided any doctor and ER visits by using their self-care guide or calling their nurse line and, if so, how many. The cost of these visits can then be determined by multiplying the number of visits avoided by the average costs of a doctor and ER visit that the company pays. This savings can then be compared with the cost of the self-care program to determine an ROI. A disadvantage of this type of evaluation is that it relies upon self-reports. Also, since there is no comparison time frame, it lacks validity.

The use of self-reports can be improved by asking participants how many doctor and ER visits they experienced in the 12 mo before implementation of the self-care program. The cost associated with these visits can once again be determined by multiplying the visit number by the average cost of a doctor and ER visit. The preintervention figures can then be compared with the postintervention figures. This type of pre- and poststudy analysis

becomes a lot more valid when actual claims data are used to determine costs. Rather than relying upon self-reports, organizations can accurately see the dollar savings from doctor and ER visits from one year to the next. Note that any type of evaluation employed will be compromised if there are changes to the benefit design that can affect utilization.

Another way to provide reliability in medical self-care research is by utilizing a quasi-experimental design that involves the use of a comparison group. The comparison group would not receive the guide and would be compared with the group that did.

Finally, the most accurate evaluation would be a true experimental design. People are randomly assigned to an experimental group that receives the guide and a control group that doesn't. This type of research would rarely be used in a corporate or managed care setting because employers are interested in providing the service to as many people as possible and in a nondiscriminatory way.

Conclusion

In conclusion, medical self-care programs are an effective way for a company to reduce its health care costs while enhancing the health and well-being of its employees. They also tend to be less expensive to implement than other types of wellness interventions, and they have the potential to produce a significant ROI. Thus, medical self-care should be a core component of any wellness program. While there are relatively few disadvantages for this strategy, there is potential for many benefits.

Chapter Review Questions

1. Is the goal of medical self-care to take care of one's own health needs without any medical guidance?
2. What are three goals of medical self-care for employers?
3. What are four methods of delivery for medical self-care programs?
4. What percent of the total U.S. population searches for health information online?
5. What promotional materials can reinforce usage of a medical self-care guide?

33

Disease Management for Employed Populations

Dennis E. Richling, MD

While *disease management* is a commonly used term among employers and health plans today, it is challenging to define. It is rooted in two very different practices, self-management in the clinical setting and population-based health education, which over time have come together to form a new approach to improving the quality of care and health of workers. For employers, cost containment is the objective of disease management. The Disease Management Association of America's (DMAA) definition for disease management is "a system of coordinated health care interventions and communications for populations with conditions in which patient self-care efforts are significant" (8; p.1665). The definition for disease management includes interventions that improve health care quality and thus health outcomes and cost containment.

Through understanding the history of disease management, an understanding of potential outcomes, opportunities for the evolution of this service, and best practices in program design is achieved. Disease management programs use evidence-based care to influence clinical practice by making the physician–patient interaction and the subsequent patient self-management more effective. Data to assist in decision support for the physician can be an additional service provided by disease management. Through an understanding of a model for care for managing the health of those with chronic disease, it is possible to develop a much clearer understanding of the value of disease management and the full potential to improve the quality of care and to shift from the disease care paradigm to a health paradigm. Self-management is a necessary component to managing chronic disease (22), and one focus of

disease management is giving patients the skills, knowledge, and motivation to better participate in managing their own health. Disease management has infrastructure and resources that can be used to contribute to significant quality improvements in the health care system if properly applied. To achieve a true health management strategy for our workforces, employer initiatives need to reach out of the walls and limits of the enterprise and create community-based health care quality improvement. So it is worthwhile to investigate the development of the self-management approach to improving health care quality that occurred outside the employer environment. At the same time, it is important to understand how innovative employer-developed health management efforts significantly contributed to the growth and development of disease management.

Because of program complexity, resource needs, and availability of choices of effective disease management programs, the employer-based health professional is far more likely to be working with an outside resource to implement programs. But it is essential that these professionals understand the inner working of disease management so they can effectively evaluate the external resources and find leverage points that help them to use the disease management resources, infrastructure, and strategic underpinnings to build an integrated health management solution for the employer. In the following pages, you will be exposed to the history of the development of the current disease management approach, to chronic disease quality initiatives supported through research, and to an in-depth look at the necessary components of a disease management program.

Complex Origins: The Development of Disease Management

Before looking closely at disease management, it is worthwhile to understand the historical perspective. Disease management has roots in clinical practice and its associated education of patients and in population health management initiatives that were started by employers. Disease management comes with a strong influence from both practices. Educating patients on the value and skills necessary to be more effective in improving their health is a long-standing practice in clinical medicine. However, three major influences required that more-disciplined approaches to providing self-management knowledge and skill be employed, particularly in the case of chronic disease. These were (1) the development of more complex and more effective clinical practices that can improve the health outcomes in chronic disease, (2) the change of patients from a passive role to an active role in managing their own care, and (3) the increased demand on the physicians' time in the clinical setting. These factors influenced the development of alternatives to provide patient education either in the clinical setting or in settings closely linked to the clinical setting, such as hospitals or community health organizations. In these settings, self-management was always offered with an understanding of the importance of the relationship between the doctor and the patient. These self-management programs were viewed as successful and grew in popularity (6). Most of these programs were focused on a single disease. Some of these clinically based programs actually became the disease management companies that we see today.

During the last 20 to 30 years, a number of employers became interested in health management as a business strategy. Most of these initiatives were founded as health promotion programs. However, many of the more recognized and long-term successful programs not only had experts in population health management but also had individuals with clinical health care backgrounds who were in significant leadership positions. Because of this, the lines demarcating primary, secondary, and tertiary prevention often blurred. Today, the stricter definition of disease management generally encompasses secondary and tertiary prevention only. But as you will see, that may be changing.

The driving force behind the current employer interest in health management as a business strategy—and thus the growth in interest in disease management—is the cost of employer-sponsored health benefits. Employers have looked to manage the inflation of health care costs through multiple strategies. But employers' involvement in providing health care to their employees is not a recent turn of events. Certain employers have a history of providing health care that dates back to the 19th century. Employers whose workers may not have access to health care, such as railroads, mining operations, and manufacturers, offered health care in company-owned or company-sponsored facilities. In this way the employer could be assured that the worker was healthy and available to perform. As time passed, this model became less likely to be the case. The story of employer-sponsored health care changed in the 1940s when employers began the widespread practice of sponsoring health benefits, and the remaining instances of company-owned facilities began to disappear. The desire to both control wage inflation and promote worker safety made the addition of low-cost health benefits an attractive alternative. The situation was further propelled by several favorable tax rulings (3). In the intervening half century, the costs of health care for employers have continued to rise. From 2000 through 2006, employment-based health insurance premiums increased 87%, compared with cumulative inflation of 18% and cumulative wage growth of 20% during the same years (16). The increased financial demand on both the employer and the employee is at a level that is creating a mandate for action.

This trend is especially important to employers in multiple ways. While employers were generally tolerant of the small inflation rate of health care benefits through the 1990s, the changes in trend that occurred at the turn of the 21st century created not only a demand for control of costs but also a recognition that cost management through contracting, discounts, and utilization management was not a long-term solution. If the near double-digit increases in health care costs continue, they will erode the net income of employers who continue to have employer-sponsored health benefits. Today employers are faced with health care cost inflation that threatens the competitiveness of American business in the global economy. To control costs, employers are addressing the burden of illness and health risk in their workforce and its effect on their bottom line. Because of this, employers are creating a demand for a broader set of strategies to reduce health care costs (12).

The IOM's *Crossing the Quality Chasm: A New Health System for the 21st Century* identified that quality failures in the health system were significant. They were contributing substantially to the costs of care and were associated with a significant safety risk to the individual (4). This report acted as the catalyst for a number of employer initiatives in an attempt to reduce costs through improving health care quality.

To quantify these costs for employers, the Midwest Business Group on Health released *Reducing the Cost of Poor Quality Health Care Through Responsible Purchasing Leadership* (15) in collaboration with the Juran Institute. The authors of the report estimated that 30% of all health costs were a result of quality failure. The causes of this failure were overuse, underuse, and misuse of medical care. This report, when inspected in unison with the IOM's health care findings, made a compelling case for employers to do something to improve the quality of care being provided to their employees, especially since it was a business practice for many employers to interact with their suppliers to improve the quality of the services and goods being purchased. Many of these initiatives were born with the desire to create solutions that would be embraced by the health care system and eventually lead to a reengineering of the health care system to achieve higher quality outcomes.

Chronic diseases were an especially fertile ground to look for opportunity to improve health care quality. There are significant variations in evidence-based care recommendations. Chart 1 shows the level of compliance with clinical guidelines for selected chronic conditions. The guideline compliance figures clearly show that there is underuse in the health care system, but the chart also demonstrates that there is variation in care. Disease management is built with the assumption that there is variation in medical practice and that this variation contributes to poor health outcomes. In response to these variations, it assumes that a system that engages individuals as better educated and skillful participants in their own care will result in better health outcomes (1,10,17,20).

Guideline Compliance Figures

Diabetes	45%
Asthma	53%
Depression	58%
Heart failure	64%
Hypertension	65%
Low-back pain	68%
Coronary disease	68%
Breast cancer	76%

Adapted from E.A. McGlynn et al., 2003, "The quality of health care delivered to adults in the U.S.," *New England Journal of Medicine* 349:1866-1868.

The assumption has been supported by research. There is evidence that health outcomes can be affected through interventions to improve quality in chronic diseases, and there is a trust that this will translate into a cost savings (22). The cost of quality from the quality failures in managing chronic disease and the demand for more effective strategies have resulted in the development of chronic disease management programs among employers.

The Opportunity for Disease Management

There are multiple reasons for the quality gap in treating chronic disease. In *Crossing the Quality Chasm,* the IOM reported that this failure of the system is not a provider problem but a system problem. The U.S. health care system is fragmented, and the system support for the average provider is not of a level to assure a systematic quality process even though most providers have the commitment to provide high-quality care (4).

In the early 1990s, a model developed from a synthesis of existing research that attempted to define a best practice to successfully manage chronic diseases. This approach is known as the *chronic care model* (22). The model emphasizes the need to empower patients by providing them with the knowledge and skills to manage their own health and health care. It also advocates for the delivery of effective, efficient clinical care that integrates self-management support into the delivery of clinical services. It also promotes clinical care that is consistent with scientific evidence and patient preferences. There are six areas of focus that support the activities: the community, the health system, the self-management support, the delivery system design, the decision support, and the clinical information system (9).

The argument for self-management is that individuals with chronic disease are constantly making decisions that affect health, some good and some poor. If individuals are unaware of the appropriate behaviors to improve their health or if they do not have the skills or motivations to practice the appropriate behaviors, they have a high likelihood of poor health outcomes. If they can become more effective in their self-management, they will see better health outcomes. This is the reason why self-management support is such an important aspect of a successful implementation of the chronic care program. Self-management support includes a wide variety of activities that empower and prepare patients to manage their health and the health care they receive. This empowerment emphasizes the patient's central role in managing health and central role in the doctor–patient interaction. Self-management also includes providing general knowledge and skill training on the assessment of needs, goal setting, action planning, problem solving, and follow-up. This support teaches skills, imparts knowledge about the condition and appropriate care, and ideally assists in creating motivation in the individual. The support may be specific to the disease state itself or may include information that complements the management of the disease, such as shared decision-making skills.

Providing ongoing self-management support to patients requires organizing community-based or clinically based resources. Much of the early self-management support began in clinical settings but not necessarily in physician offices. Hospital-based or clinically based community programs began educating individuals with chronic disease as early as the 1970s with positive results (6). Educators were placed in the clinical setting or associated with the clinical setting in many of the demonstration projects that were associated with research for Improving Chronic Illness Care (ICIC). This all builds on the value of self-management support along with the overall value of the model. It is an assumption in these educational initiatives that the patient–physician interaction is the central relationship to drive appropriate care.

The American College of Physicians (ACP) white paper on the medical home says that traditional disease management identifies the primary transaction as being between the case manager and the patient (2). This assessment of disease management may be historically accurate, but there is recognition that the self-management support does not have to occur in the health care setting. Telephone interventions have been demonstrated to be as effective as face-to-face communication for providing patient education (18). This is important, as the access to care is expanding to nontraditional settings and technology is enabling the delivery of service through multiple modes such as e-mail, blogs, video, and telephone.

If self-management education is to be provided in the clinical setting, there is a requirement for additional resources. Self-management using educators in every practice or among several physicians will become practical only if the payment system is realigned. Additionally, if there are independent educators not supported by the system, we will have a fragmented self-management approach that parallels the fragmented delivery system that currently creates some of the failure our system now experiences. However, an alternative approach is to experience self-management knowledge and skill training as an adjunct to the current care system. Through the use of outside services, several of the quality risks to a clinically based system can be avoided. Disease management can be that virtual system for the long-term practical implementation within the current system of health care delivery. However, if this is to be achieved, disease management must adhere to the fundamentals of the chronic care model and be supportive of the doctor–patient relationship.

Employers and Disease Management

Through the late 1980s and early 1990s employers implemented multiple cost control strategies that resulted in slowing the growth of health care costs for employers. While much emphasis was placed on managing costs through the use of financial and utilization controls and a managed competition strategy, there were employers who developed strategies to manage the health status of their employees (5). These initiatives improved the health of the employees through a variety of population-based approaches built on the assumption that improved health status resulted in reduced costs. In general, these initial health management efforts were structured as health promotion. There were elements of secondary prevention and even tertiary prevention, as was the case in blood pressure and cholesterol screening and treatment initiatives. These population approaches were modeled after experiences with community-based interventions, incorporating elements from education and skills training that took place in the clinical setting. Those in the employer community who were engaged in these prevention activities rarely focused only on primary prevention. Usually they also included secondary and tertiary prevention. This suggests that the earliest employer-based disease management initiatives were part of these health promotion programs.

The employers engaged in the successful worksite interventions viewed health on a continuum from a well state to a disease state. So the idea of doing disease management as a distinct entity was not a familiar situation to most employers involved in population health management. Employers such as Union Pacific Railroad, Pitney Bowes, the Dow Chemical Company, and other winners of the C. Everett Koop National Health Award demonstrate numerous examples of approaches that were successful in improving workers' health. These innovators made no significant attempt to delineate disease management, health promotion, and disability management (21). The implementations of health management were on a continuum of well to disease management.

Disease Management Fundamentals

The components that are found in most disease management programs are identification, stratification, engagement, intervention, physician engagement, and reporting. There are variations when the components are put into practice. It is useful to understand the various approaches, the risks, and the benefits.

Participation

An initial decision is the choice of allowing participants to enter the program passively or require active election to be managed by the program. The participation models are a passive mechanism, commonly known as *opting out,* or active decisions, commonly known as *opting in.* There are benefits and risks to each model. As to which model is the best may be dictated by the situation and often is the preference of the program designer.

In the opting out model, individuals are not reached or they are reached and do not exclude themselves from the program in the engagement process and are admitted to the program. The admission of this group allows those individuals to receive ongoing communications. One advantage to this approach is that individuals who are not ready to make changes in their health behaviors and are avoiding the engagement communication because they see little value or are uninterested in entering the program may receive information that may motivate them to enter the program or that may assist them in understanding the value of the interventions if their condition worsens. These outreaches may be printed materials, access to phone consultation, or face-to-face counseling.

The majority of the participants are being provided with the information, but no one is required to act. In the current environment, the materials provided are printed materials or outbound calls that are live or IVR. Because identification most often selects individuals who do not have the condition initially, as will be explained later, this approach always includes individuals in the program who are receiving communications with no actual need.

The active engagement model, or opting in, requires contact with the individual and an active decision to enter the program. This is generally done during the initial call. In this model, the participants are motivated to participate because of an active decision. A shortcoming of this approach is the exclusion of individuals who may not initially see the value of the program or be motivated to act. This weakness may be reduced by planned outreach to people at a later time, but this still misses the opportunity that is provided through ongoing communication. This approach will result in fewer but more highly motivated individuals in the program.

In each of these models there is a natural life cycle for these programs. Over time, fewer and fewer individuals will be in the program. At the initiation of the program, many individuals will be identified, and with initial engagement you will find a relatively large number of participants entering the program. However, after the initial engagement the program will only grow with the natural incidence in the diseases being managed and the new populations being added. At the same time, there is a natural dropout or graduation rate from the program. Ideally, there is a graduation criterion that allows participants to move to ever-decreasing increments of service as they become more confident in their ability to self-manage their conditions and as their clinical and utilization measures improve. In the case that there is no graduation criterion, many individuals will naturally drop out of the program by either actively asking to no longer receive the interventions or passively ignoring the communication.

Identification

Identification of individuals who have a chronic disease can occur by several different mechanisms. One of the most frequent mechanisms to identify individuals who have a chronic disease is to use health and pharmacy claims data. Medical claims data are submissions made for the purpose of the providers receiving payment. The claims data comprise disease identification codes; International Statistical Classification of Diseases and Related Health Problems (ICD-9), along with corresponding procedural codes; Current Procedural Terminology (CPT-4); and the costs of the units of service. There are standard definitions for each of these codes; however, the use of the code in any situation is dictated by the decision of the provider. Pharmacy also has standard set codes. By using these standard data it is possible to develop a uniform approach to consistently identify appropriate program participants within large populations.

It is necessary to have some logic in the review of the medical and pharmacy claims that attempts to select who in a population has a disease and who does not. There have been attempts by groups such as the NCQA to create a standard logic, but it is common to find each organization to have its own selection criteria because of a desire to match the particular characteristics of its program to its participants. There can be great variation in disease prevalence among disease vendors because of differing algorithms for the use of codes. The ideal selection criteria minimize selecting individuals without the disease, or false positives, and not identifying those who have the disease, or false negatives.

Variation in the claims data itself results in these false positives and negatives. Medical claims data are limited by source and purpose. For a variety of reasons, there is variation in the use of codes among providers. Some of this variation is very difficult to engineer out of the system and is unlikely to end. Some of this variation is also exacerbated because coding can significantly affect the reimbursement. This all means that identification through the use of medical claims can be very useful, but it also has inherent variability.

In addition to claims data, self-reported health assessments and other referral sources are used to identify participants. There is a gap in self-reported disease prevalence and claims-identified disease prevalence (3). There are several reasons for the gap, including individuals who currently have very little medical utilization and individuals who just recently have been identified. So it is useful to use self-reported data to engage participants before they have significant problems with managing their disease. The other sources that can assist in identifying participants who have not been identified through the analysis of claims data are referrals from physicians, case management vendors, disability management vendors, and so on.

Stratification

Once participants have been identified, it is useful to determine who has the greatest need. This stratification allows for prioritization of the engagement process or for setting the intensity of intervention. Stratification can be achieved through the analysis of the claims data and by using statistically based risk modeling. Another approach is to use information collected in the initial outreach of the care managers. The initial assessment may include biometric measures, missed clinical testing, gaps in the evidenced-base clinical care, behavioral assessment, a self-efficacy assessment, or social factors.

Stratification is a means to prioritize and allocate resources to individuals. In this way those with the greatest opportunity to avoid future utilization and worsening of the disease state receive the necessary interventions first. The claims-based stratification can be an effective predictor of future utilization using statistical algorithms and models. The clinical model of stratification attempts to predict variance from best practices or expected clinical outcomes as a predictor of poor health outcomes with the assumption that there will be increased utilization. Each method has strengths, and probably a combination of both will give the best stratification approach.

Engagement

Engagement of participants is one of the most important steps in the process, for it is through participation that the individual receives the interventions. The typical transaction is by phone or, less frequently, by face-to-face intervention with the identified program participant. For this to happen, the individual must connect with the care specialist. In some program designs, participants call in after receiving program information by mail. Participation in this call-in approach is not as high as participation in an engagement using outbound calling. Outbound engagement is a telephone-based outreach supported by mail or e-mail notification. There are several different options for the outbound telephone call. The call could be made by a nonclinical engagement specialist or by a clinical specialist, such as a nurse. While there are pros and cons for each of these approaches, there is no clear perfect solution. Engagement may be better done by specialists with training and experience in telephone solicitation and sales. On the other hand, a model that uses the credibility of the health professional to establish a relationship may result in higher participation levels.

The interest is to engage with most of the identified population, but this is not currently the usual circumstance. Individuals either don't see the value of the program or think the costs of participating are just too high. To increase participation, the best-practice programs use social and behavioral research to influence the participants to engage in the program. Incentives may be offered to members of the identified population in order to engage them in the program. Motivational training can be offered to the engagement specialists. The use of incentives for the identified population and specialized training for the engagement specialists can result in improved engagement.

Intervention

Interventions are designed to encourage compliance with evidenced-based care or the avoidance of inappropriate utilization. The interventions attempt to provide the awareness and knowledge, skills, and motivation and support that are needed to successfully manage chronic conditions.

The necessary components for the interventions are the care manager, a process, the supporting script, an assessment, the educational content, and the clinical decision support. The care manager is the person who interacts with the participant. Care managers may have a variety of backgrounds, which should be matched to the clinical requirements of the individual. There are differences in staffing this position. One approach is to have a primary contact, a single person who makes contact with the participants. This has the advantage of creating familiarity and the potential for developing a trusting relationship with the participants. It also has more complexity in managing participants who may call in and require some form of scheduling to assure the care manager is available. Another approach is to have no requirement for continuity in the care. The schedule is driven by the participant's availability and the predetermined schedule of calls. This approach has less opportunity to establish the personal relationship with the participants.

The care manager is supported by a process. The process includes a script that assures that the necessary information is consistently communicated to the participant. There is also a requirement for an assessment to evaluate the clinical status of the participant to determine needs for education skills training. This assessment also evaluates the psychosocial and behavioral issues of the participants. The assessment is used to develop a plan supported by a predetermined structured intervention or an unstructured plan that is driven by the decisions of the care manager. In some circumstances, both approaches may be used to form the plan.

Providing information to the participants requires a support infrastructure to provide evidence-based information. There is a need to find an original source of evidence. One of the sources used involves condition-specific clinical guidelines. The challenge is that there are often multiple clinical guidelines governing a particular condition. The guidelines need to be periodically evaluated and monitored for updates. There also needs to be a mechanism to choose which guidelines will be used, since there are often multiple guidelines for the same condition. The variation in the guidelines requires interpretation by a clinical expert. To add to this complexity, the guidelines are written to support the clinical setting. Because of this there is a need to translate the clinical guidelines for use disease management programs. For instance, guidelines may be nonspecific, such as to administer Pap smears every 1 to 3 y based on the type of test used, the age of the patient, and the past test results.

In a discussion on the use of guidelines, it is important to note that evidence-based medicine is more than guidelines. In evidence-based clinical practice, the clinician is aware of the evidence that bears on the clinical practice. It is not the adherence to the guideline that is emphasized but rather the awareness of the guideline and the incorporation of the evidence into the decision process [11]. But even more importantly, in evidence-based care the physician uses evidence, in consultation with the patient, to decide on the option that most closely aligns with the patient's needs [19]. This definition further expands evidence-based care by the incorporation of the needs of the patient into the decision process. The disease management coach and the system support can provide the evidence from the guidelines to the participant. But the disease management system has to be able to help participants integrate the guideline into understanding effective care strategies that may vary from a guideline. The clinical process can be very complex, particularly in individuals with multiple comorbidities, and the disease management care managers must support the physician–patient interaction.

Interventions have three deliverables: knowledge, skills, and motivation. Often the ability for the care manager to support the motivation to change is not appreciated. It is vital to incorporate an evidenced-based approach into achieving changes in health behaviors. The trusting relationship between the clinical educator and the participant is an effective motivational factor. If the health coaching is performed through the primary nursing model, one single nurse is responsible in most outbound situations for contacting the participant. Through ongoing interactions the nurse develops trusting relationships with patients. It is not uncommon in the primary nursing model to have participants share personal pictures of family, friends, and even pets with the nurse. The importance of establishing this trusting relationship is the value of using this relationship to enhance motivation to change. In the discussions with participants, the nurse can learn what is important to the individual.

The frequency and duration of interventions are driven by the participant's needs. There is variability structured into a process that has the flexibility to adapt to the need of the individual. In a disease management program, it is simpler to control for quality and consistency of the interventions and the whole cluster of interventions that may be associated with a managed disease if there is a tight process and little allowance for variation. The care managers are supported by processes that set the level of engagement with the participants. In approaches that allow for the clinical factors and individual participant's needs to dictate the intensity of the intervention, there are greater challenges to maintaining consistency and quality in the process. This is not to say that consistency and quality need be disrupted—only that it is more difficult to measure the process and to monitor the performance. But greater customization to the participant brings greater opportunity for behavioral change. Regardless of the method by which the call schedule is established and regardless of the number of interventions established, there is an expectation that a minimum number of interventions exist depending on the need. The higher the level of risk, the greater the number of interventions required.

While many programs focus on education about the disease states, disease management interventions must go beyond the disease states to provide information and skills that promote the development of participants who are truly able to participate in their overall health care decisions. As mentioned in an earlier discussion, evidence-based medicine occurs when the patient engages in the decision process for appropriateness of care. In our current environment, there are many barriers for patients to behave in this manner. Some participants are unable to communicate because the disease has affected their judgment to the point where they defer to the personal style of the physician. The disease management coach can assist the individual by evaluating barriers to effective communication in the physician–participant interaction. Then, by teaching some basic communication skills and coaching individuals to improve their interaction, participants can share in the decisions as they relate to their care (7).

Physician Engagement

Physician engagement is the outreach from the disease management organization to the participants' physicians. There are a variety of mechanisms to try to coordinate the interventions with the physician's plan of care and to provide feedback to the physician on compliance with evidence-based guidelines. Most often reports are either mailed or faxed to the physicians' offices. Some reports may give an overview of all the patients that the physician has in his or her practice; others may provide patient-specific information.

In the review of the claims data or in the care manager's discussion with the participant, it may be identified that the participant is not complying with the prescribed care. Providing this information to the provider is of value to improve compliance with medication or treatment plans.

In some cases, physicians or their office staff may be contacted directly to discuss the care plan of the individual. In those circumstances, the most effective discussions are those that do not try to direct a physician's clinical process and instead provide information in a collaborative manner that will assist the clinician.

Careful consideration needs to be given to any direct contact made with the physician, for the purpose of the disease management model is to help participants be effective in the self-management of their health. It is the goal of the interventions to empower the participants to be more effective in the management of their disease and to be more effective when communicating with the physician. In some circumstances, direct physician contact is necessary to ensure safety or to achieve better health outcomes for the participants.

A significant opportunity is in the use of the integrated database of the disease management company to supply performance data that may be used by the physicians to improve the quality within their practices. Databases of practice behaviors and guideline compliance, known as *registries,* are expensive and difficult to maintain in most practices today, especially since the practical EMR remains a future innovation. The disease management integrated database can act as a surrogate for the registry if the appropriate collaboration can be established.

Reporting

Lastly, the disease management program needs to be able to monitor its operational effectiveness. The ideal is to have one metric to determine if disease management programs are effective, but this is not the case in real life. As in almost any health management activity, no single number defines whether the program is functioning as designed.

In the discussion of disease management performance, the first step is to define the metric for success. Is success the improvement of clinically based outcomes? There seems to be substantial evidence that the improvement in clinical outcomes occurs. Is success the ROI of the program? There is less compelling evidence that a positive ROI occurs (13). The methods used to calculate savings are under much debate at this time. It is beyond the scope of this discussion to explain the various ROI methods and the pros and cons of each. But some general comments are needed to truly understand the effectiveness of disease management interventions.

In cost-saving demonstrations, one of the most important factors that may bias the outcomes is regression to the mean. This describes the natural flow of chronic diseases: Following a time of high utilization, utilization decreases by natural causes. The practical example of this is an individual who has a heart attack. When the heart attack occurs, the participant will experience high utilization. However, once the heart attack has resolved, utilization will be lower for a time because the acute issue has resolved. While one can argue that the disease management intervention kept the utilization down, utilization still goes down to some extent without intervention.

This discussion is not suggesting that ROI is not important—only that limitations clearly exist related to its ability to be the single evaluation tool used to measure the effectiveness of disease management. There is a need to look at a comprehensive set of measures. First, it is valuable to see if operational measures demonstrate that the program is working as expected. These operational measures include the number of phone calls, both outbound and inbound; the call desertion rates; the speed to pick up calls; and many other measures that demonstrate that the operation is working. Another set of measures vital to evaluation are the clinical measures. These include the rates of medication being used by a participant, compliance with screening tests, and a variety of clinical measures based on evidence-based guidelines. The next measure is the utilization rates of services. This measure includes hospitalization rates, surgery rates, imaging procedure rates, and emergency room rates. If all of these measures demonstrate that the program is working, then there is greater assurance of receiving value from the program. Because there is no single metric that demonstrates success of the program, it is important to understand the overall value of the program by looking at the multiple metrics and deciding if those measures define value for your organization.

The Future of Disease Management

There are two stories for disease management. The first is disease management as it has functioned and has been defined. But the other story is the potential of disease management. There will be continued evolution of disease management. Major areas of development are the participant–physician engagement and integration of disease management services into clinical practice; a broader definition of engagement that includes targeted mailings, e-mails, and other media and not just coach contact; the introduction of management of productivity; and the rising demand for integration of all health management strategies into a single health strategy in an overall human capital management strategy. This will continue to be a dynamic strategy for controlling health costs. More importantly, its role in supporting the quality of the health care system will be important to watch and nurture.

Conclusion

This chapter has provided an overview of disease management applied to the worksite setting. Specifically, the need and demand for management of chronic illness is significant among employees. Optimally, disease management should connect closely to the clinical care delivery setting, and the Chronic Care Model provides a good framework to make that happen. Disease management programs tend to be organized around components that are consistently implemented in the industry and include identification, stratification, engagement, intervention, participation, physician engagement, and reporting.

Chapter Review Questions

1. Define the term *disease management*.
2. What is the major driver behind employers' interest in disease management solutions as part of a business strategy related to health management?
3. Discuss the chronic care model and its components.
4. Name and discuss the major components of disease management programs.
5. Compare and contrast the opt-in and opt-out models of participation.

34

From the Basics to Comprehensive Programming

Mary M. Kruse, MS, ATC

Whereas different chapters in this book address various issues related to employee health management or health promotion, these chapters do not outline or describe what an entire program plan looks like and what kinds of activities should take priority over others. Once practitioners or program administrators are asked to plan, design, implement, and sustain an employee health management program, there is an enormous amount of information to comb through and consider. However, it always comes to a point where you have to decide what to include, what to put on hold, and what to let go—especially in the context of available resources. As a result, this chapter is designed to provide an outline of a suggested approach to implementing a program that includes components that lay a solid foundation, allow for continued program growth and development, and represent a fertile soil for long-term sustained program success. Detailed information on the components discussed in this chapter is provided in other chapters of this book. In fact, just about every other chapter has something to contribute to the contents of this chapter. Information here is outlined with the purpose of working the approach as opposed to explaining the whys, whats, or how-tos. This chapter is organized into five main sections:

1. Before you start
2. Building the infrastructure
3. Integrating the core program components
4. Pulling it all together
5. Building a sustainable program

Before You Start

The first step in launching a comprehensive health promotion program is ensuring that your key resources are in place. This gives you a strong foundation from which to build. Keep in mind that programs formed without thorough planning are destined for rapid failure. Strong programs should take time to ensure that

- a budget has been outlined and approved,
- a program owner has been designated,
- a senior leader has committed to act as program champion,
- all health improvement departments are represented, and
- a summary of benefits offerings has been compiled.

Budgeting

When you obtain support for a health promotion program, usually the first questions you hear will are, "How much is it going to cost?" and "What outcomes can we expect?" As you pull together the business case for your program, start by reviewing what is known based on the experience of other companies and research studies. For example, in a review of 56 different studies, Chapman (2) analyzed the economic effects of absenteeism, health care costs, workers' compensation, and disability management as well as the cost-benefit ratio or ROI. This meta-analysis, in combination with your own knowledge of your company's situation, can help you build a financial case for your program, especially when you take into consideration the continuing rise in health care costs and economic costs associated with health-related productivity losses due to absenteeism and presenteeism.

As you build a budget, keep in mind that costs vary depending on the depth of the program and the economics of an ever-changing market. A 2006 WELCOA report (www.welcoa.org) suggested that companies that invest $100 to $150 U.S. per employee per year for effective wellness programs are the ones that enjoy positive returns on their investment. The financial determinants depend on the size and demographics of your company (purchasing power may influence this), the depth and types of programs offered, the number of worksite locations, and the regions of the country worksites are located in. The best way to grasp the per-employee cost is to outline your program and then distribute a request for proposal (RFP) to vendors asking them to bid on the services. Once the RFP is returned, you will have a better idea of what the per-employee cost will be as well as what that cost will provide in terms of health programs and services.

Although this initial investment may seem high, the current literature suggests that when you figure health care benefits, absenteeism, attendance, and short- and long-term disability into the equation, ROI ranges between 3:1 and 6:1 (2,3). Thus, for every dollar you spend, you may expect to get approximately $3.00 to $6.00 U.S. in return. This return, however, is associated with a comprehensive program implemented and sustained over 3 to5 y.

The types of programs offered tend to be the most influential factor in driving the budget. For companies that start with more awareness-based programming such as health fairs, newsletters, and educational seminars, the cost will be much less than the costs for companies that include health risk assessment, health screenings, and high-risk coaching. Realize that the types of programs offered have direct effects on the extent of behaviors changed and thereby affect the ROI achieved. The more comprehensive the program, the more effect the company will see culturally, individually, and financially. Hence, to consider the budgetary needs associated with a comprehensive program, an understanding of what constitutes comprehensive programs is needed. According to *Healthy People 2010*, comprehensive programs are those that encompass health education, supportive physical and social environments, integration of the program into organizational structure, linkage to related programs, and inclusion of screening services (4). The following cornerstone services align with this definition and directly affect budget:

- *Health assessment (HA) questionnaire*—Assessment is offered to all employees and often their dependents.

- *Health screenings*—Screenings gather information on height, weight, BMI, blood pressure, and blood profile (cholesterol, HDL, and glucose are most often recommended). They are offered to all employees and occasionally spouses and domestic partners.

- *Coaching (phone-based)*—In particular, coaching is useful for employees identified as having elevated health risk factors.

- *Lifestyle behavior change programs*—These programs are geared toward the entire population and encompass physical activity, nutrition, stress management or weight management.

- *Environmental interventions*—These interventions involve food service, tobacco policy, and on-site fitness centers, among other things.

As you plan your budget, keep in mind that expenses may ebb and flow from year to year depending on the type of programming you have. Use of services already included with the health plan or benefits package should be promoted—from a budgetary perspective there is no need to duplicate services and incur unnecessary expenses. Depending on the type of health plan or benefits package you have purchased, HA and high-risk coaching may be included or offered at a reduced rate. Similarly, financial incentives designed to stimulate participation may be an added expense to your budget, although integrating incentives into the health care benefit can avoid this additional cost to your operational budget (see chapters 8 and 28 for additional insights into alignment with health benefits design and the use of incentives). However, whether the incentive rewards are driven through the health promotion budget or benefits budget, you will still need to provide cost projections and participant estimations.

Budgeting Template

The template depicted in table 34.1 is a starting point for designing a budget. This template is a sample of a first-year comprehensive program for a company with 1,500 employees in three locations. Larger companies have more costs around program consultation and delivery but often get volume pricing on products and services so that the overall per-participant cost is usually lower.

Program Ownership and Support

A designated champion for your program and a program owner are two different roles. A champion should be someone who is influential within the organization and is a senior leader or has a direct conduit to senior leadership. The role of this person is to ensure that there is ongoing support from and communication with the top. The other crucial role the champion serves is to act

Table 34.1 Budget Template

		Estimated units	Cost per unit	Total
Program consultation	Start-up	60 h		
	Monthly	4 h		
Health screening	Nonfasting finger stick			
Estimated 40% total participation	Per-person total cholesterol, HDL, glucose, blood pressure	600		
Health assessment	Online HRA for eligible population	1,200		
Estimated 40% total participation	Paper	300		
	Setup fee	1		
	Data management fee			
Lifestyle campaigns	Campaign	1		
Estimated 50% participation	Materials	750		
	Prizes	750		

Program is priced for an estimated total population of 1,500 employees. Screening and HRA participation is estimated at 40% of total population.

as the company cheerleader—it's essential that employees see and hear leadership's involvement and support in the program. The most powerful catalyst for program support is when employees see their leaders participating. It moves a program from the realm of lip service into the realm of being an important business strategy.

The program owner's responsibility is to make sure the program succeeds. The owner needs to ensure that

- a sound infrastructure is built so the program will sustain itself over time,
- a strategic plan with short- and long-term goals and objectives is drafted,
- the programming meets the needs of both the employee and the employer,
- there are metrics and measurement tools in place, and
- leadership is kept abreast of the annual calendar and program outcomes.

The responsibilities of the program owner need to be written into the scope of this person's job, and the expectation must be set that this person is the lead. Often, health promotion programming becomes just another job task within a list of responsibilities and is not designated as a key priority. When the program is new and fresh, the priority is high and things get accomplished. But, as time goes on, other tasks take priority and

the health promotion initiatives slide to the back burner. By the second or third year the program quickly wanes. By writing the health promotion duties into a job description and setting program outcomes as part of personal performance goals, you ensure that the health promotion program has the support it needs to succeed.

The same recommendations hold true if your program is going to be driven by a committee. Someone needs to be designated as the Chair, and both the Chair and the committee need direction and support from senior leadership. It needs to be understood clearly that health promotion is more than a voluntary task—it needs to be part of ongoing job responsibilities. Many programs fail because leadership expects an employee to lead a program in addition to fulfilling current job responsibilities. This is an unrealistic expectation and fosters burnout.

Integrating Departments

Soliciting representation and support from all company departments that have a vested interest in employee health is a key factor in building a solid foundation for the program. These departments usually include human resources, benefits, safety, risk management, medical, or employee health and training and development. Although each of these departments may have a different area of focus, many of the programs and outcomes overlap and support one another.

The more health initiatives are integrated into departments, the more embedded they become in the operations of the organization. The analogy of a taproot drives home this point. A weed with a single root is easy to pull out. The root may break, leaving a remnant behind, but most of the plant is gone. In other words, the health promotion program is dismantled, while one or two high-profile items are left behind. A weed with an ancillary root system, however, is difficult to pull out, and huge clumps of dirt come along with the roots. Thus when programs are woven together it is difficult to pull one without interrupting the integrity of all.

One way to consider integration is by having each department represented on a wellness committee. This ensures that similar programs are not being run out of different departments and that like initiatives are in accordance with each other. For example, if the safety department has a program focused on back injuries, then the health promotion group can tie that program into the next population-focused physical activity campaign and reiterate the message. Regardless, the more closely each department is tied to the others and the better informed each department is on the actions of other departments, the more powerful the overall message will be to employees.

Maximizing Your Current Benefits Offerings

Integrating health promotion initiatives among departments also provides greater insight into products and services the company may already be purchasing. As you assimilate your budget, you need to research what programs and services are already available. Most often these services are part of a health plan, benefits, or EAP package. It is helpful to consolidate all the services into one spreadsheet for quick reference. Make sure to include those that are free and those that may have an extra cost. The goal is to have a central spot where all department resources can be cross-referenced.

Health plans or health insurance brokers typically offer a variety of health promotion and disease prevention services as well as educational services, including HA, coaching, and health fairs. In addition, the clinical preventive services that are part of the covered benefits should be considered in terms of health promotion objectives related to early detection of health issues. The benefit of utilizing these services is the signifi-

cant savings you may incur. Some plans can also integrate HA data with claims data to provide a more comprehensive report. These cost savings are typically offered to organizations that are fully insured. If the case of self-insurance, health plans will pass on costs to the employer, although integration of these services and their data will certainly provide additional value. There are two points to consider when using a health plan's HA. First, if you change plans you risk loosing all the data you have collected. Second, if you have multiple health plans there is a high probability that you will not be able to merge the data. In either case you may want to consider an independent HA vendor.

The Role of a Consultant

Hiring a health promotion consultant to guide you through the program planning, launch, and implementation is often money well spent. Time and again wellness committees waste precious time, energy, and resources trying to get things underway. They tend to work on one program at a time, living month to month—a process that is draining and time consuming and lacks focus and outcomes.

Unless you have staff with health promotion experience, hiring an experienced consultant will provide your program with the strategies and planning needed to ensure that a sound infrastructure is built and that momentum stays at a sustainable pace. The initial launch of a program sets the tone for what is ahead—it is imperative to start out right.

When choosing a consultant, look for expertise in facilitating groups and in-depth knowledge and experience in health promotion programming. A strong consultant will ask questions, gather information, and begin shaping your program by balancing needs, wants, and best practices. A consultant needs to consider the company culture and the main drivers and operations of your business. The consultant should work with you to build a program that is within your budget and that meets your organization's unique requirements.

Be cautious of canned or turnkey programs and vendors with a mind-set of one size *can* fit all. Yes, turnkey programs are easy to drop in, and they work fine within the context of a multicomponent program. But if they are the only program offering, they tend to fizzle after a while because they do not adjust and grow to meet the unique and ever-changing needs of a company's culture. Strong health promotion programs become embedded in the culture because they meet the distinct qualities, needs, and wants of the given employee population.

Health promotion programs that withstand the test of time are those that start with a thoughtful planning process that includes input, guidance, and buy-in from a cross-section of employees and leaders. Successful health promotion programs also maintain this connection to the key stakeholders over time.

Choosing a Vendor

When choosing a vendor there are three factors to consider: cost, value, and service. Cost information is the easiest to obtain and the most objective to make a decision. But cost should not be the only driver in the decision. When purchasing a service, such as screenings or health coaching, other factors such as customer service, experience, staff credentials, reporting, and satisfaction should all be included in the decision process. This is differ-

ent from purchasing a product, such as brochures or prizes, in which cost may be a primary driver. When purchasing a service that allows cost to override value, be aware that you put the integrity of your program at risk. It is tough to win trust back once it is breached.

Table 34.2 provides an overview of major points and questions to consider when assessing the value and service a vendor will provide.

Performance Guarantees

Building in performance guarantees is becoming a more common practice in purchasing high-volume, higher-cost services. Performance guarantees are a safety net to ensure that the vendor delivers the service promised. A performance guarantee is written into the business contract and typically revolves around participation, participant satisfaction, quality of service, and program outcomes.

Table 34.2 Selecting Vendors: Topics and Questions

Topic	Questions
Customer service	How quickly are inquiries answered? How much does vendor support the implementation and delivery process? Does vendor have tools available to help you; how are complaints handled? Will you have a designated person assigned to your account? Are the fees for services clear with no hidden costs? What is the turnaround time on reports and documents?
Experience	Vendor: What is the average number of years the staff has been in the health promotion field? How many clients does the vender work with per year; does vendor have a diverse list of references to contact? How long has vendor been in the business? Does vendor have affiliations or subcontractors that deliver part of their services? Staff: What are staff credentials? How are screening and coaching staff trained? What are requirements for continuing education? Does staff act in a friendly and professional manner? What kind of customer satisfaction statistics is there on staff performance?
Confidentiality and liability	Are you HIPAA compliant? What processes are in place for handling and storing personal information? Do you have a compliance officer? How do you handle communication of personal information at screenings and health fairs to ensure confidentiality? What is your liability coverage? How do you transmit personal information? Do you have business agreements with all vendors to ensure personal information is handled appropriately?
Satisfaction (participant and customer)	What type of participant satisfaction documentation do you have for screenings and programs? (For example, was the process implemented smoothly, did participants feel comfortable, was confidentiality maintained, and was the staff knowledgeable?) How satisfied have other clients been with performance? How easy is the vender to work with? Is the vendor in tune with details? Does the vendor make the company contact's job easy?
Metrics and evaluation	What kind of evaluations (satisfaction, participation, behavior change) do you provide for a program? Do you compile a year-end report of all metrics collected? Will you work with the health plan or insurance broker to integrate information?
Account management	What is the account manager's experience? How much guidance does the manager provide? How involved is the manager in planning and operations? Who supports the manager? What type of professional resources can the manager turn to for advice, to bounce ideas off of, and to share information?

Building the Infrastructure

Programs that withstand the test of time take the time needed to lay groundwork and build an infrastructure. A solid infrastructure is built when

- support is obtained from leadership,
- a committee is formed,
- a mission or vision statement is written,
- the program has a name and branding,
- the program goals and objectives are defined,
- a first-year plan is developed,
- a communication plan is outlined, and
- year one outcomes and metrics are defined.

Too often companies are so excited about starting a program that they push aside the critical planning cycle just so they can start doing something. By sliding into the fast track, the program lacks thought, dimension, and strategic direction and develops a flavor-of-the-month approach. Lack of planning leaves staff struggling each month just to get it out. This lack of preparation becomes apparent through fast-track communications, poor program connection, and, ultimately, meager participation and receptivity.

Take time to plan. Minimally, a program takes 2 to 3 mo of planning depending on the frequency of the meetings, the size of the company, and the scope of the program. As discussed earlier, this is the time to invest in a consultant who can accelerate the planning process by providing clear direction and offering sound planning tools. Remember, the tone of the entire program will be set by the way it is launched, the thoroughness of the communication, and the continuity of the first year's program offerings. By taking time for critical planning, you will ensure that your program has the basis not only to succeed the first year but also to build a foundation for a solid future.

Leadership Support

It has been stated numerous times what a crucial role leadership plays in the success and outcomes of a health promotion program. Gaining such support starts by building a solid business case from which leaders can make strategic business decisions and then expands by engaging leaders in the planning and delivery whenever possible. Ongoing communication regarding outcomes data, participation, and personal success stories is critical to keep leadership abreast of what is happening. As stated earlier, the most powerful catalyst to a successful program occurs when employees see their leaders participating. See chapter 26 for more on leadership.

Committee Formation

Whether you have a dedicated health promotion person, a large or small company, many sites or only one, consider forming a wellness committee. Wellness committees have numerous benefits:

- They help to build ownership across the company.
- They allow the unique characteristics of a company to come forth.
- They are the voice of everyone.
- They are the frontline cheerleaders.
- They help balance needs and wants.
- They provide insight into and direction for program planning.

When forming a committee, a manageable size is 8 to 12 people. You want enough people to disseminate the work but few enough to make a decision. A volunteer committee is the easiest to establish and typically draws interest from employees who value health and want to make a difference. Some departments, such as the benefits and safety departments, may assign a dedicated staff since they have a vested interest in employee health. As you start recruiting for the committee, try to get cross-representation of the company by including executive management as well as frontline employees and any other company level in between. If the company has multiple locations or many business units, consider supplementing the committee by adding *site coordinators*. If the company has multiple shifts, consider adding *shift coordinators* and schedule meetings so as to accommodate all shifts.

Branding the Program

Like any product that strives for high visibility, a program needs a name and logo that will provide instant recognition. A brand for the program conveys value and meaning. It also states that the company is serious about the program. However, deciding on a program name and brand is far from simple. Here are some rules you should consider when choosing a name:

- Keep it short—1 to 3 words.
- Try to be all encompassing and avoid topics that are single focused.
- Keep it nonoffensive.
- Try to represent the program's vision and mission.

Consider letting the employees name the program. Doing so is a great way to introduce and build excitement about a new program. Consider holding a contest to find a name for the program. Holding a contest is pretty simple—publicize the rules just listed, set a timeline for turning in names, and offer a prize to the winner.

Logos provide visibility and instant recognition that allow you to brand all your communications and materials. Often the in-house communications or marketing department takes on designing the logo. If you want to engage employees in this process, you can put the final two logos up for a vote. A fun way to launch the first program is combining program sign-ups with the unveiling of a new logo.

Mission and Vision Statement

Programs that tie into the corporate mission and support the core business objectives will create longevity (see chapter 24 for more on this topic). This is why it is so important to develop a mission or vision statement for your program. Mission and vision statements provide purpose and meaning to the program, give it direction, and act as a foundation from which it can grow. Mission and vision statements should provide employees the answer to, "Why are we doing this?" A mission statement tells about the present, defines the customer (employee), and describes the desired level of performance. A vision statement defines where the program wants to be in the future, acts as a source of inspiration, and provides clear decision-making criteria.

Not all programs choose to have both a mission and a vision statement, but it is important that you have at least one of the two. Since companies vary in their approaches to writing vision and mission statements, use the process that best suits your company's style. When writing your program's mission or vision statement, start by having the company's mission and vision visible. Then have your wellness committee, or other group, brainstorm a list of answers to these two questions: Why are you doing this? What do you want to accomplish? The list might look something like the following:

Why Are You Doing This?

- **To decrease health care costs**
- **To empower employees to take care of themselves**
- To improve morale
- To improve the safety record
- To recruit highly talented employees
- To retain good employees
- **To support good health**
- It is the right thing to do

What Do You Want to Accomplish?

- **Healthier, more productive employees**
- Good health to enjoy retirement years
- Family participation
- **A culture that supports health**
- Programs to help employees change
- Supervisor and management participation
- Happier work environment
- **Support for work–life balance**

Once the list is developed, rank the three most important issues in each of the sample lists (these are bolded in the list provided above). Combine the resulting six issues to guide you in creating your mission and vision statements. Following are a sample mission statement and vision statement created from the six bolded bullet points in the sample list.

- Sample mission statement: To manage health care and productivity costs by developing a culture that embraces good health and an attitude that we are responsible for our own health and well-being.

- Sample vision statement: To lead our industry in innovation by developing healthy and productive employees through education, resources, and programs that support healthful behaviors and embrace balance between work and family.

Program Design and Integration

At this point, the program infrastructure should have all the key components in place, and it is now time for creativity and fun in designing the program. This is where all the program components are outlined and aligned and the goals and objectives of the program are defined. At this point, special emphasis should be placed on integration, as integration can be successfully accomplished at the program design stage. Additionally, when considering best practices and benchmark programs (see chapter 12 for more information on this topic), there are six core areas that are of particular interest: HA (both population and organizational assessment), program visibility, targeted initiatives, behavioral change programs, environmental enhancements, and program metrics and outcomes.

Assessment Information

This is a review of data that provides insight into the overall health of the organization. These data help drive decisions about program offerings. Examples of assessment data include health risk appraisal aggregate reports, claims data, risk management information, safety statistics, and any other relevant corporate surveys. See chapters 10 and 16 through 20 for more information on assessment.

Visibility and Communications

Tools and resources that help to keep the program high profile are newsletter articles, weekly e-mails, posters, educational displays, bulletin boards, seminars, special events, and health fairs. See chapters 12, 21, 28, and 30 for additional information.

Targeted Initiatives

These interventions are designed to address high-cost, high-risk employees and have a pretty narrow focus. Individualized phone-based coaching is the most common intervention that companies use for reaching employees with elevated health risks. Other targeted programs might include special interest groups such as a cancer support network, a weight management program, a monthly blood pressure check, or a tobacco cessation program. See chapters 13, 24, 25, 27, 29, 30, 32, and 33 for additional information.

Behavior Change Programs

These programs are designed to reach the entire population; their intent is to increase knowledge and change behavior. To change behavior, programs need to last a minimum of 4 wk and often longer depending on the behavior targeted for change. For example, a nutrition campaign might last 4 wk, whereas a physical activity program has the greatest effect when it lasts 6 to 8 wk. These programs can take the form of campaigns, may be introduced in a class format, or may be implemented using the Internet. The goal is to reach all employees, all shifts, and all sites and provide a framework and support system to help them adopt healthier lifestyles. See chapters 3, 8, 12, 13, 21, 23, 25, 27, 28, 29, 30, 32, and 33 for additional information.

Environmental Enhancements

Building a culture that nurtures health starts with a supportive environment. This environment can be created in a number of ways, including the following:

- Making policy changes, such as implementing a tobacco-free campus or offering flextime to allow for attendance at classes or a lunchtime workout
- Enhancing options for vending, food service, or catering
- Enriching the facility itself by adding showers or a fitness center
- Improving the grounds by adding walking paths, bike racks, or basketball hoops

See chapters 17, 23, 25, 26, 27, 30, and 31 for additional information.

Metrics and Outcomes

For your program to endure, you will need to show positive outcomes. The first step is to identify the outcomes you want to measure and then develop the process and tools to track those outcomes. The simplest, but by no means least important, metrics to start with are process measures such as program participation, participant satisfaction, and behavioral change. However, eventually you will need to be prepared to show outcomes such as cost reductions or productivity increases directly related to the program. See chapters 8, 12, and 15-19 for additional information on this topic.

Pulling It All Together

The infrastructure is built, the program design is outlined, the goals and objectives are defined—it's time to develop an annual plan and to outline your program launch.

Annual Planning Calendar

The annual plan pulls everything together and provides the direction for a well-thought-out implementation. Your calendar should reflect programming and communications for the year and include other department initiatives that you want to support, such as a benefits fair or safety campaign. The objective for the calendar is to provide a quick reference to the offerings for the year while tying together the core components of the program (communication, programs and events, relapse prevention and targeted follow-up, and environmental programs). When laying out the calendar, the goal is to keep the program visible at all times. The number of programs and events

need to be balanced so that there are enough to provide support and effect but not so many that you burn out yourself, the committee, and the participants. Figure 34.1 provides an example of an annual calendar.

Program Launch

The program launch sets the first impression for what's ahead—make it first rate! A solid launch starts with a well-designed communication plan and a big event to kick it off. Some kickoff events that will make a statement are a HA and screening activity, a health fair, or a lifestyle campaign (e.g., a physical activity or walking program). Other supportive events include seminars, a potluck lunch,

Sample — Physical activity annual initiative

	January	February	March	April	May	June
National observance	Blood donor	Heart health	Nutrition	Cancer control	Osteoporosis	Home safety
Communication	• Program launch communication • Promotional launch communication	• Supervisor update • Campaign promotion	Email/article #1	• Email/article #2 • Contemplator poster 1	Email/article #3	• Supervisor update • Email/article #4 • Contemplator poster 2
Programs/events	Pre-baseline survey	Seminar #1 : Exercise and motivation PA campaign #1 (8 weeks) ———→		Seminar #2	NEHFD event Design your own walking path campaign	Seminar #3
Relapse prevention/ targeted	(HRA high risk phone starts →)		(NRA results initiative BP program)		Step check #1	Tobacco cessation program
Environmental		Complete environmental checklist	Environment #1– Stair signage up	FC open house	Walking club	Promote walking path maps
	July	August	September	October	November	December
National observance	Sun safety	Immunizations	Cholesterol	Breast cancer	Diabetes	Drinking and driving
Communication	• Email/article #5 • Contemplator poster 3 • Calendar promotion	• Campaign promotion • Contemplator poster 4	• Supervisor update • Campaign article • Contemplator poster 5	Email/article #6	• Email/article #7 • Contemplator poster 6	• Report to manager • Email/article #8
Programs/events	Family PA calendar creation		PA campaign #2 (8 wks) ———→ Seminar		Seminar #4: Dodging hibernation	Post-baseline survey
Relapse prevention/ targeted	Step check #2		(HRA results initiative)		Frequent flights	Step-up your holidays
Environmental	Walking meeting promotion	Environment #2 initiative		FC membership drive	Environment #3 initiative	

Figure 34.1 Sample annual calendar. FC = Fc receptor related to breast cancer burden and prognosis; BP = Blood pressure HRA = Health Risk Appraisal; NEHFD = National Employee Health and Fitness Day; PA = Physical Activity.

a walk with senior leaders, a box of fruit in break areas, a putt-putt golf contest, a chair massage, or any number of creative ideas. The key is to make the kickoff fun, festive, and nonthreatening and to promote, promote, promote.

As you outline the communication plan make sure you allow at least 4 to 6 wk to roll it out. Following is a sample timeline:

- *Week one:* Begin with senior leadership announcing the new program.
- *Week two:* Introduce the vision and mission statements and announce the contest to name the program.
- *Week three:* Announce the big kickoff event and start sign-ups if appropriate.
- *Week four:* Unveil the program name and logo and continue to promote the big event.
- *Week five:* Remind employees about the big event and tell them this is their last chance to sign up.
- *Week six:* Start the big event.

Long-Term Strategic Plan

Once you have the strategies in place for year one, the next step is to outline a long-term strategic plan. A conventional plan starts with 2 or 3 y. Again, the recommendation is to pull together your committee, or key people engaged with the wellness program, and take a half day to hammer through all the details. A consultant can also be very helpful with this process. Normally, a strategic plan includes 4

to 6 goals with tasks and measurements assigned to each goal. Goals should be high level and cover the main objectives you want to accomplish. Include 4 to 6 tasks for each goal. The tasks are the items you want to achieve. Accompanying each task should be an evaluation metric. Next, record a specific individual who will be responsible for making sure a task is completed. Last, include the quarter and year in which the task will be completed. Table 34.3 outlines a sample template for long-term strategic planning.

Building a Sustainable Program

Programs that withstand the test of time work diligently at doing so. The program owners realize that their program needs to be as strong in the fourth year as it was in the first year, if not stronger. And that takes thorough planning, persistent communication, creative programming, sharing outcomes, and providing recognition.

Communicate, Communicate, Communicate

The demise of a program usually begins when regular communication dwindles. The critical link to keeping your program alive is a well-executed communication plan. One of your best resources for maintaining communication is a staff person from the communications department or the person responsible for internal communications.

Table 34.3 Long-Term Strategic Planning Template

Goal	Task	Metric	Who	When
Create an infrastructure to sustain a successful program.	Create a viable committee. Engage management through regular monthly updates. Engage supervisors and managers.	Monthly meeting Monthly reports to senior leaders Attendance at monthly staff meetings	Jan Dave Don	1Q-08 2Q-08 4Q-08
Offer lifestyle programs that support behavioral change.	Implement an 8 wk physical activity campaign. Offer Weight Watchers programs. Implement a 5-a-day program.	Number of participants and behavior change Pounds (kilograms) lost Number of participants	Lisa	3Q-08 1Q-09 3Q-09
Create an environment that supports good health.	Have healthy options in all vending machines. Map out a 10 and 20 min walking path. Implement smoking policy.	Number of healthy choices purchased Promotion of walking paths	TBD	2Q-09 3Q-09 1Q-10
Offer targeted programs for employees with elevated health risks.	Offer quarterly blood pressure checks. Start no numbers campaign. Offer smoking cessation class.	Number of participants	Don	2Q-08 3Q-10 4Q-09 2Q-10

Keeping the program visible is more than promoting the big events. It means that every few weeks there is something about wellness that is visible to employees. The range of options is vast; the visual reminder can be an article appearing regularly in the weekly corporate newsletter, a Web site with information and resources, posters in the lunchroom, or ongoing wellness messages at safety meetings. Be resourceful, creative, and persistent to keep the message of wellness at the forefront of your employees' awareness.

Communication also means providing results and information about outcomes to both leadership and employees. Keeping leaders abreast of program outcomes keeps them engaged and in tune with the program progress. Promoting individual success stories is also a way to bring the real story home and may be very inspiring and motivating.

Program Goals: Years One Through Three

The first 3 y of the program are the building years. You want to collect objective data through an HA and screening program that will provide baseline metrics from which to measure progress over time. A foundation should be laid to build upon the six key features or services that align with a comprehensive program: assessment, program visibility, targeted initiatives, behavior change campaigns, environmental enhancements, and program metrics and outcomes. If you are considering integrating an incentives program, this is the time to lay the groundwork. The first 3 y should be spent weaving wellness into the culture of the organization and providing employees with tools to make changes.

Program Goals: Year Four and Beyond

The real test begins in the fourth year. The newness has worn off, and you feel like you have done just about everything. At year four you need to step back and reevaluate the program goals and objectives, revisit the mission and vision statements to make sure they are still valid, and redo the 3 y strategic plan. It is time to really dig into your data (claims, pharmacy, health risk assessment, risk management) and analyze them to see if there has been any movement since program inception. It is important to stop and reflect and to ask for employee input. Then start fresh with a new strategic plan and outlook on programming.

Once again, this is where a consultant can provide an innovative viewpoint.

Program Recognition

Sustaining the infrastructure of the program becomes another challenge as the longevity of the program progresses. Maintaining a viable committee, management support, and employee enthusiasm takes work—it will not just happen (1). Making recognition a formal part of your strategic plan will help to ensure it does not become forgotten. There are four areas your program should address: Recognize the committee, recognize personal achievements, recognize program goals and success achieved, and apply for awards. These four areas are briefly described below.

1) Recognize the Committee

A formal thank-you lunch or gift says a lot. Publish committee names on the Web site or in a newsletter at least twice a year. Send a letter of thanks from a senior leader to each committee member.

2) Recognize Personal Achievements

Be on the alert for employees or groups who have met a personal milestone or tried something new. There is a fine line when publicizing an accomplishment to ensure that you do not breach a personal boundary or infringe on HIPAA regulations. However, when appropriate, personal testimonies go a long way in promoting your wellness efforts.

3) Recognize Program Goals and Success Achieved

Communicate outcomes of programs quarterly. Outcomes such as participation, satisfaction, and behavior change need to be shared with both employees and senior leaders. Communicate your message to senior leaders by formally presenting outcomes once or twice a year. It is also appropriate to include safety information, productivity changes, or other measures that may have been affected by the wellness initiatives. Promoting program success can serve as an excellent recruitment tool for future initiatives.

4) Apply for Awards

There are several prestigious awards that you can apply to for high-caliber recognition. The C. Everett Koop National Health Award (http://health-project.stanford.edu/) and the WELCOA Well

Workplace Awards (www.welcoa.org/presskit/well_workplace.php) are two notable examples. There are also awards offered at the local level that are worth pursuing. Any type of formal recognition outside of your organization raises the visibility and recognition of your program to a new level.

Develop an Annual Scorecard: Metrics and Evaluation

Generally speaking, in years three to five you should start seeing an ROI. However, this will become evident only if you have included the proper metrics and tracking throughout the program. Without establishing solid evaluation tools and a scorecard to report results, it is difficult to derive at the outcomes necessary to generate a strong ROI. See chapters 8, 15, 18, and 19 for additional information on this component.

Conclusion

In closing, this chapter has outlined a practical reality about starting an employee health management program, generating ongoing excitement for program implementation, and sustaining a program over time. Whereas other chapters in this book provide much more detail on any given component, this chapter provides a template that any program administrator or practitioner may be able to use to guide initial and ongoing planning and implementation efforts. While there are numerous important pieces that have to be addressed, there are four relatively simple steps that warrant special attention in order to be successful. First, take time to plan. Second, promote and promote some more. Third, keep the program visible. And fourth, recognize accomplishments.

Chapter Review Questions

1. What five areas need to be addressed before you start your program?
2. What is the average ROI expected for a comprehensive program that is in its fifth year?
3. When you are building the infrastructure for your program, what are key areas you should include in the planning cycle?
4. List four things that can lead to the demise of a program.
5. When designing a program, what six core areas should you include to meet best practices?

Part
V
Case Studies

Case studies provide real-world examples of companies that have implemented worksite health programs in a certain manner and, along the way, collected sufficient data and information to allow for a detailed account of their experiences. Part V is designed to use the case study methodology to illustrate what several companies have been able to achieve in their attempts to improve worker health, better manage productivity, and reduce medical care cost trends.

Four carefully selected case studies are presented in this section. Collectively, they represent self-employed, medium, and large employers. They represent companies from Canada, the United States, and the United Kingdom operating as self-employed individuals, or as complex organizations in the context of a global environment. Three case studies report on comprehensive, multi-component programs while one focuses on a participatory process methodology to ensure most appropriate implementation at a later stage. Interventions range across individual, inter-individuals, organizational, and environmental levels of a social-ecological model with outcomes in the health, productivity, and

financial domains. Regardless of the company profiles, geographic location, interventions options, or incentives deployed, all case studies have worker health improvement as the focal point of their initiatives.

Chapter 35 presents an innovative program design based on sport science that addresses injury reduction and worker performance among tree planters in the Pacific Northwest. Chapter 36 reports on a multi-year employer–health plan partnership which uses benefits-integrated incentives to generate high levels of health assessment and program participation. Chapter 37 describes a pilot evaluation of a health promotion program designed to address a global health and productivity initiative in a multi-national company. Finally, Chapter 38 presents and in-depth discussion of a large global organization's applied research efforts to address obesity at the worksite through environmental interventions for which new processes and methods are needed to be designed, developed, and tested. As a group, these four case studies provide insight to a rich set of real-world experiences that will hopefully prove useful to others in the field.

◄ 35 ►

The Occupational Athlete
Injury Reduction and Productivity Enhancement in Reforestation Workers

Delia B. Roberts, PhD, FACSM

Many occupations are subject to high injury rates with ensuing social and monetary costs; however, workplace wellness programs based on sport science previously have not been developed. This case study investigated the efficacy of a preseason work task–specific fitness program and improved nutritional practices on productivity, injury rates, and biochemical stress markers in tree planters. Matched planters were assigned to either a progressive design 8 wk fitness program or a control group. Trained planters increased aerobic power (from $\dot{V}O_2$max of 47.2 ± 7.9 to $\dot{V}O_2$max of 55.9 ± 5.5 ml $\cdot$ kg^{-1} $\cdot$ min^{-1}) and demonstrated a higher daily production (trained group planted $2,088 \pm 502$ trees per day versus control group, which planted $1,867 \pm 428$ trees per day), no slowing of planting rate in the afternoon (trained group took $1\% \pm 5\%$ longer to plant 50 trees versus control group, which took $13\% \pm 5\%$ longer to plant 50 trees), enhanced hand agility (trained performed 5 ± 6 more claps per person per 30 sec versus control group, which performed 1 ± 4 more claps per person per 30 sec), and fewer injury and illness incidents (trained group had 0.9 ± 1.0 incidents per planter versus the control group, which had 2.4 ± 1.7 incidents per planter). Early season postplanting levels of interleukin-6 (IL-6) were not different between groups; however, levels following planting late in the season were significantly higher in control planters (74.9 ± 85.4 mg/L) than in the trained group (249.9 ± 109.1 mg/L), suggesting that the disruption of muscle was more severe in the control group. These findings indicate that a preseason work task–specific training program can help decrease injury and illness events and increase productivity in reforestation workers. The Fit to Plant program was developed from the findings of this study and current sport nutrition practices. Over 5 y of implementation by all Weyerhaeuser Company silviculture contractors across Canada, injury rates in tree planters have dropped from 22% to less than 5%. Furthermore, the program has spontaneously crossed over into other industries.

Company Description

Two companies participated in this project. Both were small silviculture companies of up to 200 seasonal and 5 permanent employees. Engaged in the reforestation of industrial cut blocks in western Canada, each of these companies contracts to plant more than 7 million seedlings annually. Forest licensees in Canada are mandated to replant cut blocks following harvesting of an area, and these two silviculture companies were contracted to Weyerhaeuser Company. As a result of this initial case study, the Fit to Plant program was created. Currently, all silviculture contractors employed by Weyerhaeuser Company are required to offer the Fit to Plant program to their planters.

Acknowledgments: This project was funded by the Forest Resource Improvement Association of Alberta and by the Forest Engineering Research Institute of Canada. In addition, product was supplied by the Thera-Band Academy. The study findings do not constitute endorsement of any of these products by the author or by the ACSM.

Program Aims

Manual tree planting is extremely strenuous piece-work, often performed under inclement conditions (see figure 35.1). Furthermore, it has traditionally relied on a population of young seasonal workers who are given very little instruction as to the physiological consequences of the work being done. As a result, this occupation has had past injury rates as high as 22% (7). Silviculture contractors and the licensee, Weyerhaeuser Company, were concerned with the high social and economic costs associated with this injury rate. Thus, the aim of the study was to determine if a specific fitness and nutrition program could reduce injury rates in tree planters. Furthermore, as sport science has clearly shown that an increase in fitness and proper nutritional practices can have an ergogenic effect in athletic endeavors, it was reasonable to hypothesize that these changes would also lead to increased worker productivity.

Population

There are approximately 750 tree planters working across Canada for 12 silviculture companies contracted to Weyerhaeuser Company. Subjects were recruited from two of these planting contractors. Informed consent was obtained and rights and privileges observed in accordance with the Declaration of Helsinki of the World Medical Association. For this study, 23 planters who were living at a stable address were assigned to the training group. This selection requirement was necessary because tree planting is seasonal work and planters include university students as well as individuals who travel or engage in seasonal activities in other locations during the winter. Hiring begins in February but is often not completed until a few weeks before the start of the contract in May. In order to complete the testing and pre-season training program, planters hired in February were assigned to the training group. Regular contact was made to ensure compliance and that the training program was appropriate for current fitness level, lifestyle, exercise preferences, and any previous injuries. Training was recorded in detail on a daily basis. Of the 23 subjects assigned to the training group, 18 completed the 8 wk of training; 4 dropped out due to a change in employment and 1 declined to participate. There were 20 additional planters who acted as a control group. The distribution of planters between control and training groups was matched for contractor, age (24 ± 3 and 22 ± 2 y, respectively), sex (60% male and 55% male, respectively), planting experience (2.2 ± 1.6 and 2.9 ± 2.4 y, respectively), and smoking behavior (45% and 38%, respectively).

In total, 38 subjects were tested at the beginning of the season. Subsequently, 2 changed employment, 1 declined to participate, and 4 couldn't plant due to infection or injury; the remaining 32 subjects completed the study.

Methods

This section presents an overview of the training protocol, the study design, physiological parameters considered, blood profiles, and statistical analysis. Each section of the methods is described briefly.

Training Protocol

The training program consisted of an 8 wk progressive design, with two high-intensity interval programs and one longer fartlek program each week (15). Three resistance workouts were also executed weekly on alternate days to the aerobic session. Resistance training used elastic banding and 1.75 in. (4.45 cm) FlexBars (Hygenic Corporation, Akron, OH) to simulate planting movements with both concentrically and eccentrically loaded resistance. Planters were also provided with a small weighted sack of 6.6 ± 0.2 oz (187.1 ± 5.3 g) for men and 5.8 ± 0.1 oz (164.6 ± 3.6 g) for women for complex training of the wrist joint (15).

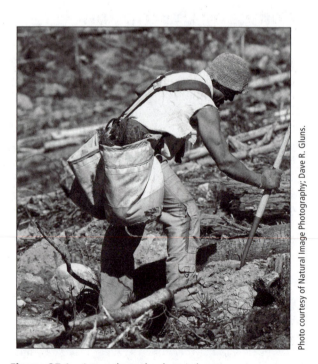

Figure 35.1 A tree planter hard at work.

Photo courtesy of Natural Image Photography; Dave R. Gluns.

Study Design

Nine weeks before the beginning of the season, body composition, grip strength, and predicted maximal oxygen consumption ($\dot{V}O_2max$) were assessed for planters assigned to the training group. These measures were repeated with trained and control subjects early in the planting season, following 11 ± 2.7 d of planting. At this time blood samples were collected before breakfast and then again, along with handgrip and hand agility, within the final hour of planting on testing days. Each planter recorded heart rate curves during planting on 3 separate days (approximately 1 wk apart) between the early season testing session and the end of the contract. Productivity data were collected throughout. The final sampling time was during the final shift of the contract, following 33 ± 5.0 working days. All of the measures performed at the early season testing were repeated. Field data collections were made while planters were working. Ambient conditions were not significantly different during the two testing sessions—early season conditions were $65.7 \pm 6.3\ °F$ ($18.7 \pm 3.5\ °C$), $44.8\% \pm 35.4\%$ humidity, and $3,609 \pm 656$ ft ($1,100 \pm 200$ m) elevation, and late-season conditions were $74.5 \pm 8.1\ °F$ ($23.6 \pm 4.5\ °C$), $58.6\% \pm 33.6\%$ humidity, and $4,265 \pm 656$ ft ($1,300 \pm 200$ m) elevation.

Physiological Parameters

Body composition was estimated from the sum of skin folds according to the protocol of Yuhasz (22). Heart rates were collected every 15 s by telemetry (Polar S610, Polar Electro Oy, Kempele, Finland) for three planting shifts between the early season and the late-season testing sessions. Handgrip strength was measured using the Smedley III Digital Grip Strength Tester (Creative Health Products, Plymouth, Michigan) according to the method of Ashford and colleagues (1). Hand agility was evaluated using a clinical protocol for the assessment of dysdiadochokinesis (20). This test is performed with the subject seated with the back supported and the nondominant hand resting supine on the ipsilateral thigh. The dominant hand is touched to the contralateral palm, with one clap being the successive dorsal-ventral slapping sequence. If the same surface is slapped twice in a sequence the event is not counted. Subjects attempt to complete as many claps as possible in 30 s. Maximal oxygen consumption was predicted by the progressive multistage run (2) and corrected by a factor of 1.15 for the increased metabolic load of running on an uneven, gravel, or grassy surface (18).

Subjects were questioned regarding the incidence and intensity of pain associated with chronic or acute trauma as well as any occurrences of infection or illness such as fever, sore throat, nasal congestion, cough, gastrointestinal symptoms such as vomiting or diarrhea, or wounds with delayed healing. The illness and injury history was assessed at all testing sessions. This information was compared with the injury logs kept by camp first aid attendants as well as the records of near misses. An injury composite was generated, with each separate injury or infection assessed a value of 1. An additional point was awarded for each of the following criteria: icing or the use of anti-inflammatory drugs for more than 3 d, a day of rest or alternate duty, or a doctor's visit. Illness was also graded using similar criteria; points were awarded for cough or nasal congestion lasting more than 3 d, for 2 d of gastrointestinal distress, for doctor's visits, or for a course of prescribed antibiotics.

Productivity was assessed by recording the number of trees planted by each worker on a daily basis. In addition, the time required to plant 50 trees in the morning (before 11:00 a.m.) was compared with the time required to plant 50 trees in the late afternoon (after 3:00 p.m.) of the same day. Terrain (ground strength, ground roughness, and slope) and environmental conditions (elevation, temperature, and humidity) were similar for morning and afternoon plantings. Timing data were collected at least five separate times for each planter and normalized using the mean change in time to complete the task from morning to afternoon.

Blood Collection and Analysis

Blood samples were collected from an antecubital vein at rest (immediately upon rising, between 5:50 and 6:30 a.m.) and again within the final hour of planting (between 5:00 and 6:00 p.m.). Serum was analyzed for markers of stress. The overall level of inflammation was evaluated using C-reactive protein (CRP) by high-sensitivity ELISA (Diagnostic Systems Laboratory, Webster, Texas). The stress hormone cortisol was analyzed on the TDxFLx system (Abbott Labs, Mississauga, Ontario), and the level of muscular stress was evaluated using the markers creatine kinase (CK), analyzed with the Vitros 950 analyzer (Ortho Clinical Diagnostics, Raritan, New Jersey), and IL-6, analyzed by ELISA (Beckman Coulter Immunotech, Mississauga, Ontario).

Statistical Analysis and Reporting of Data

All means are reported as a ±1 standard deviation (SD). Major parameters were analyzed by regression analysis or by two-factor ANOVA with replication. Identification of significant differences was made using the Bonferroni t procedure with significance taken as $p \leq .05$.

Results

There was no difference in pretraining $\dot{V}O_2$max levels for the trained and control groups. In contrast, following completion of the 8 wk program, the trained group achieved significantly higher $\dot{V}O_2$max values (see table 35.1). Neither group showed any change over the planting season. There were also no differences in body mass between groups; however, significant losses in total mass and fat mass were observed over the planting contract in both groups (table 35.1). Productivity was correlated to $\dot{V}O_2$max $(r = .34, p < .02)$, with the trained group demonstrating a significantly greater mean daily production (see table 35.2). Planting time was significantly slower in the afternoon than in the morning for the control group but not for the trained group (see figure 35.2).

Table 35.1 Physical Characteristics of the Tree Planters

	Body mass, lb (kg)			Body fat, %			$\dot{V}O_2$max, ml · kg^{-1} · min^{-1}			Max HR, beats/min
	PreS	EaS	EndC	PreS	EaS	EndC	PreS	EaS	EndC	
Control										
Mean		162.0 (73.5)	*157.0 (71.2)		15.6	*13.7		46.3	48.7	194.1
SD		22.0 (10.0)	19.8 (9.0)		8.7	7.6		8.2	6.9	11.9
Training										
Mean	165.3 (75.0)	171.3 (77.7)	*163.1 (74.0)	14.9	13.4	^*12.1	47.2	^+55.9	52.9	197.0
SD	20.1 (9.1)	26.0 (11.8)	20.9 (9.5)	7.1	5.7	4.6	7.9	5.5	6.9	4.2

PreS = preseason; EaS = early season; EndC = end contract; HR = heart rate.
* = Significantly less than EaS; ^ = significantly different from PreS; + = significantly greater than control group, $p < .05$.

Table 35.2 Physical Measures of Fatigue

Mean ±SD	Handgrip, lb (kg)					Change in hand agility test, rest to postplanting		Bag weights, lb (kg)		Injury score (incidents per planter)	Mean daily production (trees)
		EaS		EndC							
	PreS	Rest	Postplanting	Rest	Postplanting	EaS	EndC	EaS	EndC	EndC	
CG		* 88.4 (40.1)	*90.4 (41.0)	98.3 (44.6)	*95.2 (43.2)	*−1	*1	40.6 (18.4)	43.2 (19.6)	*2.4	*1,867
		22.3 (10.1)	23.1 (10.5)	23.6 (10.7)	23.4 (10.6)	4	4	7.7 (3.5)	2.6 (5.7)	1.7	428
TrG	95.2 (43.2)	^107.8 (48.9)	112.2 (50.9)	111.6 (50.6)	112.2 (50.9)	7	5	44.8 (20.3)	41.0 (18.6)	0.9	2,088
	35.1 (15.9)	30.4 (13.8)	27.6 (12.5)	22 (10)	19.6 (8.9)	5	6	7.7 (3.5)	9.3 (4.2)	1	502

CG = control group; TrG = trained group; PreS = preseason; EaS = early season; EndC = end contract.
^ = significantly higher than pretraining, $p < .01$; * = significantly different from trained group, $p < .05$.

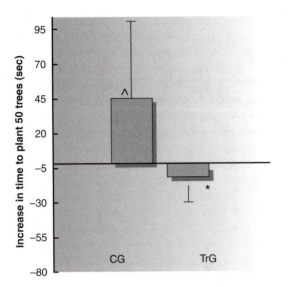

Figure 35.2 Difference in the time required to plant 50 trees in the morning and after 3:00 p.m. on the afternoon of the same day. CG = control group. TrG = trained group. * = significantly faster than the control group, $p < .02$. ^ = significantly slower in the afternoon than in the morning, $p < .03$.

The mean times spent in low-, moderate-, and high-intensity heart rate ranges are shown in figure 35.3. Time spent above 125 beats/min was $40\% \pm 23\%$ and $54\% \pm 16\%$ of the workday, respectively, for the control and trained groups, with an average of 5.9 ± 2.9 h (62% of the total workday) spent between 40% and 70% of $\dot{V}O_2$max. In addition, planters carried a mean of $26.3\% \pm 5.3\%$ of body weight (table 35.2) in their planting bags. There were no differences between groups for bag weights or time in different heart rate zones. However, the mean daily heart rate of the trained plant-

ers (126 ± 8 beats/min) was significantly higher than that of control planters (113 ± 11 beats/min). A representative heart rate recording for each group is presented in figure 35.4. Handgrip strength was not different between groups before training but was significantly higher in trained planters following the training program; there were no observable changes for either group from rest to postplanting (table 35.2). In contrast, there was a trend for the hand agility test score to be higher in the trained group following planting (table 35.2). Furthermore, the control group accrued a significantly higher injury and illness score than the trained group accrued (table 35.2).

Biochemical changes are presented in table 35.3. Increased levels of the stress markers CK, CRP, and IL-6 were observed following planting in both groups, with the magnitude of change being greater late in the season for IL-6. Postplanting values for IL-6 were higher in control planters than in trained planters at all times. In addition, there was a trend for both resting and afternoon values of cortisol to be higher in the control group late in the season than they were at the start.

Discussion

Sport science has identified effective ways of developing strength and fitness; however, this knowledge generally has not been applied to the many workers chronically exposed to physical or mental stress. An increase in the ability to sustain work output and concentration over extended durations of high workload may lead not only to increased performance, as it does in the case of athletics, but also to injury reduction

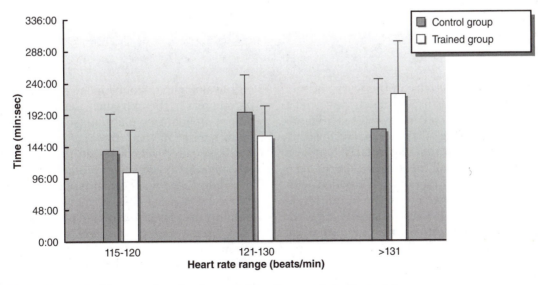

Figure 35.3 Mean ± SD of time spent in various heart rate intensity zones during the workday.

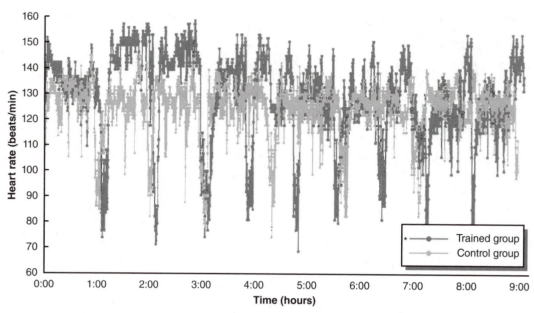

Figure 35.4 Representative heart rate curves during planting. * = significantly higher average heart rate, $p < .05$.

Table 35.3 Serum Chemistry, Data Presented as Mean ± SD

	Serum Cortisol (mmol/L)				C-Reactive Protein (ng/L)			
	EaS Rest	Post	EndC Rest	Post	EaS Rest	Post	EndC Rest	Post
CG	636±116	357±158	743±278	447±160	<5.0	^6.4±3.8	5.1±0.4	^6.8±3.6
TrG	580±82	384±126	627±243	353±128	<5.0	^5.7±2.7	<5.0	^6.5±2.9

	CK (U/L)				IL-6 (mg/L)			
	EaS Rest	Post	EndC Rest	Post	EaS Rest	Post	EndC Rest	Post
CG	144±86	^292±156	136±64	^277±85	1.0±2.5	^11.2±11.0	1.3±1.6	^*249.9±109.1
TrG	138±57	^253±97	155±59	^318±158	1.8±1.0	^11.5±7.9	1.2±3.1	^*74.9±85.4

CG = control group; TrG = trained group; EaS = early season; EndC = end contract.

* = significantly greater than at EaS, $p < .001$; ^ = significantly greater than resting, $p < .05$; # = significantly greater than trained group, $p < .001$.

and increased productivity in the workplace. In various studies, lower fitness levels have been associated with increased injury rates in firefighters (6), infantry soldiers (11), manufacturing facility employees (12), and manual material handlers (8). Although several of these studies included a treatment wherein workers were provided with access to a wellness program, none reported levels of biochemical markers for stress following work tasks or investigated fitness training programs specifically designed for the tasks performed. This case study examined the effect of an 8 wk work task–specific preseason training program

on physiological, biochemical, and performance parameters in the extremely demanding occupation of manual tree planting (see figure 35.2). As hypothesized, it was found that increased fitness was associated with reduced fatigue and injury rates as well as enhanced productivity.

While there were no differences in physical fitness measures between the two groups before training, measures for trained planters after 8 wk of training were higher for $\dot{V}O_2$max and handgrip strength (table 35.2), confirming the efficacy of the training program. The observed increase of 10% to 15% in aerobic capacity is comparable to the level of improvement seen for previously untrained subjects (21). Work performance was also enhanced in the trained group members, who demonstrated a higher daily production rate and the absence of a slowing of the planting rate that was observed in the control group late in the afternoon (table 35.2, figure 35.1). Trained planters were able to sustain a higher work intensity throughout the day as indicated by a higher average daily heart rate (figure 35.4), which was likely to have contributed to the higher production observed in this group. Planters are paid per tree planted and hence there is strong motivation to work at the highest possible intensity.

The handgrip task was not reflective of fatigue from tree planting, as no differences were observed from pre- to postplanting in either group. Although this test is thought to evaluate strength associated with the hand and forearm (1), its use for evaluation of repetitive tasks such as tree planting may not be appropriate. In contrast, the hand agility test involved a high degree of neuromuscular activation (20), which appeared to be more sensitive in the current study. Trained planters demonstrated an increase in the number of claps performed in 30 s in the afternoon, while this effect was absent in the control group (table 35.2). Neuromuscular facilitation has been previously described following *non*exhaustive exercise (9) and most likely explains this observation.

One concern with the study methodology is the absence of preseason fitness data for the control group, an omission due to subject unavailability. Many planters travel or are seasonally employed elsewhere, and hence they were not available at the time of preseason fitness testing. It is possible that these planters improved their fitness status before the start of the season without participating in the training program performed by the trained group. However, the study findings can still be considered to be valid because the preseason fitness level of the trained group (47.2 ± 7.9 ml · $kg^{-1} \cdot min^{-1}$) and the early season fitness level (46.3 ± 8.2 ml · $kg^{-1} \cdot min^{-1}$) of the control group were very similar. Furthermore, this level of fitness was found to be very similar to that seen in a previous study (14) of untrained planters (47.3 ± 6.0 ml · $kg^{-1} \cdot min^{-1}$). The trained group members clearly increased their fitness level (to 55.9 ± 5.5 ml · $kg^{-1} \cdot min^{-1}$) following the 8 wk program, and this group demonstrated less fatigue during planting (figure 35.3, table 35.1).

In addition to lower fatigue and enhanced performance, the increased fitness following training appeared to provide an extremely important protective effect. Other studies have shown that lower fitness is associated with higher injury rates (6,8,11,12), and this finding was demonstrated in the current study by the decreased injury and infection rates found in the trained group. Given the high monetary and social costs associated with workplace injuries (7,12), this finding is significant.

Of the measured biochemical changes (table 35.3), only IL-6 was significantly lower in trained planters than in control planters. This was demonstrated by the smaller increase in postplanting IL-6 values observed in the trained group late in the season; however, observed values for postplanting IL-6 were extraordinarily high in both groups (249.9 ± 109.1 mg/L and 74.9 ± 85.4 mg/L, respectively, for control and trained planters). IL-6 is released from skeletal muscle following prolonged exercise (16), in proportion to muscle damage (5), or with glycogen depletion (10). It is likely that the severity of the work and the depletion of glycogen stores were both contributing factors to IL-6 production in the current study. Planters spent an average of 5.9 ± 2.9 h (62% of the total workday) between 40% and 70% $\dot{V}O_2max$ (figures 35.3 and 35.4). In addition, they carried a mean of 26.3% ± 5.3% of body weight in their planting bags (table 35.2). Although muscle glycogen levels were not measured in this study, tree planters have been reported to demonstrate hypoglycemia and to have inadequate dietary carbohydrate intakes (14). Taken together with the loss of body mass observed during the time course of the study (table 35.1), these data suggest that muscle glycogen stores were likely to have been depleted by the work. The physiological consequences of extremely high IL-6 values are unknown in an otherwise healthy population and warrant further investigation, as severely elevated IL-6 levels are considered to be the most consistent marker of pathological hyperinflammation and infection (4).

Other markers of muscle damage and inflammation, CK and CRP, were also increased following planting (table 35.3). However, both groups demonstrated recovery from day to day, as values were not increased late in the season, and this finding taken together with large differences among subjects may be why no differences were observed between the control and the trained groups. The early season values for these parameters were very similar to those seen previously for planters (14) and are the types of changes observed following moderate physical activity (19). Previous reports of tree planting had indicated a lack of recovery late in the season (3,14); however, these previous studies were executed in terrain that was more mountainous than the terrain in the current study. When working at elevation on steep slopes the rate of planting is slower, but access to food and drink is more restricted, and this has been shown to exacerbate the stress on muscle during exercise (17). Furthermore, there is a higher degree of eccentric load when working on steep terrain, such as was the case in these previous studies. Eccentric contractions have long been known to result in a greater degree of muscle damage and CK release (13).

Program Scalability and Sustainability

In the year following completion of this study, training materials were created that were culture specific to planting. These included a video and handbook illustrating the 8 wk preseason training program; an abbreviated booklet of good practices and a more in-depth manual providing information on nutrition, hydration, and fitness; and a poster to remind planters to make healthy food choices (15). These materials strongly emphasized that in addition to following a program of physical preparation before planting, following a regime of good hydration and adequate caloric consumption

during planting was very important. Suggestions for high-carbohydrate, low-fat protein snacks before, during, and after planting were provided. The training materials were launched early in the season at a regional conference for silviculture contractors, where the program materials were distributed free of charge. Since then, silviculture contractors planting for Weyerhaeuser Company have been required to offer the program to planters at the time of hiring. Information is disseminated either in hard copy or via the silviculture contractors' Web sites and is also available on a public access Web site (15). In addition, short oral information sessions are presented to planters within the first week of planting. Table 35.4 presents the declining number of recordable incidents observed over 5 y with the implementation of this program among Weyerhaeuser Company silviculture contractors in Canada.

Conclusion

In conclusion, 8 wk of work task–specific training resulted in increased fitness levels in tree planters. The trained group demonstrated lower infection and injury rates as well as higher productivity and greater resistance to fatigue over the course of the planting season when compared with a control group with lower fitness levels. This finding is significant in that it demonstrates that a work

Table 35.4 Summary Data for Recordable Incidents (RI), 2000 to 2007, for All Weyerhaeuser Silviculture Operations in Canada

Year	Number of planters per year	Total trees planted per year	Total hours worked per year	RI per year	RI per 100 persons per year	RI per worker × 10⁻²
2007	476	24,278,458	83,228	9	4.8	1.9
2006	734	30,690,719	164,622	15	4.1	2.1
2005	736	23,522,247	98,538	12	5.4	1.6
2004	748	24,179,061	144,803	11	9.4	1.5
2003[1]	768	23,306,852	124,589	26	3.4	3.4
2002[2]	755	24,647,963	199,034	40	9.4	5.3
2001	742	22,458,601	96,322	47	9.1	6.3
2000	700	21,852,449	104,832	50	22.1	7.1
Mean	707	24,367,044	126,996	26	8	3.7
SD	89	2,547,401	37,225	16	6	2

[1]First year of program implementation; [2]year of the investigative study.

task–specific physical fitness regimen was an effective program for reducing workplace injury and enhancing productivity.

Chapter Review Questions

1. What measures were used to quantify the physical load of tree planting?

2. Why were measures of work performance important to include in this study?

3. Were there any indications that increased fitness was beneficial to the workers planting the trees?

4. Which sport science training principles were incorporated into the fitness program prescribed to the training group?

◄ **36** ►

Employee Health at BAE Systems
An Employer-Health Plan Partnership Approach

N. Marcus Thygeson, MD; Jason M. Gallagher, MBA; Kathleen K. Cross, RN, CANP; and Nicolaas P. Pronk, PhD, FACSM

This chapter describes a multiyear employer–health plan partnership between BAE Systems and HealthPartners Health Behavior Group that was set up with the goal to promote, in a cost-effective manner, healthy lifestyles and better chronic condition management for BAE Systems employees and their spouses. The approach involved the implementation of an annual health assessment (HA) program and appropriate interventions to support health risk reduction needs of the population. Participation in the program was rewarded with a reduction in co-payments for medical services or a reduction in the annual deductible. This partnership resulted in substantial and sustained improvements in healthy lifestyles. Furthermore, significant medical care cost savings were experienced for BAE Systems, resulting in an ROI of 3:1 and a reduction in average annual medical claims of approximately 3.3% per year during the first 3 y of the program.

Company and Partnership Description

BAE Systems is a defense contractor with worldwide locations. The BAE Systems facility in Minnesota is a high-tech manufacturing and engineering plant located in a suburb of the Twin Cities. The plant employs approximately 1,300 benefits-eligible employees. Before 2004, BAE Systems offered a fully insured health plan product administered by HealthPartners and a self-insured plan administered by another vendor. Effective January 1, 2004, HealthPartners became the sole insurance carrier. Concurrent with this change, BAE Systems and HealthPartners collaborated to launch a new

health and wellness initiative combining the following components into an integrated program:

- A multimedia and comprehensive communications campaign
- Strong benefits-based program participation incentives
- HA, health promotion, and disease management programs
- A strong worksite wellness program with a variety of on-site health promotion activities

This chapter reports on the experience between January 1, 2004, and December 31, 2006—a 3 y experience described using four data points.

Program Goals and Objectives

The goal of the program was to improve the overall health of the BAE Systems population in a cost-effective manner. The objectives were to initiate positive behavior changes across the population and to alter the trajectory of health care cost trending by providing information, self-help tools, and intervention programs to BAE systems employees.

Population

The BAE Systems population includes approximately 1,300 benefits-eligible employees and their spouses, totaling 1,800 to 1,900 program eligibles per year. Approximately 7% of BAE Systems employees are union members. Demographic information of those who completed the HA indicates that the majority of the population may be characterized as middle-aged (average age 43.7 y), White (91.8%), non-Hispanic origin (89.9%), male (54.6%), highly educated (92.2% educated beyond high school and 62.7% with college or graduate degrees), and in a professional or managerial job type (67%).

Program Implementation and Interventions

In June of 2003, BAE Systems initiated the early stages of a worksite health promotion program with the implementation of a comprehensive initiative called *Setting Our Sights on Fitness*. BAE Systems established a multistakeholder Wellness Steering Committee led by a dedicated program manager and hired an external consultant to conduct a strategic planning process. For each of the following 3 y, the steering committee chose a specific focus based on the results of the HA. In the first year (2004) the focus was on increasing physical activity. In subsequent years the focus was on nutrition and life balance. The steering committee adopted a worksite health promotion model with the following components: assessment, awareness, population-based programs, relapse prevention, environmental changes, and data management and evaluation. HealthPartners partnered with BAE Systems by providing the assessment, targeted programs, and evaluation.

Each year, BAE Systems employees were given the opportunity to participate in four categories of health-related activities: surveys (pre- and postparticipation), wellness seminars, wellness activities (e.g., working out at the on-site gym), and special activities (heart walk, local races, and so on). If they completed two activities in each category, they received a $100 U.S. cash incentive.

In addition to the worksite program, a new benefits design for the calendar year 2004 was introduced by HealthPartners during open enroll-ment in the fall of 2003. BAE Systems presented two different benefits plans for its employees: (1) a co-payment plan and (2) a deductible and coinsurance plan. Effective January 1, 2004, employees were offered two different benefits options for each plan design—a richer plan design (lower co-payment or deductible) and a leaner plan design (higher co-payment or deductible). Table 36.1 presents an overview of these options. To be eligible for the richer design, BAE Systems employees and their spouses needed to complete the HA before the end of the open enrollment. Additionally, in order to continue to receive the richer design in subsequent years, employees and their spouses needed to continue to complete the HA each year and, if found to be at high risk for disease development or already diagnosed with a chronic condition, to complete at least one qualifying health improvement activity each year before open enrollment. The benefits designs offered to BAE Systems employees did not change during the time of this initiative.

Employees were provided the choice of opting out of this program—either by not completing the HA or, if found to be at high risk, by not completing a qualifying health improvement activity. In cases where criteria for the richer design were not met, benefits-eligible participants were assigned to the leaner design in the plan design of their choice. However, waiver criteria were established so that for those whose participation in the program was medically contraindicated, eligibility for the richer design was maintained.

Both BAE Systems and HealthPartners provided qualifying health improvement activities for the employees and spouses. An overview of the programs provided at the worksite as well as by telephone or Internet is outlined in table 36.2. Over the 3 y of the health promotion initiative, an increasing number of qualifying activities were made available to the population in order to offer an ever-expanding variety of options and to reduce the risk that a member would feel compelled to repeat an unwanted activity or program just to qualify for the richer benefits set.

Table 36.1 Health Plan Benefits Design Options by Year of Program Implementation

Plan design options	Participant	Nonparticipant
Co-payment plan	$10 U.S. co-payment	$45 U.S. co-payment
Deductible and coinsurance plan	$250 U.S. deductible	$500 U.S. deductible

Table 36.2   Intervention Choices Provided for BAE Systems Employees and Spouses

Program	On-site delivery	Delivered by health plan	Qualifying for richer benefits
HA (online or print)		X	X
Employee interest survey	X		
Lunch and learns	X		
Health-related seminars	X		
On-site physical activity programs	X		X
Weight Watchers	X		X
Relapse prevention activities*	X		
Web-based programs			
Physical activity		X	X
Telephone-based coaching or counseling programs			
Healthy nutrition		X	X
Physical activity		X	X
Tobacco cessation		X	X
Diabetes risk reduction		X	X
Managing cholesterol		X	X
Managing high blood pressure		X	X
Managing weight		X	X
Disease management programs			
Diabetes		X	X
Coronary Artery Disease		X	X
Chronic obstructive pulmonary disease		X	X
Heart failure		X	X
Asthma		X	X
Rare and chronic conditions		X	X
Depression		X	X

*Brief programs designed to reinforce previous interventions.

Outcomes and Results

The partnership between BAE Systems and HealthPartners was designed to align the interests of the key stakeholders involved—the employees and their spouses, the employer (and purchaser of health care), and the health plan (and payer of health care). All three stakeholder groups received benefits and achieved outcomes as illustrated by documented health improvement, medical cost savings, and reduced productivity loss. These outcomes are described in more detail and organized into the following sections: program participation, behavior change, and financial effect. The latter includes both direct medical cost savings and increased workplace productivity.

Program Participation

High participation rates in HA and intervention programs were considered a proximal outcome in this project because in other settings participation

has been observed to be directly related to financial effect, a distal outcome (10). The HA was positioned as the main program entry point, and thus HA participation was considered critical. Before the program rollout, HA participation rates were less than 1% (in 2002 and before). Integrating the HA into a benefits-related incentive structure yielded a 96% participation rate in 2003, and rates of 89% and higher were maintained in subsequent years.

A high HA participation rate (89% and above) allowed for a very good representation of the total BAE Systems adult population in all of the four measurement times. In addition, a high response rate resulted in a high percentage of the employee population taking the HA in multiple years. In fact, of the members who took the HA each year, between 70% and 75% were responders in each and every year of the program. This confirmed that the HA itself served a dual purpose in being both an evaluation tool and a risk identification tool, and repeat responses allowed for the use of a paired analysis (repeated measures) that could

Table 36.3 Program Participation Overview

HA participation	2003 baseline	2004	2005	2006
Number of participants	1,734	1,782	1,685	1,654
Participation rate	96%	95.3%	89.0%	90.2%
Paired responses	1,240	1,240	1,240	1,240
Paired response rate	71.5%	70.0%	73.6%	75.0%

Program participation	2003 baseline	2004	2005	2006
10,000 Steps physical activity	682	196	231	236
Weight management	151	104	36	31
Reducing diabetes risk	93	37	0	0
Tobacco cessation	28	12	7	4
Managing cholesterol	57	16	54	30
Managing high blood pressure	0	10	44	12
Worksite programs (completed)	NA	350	201	171

Program completion	All courses	Nontobacco courses	Tobacco cessation
Completed course	74%	75%	43%
Remains active	17%	18%	0%
Discontinued	8%	7%	49%
No show	1%	1%	8%

NA = not applicable

track longitudinal behavior change and cost outcomes over the entire 3 y of the program.

Participation in the programs was also very strong. In 2003, the 10,000 Steps physical activity program was the most utilized program, accounting for 67% of all 2003 course participation. In subsequent years, the 10,000 Steps program remained the most popular program option, but employees and their spouses also utilized the more intensive telephone-based counseling programs for health improvement topics such as weight management and diabetes risk reduction. By 2006, telephonic programs accounted for 35% of all participation. Through 2006, employees and spouses had participated in 2,071 unique courses.

Across all courses, 74% of the members who signed up for a particular course also completed it (completion is defined as attending all course sessions and completing the postprogram evaluation). Another 18% were still actively engaged in programs at the time of this analysis. Only 9% of the population who signed up for a course ultimately opted out. Most courses had similar completion rates, with the exception of the tobacco cessation course, which had a 43% completion rate. Table 36.3 presents an overview of program participation statistics.

Participation in the worksite program Setting Our Sights on Fitness was also strong, although it declined over time. The number of employees who received the cash incentive for completing at least two activities in each of the four program modules each year is shown in table 36.3. Over the 3 y, 30% of the employees who enrolled in this program were able to complete it.

Behavior Change

Program participation was anticipated to result in successful behavior changes based on previously quantified outcomes of the selected programs and services. These included the HealthPartners 10,000 Steps (3,11), tobacco cessation (2), and telephonic weight management outcomes (1), among others. Table 36.4 presents the predominant health factors addressed by various intervention programs during the 3 y (for the population subset with repeated measures).

Table 36.4 Health Factors Addressed and Prevalence By Year (Repeated Measures Analysis)

Program participation	2003 baseline	2004	2005	2006	Overall absolute improvement	Overall relative improvement
Tobacco use	8.3%	6.2%*†	5.6%†	5.2%†	3.1%	37.4%
Physical activity meeting U.S. Surgeon General guidelines	51.9%	79.3%*†	79.4%†	81.9%*†	30%	57.8%
≥5 servings of fruits and vegetables per day	15.1%	24.8%*†	27.2%*†	28.5%†	13.4%	88.7%
≥5 breakfasts per week	75.9%	82.7%*†	86.3%*†	87.5%†	11.6%	15.3%
≤3 added sugar items per day	94.9%	98.6%*†	98.8%†	99.0%†	4.1%	4.3%
Overweight or obese	59.8%	59.4%	60.0%	59.8%	0%	0%
Obese	22.5%	20.8%*†	21.0%†	20.4%†	2.1%	9.4%
Average BMI (kg/m²)	27.1 kg/m²	26.8 kg/m²*†	26.8 kg/m²†	26.8 kg/m²†	0.3 kg/m²	1.1%
MHPS (points)	414.8 points	431.0 points	435.7 points*	440.1 points*	25.3 points	6.1%

n = 1,240.

The 2003 HA version did not provide an MHPS. Hence, no statistical significance is applied to that year, although aggregate estimate for 2003 was established based on common questions between the versions.

* = a statistically significant improvement from the previous year; † = a statistically significant improvement from the 2003 baseline.

Statistically significant reductions in risk behavior prevalence were achieved in each year compared with the baseline in each measured risk factor, with the exception of the proportion of members identifying as overweight. In addition, year to year statistically significant improvements were made in dietary changes between 2004 and 2005 and in physical activity between 2005 and 2006.

In addition to evaluations of the program effects on individual behavioral risk factors, an aggregate measure of behavior-related health potential called the *modifiable health potential score (MHPS)* was leveraged. The MHPS is a measure developed by HealthPartners for use with the HealthPartners HA. The measure assigns a composite value based on answers to questions related to modifiable behaviors. The MHPS can range from 0 to 512 points, with 512 being a person who has reached maximum health potential according to self-reported behaviors. This aggregate measure is particularly useful for understanding the effects of behavior change on costs, as the measure has been found, in separate analyses, to be inversely related to and predictive of health care costs and health-related productivity losses. For BAE Systems, the change in the MHPS across all 3 y of the program showed a 6.1% improvement (25.3 points) in health potential achieved. Whereas individuals

may improve or reduce their own personal MHPS in any given year, this change indicates that, as a population, BAE Systems improved its population's health each successive year. Thus, despite the general leveling off of significant improvement for specific risk factors (see table 36.4), the overall health of the population as measured by the MHPS improved every year.

Financial Effect

Strong participation and demonstrated behavior changes set the table for a financial value analysis of the program. Specifically, the effects on direct medical and pharmacy claims costs as well as the effects on workplace productivity were analyzed.

Direct Medical Costs

There are some important considerations to make when selecting the pathway for an analysis of claims data. First, medical and pharmacy claims on a per-person basis can be highly variable. Accidents and illnesses can occur and develop acutely, and one more or one less catastrophic case can disguise the real effect of the program. For this reason, claimants' costs were truncated at $25,000 U.S. annually, and employees with maternity-related services at any point were excluded due to the high cost and unpredictability of such care. Employees also needed to have 9 or more months of health plan membership in each year to ensure that their annual costs would be representative of annual expenditures. A second issue that presents itself in a claims-based analysis is that across a population there will be a subset of individuals who will utilize no health care services during a given time frame and hence will incur no medical care costs. In order to treat such cases from an analytical perspective, advanced statistical techniques are needed in order to avoid misleading results. Although these methods go well beyond the scope of this chapter, it is important that several analytical pathways be explored to lead to a conclusion that is reliable and scientifically sound.

The first step in assessing financial effect is to develop an understanding of the relationship between behaviors and medical expenses. There are several examples in the literature that provide associations between healthy behaviors and cost (4,8). In general, the BAE Systems employee population was studied in a similar manner using regression analysis. However, instead of the association between individual risk factors and cost, the MHPS was used. Examining the relationship of this score to cost on a per-person level, while controlling for demographic factors such as age, sex, and previous year cost, allows for modeling of what might be expected to happen to costs as the modifiable risk score changes.

The parameters of the regression analysis can be found in table 36.5. All were significant at $p < .10$. Table 36.5 highlights that the average male aged 45 y who has no healthy behaviors and who was in the lowest 25% of costs the previous year can be expected to have an annual total cost of care of $3,504 U.S., or $292 U.S. per member per month (a usual method of claims cost reporting). As this individual exhibits more healthy behaviors, the

regression equation highlights that fewer costs are expected. In this way, a person exhibiting a perfect MHPS of 512 and previously low cost is expected to cost $392 U.S., which coincidentally is less than the average cost of just two routine care visits for a 40+ y male ($257 U.S. each). It should be noted that to get a more accurate representation of an individual's costs and to explain more of the variation within a given population, a much more complex regression model is warranted. This complex model would likely need to include additional predictors. However, this equation is intended to simply quantify the amount of annual cost associated with 1 point's worth of modifiable health behaviors. In this case, $6.08 U.S. less cost is expended per point achieved.

Assuming that in the absence of a health improvement program the average MHPS in the BAE Systems adult population would have remained stable at approximately 414.8 points (the 2003 MHPS), the direct medical savings in each year of the program can be estimated using the following formula:

$$(M_i - M_b) \times P_i \times \$6.08,$$

where M is the MHPS, P is the number of participants, i is the intervention year, and b represents the baseline. This equation can be summed over the 3 y of the program using the following equation:

$$\sum_{i=1}^{3} (M_i - M_b) \times P_i \times \$6.08.$$

For BAE Systems, this equation has been applied. The results are depicted in figure 36.1. In aggregate, during the 3 y of the program,

Table 36.5 Results of the Regression Analysis (Coefficients and Significance)

Parameter	Coefficient	Significance
Intercept	4,783.213	<.01
MHPS	−6.0783	.07
Low-cost quartile previous year	−1,279.48	<.01
High-cost quartile previous year	6,045.379	<.01
Age (centered on 45 y)	62.9306	<.01
Gender (female = 1)	326.169	<.01

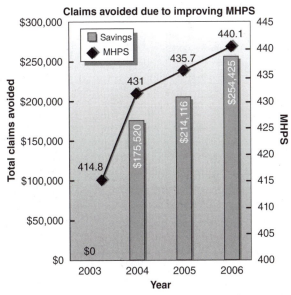

Figure 36.1 Direct medical savings based on MHPS improvements. U.S. dollars are shown.

nearly $644,061 U.S. less in medical expenses was expected due to the net behavior changes in the population, which were manifested by the increased average MHPS.

Another approach to understanding the financial value of the program was to explore what happens to costs of population subgroups who positively change their behaviors compared with costs of those who do not. Each person's change in MHPS was evaluated between 2004 and 2006. (Individual-level 2003 MHPS were unavailable due to changes made to the HA between 2003 and 2004.) Each member was categorized as improving or not improving health-related behaviors based on $MHPS_{2006} - MHPS_{2004}$. The results of this analysis are shown in figure 36.2. As illustrated, the trend in costs for the population that did not improve the MHPS was 16.8% between 2004 and 2005 and 21.2% between 2005 and 2006. Projecting those same trends on the population that improved behaviors shows actual average costs that are substantially lower than expected—6.9% between 2004 and 2005 and 10.4% between 2005 and 2006. Also note that for the subgroup that improved behavior, the cost trend leveled off and decreased slightly in 2006. These savings are not only directionally the same, as illustrated in the first analysis approach, but also roughly of the same or even greater magnitude.

Each of the two described methods yielded similar results, a fact that strengthens the confidence in the overall conclusions. However, additional analysis of the actual BAE Systems claims experience was performed to establish the *plausibility* of the savings calculations. This was done by analyzing the claims experience of the entire covered BAE Systems population (all plan members regardless of participation, kids, and so on) and, after adjusting for the illness burden (health status) of the populations studied, comparing it with the aggregate claims experience of a group of employers with similar populations that did not implement the program. Using the same catastrophic case threshold used by the MHPS methods described earlier of $25,000 U.S., net claims per member per month were calculated across the entire population. An expected net claims cost for BAE Systems was then calculated by multiplying the ratio of the BAE Systems illness burden to the comparison group illness burden by the comparison group's net claims. Illness burden was calculated using the Johns Hopkins ACG Case-Mix System.

The results are presented in figure 36.3 and show that with each successive year the difference between actual and expected net claims increases, with actual net claims being less than expected in all 3 y, 2004 through 2006. The cumulative difference between actual and expected net claims during these 3 y is $965,000 U.S. Nearly half of these savings could be attributed to lower-than-expected rates for medical and surgical bed admissions, another indicator to support the financial effectiveness of the program. As expected, this savings number is greater than the savings estimated via the MHPS, as this method is broader in scope. For example, the program also included disease management components that generate

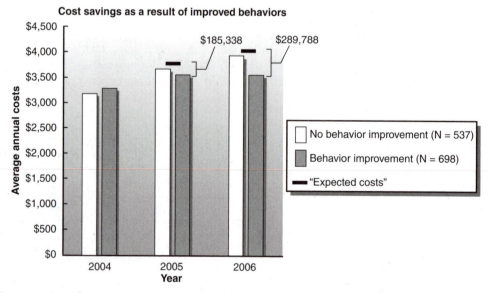

Figure 36.2 Comparison of costs between improved and nonimproved subgroups. U.S. dollars are shown.

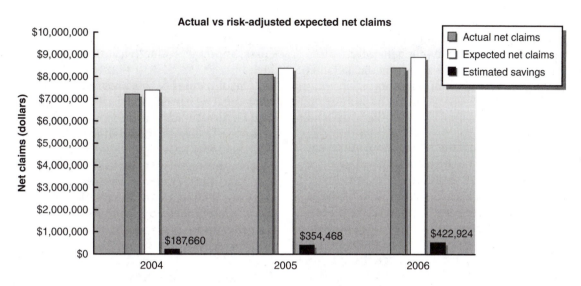

Figure 36.3 Actual versus risk-adjusted expected net claims for BAE Systems compared with those of other employers. U.S. dollars are shown.

additional value through increased medication compliance and other non-behavior-related interventions that improve chronic condition care and help to prevent inpatient admissions that are not measured by the MHPS. In addition, these reported savings may include participants who did not participate in a subsequent year but whose costs reflect the health benefits of earlier program participation or participants who were excluded from the evaluation for being pregnant at any point during the program or for not having enough membership months. Finally, these claims differences also include differentials for the population members who were not eligible for the program, such as children and other dependents.

Regardless of the method selected for analyzing the effects on direct medical care costs, the directionality of the results is the same. Moreover, results of three different analyses converge onto a relatively similar set of results, and thus this triangulated approach increases confidence in the results. Perhaps even more important, the savings appear to be increasing steadily with each subsequent year, which is also consistent with a consequence of healthier behavior, in that the benefits of sustained improvements in healthy behavior can be expected to compound over time.

Workplace Productivity

In addition to the estimated reduction in direct medical costs resulting from healthier behaviors, it was expected that there would be a concurrent reduction in work impairment (i.e., increased productivity) among BAE Systems employees. Previous research has shown that direct medical costs account for only a fraction of the total losses experienced with health-related issues, with the majority of losses being due to presenteeism, absenteeism, short-term disability, workers' compensation, and employee turnover (5,6,7). Of the HA respondents, 62% were actual employees; the rest were spouses. For employee members, we can estimate the effect of health improvement on productivity by establishing a relationship between MHPS and work impairment using regression techniques similar to the method used in the analysis for direct medical claims costs. Correlation of the MHPS with work impairment, as defined by the WPAI questionnaire (9), yields a coefficient for MHPS that indicates that for every increased point in MHPS, work impairment decreases by 0.04%. In this way, the 12.8-point increase in MHPS from 2003 to 2004 translates to a 0.51% decrease in work impairment for the average participant. Assuming a conservative estimate that the average total annual compensation of a BAE Systems employee was $50,000 U.S. during this time frame, and assuming that this amount is equivalent to the value of the employee's position, the increase in MHPS from 2003 to 2004 constitutes an additional $256 U.S. in productive output per employee per year. Thus, it can be estimated that BAE Systems experienced approximately $283,000 U.S. in productivity gains in 2004 from employees who participated in the program and improved their lifestyle behaviors. Repeating the calculation for 2005 and 2006, the total productivity gains result in a total of $1.12 million U.S. across all years of the program. For BAE Systems, this result demonstrates that productivity savings generated by this program were 2.8 times the direct medical claims savings for the employee population.

Conclusion

This case study illustrates a successful multiyear employer–health plan partnership experience designed to improve population health, lower medical health care cost trends, and address excess health-related work productivity loss. High rates of employee and spouse participation in both HA and lifestyle improvement programs were achieved, resulting in significant improvements in health status as quantified by the HA. These interventions resulted in significant medical care cost savings that accumulated over the 3 y of the program and were estimated at $965,000 U.S., or 3.3% of overall expected medical care costs. Considering the costs of the program (calculated at $100,000 U.S. per year or $58.82 U.S. per employee per year using an average of 1,700 employees), an overall ROI of 3:1 was achieved. (The ROI is closer to 2:1 if we use the estimated savings calculated from the observed change in the population MHPS.) Finally, estimated savings from reductions in work productivity loss over the 3 y were in excess of $1 million U.S. These results indicate that a partnership model designed to meet the needs and interests of all stakeholders can generate health improvement, reduce medical costs, improve productivity, and create a positive ROI.

The outcomes of this program may have been influenced by or dependent on a variety of contextual factors, including the nature of the industry (manufacturing), the population (older employees with higher-than-average education and income levels), the quality of worksite program leadership, and the culture of wellness present in the worksite. The nature of the relationship between these contextual factors and the outcomes of this program appears to be a worthwhile subject for future research.

Chapter Review Questions

1. What are the four key components of an effective worksite-based health improvement program?

2. What were the three different approaches used to measure the effect of the program on direct medical costs?

3. Why is it important to use multiple methods to measure the value of the program?

4. What are some of the challenges that can be expected in trying to maintain this program, and how might you address them?

37

Health Promotion, Participation, and Productivity
A Case Study at Unilever PLC

Peter Mills, MD, and Jessica Colling, BSC, MSC

> *"If we leave the human factor out of our business calculations we shall be wrong every time."*
>
> –William Hesketh Lever, founder of Lever Brothers

The link between health status and productivity may seem old news, but, to date, there has been limited evidence that health promotion in the workplace can affect both productivity and health risk status (1,2,5,8). The aim of this applied research project was to analyze this effect (7).

A pilot intervention group from Unilever PLC and a matched control group were followed over 12 mo. All participants were asked to complete an online health risk appraisal (HRA) and the work performance section of the WHO Health and Work Performance Questionnaire at the beginning and end of the study (4,6).

Participants in the intervention group received a personal health report and advice from their HRA, access to a health and well-being Web portal, e-mail communications every 2 wk, printed packs of information, and access to on-site seminars. The control group received no report or interventions.

Over the study, improvements in the number of health risk factors, monthly absenteeism days, and work performance were seen in the intervention group compared with the control group. Economic analysis showed an ROI of 6.21:1 (7).

Company Description

All the participants in the intervention group of the program were employees of Unilever PLC, a multinational manufacturer of foods (e.g., Flora margarine, Lipton tea, Ben and Jerry's ice cream), home care products (e.g., Cif cleaning products, Comfort softener, Domestos bleach), and personal care products (e.g., Dove, Lux, and Ponds beauty products; Signal toothpaste).

Three pilot sites were chosen to participate in the study. These were based in Kingston Upon Thames, Surrey; Walton Upon Thames, Surrey; and St. David's Park, Chester, all in the United Kingdom.

Program Aims

Unilever has a strong tradition of investing in employee well-being. This tradition dates back to the 1880s when William Hesketh Lever (figure 37.1), one of the founders of Lever Brothers, also built homes for his factory workers when he built a new soap factory (figure 37.2). The building maintenance and upkeep of the village were subsidized

Acknowledgments: The authors would like to thank Dr. John Cooper of Unilever for his help with implementing this study and his assistance in the review of this chapter.

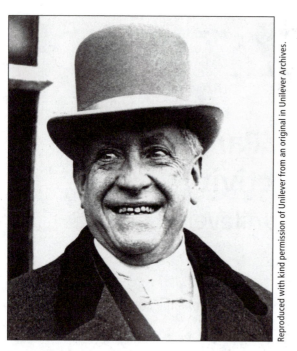

Figure 37.1   William Hesketh Lever

with a portion of the profits from Lever Brothers (figure 37.3). He also personally financed a church, technical institute, and art gallery; set up schemes for welfare, education, and entertainment; and made sure the workers all had access to health care—not such an easy task in the 1890s! This village and factory site became known as *Port Sunlight* after the soap that it produced. Only in the 1980s were the houses first sold privately to non-Unilever employees.

This tradition of social responsibility and investment in employee well-being has been maintained. Unilever has been an early adopter in the field of health and well-being at work.

To date, most research on the effect of health promotion at work has been U.S. based. As a result, vielife, Unilever, and IHPM were keen to see if similar findings were seen in a U.K. population.

This study aimed to evaluate the effect of health promotion in the worksite on individual health risk and productivity status. It has been hypothesized that employees with fewer health risks are more

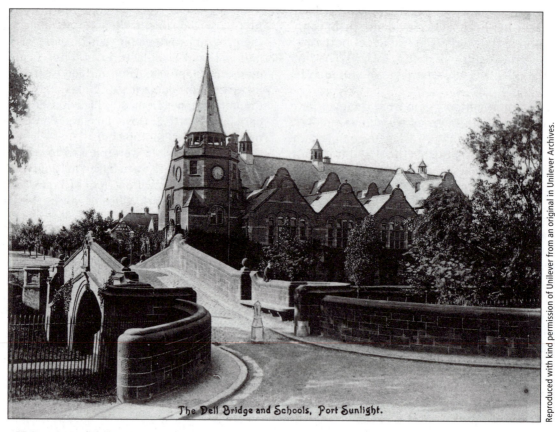

The Dell Bridge and Schools, Port Sunlight.

Figure 37.2   Port Sunlight Works

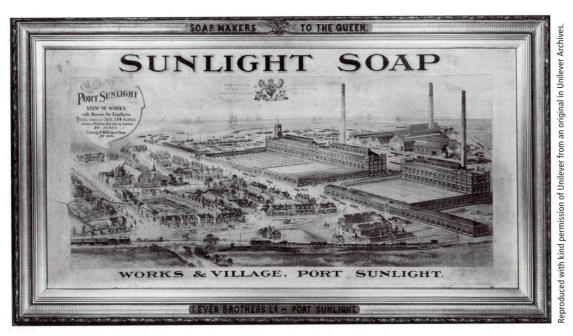

Figure 37.3   Port Sunlight Village

productive at work, and this study aimed to investigate the validity of this hypothesis in an employed population in the United Kingdom.

Population Intervention Group

There were 618 full-time Unilever employees in the intervention group of the program. The entire intervention group was asked to complete a secure online survey about health and performance at the start of the program—the baseline—and then again after 12 mo.

Of the intervention group, 84% (n = 519) completed the survey at the baseline, and 43% (n = 266) completed the survey at follow-up. Men made up 46% and women made up 54% of the intervention group and the mean age of the group was 34.3 y. Effect analyses were conducted on the 43% (n = 266) employees who completed both the baseline and 12 mo HRA. All of the intervention group members had access to an online health portal, on-site seminars, and printed health packs, irrespective of whether they had taken the online survey.

Control Group

For this research study, 2,500 people were invited to participate as controls. Participants were invited through a market research organization, and of those invited, 67.2% (n = 1,679) completed the initial baseline questionnaires (the HRA and the work performance section of the WHO Health and Work Performance Questionnaire).

In addition, 49% (n = 1,242) of the control group also completed the questionnaire at the end of the study. Men made up 54% and women made up 46% of the control group, and the mean age of this group was 34.5 y. Control participants were matched to the intervention group in employment status and baseline salary.

Approach to Implementation

To engage the intervention group in the program, a collaborative approach between vielife and Unilever was used. On the vielife side there was a dedicated project manager who arranged the implementation of the program, liaised with the key Unilever contacts, and planned events at each of the three sites. The project manager also worked with the internal communications team at vielife to schedule communications campaigns and deliver appropriate material.

At Unilever, the occupational health team took the lead at each of the three sites, organizing on-site events and galvanizing interest in the project.

The intervention program was also used to highlight services available within the company that employees may not have been aware of. Support for the program from senior management was strong; the chairman at the time, Niall Fitzgerald, was a vocal advocate for taking responsibility for one's own health and well-being, and all of the senior management team had previously been offered a personalized wellness program—the Senior Leaders' Health Initiative—that had produced some impressive results. This experience led to extensive support and encouragement from key staff members. This pilot intervention program also tied in closely to Unilever's vitality mission statement, "To add vitality to life," which is reflected in the company's attitude toward consumers as well as employees.

Program Launch

A coordinated approach was used to launch the program simultaneously at the three sites. Posters, printed fliers, and e-mails were used to inform people about the program, when it was launching, and how they could get involved. All of these communications were co-branded to introduce vielife to the population and show endorsement by each business unit for the project.

On each site a number of launch days were held, during which employees could come to a designated place, see a short movie about the service, ask questions of vielife staff members, and register online with the health promotion portal. There was also the opportunity to have basic biometric measurements taken (height, weight, body fat percentage, blood pressure).

All participants who came to the launch were also encouraged to take the HRA. Desk-drop fliers were given to any individuals who were not able to come to the launch events in order to inform them how to register for the site and how to access the HRA. E-mail support was also available to any participants who had difficulty registering or completing the HRA.

All employees on the three sites were eligible to join the program and were encouraged to participate. E-mails were sent by each business unit to encourage participation, and once participants had registered with the online service, they received e-mail communications every 2 wk from vielife.

Following the on-site launch of the program, there was a 4 wk communications campaign to encourage more people to register and to encourage registered users to take the HRA. This com-

munications campaign included a targeted e-mail campaign, posters, fliers, and countdown imagery on the vielife Online site showing people how long they had left to take the HRA to make their voice heard in the research project. Individuals were also incentivized to take the HRA through a prize draw.

Everyone in the intervention and control group was informed of the research behind the pilot project and all participants had to sign an electronic consent form agreeing to allow their personal data to be used for research purposes before beginning the baseline survey. All data collection, storage, and utilization were fully compliant with the 1998 U.K. Data Protection Act.

Control Group Engagement

The control group of participants was recruited by Interactive Prospect Targeting (IPT), a market research company. IPT contacted 2,500 employed people to participate in the research. The purpose of the project was explained to all individuals, who were incentivized to complete the questionnaires by participation in a prize draw. All participants were recruited by e-mail and were employed in the service sector.

Participants needed to complete both sections of the research project to be eligible for the prize draw. As in the intervention group, all participants had to sign an electronic consent form agreeing to allow their personal data to be used for research purposes.

Interventions

The intervention included several components including HRA feedback reports, online program access, e-mail communications, health campaigns, and health fairs. Each of these components is described briefly below.

Health and Well-Being Report

The first health promotion activity that all the intervention group participants received was a personal health report from their HRA. The health and well-being report gave people an overall wellness score and individual scores for 13 health risk elements: medical health, pain, sleep quality, body weight, nutritional balance, physical activity, stress management, life load (the amount of responsibility that someone has), risk behavior, perception of general health, perception of effectiveness, job satisfaction, and mood. Each element was color coded and given a score out of 100 to denote high-, medium-, or low-risk status. The report then provided information and advice based on participants' health risk areas and their readiness to change health-related behaviors. This personalized report gave detailed recommendations for positive health behavior change and further reading on the vielife Online health and well-being Web portal.

Individuals were able to take the assessment multiple times during the program so they could evaluate their own progress. A feature of this HRA is that it allows users to see how their score has changed in each area in a graphical form, so in addition to an overall score change, the effect on individual components of health status can be observed. For reporting purposes, only the baseline and end point assessment scores were evaluated.

Vielife Online

Throughout the program, all Unilever employees at the pilot sites had access to the vielife Online health and well-being Web portal. This site contained over 250 consumer-focused articles on health and well-being. The site concentrated on the areas of sleep, stress, nutrition, and physical activity, but there were additional topic areas on travel health and musculoskeletal health, including ergonomic workstation setup. There were also five additional health assessments (sleep, stress, nutrition, physical activity, back health, and joint health) that provided detailed personalized reports in the specific topic. On top of this, there were trackers to log biometric information such as weight, blood pressure, and cholesterol. The site was also completely searchable by key word and was regularly updated with health news and new articles.

E-Mail Communications

All participants who registered with the site received an e-mail communication every 2 wk on a particular health topic. E-mails were tailored to an individual's personal health profile and could vary by age, gender, and health risk status or could address a general health interest topic. E-mails were designed to provide practical health tips and encourage use of the vielife Online portal by linking participants to new articles on the site.

E-mail communication was also used to tell participants about other interventions that were being launched on-site and was used to drive par-

ticipation in the research study. Participants were able to choose the format of their e-mails so that they either received colorful, branded e-mails with related imagery or received a plain text format.

Health Campaigns

Targeted interventions were identified using the results of the HRA data of the intervention group participants. The 13 areas of health risk examined by the HRA allowed an aggregated report to be produced that provided an overall group risk profile. The most prevalent health risks across the population were found to be poor nutritional balance, lack of physical activity, poor stress management, and poor sleep quality. A number of interventions were put in place to address these issues.

Four paper-based packs were developed to address these key health risks. Each pack contained a newsletter and health promotional literature. The first area to be addressed was stress management, the second sleep improvement, the third nutritional balance, and the fourth physical activity. These packs were distributed throughout the year to staff at each site, and focus was directed to one health risk issue at a time.

These paper-based interventions were supported by on-site seminars. All seminars were delivered by a health professional (physician, dietitian, physiologist, or physical therapist) and were tailored to specific issues facing a working population. Each seminar lasted approximately an hour and included time for questions at the end. Seminars were run a number of times during the day to allow the maximum number of people to attend. Seminar titles included Strength and Resilience; Improving Stress Management; Eating for Energy; and Sleep Better, Feel Better, Live Better. All of the seminars and the messaging around health and well-being focused on meeting goals for positive well-being rather than managing a specific issue. The rationale for this approach was to encourage maximum participation from the entire group.

In addition to the seminars and information packs, a number of health behavior change campaigns were launched that allowed participants to sign up to achieve a specific goal. These included brief interventions such as the 2 wk hydration campaign. Water bottles were distributed to all employees, and posters in common areas were used to publicize the program. This was run in conjunction with the launch event to engender participation in the project. Most people don't drink enough fluid during the day, and even sub-clinical levels of dehydration can potentially have an effect on concentration, coordination, decision-making skills, and feelings of fatigue. This simple, light-hearted campaign was used to draw people into the project and also reflect one of the key messages of the vielife service: Lifestyle changes don't have to be huge; small, simple steps can have an effect on personal well-being. This gentle intro-duction to the service, with an easy-to-achieve target, helped encourage participation in some of the longer programs and initiatives.

A longer campaign was the Look Good, Feel Better healthy eating campaign, which was an 8 wk online campaign consisting of weekly e-mails, printed communications, and on-site seminars. The program was designed to concentrate on the basics of healthy eating for lifelong nutritional improvement. The program wasn't designed to specifically enable weight loss, because anyone at the Unilever pilot sites was able to participate (including those who didn't need to lose weight); however, improving eating habits had an effect on body weight for some participants.

Health Fairs

At each site, a number of health fairs were held during the year where individuals could have their biometric measurements taken, have a free back massage, or talk to a dietitian about their own dietary needs and eating habits. These days were popular, particularly the massages and dietitian appointments. All the appointment slots for each health fair (40 massages and 20 dietitian appointments a day) were booked within the first 2 h of communication. They also allowed the occu-pational health team to promote the services it offered on-site that many employees were unaware of. Integrating the events with the occupational health team was also important for facilitating follow-up with any individuals whose biometric measurements conferred increased risk.

Results and Effects

The three main outcome measures used in this study were the differences between the interven-tion and control groups in (1) the number of health risks identified by the HRA, (2) the quantity of workplace absenteeism, and (3) the level of work performance in the preceding 4 wk, the latter two being assessed by the WHO Health and Work Performance Questionnaire. Because the control group was not completely comparable with the intervention group at baseline, a weighting adjust-ment was made to correct for these difference using propensity scores (3). The results discussed here are based on those weighted data.

Linear regression analysis was used to analyze the weighted data to estimate the significance of differences in changes in the outcomes between intervention and control respondents. The second-ary outcomes were an estimate of the likely value of any observed change in health risk status in the form of an ROI calculation for Unilever and an assessment of the effect of the intervention upon the individual health risk factors captured by the HRA. Health care utilization data were not avail-able for the study population, so calculations of financial benefit were limited to attributing value to improvements in absenteeism and presenteeism based on salary costs.

Baseline Data

Gender, but not other variables, differed sig-nificantly between the two groups; however, the effects of gender were controlled in the regres-sion analysis. The baseline data are presented in table 37.1.

There were no significant differences in terms of gender, baseline work performance, or absen-teeism among those individuals who completed the baseline survey but not the survey at the end of the study. However, those individuals who were lost to follow-up tended to be younger and

Table 37.1 Baseline Data

Population	% Male	Mean age	Mean health risk factors	Mean number of absence days in previous month	Mean work performance rating (0-10 scale) in previous month
Intervention group (n = 266)	46	34.3	2.9	0.4	7.6
Control group (n = 1,242)	54	34.5	2.7	0.6	7.5

have fewer health risk factors than those who completed the following assessment, in both the intervention and control samples.

Program Usage

Individual utilization of the various elements of the health promotion program was not tracked. But, group usage data for the online portal (vielife Online) showed regular engagement across the intervention group. Over the 12 mo of the study, logins to the portal showed cyclical peaks, with increased use after the e-mail communications sent every 2 wk.

Outcome Measures

Key outcomes were measured across several domains including health risk factors, work performance, absence, other indicators of productivity, and ROI. Each of these outcomes is discussed below in more detail.

Health Risk Factors

The average number of health risk factors assessed in the HRA decreased significantly in the intervention group between baseline and the 12 mo follow-up. The study showed that in the intervention group there was a mean decrease of −0.48 health risk factor over the course of the study. No significant change in the number of health risk factors was observed in the control group. Regression analysis showed that there was a greater reduction of nearly half a health risk factor (0.45) in the intervention group as compared with the control group.

Work Performance

The average score on the work performance scale increased significantly in the intervention group. This mean score increased by 0.61 point (from a baseline mean of 7.6). As with health risk factors, no significant change was observed in work performance in the control group. The regression analysis found close to a 1-point improvement (0.79) on the 0-to-10 scale of work performance for the intervention group compared with the control group.

Absence

The regression analysis on the absence data found an improvement of more than one-third of a monthly absenteeism day (0.36) between the intervention group and the control group. However, although a significant effect, this was due more to an increase in absenteeism in the control group rather than to a decrease in the intervention group. Assuming a linear improvement, this equates to 2.16 fewer days of absence across 12 mo.

Return on Investment

The monetary value of the observed 0.36 d less of absenteeism and the 0.79-point (10.4%) productivity improvement in the previous month can be crudely quantified by calculating the annual salary cost of this extra productive time. For these calculations it is assumed that the improvements have occurred in a linear fashion over the 12 mo of the study and that absenteeism and presenteeism remain unchanged within the nonparticipant group (both for those who did not engage and those who engaged at the beginning but not the end).

The average pretax employee salary of the intervention group was £35,000 (approximately $70,000 U.S.). This is equivalent to a daily employment cost of £145.83 for a 48 wk work year and an hourly cost of £18.23 for an 8 h day.

The cost of the full yearlong program to Unilever was £70 ($140 U.S.) for each of the 618 eligible employees.

Productivity

Productivity indicators included both absenteeism and presenteeism as well overall ROI. Each of these indicators is discussed below.

Absenteeism

With this base cost and the observed annual improvements in absenteeism of 2.16 d less absence a year for the participant group, there is an ROI of 1.94:1 in salary costs alone.

Presenteeism

Calculating the monetary effect of improvement in work performance is more difficult. If the 0.79-point improvement in work performance score is considered linear, this represents an additional 7.9% of working time over a 4 wk time frame. However, it is unrealistic to presume that this time was previously spent idle; it is more probable that it was spent at less than optimal performance.

If we presume that before the beginning of this program this time was spent working at 50%

capacity, then a monetary value based on salary costs can be calculated for improvement in work performance.

At a 50% improvement level, an additional 6.32 h of fully productive working time has been gained over 4 wk (160 h × 0.079 × 0.5). Within the study group this has a value of £115.21 ($230.42 U.S.) for the 4 wk. Because this is assumed to be a linear improvement, it is equivalent to a return of £691.26 per engaged employee over the working year. This translates into an ROI of 4.25:1 in salary costs for increase in productivity.

Overall Return on Investment

Combining the return of both the absenteeism and the work performance calculations yields an ROI of 6.19:1.

Discussion

There are of course some limitations to the study. Using self-reported information, rather than relying on medical examinations to assess the presence of disease or health risk factors or administrative records to document absence or work performance, could lead to bias. However, previous longitudinal research has shown that self-reported data correlates with medical claims data, payroll records, and work performance records.

Another limitation is the possibility that there is an upward bias in the estimate of positive change among the individuals who were studied. It is possible that the baseline intervention group respondents who didn't participate in the interventions were less likely to complete the follow-up survey. Site usage data would also support this suggestion: Engagement with the online component of the intervention was less by those who didn't complete the follow-up survey. Average log-ins for the whole eligible population was 28% lower than for those who completed both surveys. But, the improvement in work performance in the intervention group was so large that it remains statistically significant even if there is assumed to be no effect on the survey nonresponders in the intervention group.

The Next Steps

What the research has found is that a well-implemented multicomponent health program can improve health status and work performance. For Unilever, this provided a strong business case that

complemented the core vitality value of the business. These factors, combined with an element of good timing, have enabled Unilever's health and well-being strategy to go global.

With strong support from the board and senior managers, the Senior Leaders' Health Initiative has been deployed in five Asian countries, seven African countries, and seven Latin American territories, as well as various countries in Europe and states and provinces within North America. But, as with the pilot project, the aim is not just to reach out to the senior management team.

The fact that there are many ways to view the benefits of a health intervention program—as a way of improving productivity, the right thing to do, a way to increase engagement, and so on—allowed different managers to implement the program in different ways.

Within the Indian group, the team has already managed to cascade the program to 14,000 employees over the course of a year (November 2006-2007). This has touched people at all levels of the business from office workers to manufacturing staff to shop floor employees. Specific interventions suitable for the audience have been implemented, including distributing CDs containing success stories and advice from the doctor alongside biometric measurements for BMI, cholesterol, glucose, and blood pressure.

Going Global

The key entry point to launching a global wellness strategy has been through the human resources team, and in October 2007 a vitality charter was presented to the human resources leadership team. This outlined mandatory health and well-being programs that should be available to all staff within the organization. This charter is now central to Unilever's business strategy and all sites have been tasked with providing well-being solutions that address three key areas: exercise, nutrition, and mental resilience.

Choosing how to deliver these initiatives has been left to each individual business unit, which must devise the strategy most suitable for their population, with regional occupational health teams working with the human resources department to create this strategy. Options available include an online solution, such as vielife Online, a version of the senior leadership health initiative; using internal health services to deliver activities; or using external organizations to provide the skill sets not present in-house. The key factor is that each unit within the business must have its own strategy so that health and well-being programs can be cascaded through the organization over the next 2 to 3 y.

Aligning health and well-being programs with Unilever's vitality mission has made this more than just a health initiative. Health and well-being at work are central to Unilever's business focus, and this pilot project played a central role in delivering the business metrics that drove this strategy.

Conclusion

This applied research project involved an intervention designed to be scalable and sustainable across the entire population of Unilever PLC, a multinational company. Results indicated improvement in the health domains as well as across various indicators of productivity. Financial impact of the project indicated a strongly positive ROI. Based on this initial pilot, increasing the reach of the program appears to be a sound strategy from both a health and financial perspective.

Chapter Review Questions

1. Based upon the Unilever and vielife experience, describe how companies can work effectively with health promotion vendors to create integration experiences for employees.

2. Briefly describe the intervention components of this applied research study that differ between the two study groups and outline other characteristics that you would consider important variables in terms of study outcomes but that are not being changed or manipulated as part of the study.

3. Describe the overall communications and marketing campaigns designed to draw people into the HRA program and discuss how these campaigns differ from communications specific to intervention options.

4. Describe the steps and process that moved this program from a pilot project to a global strategy for health and productivity for Unilever.

◄38►

Introducing Environmental Interventions at the Dow Chemical Company to Reduce Overweight and Obesity Among Workers

Ron Z. Goetzel, PhD; Jennie D. Bowen, MPH; Ronald J. Ozminkowski, PhD; Cheryl A. Kassed, PhD, MSPH; Enid Chung Roemer, PhD; Maryam J. Tabrizi, MS, CHES; Meghan E. Short, BA; Shaohung Wang, PhD; Xiaofei Pei, PhD; Heather M. Bowen, MS, RD, LD; David M. Dejoy, PhD; Mark G. Wilson, HSD; Kristin M. Baker, MPH; Karen J. Tully, BS; John M. White, PhD; Gary M. Billotti, MS; and Catherine M. Baase, MD

This chapter presents a case study of the Dow Chemical Company (Dow) and its involvement in a multiyear, federally funded research study to examine the health and economic benefits of introducing environmental interventions into the workplace in order to address overweight and obesity among workers. Today, business leaders are becoming increasingly aware of the human and economic toll that poor health imposes on workers and their companies' competitiveness (16). There is growing interest in changing the physical and social spaces of the workplace and introducing work policies that support employees' efforts to lead healthy lifestyles. This chapter describes Dow's efforts at implementing two levels of environmental interventions directed at reducing overweight and obesity among its workers: (1) a moderate-level intervention that introduced an array of inexpensive environmental changes focused primarily on the physical environment and (2) a more intensive intervention that established a higher level of organizational commitment, especially among managers. We describe how the research team and Dow established a baseline of experi-

ence before the start of the study and conducted formative research to collect quantitative and qualitative data about Dow's physical and social environment. We conclude with a discussion of the interventions begun as part of this 4 y effort and the learning gained from that experience.

Introduction

Business leaders are growing increasingly aware of the human and economic toll that poor health imposes on their workers and their company's ability to compete (16). Many employers have invested in health promotion and disease prevention programs aimed at reducing the prevalence of obesity in the workplace through encouragement of physical activity, healthy diet, and improved management of health risk factors (14). However, in many cases, individually directed weight management health improvement programs are not enough. Consequently, many employers are seeking innovative and evidence-based interventions that go beyond individual approaches to address the growing obesity epidemic and its adverse effects on worker productivity (13).

Funding for this study was provided by the National Heart, Lung, and Blood Institute (grant # r01 hl79546). However, its contents are the sole responsibility of the authors and do not necessarily represent the official views of the NHLBI.

Preliminary evidence suggests that altering the workplace environment can promote increased physical activity (1,3,4,8,17) and change dietary habits (2,8,9,11,12,18,20). For example, signs that prompt stair use have been shown to significantly increase such use in a train station (3,4), shopping mall (4), and library (17). Furthermore, an intervention to reduce the price of healthy foods in vending machines increased sales of those foods by 78% (10), and interventions to reduce the price of healthy foods in cafeterias produced similar results (2,9,12). Interventions in which food labels were included in cafeterias produced a 5% decrease in caloric intake (20) and a 5% reduction in fat consumption (18). Nonetheless, there is still sparse research on the effects of environmental and policy changes at the workplace and whether they can produce a substantial effect on such outcomes as improving health, reducing utilization of health care services, and improving productivity.

NHLBI Research Focused on Obesity Prevention at the Worksite

Responding to this gap in knowledge, the NHLBI funded seven research centers to study the effect of innovative workplace interventions that emphasize environmental approaches or a combination of environmental and individual approaches to prevent or manage obesity in adult workers. One of these centers, housed originally at Cornell University and now at Emory University, is evaluating the effects of environmental interventions initiated at Dow. The research team includes staff members from Thomson Healthcare, the University of Georgia, Dow, and the National Business Group on Health and also includes an external consulting economist. The 4 y study tests two levels of environmental interventions: (1) a *moderate-level* treatment that introduced an array of inexpensive environmental changes focused primarily on the physical environment and (2) an *intense-level* treatment that reflected a higher level of organizational commitment, especially among managers, to achieving an effect on workers' health status.

A Profile of Dow

Dow is a diversified chemical, science, and technology company headquartered in Midland, Michigan. It has 171 manufacturing sites in 35 countries and employs more than 65,000 workers worldwide, of whom 26,000 are in the United States. A profile of Dow employees shows that their average age is 43 y and about 75% are male. There is very low turnover at Dow (less than 1% per year). The racial composition of the workforce is 82% Caucasian, 8% African American, 6% Hispanic, 3% Asian, and about 1% other. In terms of job categories, 54% are laborers or clerical or technical workers, 44% are professional or managerial workers, and 2% are in sales.

Dow is an acknowledged leader in the health and productivity management (HPM) field. Under the guidance of its medical director, Dr. Cathy Baase, the company has provided state-of-the-art individually based health promotion programs to its employees for many years. However, even though Dow has consistently committed a relatively large amount of staff and resources to health improvement and obesity prevention programs, about three-quarters of its employees remain overweight or obese.

Establishing a Business Case for Health Improvement at Dow

In order to conduct this research, Dow's health services staff made the case to senior leaders that allocating resources toward employee health was a meaningful investment. In 2004, Dow began an ambitious project to determine whether the introduction of additional programs, including environmental changes to the organization's physical and social structure, would exert a positive influence on employees' health risks while saving money for the company. Dow's Environment, Health, and Safety (EHS) staff laid the groundwork for the company's health improvement programs through a series of focused cost burden, benchmarking, and ROI studies. For example, in 1999, with help from Thomson Healthcare researchers, EHS staff estimated that Dow United States could potentially save $30 million U.S. annually if it were to adopt best-practice integrated HPM programs that other companies were implementing. Savings would be realized in reduced health-related expenditures and lower costs associated with absenteeism, workers' compensation, disability, and other human resource spending (10).

EHS staff also showed senior management that long-term investment in employees' health could produce a significant ROI for the company. In a 10 y ROI projection study, staff demonstrated that an aggressive and effective health promotion program that produced a significant reduction in employees' health risks (i.e., an annual 1%

reduction across 10 risk factors) could save about $3.00 U.S. for every dollar spent on the program (10).

By establishing a strong business case for investment in health promotion, Dow's EHS staff was well positioned to gain senior management support for the Dow Global Health Strategy, a major corporate initiative that contained elements addressing the reduction of health risk factors among all employees and the reduction in the incidence and prevalence of chronic diseases. As a result, when the NHLBI study opportunity was presented, EHS staff and Dow's management were open to and excited by the idea of experimenting with innovative programs that might improve employees' health and produce cost savings. Dow supported the researchers in their grant application, and, through the competitive NIH grant review process, funding was secured.

Study Design

The aims of the NHLBI-funded research were to (a) design and demonstrate the feasibility of implementing moderate and intensive environmental interventions directed at preventing overweight and obesity at major Dow worksites; (b) test the multifaceted hypothesis that, relative to individual interventions, environmental interventions reduce the prevalence of obesity and overweight and an array of other weight-related risk factors, reduce health care utilization and expenditures, and improve employee productivity; and (c) conduct an analysis of the value of the intervention to the employer and the employee relative to its cost.

The research team and Dow staff chose 12 sites in Texas, Louisiana, New Jersey, and West Virginia to participate in the study: 8 manufacturing facilities, 2 sites focused on research and development and administrative functions, and 2 sites housing manufacturing, research and development, and administrative staff. Most of the sites were very large (57-5,000+ acres, or 0.2-20+ km²) and housed multiple business units. Since the interventions were directed at organizational and environmental changes, all of the employees at the study sites were designated as participants in the study.

The quasi-experimental study design placed each of the 12 study sites into intervention or control conditions. The intervention conditions aimed at increasing employees' physical activity, improving their diet, and managing their weight at two levels of intensity, while the control condition did not introduce any new environmental interventions to the worksite.

Of the 12 sites, 4 provided *moderate* environmental interventions in addition to Dow's standard individually focused health promotion programs. These activities focused on changing the employees' environment rather than focused primarily on their individual behaviors. Interventions included providing healthy eating choices in the vending machines and cafeterias and at all company-sponsored meetings, establishing marked walking paths at the sites, disseminating targeted messages that encouraged healthy eating and physical activity, and developing an employee recognition program that focused on healthy lifestyles.

Of the 12 participating sites, 5 were assigned to the *intensive* environmental intervention group. The intensive interventions included all of the interventions found at moderate sites and added programs designed to highlight and increase a healthy organizational culture and leadership commitment to employee health. Importantly, the intensive interventions reflected a significant level of organizational commitment to a culture of wellness and included embedding health targets within each site's business goals (5).

For example, the intense-level interventions included establishing site-level health goals as part of the site's management plan, training site leaders on health promotion topics, reporting site progress to senior corporate leadership, establishing and training leaders at the work group level (named *Healthy Culture Focal Points),* and recognizing and rewarding leaders and individual workers for their health promotion activities. These interventions were designed to garner strong leadership support, integrate the interventions into the company's established business practices, build a support structure, hold individual managers accountable for health improvements, and reward employees for progress toward their goals. In short, the intensive intervention sites sought to promote the integration of health promotion and business goals.

Finally, 3 sites assigned to the *control* condition did not alter the way they normally delivered Dow's core health promotion programs. These programs were a coordinated set of individually oriented interventions designed to influence health behaviors through a combination of awareness raising, education, and individual health coaching. Even though the control sites did not receive any new interventions, they agreed to more extensive health data collection from employees at their sites to mirror the data collection efforts at the intervention sites.

Of the roughly 26,000 Dow employees throughout the U.S., 10,618 were employed at the 12 study sites. Of these, 8,198 were located at moderate or intense intervention sites and 2,420 were at control sites.

Availability of Historical Archival Data From Dow

Fortunately, bountiful archival data were available at the start of the study, which proved useful for establishing a baseline. The first year of the study was spent gathering baseline data and conducting formative research to finalize the interventions and ensure that they were appropriate to the settings and acceptable to Dow employees and managers. Formative research was conducted using quantitative and qualitative data collection methods (19). Quantitative data analysis involved the aggregation and analysis of available employee health risk, biometric, medical care utilization and cost, and absenteeism utilization and cost data.

Dow collects health risk assessment (HRA) data on most employees as part of its routine screenings, so the following data elements were available for analysis at baseline: height, weight, and BMI; total and HDL cholesterol; blood pressure; blood glucose; eating habits; physical activity levels; smoking status; alcohol consumption; stress; and general well-being. Historical administrative health care claims data and absenteeism records for hourly employees were also available.

Data from Dow's 2004 HRA revealed that many employees at the 12 study sites had significant health challenges. At the intervention sites, 85% of the employees were classified as overweight or obese (BMI > 24 kg/m^2) compared with 81% at the control sites. About 50% of screened employees at the 12 study sites had total cholesterol levels of 200 mg/dl or greater. Three-fifths said they exercised less than three times a week, one-quarter had high blood glucose levels, one-quarter had high blood pressure, and 20% smoked (19).

Analysis of administrative health care claims and absenteeism data found that medical and pharmacy costs averaged approximately $2,500 U.S. per employee in 2003-2004 (excluding outliers, patients whose annual expenditures exceeded $50,000 U.S.). Absenteeism-related costs for non-exempt employees ranged from $945 to $1,744 U.S. per person per year (19). Overall, baseline employee health risks, medical and pharmacy costs, and absenteeism were sufficiently elevated to attract the attention of senior leadership. They understood the value of establishing a baseline snapshot of the employee population against which future results could be compared in order to determine whether programs of varying intensity were effective. This recognition created support for the Dow Global Health Strategy.

Assessing the Physical and Social Environment at Dow

Since increasing organizational and management support for health promotion was one of the primary aims of the study, we needed a set of instruments and tools to measure these factors. A review of the literature uncovered several instruments designed to measure management commitment to worker safety but few of them focused on health promotion. We eventually found an instrument developed by the Partnership for Prevention, called the *Leading by Example (LBE) questionnaire,* and, with permission, adapted it as our foundation for assessing leadership support and commitment to health promotion (7).

The LBE was administered to three leadership groups at each participating site: (1) the site manager and his or her leadership team, (2) a cross-discipline team that was made up of representatives from all levels of the organization and that served as an advisory and policy-making panel to the leadership team, and (3) health services staff members, including occupational physicians, nurses, and health educators who manage health service operations at each site's medical clinic.

At baseline, mean LBE scores varied widely, ranging from 2.62 to 3.30 (on a 1-5 scale where higher scores indicate greater organizational support for health improvement initiatives). Site scores were inconsistent across categories and organizational group (site leaders, cross-discipline teams, and health services). Health services staff tended to perceive higher levels of support for health improvement than did site leaders or cross-discipline teams (7).

To objectively assess Dow's physical and social environments and the extent to which they supported health improvement, we also developed another instrument named the *Environmental Assessment Tool (EAT),* an adaptation of the Checklist of Health Promotion Environments at Worksites (CHEW) instrument (15). The EAT consisted of two sections: one completed by site staff and the other completed by independent observers who toured the site and recorded their observations (6).

The EAT had several components. The *physical activity* component assessed on-site physical activity areas, stairways and elevators, hallways, parking lots, bicycle accessibility and use, showers and changing facilities, and signage and bulletin boards. The *food choices and weight management* component examined the site's cafeterias (if present), vending machines, food served at company meetings and events, and signage and bulletin boards. Finally, the *organizational characteristics and support* component included questions about access to safe walkways and open space; distance to restaurants, grocery stores, and the closest town; presence of kitchenettes or refrigerators; work rules allowing employees access to on-site or off-site facilities; community resources that could support physical activity such as health clubs and parks; written policies; and ongoing health promotion programs related to physical activity, diet and nutrition, and weight management (6).

EAT scores ranged from 0 to 100 depending on the presence of environmental supports encouraging healthy eating and physical activity, with higher scores denoting greater environmental support. These scores also varied across sites. At baseline, we found that research and development and administrative sites tended to score higher on the EAT than did those sites that were primarily manufacturing. We also found that support for physical activity was higher than support for healthy eating and weight management (6).

Gathering Qualitative Data From Dow Employees

To help structure the interventions and capture focused insights on elements of successful interventions, researchers held *focus group meetings* with health services staff, multidisciplinary employee groups, and site leaders. These meetings proved fruitful. Focus group participants identified eight physical activity and seven nutrition and weight management strategies deemed promising at their worksites, some of which were eventually adopted and others not.

Suggestions for increasing environmental support for physical activity included (in order of frequency) the following: (1) introducing competitions, (2) conducting physical activity education programs, (3) creating safe walking areas, (4) designating company time to exercise, (5) building a fitness center on the site or providing off-site fitness center reimbursement, (6) having health

promotion personnel conduct stretching sessions in control rooms, (7) installing cardiorespiratory fitness equipment, and (8) encouraging more on-site bicycle use to get from one building to the next (19).

Suggestions for environmental supports for nutrition and weight management included the following: (1) educating employees about cooking healthy meals (including demonstrations in control rooms), (2) labeling the nutrition content of items in vending machines and cafeterias, (3) increasing healthy eating choices in vending machines and cafeterias, (4) requiring company-sponsored events to serve only healthy foods, (5) providing a mobile food cart that offers healthy foods at moderate prices, (6) having healthy prepared meals available for employees to purchase and take home after their shifts, and (7) offering promotional pricing for healthy options in vending machines and cafeterias (19).

Discussions were also held with Dow's senior leaders at corporate and regional offices. These discussions were intended to educate senior managers about the study, solicit their feedback about the approaches being contemplated, and ask for their support and championing of the initiative.

Conversations with senior managers highlighted elements of Dow's culture that were critical to the success of this initiative. Dow places a strong emphasis on improving products and processes using Six Sigma tools.* Furthermore, leaders are constantly searching for new techniques to improve productivity and profitability. Dow's culture emphasizes goal setting and measuring progress toward achieving goals. Employees and managers are rewarded for achieving specific goals, which are developed by small, local business teams, resulting in a relatively flat organization structure that relies on peer leaders. During the discussions, Dow senior managers emphasized the importance of building the health improvement program into these core principles (19).

Individual workers indicated that active leadership participation in health promotion initiatives was key. When asked what led to the success of previous health improvement initiatives, the majority of respondents indicated that leadership support and involvement were the most important factor, followed by use of incentives, ease of access to programs, and promotional activities. Employees and leaders reported that the most

*Six Sigma is a business improvement methodology based on the DMAIC model for process improvement. DMAIC is an acronym that stands for *d*efine opportunity, *m*easure performance, *a*nalyze opportunity, *i*mprove performance, and *c*ontrol performance. See, for example, www.motorola.com/content.jsp?globalObjectId=3088.

common challenges to such programs were time constraints, current workload (especially due to the amount of daily task, overtime work, and shift work), and low perceptions of the relevance of health to business objectives. Suggested strategies for overcoming these challenges included incorporating healthy activities into work duties (e.g., walking rounds) and daily routines (e.g., offering healthy foods in the cafeteria and vending machines; 19).

Conclusion

Our research at Dow is currently underway. We are processing year one results from the interventions and expect to publish these findings shortly. Preliminary data appear promising. We are also engaged in a final round of data collection to determine whether the effects shown after 1 y are maintained over a longer duration. Many data elements are being examined, including several process measures (e.g., measures of treatment dose and fidelity) and health and financial outcomes. At the conclusion of the study we hope to be able to answer the following question: Does the introduction of environmental changes to the worksite produce positive health and financial outcomes that are above those achieved through individually oriented health promotion programs?

A key success of the project has been the introduction of several new evidence-based environmental interventions to reduce overweight and obesity at the workplace. These include providing increased access to healthy food choices. For example, vending machine suppliers and cafeteria operators are required to offer healthy food choices, nutritional labeling of food choices is apparent, health education materials related to healthy eating are distributed, sites have become more saturated with nutrition messages supporting healthy eating, and healthy foods are now always offered at company-sponsored meetings and events.

In addition to these required infrastructure and policy changes, site leaders are given the option of developing promotional pricing agreements for healthy food with their local cafeteria and vending machine partners, establishing healthy food cupboards in work group areas, setting up healthy food and nutrition carts in heavy traffic areas, and providing scales in workplace areas.

Dow now also provides increased access to physical activity for its workers. For example, EHS identified and labeled walking paths and routes at each of the treatment sites. Dow also introduced a new Why Weight program that combines education, weight tracking, goal setting, and pedometer distribution. Optionally, site leaders are encouraged to build or improve upon existing fitness facilities and programs, to provide cardiorespiratory fitness equipment in work areas, and to offer community fitness center subsidies.

At intensive sites, the study prompted leaders to establish site-level goals for participating in health improvement programs and achieving site-wide behavior change targets as part of the site's performance management plan (for which site leaders are held accountable and rewarded). Also introduced were training programs for site leaders on various health improvement strategies and means of encouraging employee participation in programs. Furthermore, site-level achievements were reported to senior corporate leadership during management reviews, which led to recognizing and rewarding site leaders, work groups, and Healthy Culture Focal Points that achieved their goals.

Our experience at Dow reinforced realities experienced by many worksite health promotion practitioners and researchers. Like many organizations, Dow faces global competition and must adapt its business operations to address emerging challenges. In light of this, Dow has adopted a mind-set that providing health improvement programs to its workers is an investment in the company's future rather than a growing expense that needs to be lowered. At the site level, gaining support and participation from local leaders and employees for activities not directly related to their day-to-day job responsibilities can be difficult under the best of circumstances. Although challenging, gaining support from local leadership and middle management is key to the success of any initiative, health-related or otherwise. It proved to be true that achieving leadership engagement at the local level was as important as gaining support at the corporate level.

Having worked closely with Dow's staff in the design and implementation of this multiyear study, we learned a great deal about the fine line that separates academic and business interests in the conduct of applied research. Researchers aim to design methodologically rigorous studies that clearly define treatment and control conditions, to attain treatment fidelity, to collect voluminous data, and to maintain a healthy distance between themselves and their subjects (Dow employees in this case). Business leaders, on the other hand, are not interested in research for research's sake. They require practical solutions to the business problems they face. Fortunately, many of the business leaders and employees at Dow are also scientists, researchers, and engineers who are comfortable with data and metrics and conducting scientific research aimed at answering important but complex questions.

As our study progresses, we expect to learn much more about the factors that facilitate or hinder the introduction of environmental interventions at the workplace. We also expect to learn how these interventions may influence employee health and the financial health of the organization.

Resources

Pratt, C.A., Lemon, S.C., Fernandez, I.D., et al. Design characteristics of worksite environmental interventions for weight control and obesity prevention. *Obesity.* 2007;15(9):2171-80.

Selko, A. Are health care costs making you sick? Manufacturers are discovering that a healthy workforce is a cost-effective workforce. *Industry-Week* [serial online]. January 1, 2008. Available at: www.industryweek.com/ReadArticle.aspx?ArticleID=15505.

Chapter Review Questions

1. What are some of the challenges involved in conducting applied research in a corporate setting?

2. How did Dow's EHS staff pave the way for the company's participation in this study and ameliorate some of the potential challenges?

3. In what ways was it helpful that the research team spent the first year of the study conducting formative research and collecting baseline data?

References

Chapter 1

1. Aristotle. *Nicomachean ethics book II.* In: Barnes, J., ed. *The complete works of Aristotle.* Princeton, NJ: Princeton University Press; 1984.

2. Buck Consultants. Working well: A global survey of health promotion and workplace wellness strategies. October 2007. Available at: www.bucksurveys.com.

3. Chapman, L. Expert opinions on "best practices" in worksite health promotion (WHP). *The Art of Health Promotion.* 2004;July/August:1-6.

4. Collins, J. *Good to great.* New York: HarperCollins Publishers; 2001.

5. Eby, F., and Arrowood, C.F. *The history and philosophy of education, ancient and medieval.* Englewood Cliffs, NJ: Prentice Hall; 1940.

6. Goetzel, R.Z., Guindon, A., Humphries, L., et al. Health and productivity management: Consortium benchmarking study best practice report. Houston: American Productivity and Quality Center International Benchmarking Clearinghouse; 1998. www.apqc.org.

7. Goetzel, R.Z., Shechter, D., Ozminkowski, R.J., Marmot, P.F., Tabrizi, M.J., and Roemer, E.C. Promising practices in employer health and productivity management efforts: Findings from a benchmarking study. *Journal of Occupational and Environmental Medicine.* 2007;49:111-30.

8. Gochfeld, M. Chronological history of occupational medicine. *Journal of Occupational and Environmental Medicine.* 2005;47(2):96-114.

9. HealthPartners Health Behavior Group. Unpublished internal analysis; 2006.

10. Herrick, D.M. Why employer-based health insurance is unraveling. November 1, 2005. Available at: http://cdhc.ncpa.org/commentaries/why-employer-based-health-insurance-is-unraveling.

11. Hook, G.E. Ramazzini: father of environmental health? *Environmental Health Perspectives.* 1995;103 (11): 982-3.

12. Institute of Medicine (IOM). *Integrating employee health: A model program for NASA.* Washington, DC: The National Academies Press; 2005.

13. Isidore, C. Doctors orders: GM, UAW, cut deal. October 17, 2005. Available at: http://money.cnn.com/2005/10/17/news/fortune500/gm_wagoner.

14. Kindig, D.A. Understanding population health terminology. *The Milbank Quarterly.* 2007;85(1):139-61.

15. Martinson, B.C., Crain, A.L., Pronk, N.P., O'Connor, P.J., and Maciosek, M.V. Changes in physical activity and short-term changes in health care charges: A prospective study of older adults. *Preventive Medicine.* 2003;37(4):319-26.

16. Musich, S., McDonald, T., Hirschland, D., and Edington, D.W. Examination of risk status transitions among active employees in a comprehensive worksite health promotion program. *Journal of Occupational and Environmental Medicine.* 2003;45(4):393-9.

17. O'Donnell, M., Bishop, C., and Kaplan, K. Benchmarking best practices in workplace health promotion. *The Art of Health Promotion.* 1997;1(1):12.

18. Podewils, L.J., and Guallar, E. Mens sana in corpore sano. *Annals of Internal Medicine.* 2006;144(2):135-7.

19. Pronk, N.P. Aligning program support with interventions for optimum impact. *ACSM's Health & Fitness Journal.* 2007;11(3):40-2.

20. Russell, P. *Waking up in time.* Novato, CA: Origin Press; 1998.

21. Schult, T.M.K., McGovern, P.M., Dowd, B., and Pronk, N.P. The future of health promotion/disease prevention programs: The incentives and barriers faced by stakeholders. *Journal of Occupational and Environmental Medicine.* 2006; 48:541-48.

22. Serxner, S., Baker, K., and Gold, D.B. Guidelines for analysis of economic return from health management programs. *The Art of Health Promotion.* 2006;20(6):1.

23. Serxner, S., Noeldner, S.P., and Gold, D. Best practices for an integrated population health management (PHM) program. *The Art of Health Promotion.* 2006;20(5):1.

24. Sigerist, H.E. *Medicine and human welfare.* New Haven, CT: Yale University Press; 1941:93.

25. Sigerist, H.E. *The university at the crossroads.* New York: Henry Schuman; 1946:127-8.

Chapter 2

1. Aldana, S.G. Financial impact of health promotion programs: A comprehensive review of the literature. *American Journal of Health Promotion.* 2001;15(5):296-320.

2. Aldana, S.G. Financial impact of worksite health promotion and methodological quality of the evidence. *American Journal of Health Promotion.* 1998;2:1-8.

3. Anderson, D.R., Whitmer, R.W., Goetzel, R.Z., et al. The relationship between modifiable health risks and group-level health care expenditures. *American Journal of Health Promotion.* 2000;15(1):45-52.

4. Ardell, D. B. *High Level Wellness: An Alternative to Doctors, Drugs and Disease.* Emmaus, PA: Rodale (1976).

5. Ardell, D. Seeking wellness—Wellness pioneer Don Ardell, PhD, speaks out on the state of wellness in the United States today. *Absolute Advantage.* 2004;4:12-8.

6. Bertera, R.L. The effects of workplace health promotion on absenteeism and employment costs in a large industrial population. *American Journal of Health Promotion.* 1900;80(9):1101-5.

7. Bly, J.L., Jones, R.C., and Richardson, J.E. Impact of worksite health promotion on health care costs and utilization: Evaluation of Johnson & Johnson Live for Life program. *Journal of the American Medical Association.* 1986;256(23):3235-40.

8. Borger, C., Smith, S., Truffer, C., et al. Health spending projections through 2015: Changes on the horizon. *Health Affairs.* 2006 Mar-Apr;25(2):w61-73.

9. *Brink, S. D. Health Risks and Behavior: The Impact on Medical Costs. Milliman & Robertson, Inc. and Control Data, 1987.*

10. Business Roundtable member's quarterly survey. March 2004. Available at: www.businessroundtable.org (accessed September 21, 2008) .

11. California Health Care Foundation. Average annual growth rate and per employee cost. Snapshot: Health Care Costs 101. Reporting on data from the Centers for Medicine and Medicaid Sources (CMS). Office of the Actuary. Available at: www.chcf.org/topics/healthinsurance/index.cfm?itemID=133630.

12. Catlin, A., Cowan, C., Heffler, S., and Washington, B. National health spending in 2005: The slowdown continues. *Health Affairs.* 2007;26(1):142-53.

13. Chapman, L. *Proof positive: An analysis of the cost-effectiveness of wellness.* 2nd ed. Seattle: Corporate Health Designs; 1995.

14. Data Watch. The benefits of leadership. *Business and Health.* 1999;17(2):52.

15. Davidson, K. Selling sin: The marketing of socially unacceptable products. Westport, CT. Greenwood Publishing Group; 2003:24.

16. Dunn, H.L. *High level wellness.* Arlington, VA: Beatty Press; 1961.

17. Goetzel, R.Z. The financial impact of health promotion and disease prevention programs—Why is it so hard to prove value? *American Journal of Health Promotion.* 2001;15(5):277-80.

18. Goetzel, R.Z., Anderson, D.R., Whitmer, R.W., Ozminkowski, R.J., Dunn, R.L., and Wasserman, J. The relationship between modifiable health risks and health care expenditures: An analysis of the multi-employer HERO health risk and cost database. *Journal of Occupational and Environmental Medicine.* 1998;40(10):843-54.

19. Harvey, M.R., Whitmer, R.W., Hilyer, J.C., and Brown, K.C. The impact of a comprehensive medical benefits cost management program for the City of Birmingham: Results at five years. *American Journal of Health Promotion.* 1993:7(4):296-303.

20. Institute for Health and Productivity Management . *IHPM's background.* Available at: http://www.ihpm.org/info/background.php (accessed September 21, 2008

21. Kessler, R.C., Barber, C., Beck, A., et al. The World Health Organization health and work performance questionnaire. *Journal of Occupational and Environmental Medicine.* 2003;45(2):156-74.

22. Leutzinger, J., Goetzel, R., Richling, D., and Wade, S. Projecting the impact of health promotion on medical costs. *Business and Health.* 1993;11(4):38-44.

23. Lynch, W., and Riedel, J.E., ed. *Measuring employee productivity: A guide to self-assessment tools.* Scottsdale, AZ: Institute of Health and Productivity Management; 2001.

24. McGinnis, J.M., and Foege, W.H. Actual causes of death in the United States. *Journal of the American Medical Association.* 1993;270(18):2207-12.

25. Mokdad, A.H., Marks, J.S., Stroud, D.F., and Gerberding, J.L. Actual causes of death in the United States—2000. *Journal of the American Medical Association.* 2004;291(10):1238-45.

26. Moore, G. The carrot or the stick? *Business and Health* 2003; 21(11):3.

27. O'Donnell, M.P. Health impact of work-place health promotion programs and methodological quality of the research literature. *American Journal of Health Promotion.* 1997;1:1-7.

28. Office of Management and Budget. Budget of the United States Government. Fiscal year 2006. 2006. Available at: www.whitehouse. gov/omb/budget/fy2006/pdf/06msr.pdf.

29. Pelletier, K.R. A review and analysis of the clinical and cost-effectiveness studies of comprehensive health promotion and disease management programs at the worksite: 1998-2000 update. *American Journal of Health Promotion.* 2001;16(2):107-16.

30. Prochaska, J.O., and Velicer, W.F. The transtheoretical model of health behavior change. *American Journal of Health Promotion.* 1997;12(1):38-48.

31. Pronk, N.P., Goodman, M.J., and O'Conner, P.J. Relationship between modifiable health risks and short-term health care charges. *Journal of the American Medical Association.* 1999;282(23):2235-9.

32. Seek Wellness. Available at: http://www.seekwellness.com/wellness/ardell_bio.htm (accessed September 21, 2008

33. The state of health care in America: 1998. *Business Health Annual Issue.* 1998:25.

34. Travis, J. *Simply well: Choices for a healthy life.* 10th ed. , Berkeley, CA Ten Speed Press; 2001:18, page 15.

35. Travis, J., and Ryan, R.S. *Wellness—small changes you can use to make a big difference.* , Berkeley, CA Ten Speed Press; 1991:4-5.

36. Wang, S., Beck, A., Berglund, P., et al. Chronic medical conditions and work performance in the health and work performance questionnaire calibration surveys. *Journal of Occupational and Environmental Medicine.* 2003;45(12):1303-11.

37. Wellness Councils of America (WELCOA). Our founder. Available at: http://www.welcoa.org/presskit/founder.php (accessed September 21, 2008)

38. Wikipeda—The Free Encyclopedia. Galen. Available at: www. en.wikipedia.org/wiki/Galen (accessed September 21, 2008).

39. Yen, L.T., Edington, D.W., and Witting, P. Association between health risk appraisal scores and employee medical claims costs in a manufacturing company. *American Journal of Health Promotion.* 1991;6(1):46-54.

40. Travis, J.W. The illness-wellness continuum: *The wellness workbook for health professionals.* 1977; Mill Valley, CA: Wellness Resource Center

41. Milliman and Roberson, Inc. *Health Risk and Behaviors: The Impact on Medical Cost.* Control Data Corporation, 1987.

42. *Healthwise Handbook, First Edition.* Healthwise, Inc. Boise, Idaho, 1976.

Chapter 3

1. Aldana, S.G. Financial impact of health promotion programs: A comprehensive review of the literature. *American Journal of Health Promotion.* 2001;15(5):296-320.

2. Beal, A.C., Doty, M.M., Hernandez, S.E., Shea, K.K., and Davis, K. Closing the divide: How medical homes promote equity in health care. Commonwealth Fund. 2007. Available at: www.commonwealthfund. org/publications/publications_show.htm?doc_id=506814.

3. Bertera, R.L. Planning and implementing health promotion in the workplace: A case study of the DuPont company experience. *Health Education Quarterly.* 1990;17(3):307-27.

4. Bertera, R.L. The effects of workplace health promotion on absenteeism and employment costs in a large industrial population. *American Journal of Public Health.* 1990;80(9):1101-5.

5. Bloom, D.E., and Canning, D. The health and wealth of nations. *Science.* 2000;287:1207-9.

6. Blumenthal, D. Employer-sponsored insurance—riding the health care tiger. *The New England Journal of Medicine.* 2006;355:195-202.

7. Brandt-Rauf, P., Burton, W.N., and McCunney, R.J. Health, productivity, and occupational medicine. *Journal of Occupational and Environmental Medicine.* 2001;43(1):1.

8. Butcher, L. The workplace doctor is in. *HealthLeaders Media Magazine* [serial online]. 2007;March. Available at: www.healthleadersmedia.com/magazine/ view_magazine_feature.cfm?content_id=87829&categoryid=153.

9. Centers for Disease Control and Prevention (CDC). Achievements in public health, United States 1900-1999: Improvements in workplace safety. *Morbidity and Mortality Weekly Report.* 1999;48(22):461-69.

10. Chapman, L. Meta-evaluation of worksite health promotion economic return studies: 2005 update. *The Art of Health Promotion.* 2005;July/August:1-10.

11. Chapman, L.S., and Pelletier, K.R. Population health management as a strategy for creation of optimal healing environments in worksite and corporate settings. *Journal of Alternative and Complementary Medicine.* 2004;19(S1):S127-40.

12. Coulter, C.H. The employer's case for health management. *Benefits Quarterly.* 2006;22(1):23-33.

13. Downey, A.M., and Sharp, D.J. Why do managers allocate resources to workplace health promotion programmes in countries with national health coverage? *Health Promotion International.* 2007;22(2):102-11.

14. Draper, E. *The company doctor: Risk, responsibility, and corporate professionalism.* New York: Russell Sage Foundation; 2003:396.

15. Edington, D.W. Emerging research: A view from one research center. *American Journal of Health Promotion.* 2001;15(5):341-9.

16. Fabius, R. The migration strategy: Building a benchmark medical presence at the workplace. *Health and Productivity Management.* 2007;6(1):4-7.

17. Forouzesh, M.R., and Ratzker, L.E. Health promotion and wellness programs: An insight into the Fortune 500. *Journal of Health Education.* 1985;January:18-22.

18. Frazee, S.G., Fabius, R., Ryan, P., Broome, R., and Manfred, J. A prescription for appropriate antibiotic usage: Physicians and pharmacists collaborate within a workplace health center. *Journal of Health and Productivity.* 2007;March:10-7.

19. Frazee, S.G., Kirkpatrick, P., Fabius, R., and Chimera, J. Leveraging the trusted clinician: Documenting disease management program enrollment. *Disease Management.* 2007;10:16-29.

20. Gochfeld, M. Chronological history of occupational medicine. *Journal of Occupational and Environmental Medicine.* 2005;47(2):96-114.

21. Goetzel, R.Z., Guindon, A.M., Turshen, I.J., and Ozminkowski, R.J. Health and productivity management: Establishing key performance measures, benchmarks and best practices. *Journal of Occupational and Environmental Medicine.* 2001;43(1):10-7.

22. Goetzel, R.Z., Ozminkowski, R.J., Bruno, J.A., Rutter, K.A., Isaac, F., and Wang, S. The long-term impact of Johnson & Johnson's health and wellness program on employee health risks. *Journal of Occupational and Environmental Medicine.* 2002;44(5):417-24.

23. Golaszewski, T., Barr, D., and Cochran, S. An organization-based intervention to improve support for employee heart health. *American Journal of Health Promotion.* 1998;13(1):26-35.

24. Hunnicutt, D. Discover the power of wellness. *Business and Health.* 2001;9(3):41-5.

25. Institute of Medicine (IOM.) *Integrating employee health: A model program for NASA.* Washington, DC: National Academy Press; June 2005. Available at: www.iom.edu/Object.File/ Master/27/358/nasa--FINAL.pdf.

26. Interstate Commerce Commission (ICC). *Fifth annual report of the Interstate Commerce Commission.* Washington, DC: U.S. Government Printing Office; 1902.

27. Kessler, R.C. The effects of medical conditions on work loss and work cutback. *Journal of Occupational and Environmental Medicine.* 2001;43:218-25.

28. Kingery, P., Ellsworth, C., Corbett, B. et al. High-cost analysis: A closer look at the case for work-site health promotion. *Journal of Occupational and Environmental Medicine.* 1994;36(9):1341-7.

29. Library of Congress, Bills, Resolutions. Healthy Workforce Act of 2007. July 9, 2007. Available at: www.healthpromotionadvocates.org/ legislative_priorities.htm

30. Loeppke, R., Taitel, M., Richling, D., Parry, T., Kessler, R.C., Hymel, P., and Konicki. D. Health and productivity as a business strategy. *Journal of Occupational and Environmental Medicine.* 2007;49:712-21.

31. Mercer. U.S. employers' health benefit cost continues to rise at twice inflation rate, Mercer survey finds. 2007. Available at: www.mercer.com/referencecontent.jhtml?idContent=1287790.

32. Richardson, E., and Fabius, R. Back to the future and beyond: Primary care at the worksite. Presentation at: IHPM Fall Conference; October 17, 2007; Scottsdale, AZ.

33. Schoenleber, A.W. Industrial health programs: Trends which indicate that industry is beginning to acknowledge its responsibility for the medical care of employees. *Industrial Medicine.* 1933;2:242-9.

34. Selleck, H.B., and Whittaker, A.H. *Occupational health in America.* Detroit: Wayne State University Press; 1962:537.

35. Serxner, S.G., Gold, D., Anderson, D., and Williams, D. The impact of worksite health promotion program on short-term disability usage. *Journal of Occupational and Environmental Medicine.* 2001;43(1):25-9.

36. Sherman, B., and Fabius, R. On the road to health and productivity management: Improving employee health through strategic integration. Presentation at: DMAA-NAM Joint Conference; September 17, 2007; Las Vegas, NV.

37. Starfield, B., Shi, L., and Macinko, J. Contribution of primary care to health systems and health. *The Milbank Quarterly.* 2005;83(3):457-502.

38. Starr, P. *The social transformation of American medicine.* New York: Basic Books; 1982:514.

39. Stempien, D.E., Milles, S.S., and O'Neill, F.N. The hidden savings of an on-site corporate medical center. *Journal of Occupational and Environmental Medicine.* 1996;38(10):1047-8.

40. Towers Perrin. Towers Perrin health cost survey projects that average annual per-employee cost for 2008 will exceed $9,300. 2007. Available at: www.towersperrin.com/tp/showdctmdoc.jsp?url=HR_Services/United_States/Press_Releases/2007/20070924/2007_09_24.htm&language_code=global&selected=home

41. U.S. Census Bureau. Population of Alleghany County, PA in 1906-1907 was between 775,058 (1900 Census) and 1,018,463 (1910 Census). Population data from United States Census, Pennsylvania population of counties by decennial census: 1900-1990. 2007. Available at: www.census.gov/population/cencounts/pa190090.txt.

42. U.S. Department of Health and Human Services. *Healthy people 2010: Understanding and improving health.* 2nd ed. Washington, DC: U.S. Government Printing Office; 2000:76.

43. U.S. Department of Labor, Mine Safety and Health Administration. Coal fatalities for 1900 through 2006. 2007. Available at: www.msha.gov/stats/centurystats/coalstats.asp.

44. Watson Wyatt. 12th annual National Business Group on health/Watson Wyatt survey report no. 2007-US-0031. Washington, DC: Watson Wyatt Worldwide; 2007.

45. Wright, D., Adams, L., Beard, M.J., et al. Comparing excess costs across multiple corporate populations. *Journal of Occupational and Environmental Medicine.* 2004;46(9):937-45.

46. Zenz, C., Dickerson, B., Horvath, E.P. *Occupational medicine.* St. Louis: Mosby; 1994:1316.

47. Smith A. *Wealth of Nations,* Raleigh, NC, Hayes Barton Press, 1956.

48. Hewitt Associates: *The road ahead: Emerging health trends, 2007.* Lincolnshire, IL: Hewitt; 2007.

Chapter 4

1. An, A.B. Performing logistic regression on survey data with the new SURVEYLOGISTIC procedure. Cary, NC: SAS Institute; October 15, 2007. Available at: www.lexjansen.com/pharmasug/2002/proceed/sas05.pdf.

2. Claxton, G., Gabel, J., Gil, I., et al. Health benefits in 2006: Premium increases moderate, enrollment in consumer-directed health plans remains modest. *Health Affairs.* 2006;25(6):w476-85.

3. Dun & Bradstreet. Million dollar databases. October 15, 2007. Available at: www.dnbmdd.com.

4. Eakin, J.M. Leaving it up to the workers: Sociological perspective on the management of health and safety in small workplaces. *International Journal of Health Services.* 1992;22(4):689-704.

5. Fielding, J.E., and Piserchia, P.V. Frequency of worksite health promotion activities. *American Journal of Public Health.* 1989;79(1):16-20.

6. Grosch, J.W., Alterman, T., Petersen, M.R., and Murphy, L.R. Worksite health promotion programs in the US: Factors associated with availability and participation. *American Journal of Health Promotion.* 1998;13:36-45.

7. Kleinbbaum, D.G., and Klein, M. *Logistic regression: A self-learning text.* 2nd ed. New York: Springer-Verlag; 2002.

8. Linnan, L., Bowling, M., Childress J, Lindsay G, Blakey C, Pronk S, Wieker S, Royall P. Results of the 2004 national worksite health promotion survey. *American Journal of Public Health 2008;98:1503-1509*

9. National Institute for Occupational Health and Safety (NIOSH). All NIOSH topics. Atlanta, GA: Centers for Disease Control and Prevention; October 31, 2007. Available at: www.cdc.gov/niosh.

10. Partnership for Prevention. Healthy workforce 2010: An essential health promotion sourcebook for employers, large and small. 2001. Available at: www.prevent.org/content/view/29/40.

11. Rao, J.N., and Scott, A.J. A simple method for the analysis of clustered binary data. *Biometrics.* 1992;48:577-85.

12. SAS Institute. *SAS 9.1.3 help and documentation.* Cary, NC: SAS Institute; 2002-04.

13. U.S. Department of Health and Human Services. *1992 national survey of worksite health promotion activities. Summary report.* Washington, DC: Department of Health and Human Services, Public Health Service; 1993.

14. U.S. Department of Health and Human Services. *1999 national worksite health promotion activities: Summary report.* Washington, DC: Department of Health and Human Services, Public Health Service; 2000:27.

15. U.S. Department of Health and Human Services. *Healthy people 2010. Understanding and improving health* and *Objectives for improving health.* 2 vols. Washington, DC: U.S. Government Printing Office; 2000:76.

16. Wilson, M.G., DeJoy, D.M., Jorgensen, C.M., and Crump, C.J. Health promotion programs in small worksites: Results of a national survey. *American Journal of Health Promotion.* 1999;13(6):358-65.

Chapter 5

1. Association for Worksite Health Promotion, Mercer WM, Inc., and U.S. Department of Health and Human Services. *1999 worksite health promotion survey.* Northbrook, IL: Association for Worksite Health Promotion; 1999.

2. Barbeau, E., Roelofs, C., Youngstrom, R., Sorensen, G., Stoddard, A., and LaMontagne, A.D. Assessment of occupational safety and health programs in small businesses. *American Journal of Industrial Medicine.* 2004;45:371-9.

3. Benedict, I., Truman, C., Smith-Akin, C.K., et al. Developing the Guide to Community Preventive Services—Overview and rationale. *American Journal of Preventive Medicine.* 2000;18(1S):18-26.

4. Butterfoss, G.D., Goodman, R.M., and Wandersman, A. Community coalitions for prevention and health promotion. *Health Education Research.* 1993;8(3):315-30.

5. Chapman, L.S. Meta-evaluation of worksite health promotion economic return studies: 2005 update. *American Journal of Health Promotion.* 2005;19(6):1-11.

6. Fielding, J.E., and Piserchia, P.V. Frequency of worksite health promotion activities. *American Journal of Public Health.* 1989;79:16-20.

7. Fronstin, P., Helman, R., and Greenwald, M. Small employers and health benefits: Findings from the 2002 small employer health benefits survey. *EBRI Issue Brief.* 2003;253:1-21.

8. Goetzel, R.Z. Essential building blocks for successful worksite health promotion programs. *Managing Employee Health Benefits.* 1997;6:1.

9. Goetzel, R.Z. *Examining the value of integrating occupational health and safety and health promotion programs in the workplace.* Rockville, MD: U.S. Department of Health and Human Services, Public Health Service, Centers for Disease Control and Prevention, National Institute for Occupational Safety and Health; 2004.

10. Goetzel, R.Z, Shechter, D., Ozminkowski, R.J., Marmet, P.F., Tabrizi, M.J., and Roemer, E.C. Promising practices in employer health and productivity management efforts: Findings from a benchmarking study. *Journal of Occupational and Environmental Medicine.* 2007;49:111-30.

11. Grosch, J.W., Alterman, T., Peterson, M.R., and Murphy, L. Worksite health promotion programs in the US: Factors associated with availability and participation. *American Journal of Health Promotion.* 2000 13:36-45.

12. Headd, B. The characteristics of small-business employees. *Monthly Labor Review.* 2000, July;13-8.

13. Heaney, C., and Goetzel, R. A review of health-related outcomes of multi-component worksite health promotion programs. *American Journal of Health Promotion.* 1998;11:290-307.

14. Linnan, L., Bowling, M., Childress J, Lindsay G, Blakey C, Pronk S, Wieker S, Royall P. Results of the 2004 national worksite health promotion survey. *American Journal of Public Health* 2008;98:1503-1509

15. McMahan, S., Wells, M., Stokols, D., Phillips, K., and Clitheroe, H.C. Assessing health promotion programming in small businesses. *American Journal of Health Studies.* 2001;17(3):20-8.

16. Minkler, M., and Wallerstein, N. *Community based participatory research for health.* 1st ed. San Francisco: Jossey-Bass; 2002:512.

17. National Small Business Association. *NSBA survey of small and mid-sized businesses.* NSBA, Washington, D.C. 2007.

18. O'Donnell, M., Bishop, C., and Kaplan, K. Benchmarking best practices in workplace health promotion. *The Art of Health Promotion.* 1997;1:12.

19. Ostbye, T., Dement, J.M., and Krause, K.M. Obesity and workers' compensation: Results from the Duke health and safety surveillance system. *Archives of Internal Medicine.* 2007;167:766-73.

20. Pelletier, K.R. A review and analysis of the clinical and cost-effectiveness studies of comprehensive health promotion and disease management programs at the worksite: Update VI 2000-2004. *Journal of Occupational and Environmental Medicine.* 2005;47:1051-8.

21. *Standard Industrial Classification Manual.* U.S. Office of Management and Budget; Executive Office of the President, Washington, D.C. 1987:12.

22. Stokols, D., McMahan, S., and Phillips, K. Workplace health promotion in small businesses. In O'Donnell, M., ed. *Health promotion in the workplace.* Albany, NY: Delmar Publishers; 2001:493-518.

23. U.S. Bureau of Labor Statistics. Employment and wages, annual averages 2004. Available at: www.bls.gov/cew/cewbultn04.htm. (Accessed September 27, 2008).

24. U.S. Department of Health and Human Services. *Healthy people 2010: Understanding and improving health.* 2nd ed. Washington, DC: U.S. Government Printing Office; 2000. Available at: www.health.gov/healthypeople.

25. U.S. Department of Health and Human Services Public Health Service. 1992 national survey of worksite health promotion activities: Summary. *American Journal of Health Promotion.* 1993;7(6):452-64.

26. U.S. Small Business Administration. Size standards. Available at: www.sba.gov/services/contractingopportunities/sizestandardstopics/index.html.

27. U.S. Small Business Administration Office of Advocacy. Rural and urban areas by firm size, 1990-1995. 1998. Available at: www.sba.gov/advo/stats.

28. U.S. Small Business Administration Office of Advocacy. Small business growth by major industry, 1988-1995. 1998. Available at: www.sba.gov/advo/stats.

29. Wellness Councils of America. *Seven benchmarks of success.* September 21, 2007. Available at: www.welcoa.org/wwp/pdf/aa_6.1_novdec06.pdf. (Accessed September 27, 2008).

30. Wells, M., Stokols, D., McMahan, S., and Clitheroe, C. Evaluation of worksite injury and illness prevention program: Do the effects of the REACH OUT Training Program reach the employees? *Journal of Occupational Health Psychology.* 1997;2:25-54.

31. Whitmer, R.W., Pelletier, K.R., Anderson, D.R., Baase, C.M., and Frost, G.J. A wake-up call for corporate America. *Journal of Occupational and Environmental Medicine.* 2003;45:916-25.

32. Wiatrowski, W.J. Small businesses and their employees. *Monthly Labor Review.* 1994, October;29-35.

33. Wilson, M.G., DeJoy, D.M., Jorgensen, C.M., and Crump, C.J. Health promotion programs in small worksites: Results of a national survey. *American Journal of Health Promotion.* 1999;13(6):358-65.

Chapter 6

1. Health Insurance Portability and Accountability Act of 1996.

2. If an employer-sponsored health plan fails to comply with HIPAA, the employer ultimately will be liable for paying civil and criminal penalties. Moreover, employees may sue the employer in its capacity as plan administrator in the event the employer breaches its fiduciary duties under ERISA by using or sharing health information in a manner that violates the privacy rules.

3. Staff health care providers often provide only first aid treatment and education. Usually, they do not perform any of the standard transactions electronically. They do not submit claims or report health care encounters to any HIPAA-covered health plan. Nor do they inquire about claim status or request eligibility information from any HIPAA-covered health plan for purposes related to the health services they provide. Although a staff health care provider might submit a first report of injury to the workers' compensation program, there is no standard in place for this transaction.

4. HIPAA defines a group health plan as an ERISA welfare benefits plan "to the extent that the plan provides 'medical care' (as defined in PPHSA Section 2791(a)(2)) to employees or their dependents. . . ." Medical care is defined as "the diagnosis, cure, mitigation, treatment or prevention of disease, or amounts paid for the purpose of affecting any structure of the body." (1) U.S. Code §213 uses this same definition and has been interpreted to consider fitness centers as organizations that merely support good health and do not treat illnesses.

5. Section 164.506(c)(5) permits covered entities that participate in an OCHA to share information for any health care operation activities of the OCHA.

6. The preamble states that the OCHA provisions "define the arrangements between health plans and health insurance issuers or HMOs as OCHAs, which are permitted to share information for each other's health care operations. Such disclosures also may be made to a broker or agent that is a business associate of the health plan." *Federal Register.* August 14, 2003;68:53217.

7. Section 164.501.

8. ERISA Section 702 and U.S. Tax Code Section 9802. A group health plan, and a health insurance issuer offering group health insurance coverage in connection with a group health plan, may not establish rules for eligibility (including continued eligibility) of any individual to enroll under the terms of the plan based on any factors related to health status in relation to the individual or a dependent of the individual—ERISA Section 702(a)(1). A group health plan or a health insurance issuer offering group health insurance coverage in connection with a group health plan may not require any individual (as a condition of enrollment or continued enrollment under the plan) to pay a premium or contribution that is greater than such premium or contribution for a similarly situated individual enrolled in the plan on the basis of any factor related to health status in relation to the individual or to an individual enrolled under the plan as a dependent of the individual—ERISA Section 702(b)(1).

9. 26 CFR Section 54.9802-1(f)(2).

10. HIPAA expressly states that the nondiscrimination rules do not require employers to provide any additional benefits and do not prevent employers from creating limits or restrictions on the "amount, level, extent or nature of the benefits or coverage for similarly situated individuals enrolled in the plan." ERISA Section 702(a)(2) and (b)(2).

11. The nondiscrimination rules state that a plan amendment that limits benefits is not considered to be directed at any individual participants or beneficiaries if (1) it is applicable to all individuals in one or more groups of similarly situated individuals under the plan and (2) it becomes effective no sooner than the first day of the first plan year after the amendment is adopted. Labor Regulation §2590.702(b)(2)(i)(C); U.S. Code §54.9802-1T(b)(2)(i)(C).

12. Americans with Disabilities Act of 1990, 42 U.S. Code §12112(a), (b).

13. *EEOC Compliance Manual,* Chapter 3, ADA Issues §I.

14. *Templet v Blue Cross/Blue Shield of Louisiana,* LEXIS 15605 (U.S. Dist. 2000).

15. 42 U.S. Code §12201(c)(1).

16. 42 U.S. Code §12201(c)(1); 42 U.S. Code §12201(c)(2), (3); See *Barnes v. The Benham Group, Inc.,* 22 F.Supp.2d 1013 (Minnesota 1998).

17. 42 U.S. Code §(d)(4)(A).

18. U.S. Equal Employment Opportunity Commission. Enforcement guidance: Disability-related inquiries and medical examinations of employees under the Americans with Disabilities Act (ADA). July 27, 2000. Available at: www.eeoc.gov/policy/docs/guidance-inquiries.html. Questionnaires about behavior, such as eating, physical activity, and sleeping habits, are not medical inquiries.

19. id.

20. U.S. Code §213(d).

21. Earles, A.C. *Legal considerations for employer-sponsored health improvement and incentive programs.* Washington, D.C., National Business Group on Health; 2007.

Chapter 7

1. Bridgman, P., and Glyn, D. *The Australian policy handbook.* Crows Nest, New South Wales: Allen & Unwin; 2004.

2. GovTrack.us. S. 1753: Healthy Workforce Act of 2007. 2007. Available at: www.govtrack.us/congress/bill.xpd?bill=s110-1753.

3. Grzywacz, J.G., Casey, P.R., and Jones, F.A. The effects of workplace flexibility on health behaviors: A cross-sectional and longitudinal analysis. *Journal of Occupational and Environmental Medicine.* 2007;49(12):1302-9.

4. Lee, T.H., and Kinga, Z. Do high-deductible health plans threaten quality of care? *New England Journal of Medicine.* 2005;(12) 353:1202-4.

5. Mahoney, J.J., and Hom, D. *BeneFIT design. Seven steps for creating value-based benefit decisions.* Philadelphia: GlaxoSmithKline; 2007.

6. Mahoney, J.J., and Hom, D. *Total Value/Total Return™: Seven rules for optimizing employee health benefits for a healthier and more productive workforce.* Philadelphia: GlaxoSmithKline; 2006.

7. Merriam-Webster Online. 2008. Available at: www.m-w.com/dictionary.

8. Partnership for Prevention. Healthy workforce 2010: An Essential Health Promotion Sourcebook for Employers, Large and Small. 2008 Partnership for Prevention, Washington, D.C.. Available at: http://www.prevent.org/images/stories/Files/publications/Healthy_Workforce_2010.pdf .

9. Partnership for Prevention. Leading by Example. Leading practices for employee health management. 2005. Available at: www.prevent.org/content/view/30/57/

10. Partnership for Prevention. Why invest? Recommendations for improving your prevention investment. 2007. Available at: www.prevent.org/images/stories/PDF/whyinvest_web_small.pdf.

11. U.S. Department of Health and Human Services. Office for Civil Rights—HIPAA. Medical privacy—National standards to protect the privacy of personal health information. 1996. Available at: www.hhs.gov/ocr/hipaa.

12. U.S. Department of Justice. Americans with Disabilities Act. 1990. Available at: www.ada.gov.

13. U.S. Department of Labor. Bloodborne pathogens and needlestick prevention. OSHA standards. 2001 Available at: www.osha.gov/SLTC/bloodbornepathogens/standards.html.

14. U.S. Department of Labor. Family and Medical Leave Act. 1993. Available at: www.dol.gov/esa/whd/fmla.

15. U.S. Department of Labor. Occupational Safety and Health Administration. 2008. Available at: www.osha.gov.

16. U.S. Department of Transportation. Office of Drug and Alcohol Policy and Compliance. 2008. Available at: www.dot.gov/ost/dapc/index.html.

17. Wikipedia. Policy: Intended effects. 2008. Available at: http://en.wikipedia.org/wiki/Policy#Intended_Effects.

18. Wikipedia. Policy: Policy cycle. 2008. Available at: http://en.wikipedia.org/wiki/Policy#Policy_cycle.

19. World Research Group. Rewarding healthy behaviors for health plans. Calculating ROI for preventive care through health risk assessments, disease management and wellness. World Research Group Conference; January 23, 2007; Grosvenor Resort, Lake Buena Vista, FL.

Chapter 8

1. Aldana, S.J., and Pronk, N.P. Health promotion programs, modifiable health risks, and employee absenteeism. *Journal of Occupational and Environmental Medicine.* 2001;43:36-46.

2. Anderson, D.R., and Staufacker, M.J. The impact of worksite-based health risk appraisal on health-related outcomes: A review of the literature. *American Journal of Health Promotion.* 1996;10:499-508.

3. Bartlett, C.J., and Coles, E.C. Psychological health and well-being: Why and how should public health specialists measure it? Part 2: Stress, subjective well-being and overall conclusions. *Journal of Publice Health Medicine.* 1998;20:288-94.

4. Bondi, M.A., Harris, J.R., Atkins, D., French, M.E., and Umland, B. Employer coverage of clinical preventive services in the United States. *American Journal of Health Promotion.* 2006;20:214-22.

5. Braithwaite, R.S., and Rosen, A.B. Linking cost sharing to value: An unrivaled yet unrealized public health opportunity. *Annals of Internal Medicine.* 2007;146:602-5.

6. Burton, W.N., Chen, C.-Y., Conti, D.J., Schultz, A.B., and Edington, D.W. The association between health risk change and presenteeism change. *Journal of Occupational and Environmental Medicine.* 2006;48:252-63.

7. Burton, W.N., Chen, C.-Y., Conti, D.J., Schultz, A.B., Pransky, G., and Edington, D.W. The association of health risks with on-the-job productivity. *Journal of Occupational and Environmental Medicine.* 2005;47:769-77.

8. Centers for Disease Control and Prevention. Task Force on Community Preventive Services. *The guide to community preventive services: What works to promote health?* New York: Oxford University Press; 2005.

9. Christensen, K.B., Lund, T., Labriola, M., Bultmann, U., and Villadsen, E. The impact of health behavior on long term sickness absence: Results from DWECS/DREAM. *Industrial Health.* 2007;45:348-51.

10. Edington, D.W. Emerging research: A view from one research center. *American Journal of Health Promotion.* 2001;15:341-9.

11. Evans, S., Huxley, P., Gately, C., et al. Mental health, burnout and job satisfaction among mental health social workers in England and Wales. *British Journal of Psychiatry.* 2006;188:75-80.

12. Fronstin, P. Health promotion and disease prevention: A look at demand management programs. *EBRI Issue Brief.* 1996;177:1-14.

13. Goetzel, R.Z., Guindon, A.M., Turshern, I.J., and Ozminkowski, R.J. Health and productivity management: Establishing key performance measures, benchmarks, and best practices. *Journal of Occupational and Environmental Medicine.* 2001;43:10-7.

14. Goetzel, R.Z., Hawkins, K., Ozminkowski, R.J., and Wang, S. The health and productivity cost burden of the "top 10" physical and mental health conditions affecting six large U.S. employers in 1999. *Journal of Occupational and Environmental Medicine.* 1999;45:5-14.

15. Hennikus, D.J., Jeffery, R.W., Lando, H.A., et al. The SUCCESS project: The effect of program format and incentives on participation and cessation in worksite smoking cessation programs. *American Journal of Public Health.* 2002;92: 274-9.

16. Hudson, L.R., and Pope, J.E. The role of health-risk appraisals in disease management. *Managed Care Interface.* 2006;19:43-5.

17. Hunt, M.K., Stoddard, A.M., Kaphingst, K.A., and Sorensen, G. Characteristics of participants in a cancer prevention intervention designed for multiethnic workers in small manufacturing worksites. *American Journal of Health Promotion.* 2007;22:33-7.

18. Institute of Medicine (IOM). *Integrating employee health: A model program for NASA.* Washington, DC; National Academies Press; 2005.

19. Kane, R.I., Johnson, P.E., Town, R.J., and Butler, M. A structured review of the effect of economic incentives on consumers' preventive behavior. *American Journal of Preventive Medicine.* 2004;27:327-52.

20. Kanner, A.D., Coyne, J.C., Schaefer, C., and Lazarus, R.S. Comparison of two modes of stress measurement: Daily hassles and uplifts versus major life events. *Journal of Behavioral Medicine.* 1981;4:1-39.

21. Karasek, R., Brisson, C., Kawakami, N., Houtman, I., Bongers, P., and Amick, B. The Job Content Questionnaire (JCQ): An instrument for internationally comparative assessments of psychosocial job characteristics. *Journal of Occupational Health Psychology.* 1998;3:322-55.

22. Leon, K.A., Hyre, A.D., Ompad, D., DeSalvo, K.V., and Munter, P. Percieved stress among a workforce 6 months following hurricane Katrina. *Social Psychiatry and Psychiatric Epidemiology.* 2007; 42(12):1005-11.

23. Lundborg, P. Does smoking increase sick leave? Evidence using register data on Swedish workers. *Tobacco Control.* 2007;16:114-8.

24. Mills, P.R., Kessler, R.C., Cooper, J., and Sullivan, S. Impact of a health promotion program on employee health risks and work productivity. *American Journal of Health Promotion.* 2007;22:45-53.

25. National Institute of Occupational Safety and Health (NIOSH). Steps to a healthier U.S. workforce. 2004. Available at: www.cdc.gov/niosh/worklife/steps/default.html.

26. Nomura, K., Nakado, M., Sato, M., Ishikawa, H., and Yano, E. The association of the reporting of somatic symptoms with job stress and active coping among Japanese white-collar workers. *Journal of Occupational Health.* 2007; 49(5):370-5.

27. Pronk, N.P. Building partnerships between mature worksite health promotion programs and managed care. In: Cox, C., ed. *ACSM's worksite health promotion manual: A guide to building and sustaining healthy worksites.* Champaign, IL: Human Kinetics; 2003:89-97.

28. Schoenbach, V.J., Wagner, E.H., and Beery, W.L. Health risk appraisal: Review of evidence for effectiveness. *Health Services Research.* 1987;22:553-80.

29. Solberg, L.I., Mosser, G., and McDonald, S. The three faces of performance measurement: Improvement, accountability, and research. *Joint Commission Journal on Quality Improvement* 1997;23:135-47.

30. Sorensen, G. Smoking cessation at the worksite: What works and what is the role of occupational health? In: National Institute for Occupational Safety and Health (NIOSH), ed. *Work, smoking, and health, a NIOSH scientific workshop.* Washington, DC: NIOSH; 2000:99-120. USDHHS (NIOSH) publication no. 2002-148.

31. Sorensen, G., Stoddard, A., Hunt, M.K., et al. The effects of a health promotion-health protection intervention on behavior change: The WellWorks study. *American Journal of Public Health.* 1998;88:685-90.

32. Sorensen, G., Stoddard, A., LaMontagne, A., et al. A comprehensive worksite cancer prevention intervention: Behavior change results from a randomized controlled trial in manufacturing worksites (United States). *Cancer Causes and Control.* 2002;13:188-97.

33. Stein, A.D., Shakour, S.K., and Zuidema, R.A. Financial incentives, participation in employer-sponsored health promotion, and changes in employee health and productivity: HealthPlus Health Quotient program. *Journal of Occupational and Environmental Medicine.* 2000;42:1148-55.

34. Storseth, F. Changes at work and employee reactions: Organizational elements, job insecurity, and short-term stress as predictors for employee health and safety. *Scandinavian Journal of Psychology.* 2006;47:541-50.

35. Turner, C.J. Health risk appraisals: The issues surrounding use in the workplace. *American Association of Occupational Health Nurses Journal.* 1995;43:357-61.

36. U.S. Department of Health and Human Services (USDHHS). *Healthy people 2010.* Washington, DC: U.S. Government Printing Office; 2000. Available at: www.healthypeople.gov./Publications.

37. Yen, L., Edington, M.P., McDonald, T., Hirschland, D., and Edington, D.W. Changes in health risks among the participants in the United Auto Workers—General Motors LifeSteps Promotion Program. *American Journal of Health Promotion.* 2001;16:7-15.

38. Zdrenghea, D., Poanta, L., and Gaita, D.. Cardiovascular risk factors and risk behaviors in railway workers. Professional stress and cardiovascular risk. *Romanian Journal of Internal Medicine.* 2005;43:49-59.

Chapter 9

1. Bhandari, M., Busse, J.W., Jackowski, D., et al. Association between industry funding and statistically significant pro-industry findings in medical and surgical randomized trials. *Canadian Medical Association Journal.* 2004;170(4):477-80.

2. Bravata, D.M., Smith-Spangler, C., Sundaram, V., et al. Using pedometers to increase physical activity and improve health: A systematic review. *Journal of the American Medical Association.* 2007;298(19):2296-304.

3. Briss, P.A., Zaza, S., Pappaioanou, M., et al. Developing an evidence-based guide to community preventive services—methods. *American Journal of Preventive Medicine.* 2000;18 Suppl. 1:35-43.

4. Brockway, L.M., and Furcht, L.T. Financial disclosure policies of scientific publications. *Journal of the American Medical Association.* 2006;296(24):2925-6.

5. Brownson, R.C., Baker, E.A., Leet, T.L., and Gillespie, K.N. *Evidence-based public health.* New York: Oxford University Press; 2003.

6. Cochrane Collaboration. The Cochrane Collaboration. 2007. Available at: www.cochrane.org/index.htm.

7. Cochrane Collaboration. *The Cochrane Library* [serial online]. 2007;4. Available at: www.cochrane.org.

8. Coulter, C.H. The employer's case for health management. *Benefits Quarterly.* 2006;22(1):23-33.

9. Fielding, J.E., and Briss, P.A. Promoting evidence-based public health policy: Can we have better evidence and more action? *Health Affairs.* 2006;25(4):969-78.

10. Friedman, L.S., and Richter, E.D. Relationship between conflicts of interest and research results. *Journal of General Internal Medicine.* 2004;19(1):51-6.

11. Guide to Community Preventive Services. The community guide. 2007. Available at: www.thecommunityguide.org.

12. Harris, R.P., Helfand, M., Woolf, S.H. et al. Current methods of the U.S. Preventive Services Task Force: A review of the process. *American Journal of Preventive Medicine.* 2001;20(3) Suppl. 1:21-35.

13. Howes, F., Doyle, J., Jackson, N., and Waters, E.. Evidence-based public health: The importance of finding 'difficult to locate' public health and health promotion intervention studies for systematic reviews. *Journal of Public Health (Oxford, England).* 2004;26(1):101-4.

14. Kohatsu, N.D., Robinson, J.G., and Torner, J.C. Evidence-based public health: An evolving concept. *American Journal of Preventive Medicine.* 2004;27(5):417-21.

15. McGinnis, J.M., and Foege, W.H. Actual causes of death in the United States. *Journal of the American Medical Association.* 1990;270:2207-12.

16. Rychetnik, L., Hawe, P., Waters, E., Barratt, A., and Frommer, M. A glossary for evidence-based public health. *Journal of Epidemiology and Community Health.* 2004;58(7);538-45.

17. Shojania, K.G., McDonald, K.M., Wachter, R.M., and Owens, D.K. *Closing the quality gap: A critical analysis of quality improvement strategies, vol 1: Series overview and methodology.* Rockville, MD: Agency for Health care Research and Quality; 2004. Technical Review 9a. AHRQ Publication No. 04-0051-1.

18. Task Force on Community Preventive Services. *The guide to community preventive services: What works to promote health?* New York: Oxford University Press; 2005.

19. The Oxford Illustrated American Dictionary. New York, NY, Oxford University Press; 1998:277.

20. U.S. Department of Health and Human Services, Centers for Disease Control and Prevention, National Center for Chronic Disease Prevention and Health Promotion, and Office on Smoking and Health. *The health consequences of smoking: A report of the Surgeon General.* Atlanta, GA, Washington, DC: Author; 2004.

21. Wilcox, R., and Knapp, A. Building communities that create health. *Public Health Reports.* 2000;115(2-3):139-43.

22. Hook, G.E. Ramazzini: father of environmental health? *Environmental Health Perspectives.* 1995;103 (11): 982-3.

Chapter 10

1. Alexander, G. Health risk appraisal. In: Hyner, G.C., Peterson, K., Travis, J., et al. ed. *SPM handbook of health assessment tools.* Pittsburgh, PA. The Society of Prospective Medicine and The Institute for Health and Productivity Management; 1999:5-8.

2. Anderson, D.R., and Staufacker, M.J. The impact of worksite-based health risk appraisal on health-related outcomes: A review of the literature. *American Journal of Health Promotion.* 1996;10(6):499-508.

3. Briss, P.A., Zaza, S., Pappaioanou, M., et al. Developing an evidence-based guide to community preventive services—methods. *American Journal of Preventive Medicine.* 2000;18 Suppl. 1:35-43.

4. Carande-Kulis, V.G., Maciosek, M.V., Briss, P.A., et al. Methods for systematic reviews of economic evaluations for the Guide to Community Preventive Services. *American Journal of Preventive Medicine.* 2000;18 Suppl. 1:75-91.

5. DeFriese, G.H., and Fielding, J.E. Health risk appraisal in the 1990s: Opportunities, challenges, and expectations. *Annual Review of Public Health.* 1990;11:401-18.

6. Gemson, D.H., and Sloan, R.P. Efficacy of computerized health risk appraisal as part of a periodic health examination at the worksite. *American Journal of Health Promotion.* 1995;9(6):462-6.

7. Goetzel, R.Z., Ozminkowski, R.J., Bruno, J.A., Rutter, K.R., Isaac, F., and Wang, S. The long-term impact of Johnson & Johnson's Health & Wellness Program on employee health risks. *Journal of Occupational and Environmental Medicine.* 2002;44(5):417-24.

8. Hanlon, P., Carey, L., Tannahill, C., Kelly, M., Gilmour, H., Tannahill, A., and McEwen, J. Behaviour change following a workplace health check: How much change occurs and who changes? *Health Promotion International.* 1998;13(2): 134-9.

9. Linnan, L., Bowling, M., Childress J, Lindsay G, Blakey C, Pronk S, Wieker S, Royall P. Results of the 2004 national worksite health promotion survey. *American Journal of Public Health 2008;98:1503-1509.*

10. Ozminkowski, R.J. Long-term impact of Johnson & Johnson's Health & Wellness Program on health care utilization and expenditures. *Journal of Occupational and Environmental Medicine.* 2002;44(1):21-9.

11. Shi, L. Health promotion, medical care use, and costs in a sample of worksite employees. *Evaluation Review.* 1993;17(5):475-87.

12. Shi, L. Impact of increasing intensity of health promotion intervention on risk reduction. *Evaluation and the Health Professions.* 1992;15(4):3-25.

13. Task Force on Community Preventive Services. The guide to community preventive services. What works to promote health? New York: Oxford University Press; 2005.

14. Wagner, E.H., Beery, W.L., Schoenbach, V.J., and Graham, R.M. An assessment of health hazard/health risk appraisal. *American Journal of Public Health.* 1982;72(4):347-52.

15. Wetzler, H. The status of health status assessment. In: Hyner, G.C., Peterson, K., Travis, J., et al., ed. *SPM handbook of prospective medicine.* Pittsburgh: The Society of Prospective Medicine and The Institute for Health and Productivity Management; 1999:17-23.

Chapter 11

1. Agency for Healthcare Research and Quality. Program announcement (PA) number: PAR-06-448. 2007. Available at: http://grants.nih.gov/grants/guide/pa-files/PAR-06-448.html

2. Aristotle. *Nicomachean ethics book VI, 1797-1808.* In: Barnes J., ed. *The complete works of Aristotle.* Princeton, NJ: Princeton University Press; 1984. Pp. 1797-1808.

3. Banthin, J.S., and Bernard, D.M. Changes in financial burdens for health care. National estimates for the population younger than 65 years, 1996 to 2003. *Journal of the American Medical Association.* 2006;296:2712-9.

4. Berwick, D.M. Continuous improvement as an ideal in health care. *New England Journal of Medicine.* 1989;320:53-6.

5. Best, A., Stokols, D., Green, L.W., Leischow, S., Holmes, B., and Buchholz, K. An integrative framework for community partnering to translate theory into effective health promotion strategy. *American Journal of Health Promotion.* 2003;18(2):168-76.

6. β-Blocker Heart Attack Study Group. The β-blocker heart attack trial. *Journal of the American Medical Association.* 1981;246:2073-4.

7. Califf, R.M., DeLong, E.R., Ostbye, T., et al. Underuse of aspirin in a referral population with documented coronary artery disease. *American Journal of Cardiology.* 2002;89:653-61.

8. Deming ,W.E. *Out of crisis.* Cambridge, MA: Massachusetts Institute of Technology, Center for Advanced Engineering Study; 1986.

9. Eckes, G. *The Six Sigma revolution.* New York: Wiley; 2001.

10. Franz, M.J., VanWormer, J.J., Crain, A.L., et al. Weight loss outcomes: A systematic review and meta-analysis of weight loss clinical trials with a minimum 1-year follow-up. *Journal of the American Dietetic Association.* 2007;107:1755-67.

11. Galuska, D.A., Will, J.C., Serdula, M.K., and Ford, E.S. Are health professionals advising obese patients to lose weight? *Journal of the American Medical Association.* 1999;282:1576-8.

12. Glasgow, R.E., Vogt, T.M., and Boles, S.M. Evaluating the public health impact of health promotion interventions: The RE-AIM framework. *American Journal of Public Health.* 1999;89:1322-7.

13. Green, L.W. Public health asks of systems science: To advance our evidence-based practice, can you help us get more practice-based evidence? *American Journal of Public Health.* 2006;96(3):406-9.

14. Green, L.W., and Glasgow, R.E. Evaluating the relevance, generalization, and applicability of research: Issues in external validation and translation methodology. *Evaluation & the Health Professions.* 2006;29(1):1-28.

15. Green, L.W., and Ottoson, J.M. From efficacy to effectiveness to community and back: Evidence-based practice vs practice-based evidence. In: National Institutes of Health, ed. *Proceedings from conference: From clinical trials to community: The science of translating diabetes and obesity research.* Bethesda, MD: National Institutes of Health; 2004.

16. Kottke, T.E., and Pronk, N.P. Physical activity: Optimizing practice through research. *American Journal of Preventive Medicine.* 2006;31 Suppl. 4:S8-10.

17. Kottke, T., and Solberg, L.I. Optimizing practice through research: A preventive services case study. *American Journal of Preventive Medicine.* 2007;33(6):505-6.

18. Lewin, K. *Field theory in social science: Selected theoretical papers.* New York: Harper & Row; 1951.

19. Lewin, K. *Resolving social conflicts: Field theory in social science.* Washington, DC: American Psychological Association; 1997.

20. National Committee for Quality Assurance. *The state of health care quality.* Washington, DC: National Committee for Quality Assurance; 2002.

21. National Institutes of Health (NIH). Overview of the NIH road map. 2007. Available at: http://nihroad map.nih.gov/overview.asp.

22. Nonaka, I., and Takeuchi, H. *The knowledge-creating company: How Japanese companies create the dynamics of innovation.* Oxford: Oxford University Press; 1995.

23. Nonaka, I., Toyama, R., and Konno, N. SECI, *Ba* and leadership: A unified model of dynamic knowledge creation. In: Nonaka, I., and Tece, D., ed. *Managing industrial knowledge: Creation, transfer, and utilization.* London: Sage Publications; 2001.

24. Plato. Theaetetus. In: Cooper, J.M., ed. *Plato: Complete works.* Indianapolis: Hacket Publishing Company; 1997. Pages 157-234.

25. Pronk, N.P. Designing and evaluating health promotion programs: Simple rules for a complex issue. *Disease Management and Health Outcomes.* 2003;11(3):149-57.

26. Pronk, N.P., Peek, C.J., and Goldstein, M.G. Addressing multiple behavioral risk factors in primary care. *American Journal of Preventive Medicine.* 2004;27 Suppl. 2:4-17.

27. Reason, P., and Bradbury, H. Introduction: Inquiry and participation in search of a world worthy of human aspiration. In: Reason, P., and Bradbury, H., ed. *Handbook of action research.* London: Sage Publications; 2001:1-14.

28. Scharmer, C.O. Organizing around not-yet-embodied knowledge. In: von Krogh, G., Nonaka, I., and Nishiguchi, T., ed. *Knowledge creation: A new source of value.* New York: Macmillan; 1999.

29. Scharmer, C.O. Self-transcending knowledge: Organizing around emerging realities. In: Nonaka, I., and Tece, D., ed. *Managing industrial knowledge: Creation, transfer, and utilization.* London: Sage Publications; 2001.

30. Scharmer, C.O. *Theory U: Leading from the future as it emerges.* Cambridge, MA: Society of Organizational Learning; 2007.

31. Senge, P.M. *The fifth discipline. The art and practice of the learning organization.* New York: Doubleday; 1990.

32. Senge, P., Kleiner, A., Roberts, C., Ross, R., Roth, G., and Smith, B. *The dance of change: The challenges to sustaining momentum in learning organizations.* New York: Doubleday; 1999.

33. Task Force on Community Preventive Services. *The guide to community preventive services: What works to promote health?* Zaza, S., Briss, P.A., and Harris, K.W., ed. New York: Oxford University Press; 2005.

34. Truman, B.I., Smith-Akin, C.K., Hinman, A.R., Gebbie, M., and Brownson, R. Developing the guide to community preventive services—overview and rationale. *American Journal of Preventive Medicine.* 2000;18 Suppl. 1:18-26.

35. VanWormer, J.J., Boucher, J.L., and Pronk, N.P. Telephone-based counseling improves dietary fat, fruit, and vegetable consumption: A best evidence synthesis. *Journal of the American Dietetic Association.* 2006;106:1434-44.

36. von Hayek, F.A. The use of knowledge in society. *American Economic Review.* 1945;35:519-30.

37. Wilbur, K. *A theory of everything: An integral vision for business, politics, science, and spirituality.* Boston: Shambhala; 2001.

38. Wilbur, K. *Sex, ecology, spirituality: The spirit of evolution.* Boston: Shambhala; 1995.

39. Sorenson, G., Emmons, K., Hunt, M.K., and Johnston, D. Implications of the results of community intervention trials. *Annual Review of Public Health.* 1998;19:379-416.

Chapter 12

1. Bandura, A. Self-efficacy: Toward a unifying theory of behavior change. *Psychological Review.* 1977;84:191-215.

2. Camp, R.C. *Benchmarking: The search for industry best practices that lead to superior performance.* New York: Quality Resources; 1989:299.

3. Clymer, J.M. *A call to action: Leading by example.* Washington, D.C. Partnership for Prevention; 2005:1-26.

4. Cox, C. *ACSM's worksite health promotion manual: A guide to building and sustaining healthy worksites.* Champaign, IL: Human Kinetics; 2003:250.

5. Goetzel, R.Z. *The role of business in improving the health of workers and the community.* Report prepared under contract for the Institute of Medicine (IOM) of the National Academy of Sciences (NAS). September 2001.

6. Goetzel, R., Guindon, A., Humphries, L., Newton, P., Turshen, J., and Webb, R. *Health and productivity management consortium benchmarking study: Best practice report.* Houston, TX: APQC; 1998:101.

7. Goetzel, R.Z., Shechter, D., Ozminkowski, R.J., Marmet, P.F., Tabrizi, M.J., and Roemer, E.C. Promising practices in employer health and productivity management efforts: Findings from a benchmarking study. *Journal of Occupational and Environmental Medicine.* 2007;49:111-30.

8. Hunnicutt, D., and Leffelman, B. WELCOA's 7 benchmarks of success. *Absolute Advantage.* 2006;6:1-29.

9. Linnan, L., Bowling, M., Childress J, Lindsay G, Blakey C, Pronk S, Wieker S, Royall P. Results of the 2004 national worksite health promotion survey. *American Journal of Public Health 2008;98:1503-1509*

10. Mercer Health & Benefits. *National survey of employer-sponsored health plans 2005.* New York, NY Mercer Health & Benefits; 2006.

11. O' Donnell, M.P., Bishop, C.A., and Kaplan, K.L. Benchmarking best practices in workplace health promotion. *The Art of Health Promotion.* 1997;1:1-8.

12. Pelletier, K.R. A review and analysis of the clinical and cost-effectiveness studies of comprehensive health promotion and disease management programs at the worksite: Update VI, 2000-2004. *Journal of Occupational and Environmental Medicine.* 2005;47:1051-8.

13. Prochaska, J.O., Redding, C.A., and Evers, K.E. The transtheoretical model and stages of change. In: Glanz, K., Frances, M.L., and Rimer, B.K., ed. *Health behavior and health education: Theory, research, and practice.* 2nd ed. San Francisco: Jossey-Bass; 1997:60-84.

14. Spendolini, M.J. *The benchmarking book.* New York: American Management Association; 1992:3-37.

Chapter 13

1. Alder, P.S., Borys, B. Two types of bureaucracy: Enabling and coercive. *Administrative Science Quarterly.* 1996;41(1):61-89.

2. Amick, B.C. 3rd, Habeck, R.V., Hunt, A., Fossel, A.H., Chapin, A., Keller, R.B., and Katz, J.N. Measuring the impact of organizational behaviors on work disability prevention and management. *Journal of Occupational Rehabilitation.* 2000;10(1):21-38.

3. Amick, B.C. 3rd, and Lavis, J.N. Labor markets and health: A framework and set of applications. In: Tarlov, A.R., and St. Peter, R.F., ed. *The society and population health reader. Volume II: A state and community perspective.* New York: The New Press; 2000:178-210.

4. Bambra, C., Egan, M., Thomas, S., Petticrew, M., and Whitehead, M. The psychosocial and health effects of workplace reorganisation. 2. A systematic review of task restructuring interventions. *Journal of Epidemiology and Community Health.* 2007;61(12):1028-37.

5. Barrientos-Gutiérrez ,T., Gimeno, D., Harrist, R., Mangione, T.W., and Amick, B.C. 3rd. Drinking social norms and drinking behaviors: A multilevel analysis on 137 workgroups in 16 worksites. *Occupational and Environmental Medicine.* 2007;64(9):602-8.

6. Belkic, K.L., Landsbergis, P.A., Schnall, P.L., and Baker, D. Is job strain a major source of cardiovascular disease risk? *Scandinavian Journal of Work, Environment, and Health.* 2004;30(2):85-128.

7. Benach, J., and Muntaner, C. Precarious employment and health: Developing a research agenda. *Journal of Epidemiology and Community Health.* 2007;61(4):276-7.

8. Beniger, J.R. *The control revolution: Technological and economic origins of the information society.* Cambridge, MA: Harvard Business Press; 1986.

9. Berggren, C. *Alternatives to lean production: Work organization in the Swedish auto industry.* Ithaca, NY: ILR Press; 1992.

10. Bongers, P.M., Ijmker, S., van den Heuvel, S., and Blatter, B.M. Epidemiology of work related neck and upper limb problems: Psychosocial and personal risk factors (part I) and effective interventions from a bio behavioural perspective (part II). *Journal of Occupational Rehabilitation.* 2006;16(3):279-302.

11. Brown, G.D., and O'Rourke, D. Lean manufacturing comes to China: A case study of its impact on workplace health and safety. *International Journal of Occupational and Environmental Health.* 2007;13(3):249-57.

12. Brunner, E.J., Chandola, T., and Marmot, M.G. Prospective effect of job strain on general and central obesity in the Whitehall II Study. *American Journal of Epidemiology.* 2007;165(7):828-37.

13. Bryman, A. Structure in organizations: A reconsideration. *Journal of Occupational Psychology.* 1976;49(1):1-9.

14. Budros, A. The mean and lean firm and downsizing: Causes of involuntary and voluntary downsizing strategies. *Sociological Forum.* 2002;17(2):307-42.

15. Campbell, S.L., Fowles, E.R., and Weber, B.J. Organizational structure and job satisfaction in public health nursing. *Public Health Nursing.* 2004;21(6):564-71.

16. Cappelli, P., and Sherer, P.D. The missing role of context in OB: The need for a meso-level approach. *Research in Organizational Behavior.* 1991;13:55-110.

17. Cascio, W.F. Downsizing: What do we know? What have we learned? *Academy of Management Executive.* 1993;7(1):95-104.

18. Clarke, S. The relationship between safety climate and safety performance: A meta-analytic review. *Journal of Occupational Health Psychology.* 2006;11(4):315-27.

19. Cullen, K.L., Williams, R.M., Shannon, H.S., Westmorland, M., and Amick, B.C. 3rd. Workplace organizational policies and practices in Ontario educational facilities. *Journal of Occupational Rehabilitation.* 2005;15(3):417-33.

20. Daft, R.L. *Management.* 7th ed. Fort Worth, TX: Thomson South-Western; 2005.

21. de Jonge, J., Bosma, H., Peter, R., and Siegrist, J. Job strain, effort-reward imbalance and employee well-being: A large-scale cross-sectional study. *Social Science and Medicine.* 2000;50(9):1317-27.

22. de Jonge, J., Mulder, M.J., and Nijhuis, F.J. The incorporation of different demand concepts in the job demand-control model: Effects on health care professionals. *Social Science and Medicine.* 1999;48(9):1149-60.

23. de Lange, A.H., Taris, T.W., Kompier, M.A., Houtman, I.L., and Bongers, P.M. "The very best of the millennium": Longitudinal research and the demand-control-(support) model. *Journal of Occupational Health Psychology.* 2003;8(4):282-305.

24. Duijts, S.F., Kant, I., Swaen, G.M., van den Brandt, P.A., and Zeegers, M.P. A meta-analysis of observational studies identifies predictors of sickness absence. *Journal of Clinical Epidemiology.* 2007;60(11):1105-15.

25. Egan, M., Bambra, C., Thomas, S., Petticrew, M., Whitehead, M., and Thomson, H. The psychosocial and health effects of workplace reorganisation. 1. A systematic review of organisational-level interventions that aim to increase employee control. *Journal of Epidemiology and Community Health.* 2007;61(11):945-54.

26. Elovainio, M., Kivimaki, M., Puttonen, S., Lindholm, H., Pohjonen, T., and Sinervo, T. Organisational injustice and impaired cardiovascular regulation among female employees. *Occupational and Environmental Medicine.* 2006;63(2):141-4.

27. Elovainio, M., Kivimaki, M., and Vahtera, J. Organizational justice: Evidence of a new psychosocial predictor of health. *American Journal of Public Health.* 2002;92(1):105-8.

28. Elovainio, M., Leino-Arjas, P., Vahtera, J., and Kivimaki, M. Justice at work and cardiovascular mortality: A prospective cohort study. *Journal of Psychosomatic Research.* 2006;61(2):271-4.

29. Fahlen, G., Knutsson, A., Peter, R., Akerstedt, T., Nordin, M., Alfredsson, L., and Westerholm, P. Effort-reward imbalance, sleep disturbances and fatigue. *International Archives of Occupational and Environmental Health.* 2006;79(5):371-8.

30. Ferrie, J.E., Head, J., Shipley, M.J., Vahtera, J., Marmot, M.G., and Kivimaki, M. Injustice at work and incidence of psychiatric morbidity: The Whitehall II study. *Occupational and Environmental Medicine.* 2006;63(7):443-50.

31. Ferrie, J.E., Shipley, M.J., Marmot, M.G., Stansfeld, S., and Davey Smith, G. The health effects of major organisational change and job insecurity. *Social Science and Medicine.* 1998;46(2):243-54.

32. Finlay, W., Marin, J.K., Roman, P.M., and Blum, T.C. Organizational structure and job satisfaction: Do bureaucratic organizations produce more satisfied employees? *Administration and Society.* 1995;27(3):427-50.

33. Flin, R., Burns, C., Mearns, K., Yule, S., and Robeertson, E.M. Measuring safety climate in health care. *Quality and Safety in Health Care.* 2006;15:109-15.

34. Frese, M., and Zapf, D. Methodological issues in the study of work stress: Objective vs. subjective measurement of work stress and the question of longitudinal studies. In: Cooper, C.L., and Payne, R., ed. *Causes, coping and consequences of stress at work.* Chichester, England: Wiley; 1988. Pp. 375-411.

35. Gimeno, D., Amick, B.C. 3rd, Habeck, R.V., Ossmann, J., and Katz, J.N. The role of job strain on return to work after carpal tunnel surgery. *Occupational and Environmental Medicine.* 2005;62(11):778-85.

36. Gimeno, D., Benavides, F.G., Amick, B.C. 3rd, Benach, J., and Martinez, J.M. Psychosocial factors and work related sickness absence among permanent and non-permanent employees. *Journal of Epidemiology and Community Health.* 2004;58(10):870-6.

37. Gimeno, D., Benavides, F.G., Mira, M., Martinez, J.M., and Benach, J. External validation of psychological job demands in a bus driver sample. *Journal of Occupational Health.* 2004;46(1):43-8.

38. Hackman, J.R., and Oldham, G.R. *Work redesign.* Reading, MA: Addison-Wesley; 1980.

39. Head, J., Kivimaki, M., Siegrist, J., Ferrie, J.E., Vahtera, J., Shipley, M.J., and Marmot, M.G. Effort-reward imbalance and relational injustice at work predict sickness absence: The Whitehall II study. *Journal of Psychosomatic Research.* 2007;63(4):433-40.

40. Herzberg, F. *Work and the nature of man.* New York: World Publishing; 1966.

41. Hunt, H.A., and Habeck, R.V. *The Michigan Disability Prevention Study research highlights: Upjohn Institute Staff Working Paper 93-18.* Kalamazoo, MI : W.E. Upjohn Institute for Employment Research; 1993. Available at: www.upjohninst.org/publications/wp/93-18.pdf.

42. Ivancevich, J.M., and Donnelly, J.H. Jr. Relation of organizational structure to job satisfaction, anxiety-stress, and performance. *Administrative Science Quarterly.* 1975;20(2):272-80.

43. Jansson, M., and Linton, S.J. Psychosocial work stressors in the development and maintenance of insomnia: A prospective study. *Journal of Occupational Health Psychology.* 2006;11(3):241-8.

44. Johnson, J.V., and Hall, E.M. Job strain, work place social support, and cardiovascular disease: A cross-sectional study of a random sample of the Swedish working population. *American Journal of Public Health.* 1988;78(10):1336-42.

45. Johnson, J.V., and Lipscomb, J. Long working hours, occupational health and the changing nature of work organization. *American Journal of Industrial Medicine.* 2006;49(11):921-9.

46. Jorgensen, E., Sokas, R.K., Nickels, L., Gao, W., and Gittleman, J.L. An English/Spanish safety climate scale for construction workers. *American Journal of Industrial Medicine.* 2007;50(6):438-42.

47. Karasek, R.A. Job demands, job decision latitude and mental strain: Implications for job redesign. *Administrative Science Quarterly.* 1979;24:285-308.

48. Kim, C.S., Spahlinger, D.A., Kin, J.A., and Billi, J.E. Lean health care: What can hospitals learn from a world-class automaker? *Journal of Hospital Medicine.* 2006;1(3):191-9.

49. Kivimaki, M., Elovainio, M., Vahtera, J., and Ferrie, J.E. Organisational justice and health of employees: Prospective cohort study. *Occupational and Environmental Medicine.* 2003;60(1):27-33.

50. Kivimaki, M., Elovainio, M., Vahtera, J., Virtanen, M., and Stansfeld, S.A. Association between organizational inequity and incidence of psychiatric disorders in female employees. *Psychological Medicine.* 2003;33(2):319-26.

51. Kivimaki, M., Ferrie, J.E., Brunner, E., Head, J., Shipley, M.J., Vahtera, J., and Marmot, M.G. Justice at work and reduced risk of coronary heart disease among employees: The Whitehall II study. *Archives of Internal Medicine.* 2005;165(19):2245-51.

52. Kivimaki, M., Honkonen, T., Wahlbeck, K., Elovainio, M., Pentti, J., Klaukka, T., Virtanen, M., and Vahtera, J. Organisational downsizing and increased use of psychotropic drugs among employees who remain in employment. *Journal of Epidemiology and Community Health.* 2007;61(2):154-8.

53. Kivimaki, M., Vahtera, J., Ferrie, J.E., Hemingway, H., and Pentti, J. Organisational downsizing and musculoskeletal problems in employees: A prospective study. *Occupational and Environmental Medicine.* 2001;58(12):811-7.

54. Kivimaki, M., Vahtera, J., Pentti, J., and Ferrie, J.E. Factors underlying the effect of organisational downsizing on health of employees: Longitudinal cohort study. *British Medical Journal.* 2000;320(7240):971-5.

55. Kompier, M.A. New systems of work organization and workers' health. *Scandinavian Journal of Work, Environment, and Health.* 2006;32(6):421-30.

56. Kompier, M.A. Work organization interventions. *Sozial- und Praventivmedizin.* 2004;49(2):77-8.

57. Kouvonen, A., Kivimaki, M., Elovainio, M., Vaananen, A., De Vogli, R., Heponiemi, T., Linna, A., Pentti, J., and Vahtera, J. Low organisational justice and heavy drinking: A prospective cohort study. *Occupational and Environmental Medicine.* 2008;65(1):44-50.

58. Kouvonen, A., Vahtera, J., Elovainio, M., Cox, S.J., Cox, T., Linna, A., Virtanen, M., and Kivimaki, M. Organisational justice and smoking: The Finnish Public Sector Study. *Journal of Epidemiology and Community Health.* 2007;61(5):427-33.

59. Lamontagne, A.D., Keegel, T., Louie, A.M., Ostry, A., and Landsbergis, P.A. A systematic review of the job-stress intervention evaluation literature, 1990-2005. *International Journal of Occupational and Environmental Health.* 2007;13(3):268-80.

60. Landsbergis, P.A., Cahill, J., and Schnall, P. The impact of lean production and related new systems of work organization on worker health. *Journal of Occupational Health Psychology.* 1999;4(2):108-30.

61. Leventhal, G.S. What should be done with equity theory? New approaches to the study of fairness in social relationships. In: Gergen, K.S., Greenberg, M.S., and Willis, R.H., ed. *Social exchange: Advances in theory and research.* New York: Plenum; 1980:27-55.

62. Liker, J. *The Toyota way: 14 management principles from the world's greatest manufacturer.* New York: McGraw-Hill; 2003.

63. Lincoln, J.R., and Kalleberg, A.L. *Culture, control, and commitment: A study of work organization and work attitudes in the United States and Japan.* New York: Cambridge University Press; 1990.

64. Marsden P.V., and Cook, C.R. Measuring organizational structures and environments. *American Behavioral Scientist.* 1994;37(7):891-910.

65. Mirabal, N., and De Young, R. Downsizing as a strategic intervention. *Journal of American Academy of Business, Cambridge.* 2005;6(1):39-45.

66. Moore, S., Grunberg, L., and Greenberg, E. Repeated downsizing contact: The effects of similar and dissimilar layoff experiences on work and well-being outcomes. *Journal of Occupational Health Psychology.* 2004;9(3):247-57.

67. Moorman, R.H. Relationship between organizational justice and organizational citizenship behaviors: Do fairness perception influence employee citizenship? *Journal of Applied Psychology.* 1991;76:845-55.

68. Murphy, L.R., and Sauter, S.L. Work organization interventions: State of knowledge and future directions. *Sozial- und Praventivmedizin.* 2004;49(2):79-86.

69. Ossmann, J., Amick, B.C. 3rd, Habeck, R.V., Hunt, A., Ramamurthy, G., Soucie, V., and Katz, J.N. Management and employee agreement on reports of organizational policies and practices important in return to work following carpal tunnel surgery. *Journal of Occupational Rehabilitation.* 2005;15(1):17-26.

70. Palmer, K.T., and Smedley, J. Work relatedness of chronic neck pain with physical findings—a systematic review. *Scandinavian Journal of Work, Environment, and Health.* 2007;33(3):165-91.

71. Parker, S.K. Longitudinal effects of lean production on employee outcomes and the mediating role of work characteristics. *Journal of Applied Psychology.* 2003;88(4):620-34.

72. Peter, R., and Siegrist, J. Psychosocial work environment and the risk of coronary heart disease. *International Archives of Occupational and Environmental Health.* 2000;73 Suppl.: S41-5.

73. Polanyi, M., and Tompa, E. Rethinking work-health models for the new global economy: A qualitative analysis of emerging dimensions of work. *Work.* 2004;23(1):3-18.

74. Printezis, A., and Gopalakrishnan, M. Current pulse: Can a production system reduce medical errors in health care? *Quality Management in Health Care.* 2007;16(3):226-38.

75. Reis, D., and Peña, L. Reengineering the motivation to work. *Management Decision.* 2001;39(8):666-75.

76. Rugulies, R., and Krause, N. Effort-reward imbalance and incidence of low back and neck injuries in San Francisco transit operators. *Occupational and Environmental Medicine.* 2007.

77. Schneider, B. Organizational climates: An essay. *Personnel Psychology.* 1975;28:447-79.

78. Semmer, N.K. Job stress interventions and the organization of work. *Scandinavian Journal of Work, Environment, and Health.* 2006;32(6):515-27.

79. Siegrist, J. Adverse health effects of high-effort/low-reward conditions. *Journal of Occupational Health Psychology.* 1996;1(1):27-41.

80. Siegrist, J. Social reciprocity and health: New scientific evidence and policy implications. *Psychoneuroendocrinology.* 2005;30(10):1033-8.

81. Siegrist, J., and Rodel, A. Work stress and health risk behavior. *Scandinavian Journal of Work, Environment, and Health.* 2006;32(6):473-81.

82. Stansfeld, S., and Candy, B. Psychosocial work environment and mental health—a meta-analytic review. *Scandinavian Journal of Work, Environment, and Health.* 2006;32(6):443-62.

83. Suominen, S., Vahtera, J., Korkeila, K., Helenius, H., Kivimaki, M., and Koskenvuo, M. Job strain, life events, and sickness absence: A longitudinal cohort study in a random population sample. *Journal of Occupational and Environmental Medicine.* 2007;49(9):990-6.

84. Vahtera, J., Kivimaki, M., Forma, P., Wikstrom, J., Halmeenmaki, T., Linna, A., and Pentti, J. Organisational downsizing as a predictor of disability pension: The 10-town prospective cohort study. *Journal of Epidemiology and Community Health.* 2005;59(3):238-42.

85. Vahtera, J., Kivimaki, M., Pentti, J., Linna, A., Virtanen, M., Virtanen, P., and Ferrie, J.E. Organisational downsizing, sickness absence, and mortality: 10-town prospective cohort study. *British Medical Journal.*2004;328(7439):555-9.

86. van Vegchel, N., de Jonge, J., Bosma, H., and Schaufeli, W. Reviewing the effort-reward imbalance model: Drawing up the balance of 45 empirical studies. *Social Science and Medicine.* 2005;60(5):1117-31.

87. Weaver, F.S. *Latin America in the world economy: Mercantile colonialism to global capitalism.* Boulder, CO: Westview Press; 2000.

88. Weber, M. *The theory of social and economic organization.* New York: The Free Press; 1966.

89. Zohar, D. Safety climate: Conceptual and measurement issues. In: Quick, J.C., and Tetrick, L.E., ed. *Handbook of occupational health psychology.* Washington, DC: American Psychological Association; 2003:123-42.

90. Zohar, D., and Luria, G. A multilevel model of safety climate: Cross-level relationships between organization and group-level climates. *Journal of Applied Psychology.* 2005;90(4):616-28.

Chapter 14

1. Chapman, L.S. Health and productivity management framework and metrics. In: Leutzinger, J., Sullivan, S., and Chapman, L., ed. *Platinum book: Practical applications of the health and productivity management model.* Scottsdale, AZ: Institute for Health and Productivity Management; 2004:74.

2. Davis, K., Collins, S.R., Doty, M.M., Ho, A., and Holmgren, A.L. Health and productivity among U.S. workers. *Commonwealth Fund.* 2005;856:1-5.

3. Evans, R.G., Barer, M.L., and Marmor, T.R. *Why are some people healthy and others not? The determinants of health of populations.* Hawthorne, NY: Aldine De Gruyter; 1994.

4. Leutzinger, J. Academy for health and productivity management. Presentation at the *Annual IHPM Conference*; 2005 Oct 5; Scottsdale, AZ. Institute for Health and Productivity Management, Scottsdale, AZ.

5. Leutzinger, J., Sullivan, S., and Chapman, L. Productivity as measured by organizations. In: Leutzinger, J., Sullivan, S., and Chapman, L., ed. *Platinum book: Practical applications of the health and productivity management model.* Scottsdale, AZ: Institute for Health and Productivity Management; 2004:14.

6. Leutzinger, J., Sullivan, S., and Chapman, L., ed. *Platinum book: Practical applications of the health and productivity management model.* Scottsdale, AZ: Institute for Health and Productivity Management; 2004.

7. Lynch, W. H&P Q&A. *Absolute Advantage.* 2003;2(8):9-13.

8. Surowiecki, J. *The wisdom of crowds.* 1st ed. New York: Anchor Books; 2005.

Chapter 15

1. Campbell, D.T., and Stanley, J. Experimental and quasi-experimental designs for research. New York: Houghton Mifflin; 2005.

2. Centers for Disease Control and Prevention. Framework for program evaluation in public health. *Morbidity and Mortality Weekly Report.* 1999;48(NoRR-11):1-40.

3. Joint Committee on Standards for Educational Evaluation. *The program evaluation standards: How to assess evaluations of educational programs.* 2nd ed. Thousand Oaks, CA: Sage Publications; 1994.

4. Scriven, M. Minimalist theory of evaluation: The least theory that practice requires. *American Journal of Evaluation.* 1998;19:57-70.

5. WHO European Working Group on Health Promotion Evaluation. *Health promotion evaluation: Recommendations to policy-makers: Report of the WHO European working group on health promotion evaluation.* Copenhagen, Denmark: World Health Organization, Regional Office for Europe; 1998.

Chapter 16

1. Alexander, G. Health risk appraisal. *Health and Productivity Management.* 2006;5(3):26-9.

2. Anderson, D.R., Serxner, S., and Terry, P. Health assessment. In: O'Donnell, M.P., ed. *Health promotion in the workplace.* 3rd ed. Stamford, CT: Delmar/Thomson Learning; 2002:232-4.

3. Anderson, K.M., Odell, P.M., Wilson, P.W., et al. Cardiovascular disease risk profiles. *American Heart Journal.* 1991;121(1):293-8.

4. Bryson, C.L., and Boyko, E.J. Review: Glycated haemoglobin A1c and fasting plasma glucose screening tests have similar sensitivities and specificities for early detection of type 2 diabetes. *Evidence-Based Medicine.* 2007;12:152.

5. Gail, M.H., Brinton, L.A., Byar, D.P., et al. Projecting individualized probabilities of developing breast cancer for white females who are being examined annually. *Journal of the National Cancer Institute.* 1989;81(24):1879-86.

6. Goetzel, R.Z., Anderson, D.R., Whitmer, W., et al. The relationship between modifiable health risks and health care expenditures: An analysis of the multi-employer HERO health risk and cost database. *Journal of Occupational and Environmental Medicine.* 1998;40(10):843-54.

7. Grundy, S.M., Pasternak, R., Greenland, P., et al. Assessment of cardiovascular risk by use of multiple-risk-factor assessment equations: A statement for healthcare professionals from the American Heart Association and the American College of Cardiology. *Circulation.* 1999;100(13):1481-92.

8. Harris, J.S., and Fries, J. The health effects of health promotion. In: O'Donnell, M.P., ed. *Health promotion in the workplace.* 3rd ed. Stamford, CT: Delmar/Thomson Learning; 2002:1-22.

9. Lab Tests Online. hs-CRP. American Association for Clinical Chemistry. 2008. Available at: www.labtestsonline.org/understanding/analytes/hscrp/test.html.

10. Moussavi, S., Chatterji, S., Verdes, E., Tandon, A., Patel, V., and Ustun, B. Depression, chronic diseases, and decrements in health: Results from the World Health Surveys. *Lancet.* 2007;370(9590):851-8.

11. Schoenbach, V.J., Wagner, E.H., and Berry, W.M. Health risk appraisal: Review of evidence for effectiveness. *Health Service Research.* 1987;22(4):553-80.

12. Strecher, V.J., and Kreuter, M.W. Health risk assessment from a behavioral perspective: Present and future. In: Hyner, G.C., Peterson, K.W., Travis, J.W., Dewey, J.E., Foerster, J.J., and Framer, E.M., ed. *SPM handbook of health assessment tools.* Pittsburgh: The Society of Prospective Medicine and The Institute for Health and Productivity Management; 1999:75-82.

13. U.S. Preventive Services Task Force. *The guide to clinical preventive services 2007.* Rockville, MD: U.S. Department of Health and Human Services, Agency for Healthcare Research and Quality; 2007.

14. Ware, J.E., and Dewey, J.E. Health status and outcomes assessment tools. In: Hyner, G.C., Peterson, K.W., Travis, J.W., Dewey, J.E., Foerster, J.J., and Framer, E.M, ed. *SPM handbook of health assessment tools.* Pittsburgh: The Society of Prospective Medicine and The Institute for Health and Productivity Management; 1999:9-16.

15. Wasserman, J., Whitmer, R., Bazzarre, T., et al. The gender specific effects of modifiable health risk factors on coronary heart disease and related health care expenditures. *Journal of Occupational and Environmental Medicine.* 2000;42(11):973-85.

Chapter 17

1. Alexander, J., Matson Koffman, D., Hersey, J., et al. Heart/Stroke Check: A worksite tool for prevention of heart disease and stroke. Poster presented at: NIOSH Worklife 2007 National Symposium: Protecting and promoting worker health; September 10, 2007; Bethesda, MD.

2. CEO Cancer Gold Standard. Welcome to the CEO Cancer Gold Standard Web site. 2007. Available at: www.cancergoldstandard.org.

3. Centers for Disease Control and Prevention. Guide to community preventive services: Worksite. 2007. Available at: www.thecommunityguide.org/worksite/default.htm.

4. Chapman, L.S. Using health risk appraisals (HRAs) in health promotion. *The Art of Health Promotion.* 2000:4(1):1-12.

5. DeJoy, D.M., and Southern, D. An integrative perspective on worksite health promotion. *Journal of Occupational Medicine.* 1993;35(12):221-30.

6. DeJoy, D.M., and Wilson, M.G. Organizational health promotion: Broadening the horizon of workplace health promotion. *American Journal of Health Promotion.* 2003;17(5):337-41.

7. DeJoy, D.M., Wilson, M.G., Goetzel, R.Z., et al. Development of the Environmental Assessment Tool (EAT) to measure organizational physical and social support for worksite obesity prevention programs. *Journal of Occupational and Environmental Medicine.* 2008;50(2):126-37.

8. Dorn, J., Golaszewski, T., Hoebbel, C., Foley, F., and Heidler, K. A comparison between corporate environmental support for wellness and individual employee health risks and behaviors. Poster presented at: Annual Conference of the American College of Sports Medicine; May 31, 2007; New Orleans, LA.

9. Fisher, B., and Golaszewski, T. Heart Check Lite: Modifications to an established worksite heart health assessment. *American Journal of Health Promotion.* In press.

10. Fisher, B., Golaszewski, T., and Barr, D. Measuring worksite resources for employee heart health. *American Journal of Health Promotion.* 1999;13(6):325-32.

11. Goetzel, R.Z., Ozminkowski, R.J., Pelletier, K.R., Metz, R.D., and Chapman, L.S. Emerging trends and productivity management. *The Art of Health Promotion* 2007;22(1):1-10.

12. Goetzel, R.Z., Shechter, D., and Ozminkowski, R.J. Promising practices in employer health and productivity management efforts: Findings from a benchmarking study. *Journal of Occupational and Environmental Medicine.* 2007;49(2):111-30.

13. Golaszewski, T., and Fisher, B. Heart Check: The development and evolution of an organizational heart health assessment. *American Journal of Health Promotion.* 2002;17(2):132-53.

14. Government of Alberta. *Alberta active living strategy.* Alberta Government, Edmonton, AB; 1997.

15. Harris, J.R., Cross, J., Hannon, P.A., Mahoney, E., Ross-Viles, S., and Kuniyuki, A. Employer adoption of evidence-based chronic disease prevention: A pilot study. *Preventing Chronic Disease.* In press.

16. Health Communication Unit. Comprehensive workplace health promotion: Catalogue of situational assessment tools. 2007. Available at: ww.thcu.ca/workplace/sat/index.cfm.

17. Marzec, M., Zuniga, E., Powers, P., Shewry, S., Golaszewski, T., and Edington, D. Worksite environment: Multiple interventions and risk status—a pilot study. Presentation at: National Prevention and Health Promotion Summit; November 16, 2007; Washington, DC.

18. McLeroy, K.R., Bibeau, D., Steckler, A., and Glanz, K. An ecological perspective on health promotion programs. *Health Education Quarterly.* 1988;15(4):351-77.

19. Oldenburg, B., Sallis, J., Harris, D., and Owen, N. Checklist of health promotion environments at worksites (CHEW): Development and measurement characteristics. *American Journal of Health Promotion.* 2002;16(5):288-95.

20. Parkinson, R. *Managing health promotion in the workplace: Guidelines for implementation and evaluation.* Palo Alto, CA: Mayfield; 1982:17-21.

21. Plotnikoff, R.C., Prodaniuk, T.R., Fein, A.J., and Milton, L. Development of an ecological assessment tool for a workplace physical activity program standard. *Health Education Quarterly.* 2005;6(4):453-63.

22. Salis, J., and Owen, N. Ecological models of health behavior. In Glanz, K., Rimer, B., and Marcus-Lewis, R., ed. *Health behavior and health education.* 3rd ed. San Francisco: Jossey-Bass; 2002:462-84.

23. Stokols, D. Establishing and maintaining healthy environments: Toward a social ecology of health promotion. *American Psychologist.* 1992;47(1):6-22.

24. Stokols, D., Pelletier, K., and Fielding, J. The ecology of work and health: Research and policy directions for the promotion of employee health. *Health Education Quarterly.* 1996;23(2):137-58.

25. The Health Enhancement Research Organization. The Health Enhancement Research Organization. 2007. Available at: www.the-hero.org/Scorecard_Version%20Two.pdf (Accessed September 28, 2008).

26. Wellness Councils of America (WELCOA). Creating well workplaces. 2007. Available at: www.welcoa.org/wellworkplace/?PHPSESSID=bb55 9fc71c8ab47338ac8fb1e33bfa16.

27. Wilson, M.G., Goetzel, R.Z., Ozminkowski, R.J., et al. Using formative research to develop environmental and ecological interventions to address overweight and obesity. Unpublished manuscript.

28. Workplace Solutions Survey. American Cancer Society. 2007. Available at: www.acsworkplacesolutions.com/assessmentandconsulting. asp.(Accessed September 28, 2008).

Chapter 18

1. Burton, W.N., Chen, C.-Y., Conti, D.J., Schulz, A.B., and Edington, D.W. The association between health risk change and presenteeism change. *Journal of Occupational and Environmental Medicine.* 2006;48:252-63.

2. Burton, W.N., Pransky, G., Conti, D.J., Chen, C.-Y., and Edington, D.W. The association of medical conditions and presenteeism. *Journal of Occupational and Environmental Medicine.* 2004;46:S38-45.

3. Brandt-Rauf, P., Burton, W., and McCunney, R.J. Health, productivity, and occupational medicine. *Journal of Occupational and Environmental Medicine.* 2001;43:1.

4. Lerner, D., Adler, D.A., Chang, H., Berndt, E.R., Irish, J.T., Lapitsky, L., Hood, M.Y., Reed, J., and Rogers, W.H. The clinical and occupational correlates of work productivity loss among employed patients with depression. *Journal of Occupational and Environmental Medicine.* 2004;46:S46-55.

5. Lofland, J.H., Pizzi, L., and Frick, K.D. A review of health-related workplace productivity loss instruments. *Pharmacoeconomics.* 2004;22(3):165-84.

6. Lynch, W., and Riedel, J.E., ed. *Measuring Employee Productivity: A Guide to Self-Assessment Tools* Scottsdale, AZ: Institute of Health and Productivity Management; 2001.

7. Mattke, S., Balakrishnan, A., Bergamo, G., and Newberry, S.J. A review of methods to measure health-related productivity loss. *American Journal of Managed Care.* 2007;13:211-7.

8. Mill, J.S. *Principles of political economy, with some of their applications to social philosophy.* 7th ed. Introduction by Ashley, W.J., ed. London: John W. Parker, West Strand; 1909.

9. Prasad, M., Wahlquist, P., Shikiar, R., and Shih, Y.-C.T. A review of self-report instruments measuring health-related work productivity. *Pharmacoeconomics.* 2004;22(4):225-44.

Chapter 19

1. Anderson, D.R., Serxner, S.A., and Gold, D.B. Conceptual framework, critical questions, and practical challenges in conducting research on the financial impact of worksite health promotion. *American Journal of Health Promotion.* 2001;15(5):281-7.

2. Bachler, R., Duncan, I., and Juster, I. A comparative analysis of chronic and non-chronic insured commercial member health care trends. *North American Actuarial Journal.* 2006;10(4):76-89.

3. Chapman, L. Meta-evaluation of worksite health promotion economic return studies: 2005 update. *The Art and Science of Health Promotion.* 2005;July/August:1-10.

4. Congressional Budget Office. An analysis of the literature on disease management programs. 2004. Available at: http://www.cbo. gov/ftpdocs/59xx/doc5909/10-13-DiseaseMngmnt.pdf (Accessed September 28, 2008).

5. Disease Management Association of America. *Outcomes guidelines report, volume II.* Washington, DC: DMAA; 2007.

6. Goetzel, R.Z., Ozminkowski, R.J., Villagra, V.G., and Duffy, J. Return on investment in disease management: A review. *Health Care Financing Review.* 2005;Summer:1-19.

7. Mattke, S., Serxner, S., and Zakowski, S. Comparing disease management evaluation methods. Disease Management Leadership Forum; September, 16-19,2007; Las Vegas, NV.

8. Pelletier, K.R. A review and analysis of the health and cost-effective outcome studies of comprehensive health promotion and disease prevention programs at the worksite: update VI 2000-2004. *Journal of Occupational and Environmental Medicine.* 2005;47(10):1051-8.

9. Serxner, S.A., Baker, K., and Gold, D.B. Guidelines for analysis of economic return from health management programs. *The Art of Health Promotion.*, July/Aug 2006, V20, I6 1A

10. Serxner, S.A., Noeldner, S.P., and Gold, D.B. Best practices for an integrated population health management (PHM) program. *The Art of Health Promotion.* May/June 2006, V20, I5 1A.

11. U.S. Department of Labor. Bureau of Labor Statistics. 2008. Available at: www.bls.gov/cpi/cpi_dr.htm.

12. Winkleman, R., and Mehmud, S. A comparative analysis of claims-based risk assessment tools (excerpt of the Society of Actuaries Research Project). *Health Watch.* 2007;September Issue 56:14-19. (see www.soa.org/library/newsletters/health-watch-newsletter/2007/september/hsn-0708.pdf. (Accessed September 28, 2008).

Chapter 20

1. Banham, R. Tracing safety problems to their source. *Treasury and Risk Management.* 2000;August:59-63.

2. Chenoweth, D. Claims data analysis: Getting what you ask for. *AWHP's Worksite Health.* 1997;Winter:40-44.

3. Chenoweth, D. Health claims data analysis: Rx for behavior risk management. *EAP Digest.* 1994;July/August:23-6.

4. Greenberg, P. Tackling costs one disease at a time. *Business and Health.* 1999;May:31-37.

5. World Health Organization. *International classification of diseases, ninth revision (ICD-9).* 1990. Available at: www.cdc.gov/nchs/about/ major/dvs/icd9des.htm. (Accessed September 28, 2008.)

6. McCarthy, R. Target your health care dollars to the root causes. *Business and Health.* 1999;December:23-7.

Chapter 21

1. Deloitte. The transparent marketplace: Harnessing the collaborative power of the consumer. 2008. Available at: www.deloitte.com/dtt/article/0,1002,sid%253D6233%2526cid%253D187066,00.html. (Accessed September 28, 2008)..

2. Hibbard, J.H., and Peters, E. Supporting informed consumer health care decisions: Data presentation approaches that facilitate the use of information in choice. *Annual Review of Public Health.* 2003;24:413-33.

3. Institute of Medicine (IOM). *Integrating employee health: A model program for NASA.* Washington, DC: The National Academies Press; 2005.

4. Kreuter, M.W., and Holt, C.L. How do people process health information? Applications in an age of individualized communication. Current directions. *Psychological Science.* 2001;10:206-9.

5. Kreuter, M.W., Oswald, D.L., Bull, F.C., and Clark, E.M. Are tailored health education materials always more effective than non-tailored materials? *Health Education Research.* 2000;15:305-15.

6. Lietz, C. How leading consumer packaged goods companies are transforming the way they market. *Fair Isaac White Paper* [series online]. 2003. Available at: http://fairisaac.com.

7. McGinnis, J.M., Williams-Russo, P., and Knickman, J.R. The case for more active policy attention to health promotion. *Health Affairs.* 2003;21(2):78-93.

8. Peppers, D., and Rogers, M. *The one-to-one future: Building relationships one customer at a time.* New York: Currency Doubleday; 1996.

9. Pronk, S., Travis, K., and Rawlings, J. *Ingenix health manager.* Eden Prairie, MN: Ingenix; 2007.

10. U.S. Department of Health and Human Services. *Physical activity and health: A report of the Surgeon General.* Atlanta: U.S. Department of Health and Human Services, Centers for Disease Control and Prevention, National Center for Chronic Disease Prevention and Health Promotion; 1996.

Chapter 22

1. Ajzen, I. The theory of planned behavior. *Organizational Behavior and Hum Decision Processes.* 1991;50:179-211.

2. Ammerman, A.S., Lindquist, C.H., Lohr, K.N., and Hersey, J. The efficacy of behavioral interventions to modify dietary fat and fruit and vegetable intake: A review of the evidence. *Preventative Medicine.* 2002;35:25-41.

3. Armitage, C.J. Efficacy of a brief worksite intervention to reduce smoking: The roles of behavioral and implementation intentions. *Journal of Occupational Health Psychology.* 2007;12(4):376-90.

4. Bandura, A. *Self-efficacy: The exercise of control.* New York: W.H. Freeman and Company; 1997.

5. Bandura, A. *Social foundations of thought and action: A social cognitive theory.* Englewood Cliffs, NJ: Prentice Hall; 1986.

6. Berry, T.R., Plotnikoff, R.C., Raine, K., Anderson, D., and Naylor, P.J. An examination of the stages of change construct for health promotion within organizations. *Journal of Health Organization and Management.* 2007;21(2-3):121-35.

7. Biener, L., Glanz, K., McLerran, D., et al. Impact of the Working Well Trial on the worksite smoking and nutrition environment. *Health Education and Behavior.* 1999;26(4):478-94.

8. Butterfield-Booth, S., and Reger, B. The message changes belief and the rest is theory: The "1% or less" milk campaign and reasoned action. *Preventive Medicine.* 2004;39:581-8.

9. Gates, D., Brehm, B., Hutton, S., Singler, M., and Poeppelman, A. Changing the work environment to promote wellness: A focus group study. *American Association of Occupational Health Nurses Journal.* 2006;54(12):515-20.

10. Glanz, K., and Seewald-Klein, T. Nutrition at the worksite: An overview. *Journal of Nutrition Education.* 1986;18 Suppl. 1:S1-12.

11. Glanz, K., Patterson, R.E., Kristal, A.R., et al. Impact of work site health promotion on stages of dietary change: The Working Well Trial. *Health Education and Behavior.* 1998;25:448-63.

12. Glanz, K., Rimer, B.K., and Lewis, F.M, ed. *Health behavior and health education: Theory, research and practice.* 3rd ed. San Francisco: Jossey-Bass; 2002:583.

13. Graham, A.L., Cobb, N.K., Raymond, L., Sill, S., and Young, J. Effectiveness of an Internet-based worksite smoking cessation intervention at 12 months. *Journal of Occupational and Environmental Medicine.* 2007;49(8):821-8.

14. Griffin-Blake, C.S., and DeJoy, D.M. Evaluation of social-cognitive versus stage-matched, self-help physical activity interventions at the workplace. *American Journal of Health Promotion.* 2006;20(3):200-9.

15. Janis, I., and Mann, L. *Decision making: A psychological analysis of conflict.* New York: Free Press; 1977.

16. Katz, D.L., O'Connell, M., Yeh, M.C., et al. Public health strategies for preventing and controlling overweight and obesity in school and worksite settings: A report on recommendations of the Task Force on Community Preventive Services. *Morbidity and Mortality Weekly Report Recommendations and Reports.* 2005;54:1-12.

17. Kwak, L., Kremers, S.P., Werkman, A., Visscher, T.L., van Baak, M.A., and Brug, J. The NHF-NRG in Balance project: The application of intervention mapping in the development, implementation and evaluation of weight gain prevention at the worksite. *Obesity Reviews.* 2007;8(4):347-61.

18. Legler, J., Meissner, H.I., Coyne, C., Breen, N., Chollette, V., and Rimer, B.K. The effectiveness of interventions to promote mammography among women with historically lower rates of screening. *Cancer Epidemiology, Biomarkers, and Prevention.* 2002;11(1):59-71.

19. Lewin, K. *A dynamic theory of personality.* New York: McGraw-Hill; 1935.

20. Marlatt, A.G., and Gordon, J.R. *Relapse prevention: Maintenance strategies in the treatment of addictive behaviors.* New York: The Guilford Press; 1985.

21. McLeroy, K., Bibeau, D., Steckler, A., and Glanz, K. An ecological perspective on health promotion programs. *Health Education Quarterly.* 1988;15:351-77.

22. Moher, M., Hey, K., and Lancasater, T. Workplace interventions for smoking cessation. *Cochrane Database of Systematic Reviews.* 2003;2:CD003440.

23. Montaño, D.E., and Kasprzyk, D. The theory of reasoned action and the theory of planned behavior. In Glanz, K., Rimer, B.K., and Lewis, F.M., ed. *Health behavior and health education: Theory, research, and practice.* 3rd ed. San Francisco: Jossey-Bass; 2002:67-98.

24. Prochaska, J.M., Prochaska, J.O., and Levesque, D.A. A transtheoretical approach to changing organizations. *Administration and Policy in Mental Health.* 2001;28(4):247-61.

25. Prochaska, J.O., DiClemente, C.C., and Norcross, J. In search of how people change: Applications to addictive behaviors. *American Psychologist* 1992;47:1102-14.

26. Prochaska, J.O., Redding, C., and Evers, K. The transtheoretical model of behavior change. In: Glanz, K., Rimer, B.K., and Lewis, F.M., ed. *Health behavior and health education: Theory, research, and practice.* 3rd ed. San Francisco: Jossey-Bass; 2002:99-120.

27. Sallis, J., and Owen, N. Ecological models. In Glanz, K., Rimer, B.K., and Lewis, F.M., ed., *Health behavior and health education: Theory, research, and practice.* 3rd ed. San Francisco: Jossey-Bass; 2002:462-84.

28. Sorensen, G., Linnan, L., and Hunt, M.K. Worksite-based research and initiatives to increase fruit and vegetable consumption. *Preventive Medicine.* 2004;39 Suppl. 2:S94-100.

29. Volpp, K.G., Gurmankin Levy, A., Asch, D.A., et al. A randomized controlled trial of financial incentives for smoking cessation. *Cancer Epidemiology, Biomarkers, and Prevention.* 2006;15(1):12-8.

Chapter 23

1. Adams, K.F., Schatzkin, A., Harris, T.B., et al. Overweight, obesity, and mortality in a large prospective cohort of persons 50 to 71 years old. *New England Journal of Medicine.* 2006;355(8):763-78.

2. Anema, J.R., Streenstra, I.A., Bongers, P.M., et al. Multidisciplinary rehabilitation for subacute low back pain: graded activity or workplace intervention or both? *Spine.* 2007;32(3):291-8.

3. Ariens, G.A.M., Bongers, P.M., Hoogendoorn, W.E., van der Wal, G., and van Mechelen, W. High physical and psychosocial load at work and sickness absence due to neck pain. *Scandinavian Journal of Work, Environment and Health.* 2002;28(4):222-31.

4. Baldwin, M.L. Reducing the costs of work-related musculoskeletal disorders: Targeting strategies to chronic disability cases. *Journal of Electromyography and Kinesiology.* 2004;14(1):33-41.

5. Blair, S.N., Kohl, H.W., Paffenbarger, R.S., Clark, D.G., Cooper, K.H., and Gibson, L.W. Physical fitness and all-cause mortality: A prospective study of healthy men and women. *Journal of the American Medical Association*. 1989;262(17);2395-401.

6. Bosma, H., Peter, R., Siegrist, J., and Marmot, M. Two alternative job stress models and the risk of coronary heart disease. *American Journal of Public Health*. 1998;88(1):68-74.

7. Carragee, E.J., Alamin, T.F., Miller, J.L., and Carragee, J.M. Discographic, MRI and psychosocial determinants of low back pain disability and remission: A prospective study in subjects with benign persistent back pain. *Spine*. 2005;5(1):24-35.

8. Centers for Disease Control and Prevention. State-specific prevalence of current cigarette smoking among adults and secondhand smoke rules and policies in homes and workplaces—United States, 2005. *Morbidity and Mortality Weekly Report*. 2006;55(42):1148-51.

9. Chandola, T., Brunner, E., and Marmot, M. Chronic stress at work and the metabolic syndrome: Prospective study. *British Medical Journal*. 2006;332(7540):521-5.

10. Chapman, L.S. Meta-evaluation of worksite health promotion economic return studies: 2005 update. *American Journal of Health Promotion*. 2005;19(6):1-11.

11. De Jonge, J., Bosma, H., Peter, R., and Siegrist, J. Job strain, effort-reward imbalance and employee well-being: A large-scale cross-sectional study. *Social Science and Medicine*. 2000;50(9):1317-27.

12. DeJoy, D.M., and Wilson, M.G. Organizational health promotion: Broadening the horizon of workplace health promotion. *American Journal of Health Promotion*. 2003;17(5):337-41.

13. Donaldson, S.I., Sussman, S., Dent, C.W., Severson, H.H., and Stoddard, J.L. Health behavior, quality of work life, and organizational effectiveness in the lumber industry. *Health Education and Behavior*. 1999;26(4):579-91.

14. Dorr, D.A., Wilcox, A., Burns, L., Brunker, C.P., Narus, S.P., and Clayton, P.D. Implementing a chronic care model in primary care using people and technology. *Disease Management*. 2006;9(1):1-15.

15. Engbers, L.H., van Poppel, M.N.M., Chin, A., Paw, M.J.M., van Mechelen, W. Worksite health promotion programs with environmental changes. A systematic review. *American Journal of Preventive Medicine*. 2005;29(1):61-70.

16. Goetzel, R.Z., Ozminkowski, R.H., Villagra, V.G., and Duffy, J. Return on investment in disease management: A review. *Health Care Financing Review*. 2005;26(4):119.

17. Goldberg, M.S., Scott, S.C., and Mayo, N.E. A review of the association between cigarette smoking and the development of nonspecific back pain and related outcomes. *Spine*. 2000;25(8):995-1014.

18. Grawitch, M.J., Gottschalk, M., Munz, D.C. The path to a healthy workplace. A critical review linking healthy workplace practices, employee well-being, and organizational improvements. *Journal of Consulting Psychology*. 2006;58(3):129-47.

19. Guo, H.R., Tanaka, S., Halperin, W.E., and Cameron, L.L. Back pain prevalence in US industry and estimates of lost workdays. *American Journal of Public Health*. 1999;89(7):1029-35.

20. Hammer, L.B., Neal, M.B., Newsom, J.T., Brockwood, K.J., and Colton, C.L. A longitudinal study of the effects of dual-earner couples' utilization of family-friendly workplace supports on work and family outcomes. *Journal of Applied Psychology*. 2005;90(4):799-810.

21. Harmon, G., Lefante, J., and Krousel-Wood, M. Overcoming barriers: The role of providers in improving patient adherence to antihypertensive medications. *Current Opinion in Cardiology*. 2006;21(4):310-5.

22. Heaney, C.A., and Goetzel, R.Z. A review of health-related outcomes of multi-component worksite health promotion programs. *American Journal of Health Promotion*. 1997;11(4):290-307.

23. IJzelenberg, W., and Burdorf, A. Risk factors for musculoskeletal symptoms and ensuing health care use and sick leave. *Spine*. 2005;30(13):1550-6.

24. Ilmarinen, J., and Rantanen, J. Promotion of work ability during aging. *American Journal of Industrial Medicine*. 1999;Suppl. 1:21-3.

25. Kappagoda, C.T., Ma, A., Cort, D.A., et al. Cardiac event rate in a lifestyle modification program for patients with chronic coronary artery disease. *Clinical Cardiology*. 2006;29(7):317-21.

26. Karasek, R.A., and Theorell, T. *Health work, stress, productivity and the reconstruction of working life*. New York: Basic Books; 1990.

27. Kerns, R.D., and Rosenberg, R. Predicting responses to self-management treatments for chronic pain: Application of the pain stages of change model. *Pain*. 2000;84(1):49-55.

28. Kivimaki, M., Vahtera, J., Pentti, J., and Ferrie, J.E. Factors underlying the effect of organizational downsizing on health of employees: Longitudinal cohort study. *British Medical Journal*. 2000;320(7240):971-5.

29. Kouvonen, A., Kivimaki, M., Virtanen, M., et al. Effort-reward imbalance at work and the co-occurrence of lifestyle risk factors: Cross-sectional survey in a sample of 36,127 public sector employees. *BMC Public Health*. 2006;6:24.

30. Krantz, G., and Ostergren, P.O. Common symptoms in middle aged women: Their relation to employment status, psychosocial work conditions and social support in a Swedish setting. *Journal of Epidemiology and Community Health*. 2000;54(3):192-9.

31. Leino-Arjas, P., Solovieva, S., Kirjonen, J., Reunanen, A., and Riihimaki, H. Cardiovascular risk factors and low-back pain in a long-term follow-up of industrial employees. *Scandinavian Journal of Work, Environment and Health*. 2006;32(1):12-9.

32. Lloyd-Jones, D.M., Wilson, P.W.F., Larson, M.G., et al. Framingham risk score and prediction of lifetime risk for coronary heart disease. *American Journal of Cardiology*. 2004;94(1):20-4.

33. Lowe, G.S., Schellenberg, G., and Shannon, H.S. Correlates of employees' perception of a healthy work environment. *American Journal of Health Promotion*. 2003;17(6):390-9.

34. Musich, S., Burton, W., and Edington, D.W. Costs and benefits of prevention and disease management. *Disease Management and Health Outcomes*. 1999;5(3):153-66.

35. Musich, S., McDonald, T., Hirschland, D., and Edington, D.W. Examination of risk status transitions among active employees in a comprehensive worksite health promotion program. *Journal of Occupational and Environmental Medicine*. 2003;45(4):393-9.

36. Musich, S., McDonald, T., Hirschland, D., and Edington, D.W. Excess healthcare costs associated with excess health risks in diseased and non-diseased health risk appraisal participants. *Disease Management and Health Outcomes*. 2002;10(4):251-8.

37. Nakasato, Y.R., and Carnes, B.A. Health promotion in older adults. Promoting successful aging in primary care settings. *Geriatrics*. 2006;61(4):27-31.

38. Pelletier, K.R. A review and analysis of the clinical- and cost-effectiveness studies of comprehensive health promotion and disease management programs at the worksite: 1998-2000 update. *American Journal of Health Promotion*. 2001;16(2):107-16.

39. Peter, R., and Siegrist, J. Chronic work stress, sickness absence, and hypertension in middle managers: General or specific sociological explanations? *Social Science and Medicine*. 1997;45(7):1111-20.

40. Pikhart, H., Bobak, M., Pajak, A., et al. Psychosocial factors at work and depression in three countries of Central and Eastern Europe. *Social Science and Medicine*. 2004;58(8):1475-82.

41. Pincus, T., Burton, A.K., Vogel, S., and Field, A.P. A systematic review of psychological factors as predictors of chronicity/disability in prospective cohorts of low back pain. *Spine*. 2002;27(5):E109-20.

42. Riedel, J.E., Lynch, W., Baase, C., Hymel, P., and Person, K.W. The effect of disease prevention and health promotion on workplace productivity: A literature review. *American Journal of Health Promotion*. 2001;15(3):167-91.

43. Rosal, M.C., Ockene, J.K., Ma, Y., et al. Behavioral risk factors among members of a health maintenance organization. *Preventive Medicine*. 2001;33(6):586-94.

44. Sauter, S.L., Brightwell, W.S., Colligan, M.J., et al. *The changing organization of work and the safety and health of working people*. Cincinatti, OH, Department of Health and Human Services. Centers for Disease Control and Prevention; 2002. DHHS (NIOSH) publication no. 2002-116. see http://www.cdc.gov/niosh/docs/2002-116/pdfs/2002-116.pdf. Accessed September 28, 2008).

45. Siegrist, J. Adverse health effects of high effort/low-reward conditions. *Journal of Occupational Health Psychology*. 1996;1(1):27-41.

46. Smith, T.W. Job satisfaction in the United States, 2007. National Opinion Center/University of Chicago. 2007. Available at: www-news.uchicago.edu/releases/07/pdf/070417.jobs.pdf (Accessed September 28, 2008).

47. Teixeira, P.J., Going, S.B., Houtkooper, L.B., et al. Exercise motivation, eating, and body image variables as predictors of weight control. *Medicine and Science in Sports and Exercise*. 2006;38(1):179-88.

48. Tuomi, K., Huuhtanen, P., Nykyri, E., and Ilmarinen, J. Promotion of work ability, the quality of work and retirement. *Occupational Medicine.* 2001;51(5):318-24.

49. Tuomi, K., Ilmarinen, J., Martikainen, R., Aalto, L., and Klockars, M. Aging, work, life-style and work ability among Finnish municipal workers in 1981-1992. *Scandinavian Journal of Work, Environment and Health.* 1997;Suppl. 1:58-65.

50. Vahtera, J., Kivimaki, M., Pentti, J., and Theorell, T. Effect of change in the psychosocial environment on sickness absence: A seven-year follow up of initially healthy employees. *Journal of Epidemiology and Community Health.* 2000;54(7):484-93.

51. van Poppel, M.N.M., Hooftman, W.E., and Koes, B.W. An update of a systematic review of controlled clinical trials on the primary prevention of back pain at the workplace. *Occupational Medicine.* 2004;54(5):345-52.

52. Vita, A.J., Terry, R.B., Hubert, H.B., and Fries, J.F. Aging, health risks, and cumulative disability. *New England Journal of Medicine.* 1998;338(15):1035-41.

53. Voss, M., Floderus, B., and Diderichsen, F. How do job characteristics, family situation, domestic work and lifestyle factors relate to sickness absence? A study based on Sweden Post. *Journal of Occupational and Environmental Medicine.* 2004;46(11):1134-43.

54. Weiss, D.S., Horowitz, M.J., and Wilner, N. The Stress Response Scale: A clinician's measure for rating the response to serious life events. *British Journal of Clinical Psychology.* 1984;23 Part 3:202-15.

55. Weissman, J.S., and Epsten, A. The insurance gap: Does it make a difference? *Annual Review of Public Health.* 1993;14:243-70.

56. Willcox, G.J., He, Q., Chen, R., et al. Midlife risk factors and healthy survival in men. *Journal of the American Medical Association.* 2006;296(19):2343-50.

Chapter 24

1. Anderson, D.R., Whitmer, R.W., Goetzel, R.Z., Ozminkowski, R.J., Wasserman, J., Serxner, S., and Health Enhancement Research Organization Research Committee. The relationship between modifiable health risks and group-level health care expenditures. *American Journal of Health Promotion.* 2000;15(1):45-52.

2. As GM battles surging costs, workers' health becomes issue. *Wall Street Journal.* April 7, 2005:A1.

3. Brady, W., Bass, J., Moser, R., Anstadt, G., Loeppke, R., and Leopold, R. Total corporate health costs. *Journal of Occupational and Environmental Medicine.* 1997;39:224-31.

4. Colliver, V. Preventative health plan may prevent cost increases / Safeway program includes hot line, lifestyle advice. *San Francisco Chronicle.* February 11, 2007.

5. Edington, D.W. Emerging research: A view from one research center. *American Journal of Health Promotion.* 2001;(5):341-9.

6. Goetzel, R.Z., Anderson, D.R., Whitmer, R.W., Ozminkowski, R.J., Dunn, R.L., Wasserman, J., and The Health Enhancement Research Organization (HERO) Research Committee. The relationship between modifiable health risks and health care expenditures: An analysis of the multi-employer HERO health risk and cost database. *Journal of Occupational and Environmental Medicine.* 1998;40(10):843-54.

7. Goetzel, R.Z., Long, S.R., Ozminkowski Hawkins, K., Wang, S., Lynch, W. Health, absence, disability, and presenteeism cost estimates of certain physical and mental health conditions affecting U.S. employers. *Journal of Occupational and Environmental Medicine.* 2004;46:398-412.

8. Kessler, R.C., Barber, C., Beck, A., et al. The World Health Organization health and work performance questionnaire (HPQ). *Journal of Occupational and Environmental Medicine.* 2003;45:156-74.

9. Lerner, D., Amick, B.C., Rogers, W.H., et al. The work limitations questionnaire. *Medical Care.* 2001;39:72-85.

10. Loeppke, R., Hymel, P.A., Lofland, J.H., et al. Health-related workplace productivity measurement: General and migraine-specific recommendation from the ACOEM expert panel. *Journal of Occupational and Environmental Medicine.* 2003;45:349-59.

11. Mercer. National survey of employer-sponsored health plans. 2006. Available at: www.mercer.com/ecomm/shopbroker.jhtml.

12. Musich, S., Lu, C., McDonald, T., Campagne, L.J., and Edington, D.W. Association of additional health risks on medical charges and prevalence of diabetes within body mass index categories. *American Journal of Health Promotion.* 2004;18(3):264-8.

13. Pelletier, K. A review and analysis of the clinical and cost-effectiveness studies of comprehensive health promotion and disease

management programs at the worksite: Update VI 200-2004. *Journal of Occupational and Environmental Medicine.* 2005;47:1051-8.

14. Serxner, S., Baker, K., and Gold, D. Guidelines for analysis of economic return from health management programs. *American Journal of Health Promotion.* 2006;20 Suppl. 6:1-17.

15. Serxner, S., Noeldner, S.P., and Gold, D. Best practices for an integrated population health management (PHM) program. *American Journal of Health Promotion.* 2006; 20 Suppl. 5:1-10, iii.

16. Thomasson, M. From sickness to health: The twentieth century development of U.S. health insurance. *Explorations in Economic History.* 2002;32:233-53.

17. Wahlqvist, P., Carlsson, J., Stalhammar, N.O., and Wiklund, I. Validity of a work productivity and activity impairment questionnaire for patients with symptoms of gastroesophageal reflux disease (WPAI-GERD): Results from a cross sectional study. *Value in Health.* 2002;5:106-13.

Chapter 25

1. Alcalay, R., Alvarado, M., Balcazar, H., Newman, E., and Huerta, E. Salud para su Corazon: A community-based Latino cardiovascular disease prevention and outreach model. *Journal of Community Health.* 1999;24(5):359-79.

2. Andersen, R.E., Franckowiak, S.C., Snyder, J., Bartlett, S.J., and Fontaine, K.R. Can inexpensive signs encourage the use of stairs? Results from a community intervention. *Annals of Internal Medicine.* 1998;129(5):363-9.

3. Andersen, R.E., Franckowiak, S.C., Zuzak, K.B., Cummings, E.S., Bartlett, S.J., and Crespo, C.J. Effects of a culturally sensitive sign on the use of stairs in African American commuters. *Sozial- und Praventivmedizin.* 2006;51(6):373-80.

4. Brown, D.R., and Alexander, M. Recruiting and retaining people of color in health research studies: Introduction. *Journal of Aging and Health.* 2004;16(5):s5-8.

5. Brownell, K.D., Stunkard, A.J., and Albaum, J.M. Evaluation and modification of exercise patterns in the natural environment. *American Journal of Psychiatry.* 1980;137(12):1540-5.

6. California Department of Health Services. California nutrition network and California 5 a day campaign issue brief: Workplace nutrition and physical activity. Available at: www.cdph.ca.gov/programs/wicworks/Documents/WIC-Training-StaffWellness-PhysicalActivityAtMeetings.doc. (Accessed September 28, 2008).

7. Campbell, M.K., Tessaro, I., DeVellis, B., et al. Effects of a tailored health promotion program for female blue-collar workers: Health works for women. *Preventive Medicine.* 2002;34(3):313-23.

8. Cooke, L. The importance of exposure for healthy eating in childhood: A review. *Journal of Human Nutrition and Dietetics.* 2007;20(4):294-301.

9. Crawford, P.B., Gosliner, W., Strode, P., et al. Walking the talk: Fit WIC wellness programs improve self-efficacy in pediatric obesity prevention counseling. *American Journal of Public Health.* 2004;94(9):1480-5.

10. DeBate, R., Plescia, M., Joyner, D., and Spann, L. A qualitative assessment of Charlotte REACH: An ecological perspective for decreasing CVD and diabetes among African Americans. *Ethnicity and Disease.* 2004;14(3 Suppl. 1):S77-82.

11. Elbel, R., Aldana, S., Bloswick, D., and Lyon, J.L. A pilot study evaluating a peer led and professional led physical activity intervention with blue-collar employees. *Work.* 2003;21(3):199-210.

12. Escobar-Chavez, S.L., Tortolero, S.R., Masse, L.C., Watson, K.B., and Fulton, J.E. Recruiting and retaining minority women: Findings from the Women on the Move study. *Ethnicity and Disease.* 2002;12:242-51.

13. Fouad, M.N., Partridge, E., Green, B.L., et al. Minority recruitment in clinical trials: A conference at Tuskegee, researchers and the community. *Annals of Epidemiology.* 2000;10 Suppl. 8:S35-40.

14. Glasgow, R.E., Nelson, C.C., Kearney, K.A., et al. Reach, engagement, and retention in an Internet-based weight loss program in a multi-site randomized controlled trial. *Journal of Medical Internet Research.* 2007;9(2):e11.

15. Grier, S., and Bryant, C.A. Social marketing in public health. *Annual Review of Public Health.* 2005;26:319-39.

16. Griffin, S.C., Barber, J.A., Manca, A., et al. Cost effectiveness of clinically appropriate decisions on alternative treatments for angina pectoris: Prospective observational study. *British Medical Journal.* 2007;334(7594):624.

17. Hammond, S.L., Leonard, B., and Fridinger, F. The Centers for Disease Control and Prevention Director's Physical Activity Challenge:

An evaluation of a worksite health promotion intervention. *American Journal of Health Promotion.* 2000;15(1):17-20, ii.

18. Institute of Medicine. *Health literacy: A prescription to end confusion.* Washington, DC: Board on Neuroscience and Behavioral Health, Committee on Health Literacy; 2004.

19. Kelley, M.A., Baldyga, W., Barajas, F., and Rodriguez-Sanchez, M. Capturing change in a community--university partnership: Si Se Puede! project. *Preventing Chronic Disease.* 2005;2(2):A22.

20. King, A.C. How to promote physical activity in a community: Research experiences from the US highlighting different community approaches. *Patient Education and Counseling.* 1998;33 Suppl. 1:S3-12.

21. Kreuter, M.W., Lukwago, S.N., Bucholtz, R.D., Clark, E.M., and Sanders-Thompson, V. Achieving cultural appropriateness in health promotion programs: Targeted and tailored approaches. *Health Education and Behavior.* 2003;30(2):133-46.

22. Laken, M.A., Wilcox, S., and Swinton, R. Working across faith and science to improve the health of African Americans. *Ethnicity and Disease.* 2007;17(1 Suppl. 1):S23-6.

23. Lara, A., Yancey, A.K., Tapia-Conye, R., et al. Pausa para tu Salud: Reduction of weight and waistlines by integrating exercise breaks into workplace organizational routine. *Preventing Chronic Disease.* 2008;5(1):A12.

24. Mahar, M.T., Murphy, S.K., Rowe, D.A., Golden, J., Shields, A.T., and Raedeke, T.D. Effects of a classroom-based program on physical activity and on-task behavior. *Medicine and Science in Sports and Exercise.* 2006;38(12):2086-94.

25. Maibach, E.W., Rothschild, M.R., and Novelle, W.D. Social marketing. In: Glanz, K., Rimer, B., and Lewis, F.M., et al., trans-eds., *Health behavior and health education.* 3rd ed. San Francisco: Jossey-Bass; 2002:437-61.

26. McCarthy, W.J., Yancey, A.K., Harrison, G.G., Leslie, J., and Siegel, J.M. Fighting cancer with fitness: Dietary outcomes of a randomized, controlled lifestyle change intervention in healthy African-American women. *Preventive Medicine.* 2007;44(3):246-53.

27. Miyashita, M., Burns, S.F., and Stensel, D.J. Exercise and postprandial lipemia: Effect of continuous compared with intermittent activity patterns. *American Journal of Clinical Nutrition.* 2006;83(1):24-9.

28. Plescia, M., Groblewski, M., and Chavis, L. A lay health advisor program to promote community capacity and change among change agents. *Health Promotion Practice.* 2006 doi:10.1177/1524839906289670 (Nov. 14, 2006).

29. Pohjonen, T., and Ranta, R. Effects of worksite physical exercise intervention on physical fitness, perceived health status, and work ability among home care workers: Five-year follow-up. *Preventive Medicine.* 2001;32(6):465-75.

30. Pronk, N.P. Designing and evaluating health promotion programs: Simple rules for a complex issue. *Disease Management and Health Outcomes.* 2003;11(3):149-57.

31. Rogers, E.M. *Diffusion of innovations.* 5th ed. New York: Free Press; 2003.

32. Rudd, R.E., Goldberg, J., and Dietz, W. A five-stage model for sustaining a community campaign. *Journal of Health Communication.* 1999;4(1):37-48.

33. Seabury, S.A., Lakdawalla, D., and Reville, R.T. *The economics of integrating injury and illness prevention and health promotion programs.* Santa Monica, CA: RAND Corporation; 2005. Working paper no. WR-243-ICJ.

34. Sorensen, G., Barbeau, E., Stoddard, A.M., Hunt, M.K., Kaphingst, K., and Wallace, L. Promoting behavior change among working-class, multiethnic workers: Results of the healthy directions—small business study. *American Journal of Public Health.* 2005;95(8):1389-95.

35. Steckler, A., and Goodman, R. How to institutionalize health promotion programs. *American Journal of Health Promotion.* 1989;3:34-44.

36. Stolley, M. Integrating contextual factors into health disparity research: Examples from obesity, asthma and cancer. *Annals of Behavioral Medicine* 2006;31(1):i-I.

37. Strecher, V.J. Keynote address: Tools for lifestyle and health risk behavior change. *Inaugural* Summit on Behavioral Telehealth. Boston, MA. 2007; May 31 – June 1.

38. Tanjasiri, S. Shared responsibility: California's state and community partnerships to promote physical activity among diverse populations. *Journal of Health Education.* 1999;30(2):S64-71.

39. Wolch, J., Wilson, J., and Fehrenbach, J. Parks and park funding in Los Angeles: An equity mapping analysis. *Urban Geography.* 2004;26:4-35.

40. Wyatt, S.B., Diekelmann, N., Henderson, F., et al. A community-driven model of research participation: The Jackson Heart Study Participant Recruitment and Retention Study. *Ethnicity and Disease.* 2003;13(4):438-55.

41. Yancey, A., McCarthy, W., Leslie, J., et al. Results of a randomized, controlled lifestyle change intervention: African-American women fight cancer with fitness. *Journal of Women's Health.* 2006;15(4):412-29.

42. Yancey, A.K. Facilitating health promotion in communities of color. *Cancer Research, Therapy, and Control.* 1999;8:113-22.

43. Yancey, A.K., Jordan, A., Bradford, J., et al. Engaging high-risk populations in community-level fitness promotion: ROCK! Richmond. *Health Promotion Practice.* 2003;2:180-8.

44. Yancey, A.K., Kumanyika, S.K., Ponce, N.A., et al. Population-based interventions engaging communities of color in healthy eating and active living: A review. *Preventing Chronic Disease.* 2004;1(1):A09.

45. Yancey, A.K., Lewis, L.B., Guinyard, J.J., et al. Putting promotion into practice: The African Americans building a legacy of health organizational wellness program. *Health Promotion Practice.* 2006;7 Suppl. 3:233S-46S.

46. Yancey, A.K., Lewis, L.B., Sloane, D.C., et al. Leading by example: A local health department-community collaboration to incorporate physical activity into organizational practice. *Journal of Public Health Management and Practice.* 2004;10(2):116-23.

47. Yancey, A.K., Miles, O.L., McCarthy, W.J., et al. Differential response to targeted recruitment strategies to fitness promotion research by African-American women of varying body mass index. *Ethnicity and Disease.* 2001;11(1):115-23.

48. Yancey, A.K., Ory, M.G., and Davis, S.M. Dissemination of physical activity promotion interventions in underserved populations. *American Journal of Preventive Medicine.* 2006;31 Suppl. 4:S82-91.

49. Yancey, A.K., Siegel, J.M., and McDaniel, K.L. Role models, ethnic identity, and health-risk behaviors in urban adolescents. *Archives of Pediatrics and Adolescent Medicine.* 2002;156(1):55-61.

Chapter 26

1. Campbell, J. *The hero with the thousand faces.* Princeton, NJ: Princeton University Press; 1973.

2. Chapman, L. Expert opinions on "best practices" in worksite health promotion (WHP). *The Art of Health Promotion.* 2004; July/August:1-6.

3. Goetzel, R.A., Guindon, A., Humphries, L., et al. Health and productivity management: Consortium benchmarking study best practice report. Houston, TX: American Productivity and Quality Center International Benchmarking Clearinghouse; 1998.

4. Greenleaf, R. *Servant leadership.* Mahwah, NJ: Paulist Press; 1991.

5. Hesse, H. *Siddharta.* New York: New Directions Publishing Corporation; 1951.

6. Hesse, H. *The journey to the East.* New York: Farrar, Straus & Giroux; 2000.

7. Karasek, R., and Theorell, T. *Healthy work: Stress, productivity, and the reconstruction of working life.* New York: Basic Books; 1990.

8. Kuhn, T.S. *The structure of scientific revolutions.* 3rd ed. Chicago: University of Chicago Press; 1996.

9. Maslow, A. *Motivation and personality.* 2nd ed. New York: Harper & Row; 1970.

10. O'Brien, W.J. *The soul of corporate leadership.* Waltham, MA: Pegasus Communications; 1998.

11. O'Donnell, M., Bishop, C., and Kaplan, K. Benchmarking best practices in workplace health promotion. *The Art of Health Promotion.* 1997;1(1):12.

12. Pronk, N.P. Aligning program support with interventions for optimum impact. *ACSM's Health & Fitness Journal.* 2007;11(3):40-2.

13. Pronk, N.P. Leadership for worksite health promotion. *ACSM's Health & Fitness Journal.* 2007;11(5):40-2.

14. Pronk, N.P. The challenge of work and family balance. *ACSM's Health & Fitness Journal.* 2005;9(3):34-6.

15. Pronk, N.P., Goldstein, M.G., and Peek, C.J. Addressing multiple health risk behaviors in primary care: A synthesis of current knowledge and stakeholder dialogue sessions. *American Journal of Preventive Medicine.* 2004;27(2S):4-17.

16. Senge, P.M. *The fifth discipline: The art and practice of the learning organization.* New York: Doubleday, 1990.

17. Silversin, J., and Kornacki, M.J. *Leading physicians through change.* Tampa, FL. American College of Physician Executives; 2000.

18. Wayne, G. Building a healthy worksite from the view of a CEO. In: Cox, C., ed. *ACSM's worksite health promotion manual.* Champaign, IL: Human Kinetics; 2003; 3-5.

Chapter 27

1. Ball, K. People, places . . . and other people? Integrating understanding of intrapersonal, social and environmental determinants of physical activity. *Journal of Science and Medicine in Sport.* 2006;9(5):367.

2. Bandler, R., and Grinder, J. *Reframing: NLP and the transformation of meaning.* Boulder, CO. Real People Press; 1982.

3. Campbell, J. *Myths to live by.* New York: Penguin Books; 1972.

4. Frank, A. *The wounded storyteller: Body, illness, and ethics.* Chicago: University of Chicago Press; 1995.

5. Freedman, J., and Combs, G. *Narrative therapy: The social construction of preferred realities.* New York: Norton; 1996:7,16.

6. Leo, P. Cell phone statistics that may surprise you. *Pittsburgh Post-Gazette* [online]. March 16, 2006. Available at: www.eng.vt.edu/newsitems/pdf/Cell%20phone%20statistics.pdf (Accessed September 28, 2008).

7. Locke, C., Searles, D., and Weinberger, D. *The cluetrain manifesto.* Jackson, TN. Perseus Publishing; 2000:xxi.

8. Madden, M. Internet penetration and impact. Pew Internet and American Life Project. 2006. Available at: www.pewinternet.org/PPF/r/182/report_display.asp.

9. Madden, M., and Fox, S. Riding the wave of "Web.2.0." Pew Internet and American Life Project. 2006. Available at: www.pewinternet.org/PPF/r/189/report_display.asp.

10. Preece, J. Sociability and usability: Twenty years of chatting online. *Behavior and Information Technology Journal.* 2001; 20(5):349.

11. Putnam, R. *Bowling alone: The collapse and revival of American community.* Online: Touchstone Books; 2000:22-4.

12. Rosch, E., quoted in Lakeoff, G. *Women, fire, and dangerous things: What categories reveal about the mind.* Chicago: University of Chicago Press; 1987:44.

13. Schwartz, B. *The paradox of choice. Why less is more.* New York, NY. HarperCollins Publishers; 2004:56-61.

14. Sofian, N., Newton, D., and DeClaire, J. Strengthen context to enhance health promotion effectiveness. *American Journal of Health Promotion.* 2003;7(1):1-9.

15. Wright, A. *Glut: Mastering information through the ages.* Washington, D.C. Joseph Henry Press; 2007:32.

16. Ong, W. *Orality and Literacy: The Technologizing of the Word.* New York, NY. Routledge; 2002.

Chapter 28

1. Abdolrasulnia, M., Collins, B.C., Casebeer, L., et al. Using email reminders to engage physicians in an Internet-based CME intervention. *BMC Medical Education.* 2004;4:17.

2. Bandura, A. *Social foundations of thought and action: A social cognitive theory.* Englewood Cliffs, NJ: Prentice Hall; 1986.

3. Chapman, L.S. Expert opinions on "best practices" in worksite health promotion (WHP). *American Journal of Health Promotion.* 2004;18:1-6.

4. Cooper, J.O., Heron, T.E., and Heward, W.L. *Applied behavior analysis.* Upper Saddle River, NJ: Prentice Hall; 1987:255-74.

5. Daniels, A. *Bringing out the best in people.* New York: McGraw-Hill; 2000:150-64.

6. Donatelle, R., Hudson, D., Dobie, S., Goodall, A., Hunsberger, M., and Oswald, K. Incentives in smoking cessation: Status of the field and implications for research and practice with pregnant smokers. *Nicotine and Tobacco Research.* 2004;6 Suppl. 2:S163-79.

7. Edwards, P., Roberts, I., Clarke, M., et al. Methods to increase response rates to postal questionnaires. *Cochrane Database of Systematic Reviews.* 2007;2:MR000008.

8. Finkelstein, E.A., and Kosa, K.M. Use of incentives to motivate healthy behaviors among employees. *Gender Issues.* 2003;21:50-9.

9. Giuffrida, A., and Torgerson, D.J. Should we pay the patient? Review of financial incentives to enhance patient compliance. *British Medical Journal.* 1997;315:703-7.

10. Green, L., and Myerson, J. A discounting framework for choice with delayed and probabilistic rewards. *Psychological Bulletin.* 2004;130:769-92.

11. Hall, R.V., and Hall, M.C. *How to select reinforcers.* 2nd ed. Austin, TX: Pro-Ed; 1998:1-38.

12. Hey, K., and Perera, R. Competitions and incentives for smoking cessation. *Cochrane Database of Systematic Reviews.* 2005;2:CD004307.

13. Janer, G., Sala, M., and Kogevinas, M. Health promotion trials at worksites and risk factors for cancer. *Scandinavian Journal of Work, Environment and Health.* 2002;28:141-57.

14. Kane, R.L., Johnson, P.E., Town, R.J., and Butler, M. A structured review of the effect of economic incentives on consumers' preventive behavior. *American Journal of Preventive Medicine.* 2004;27:327-52.

15. Kiernan, M., Phillips, K., Fair, J.M., and King, A.C. Using direct mail to recruit Hispanic adults into a dietary intervention: An experimental study. *Annals of Behavioral Medicine.* 2000;22:89-93.

16. Linnan, L., Bowling, M., Childress, J., et al. Results of the 2004 National Worksite Health Promotion Survey. *American Journal of Public Health.* 2007;29:1-7.

17. Mapstone, J., Elbourne, D., and Roberts, I. Strategies to improve recruitment to research studies. *Cochrane Database of Systematic Reviews.* 2007;2:MR000013.

18. Martinez, A., VanWormer, J., and Pronk, N. The role of incentives and communication on health assessment participation. *ACSM's Health & Fitness Journal.* 2008;12(3):41-44.

19. Moher, M., Hey, K., and Lancaster, T. Workplace interventions for smoking cessation. *Cochrane Database of Systematic Reviews.* 2005;2:CD003440.

20. Mokdad, A.H., Marks, J.S., Stroup, D.F., and Gerberding, J.L. Actual causes of death in the United States, 2000. *Journal of the American Medical Association.* 2004;291:1238-45.

21. Reitman, D. The real and imagined harmful effects of rewards: Implications for clinical practice. *Journal of Behavior Therapy and Experimental Psychiatry.* 1998;29:101-13.

22. Ryan, R.M., and Deci, E.L. Self-regulation and the problem of human autonomy: Does psychology need choice, self-determination, and will? *Journal of Personality.* 2006;74:1557-85.

23. Serxner, S., Anderson, D.R., and Gold, D. Building program participation: Strategies for recruitment and retention in worksite health promotion programs. *American Journal of Health Promotion.* 2004;18:1-6.

24. Skinner, B.F. *Science and human behavior.* New York: Macmillan; 1953.

25. Strum, R. The effects of obesity, smoking, and problem drinking on chronic medical problems and health care costs. *Health Affairs.* 2002;21:245-53.

26. Volpp, K.G., Gurmankin Levy, A., Asch, D.A., et al. A randomized controlled trial of financial incentives for smoking cessation. *Cancer Epidemiology, Biomarkers and Prevention.* 2006;15:12-8.

27. Wall, J, Mhurchu, C.N., Blakely, T., Rodgers, A., and Wilton, J. Effectiveness of monetary incentives in modifying dietary behavior: A review of randomized, controlled trials. *Nutrition Reviews.* 2006;64:518-31.

28. Warner, K.E., and Murt, H.A. Economic incentives for health. *Annual Review of Public Health.* 1984;5:107-33.

Chapter 29

1. Ahern, D.K. Challenges and opportunities of ehealth research. *American Journal of Preventive Medicine.* 2007;32 Suppl. 5:S75-82.

2. Berger, J. Economic and clinical impact of iPharmacy benefit designs in the management of diabetes pharmacotherapy. *American Journal of Managed Care.* 2007;13:S55-8.

3. Brennan, T., and Reisman, L. Value-based insurance design and the next generation of consumer-driven health care. *Health Affairs.* 2007;26(2):204-7.

4. Denelsbeck, S., Engaging employees in health and wellness: The Healthy Pfizer Program. *American Journal of Managed Care.* 2006;12 Spec. no. 12:SP40-3.

5. Devol, R., Bedroussian, A., Charuworm, A., et al. *An unhealthy America: The economic burden of chronic disease—charting a new course to save lives and increase productivity and economic growth.* Santa Monica, CA. Research Report Milken Institute; 2007:5-7.

6. Fox, S. Eight in ten internet users have looked for health information online, with increased interest in diet, fitness, drugs, health insurance, experimental treatments, and particular doctors and hospitals. Pew Internet and American Life Project. 2005. Available at: www.pewinternet.org/PPF/r/156/report_display.asp. (Accessed September 28, 2008).

7. Franklin, P.D., Rosenbaum, P.F., Carey, M.P., and Roizen, M.F. Using sequential email messages to promote health behaviors: Evidence of feasibility and reach in a worksite sample. *Journal of Medical Internet Research.* 2006;8(1):e3.

8. Kashima, S.R. Transitioning from a pen-and-paper health risk appraisal to an online health risk appraisal at a petroleum company. *Health Promotion Practice.* 2006;7(4):450-8.

9. Madden, M., and Fox, S. *Finding answers online in sickness and in health.* Pew Internet and American Life Project. 2006. Available at: www.pewinternet.org/PPF/r/183/report_display.asp. (Accessed September 28, 2008).

10. Markle Foundation. The Personal Health Working Group: Final report. 2003. Available at: www.markle.org/markle_programs/health-care/projects/connecting_for_health.php#report1.

11. McCauley, R. Managing for health and productivity. *Absolute Advantage: The Workplace Wellness Magazine.* 2004;3(5):12-7.

12. Murray, E., Burns, J., See, T.S., Lai, R., and Nazareth, I. Interactive health communication applications for people with chronic disease. *Cochrane Database of Systematic Reviews.* 2005, Issue 3. Art. No.: CD004274. DOI: 10.1002/14651858.CD004274.pub4.

13. Shetty, S., Secnik, K., and Oglesby, A. Relationship of glycemic control to total diabetes-related costs for managed care health plan members with type 2 diabetes. *Journal of Managed Care Pharmacy.* 2005;11:559-64.

14. Taylor, H. 4-country survey finds most cyberchondriacs believe online health care information is trustworthy, easy to find and understand. *Harris Interactive Health Care News.* 2002;2(12):1-3. Available at: www.harrisinteractive.com/news/newsletters/healthnews/HI_Health-CareNews2002Vol2_Iss12.pdf . (Accessed September 28, 2008.)

Chapter 30

1. Abrams, D.B. Conceptual models to integrate individual and public health interventions: The example of the workplace. In: Henderson, M., ed. *Proceedings of the International Conference on Promoting Dietary Change in Communities.* Seattle, WA: The Fred Hutchinson Cancer Research Center; 1991:173-194.

2. Abrams, D.B., Orleans, C.T., Niaura, R.S., Goldstein, M.G., Prochaska, J.O., and Velicer, W. Integrating individual and public health perspectives for treatment of tobacco dependence under managed health care: A combined stepped-care and matching model. *Annals of Behavioral Medicine.* 1996;18:290-304.

3. Aldana, S.G. Financial impact of health promotion programs: A comprehensive review of the literature. *American Journal of Health Promotion.* 2001;15:296-320.

4. Aldana, S.G., and Pronk, N.P. Health promotion programs, modifiable health risks, and employee absenteeism. *Journal of Occupational and Environmental Medicine.* 2001;43:36-46.

5. Anderson, M.A., and Stoltzfus, J.A. The 3M corporate experience: Health as a business strategy. *American Journal of Health Promotion.* 2001;15:371-3.

6. Baker, E., Israel, B., and Schurman, S. The integrated model: Implications for worksite health promotion and occupational health and safety practice. *Health Education Quarterly.* 1996;23:175-88.

7. Baker, F. Risk communication about environmental hazards. *Journal of Public Health Policy.* 1990;11:341-59.

8. Barbeau, E., Goldman, R., Roelofs, C., et al. A new channel for health promotion: Building trades unions. *American Journal of Health Promotion.* 2005;19:297-303.

9. Barbeau, E., Li, Y., Calderon, P., et al. Results of a union-based smoking cessation intervention for apprentice iron workers. *Cancer Causes and Control.* 2006;17:53-61.

10. Barbeau, E., Roelofs, C., Youngstrom, R., Sorensen, G., Stoddard, A.M., and LaMontagne, A.D. Assessment of occupational safety and health programs in small businesses. *American Journal of Industrial Medicine.* 2004;45:371-9.

11. Bettenhausen, K., and Murnighan, J.K. The emergence of norms in competitive decision-making groups. *Administrative Science Quarterly.* 1985;30:350-72.

12. Blewett, V., and Shaw, A. Health promotion, handle with care: Issues for health promotion in the workplace. *Journal of Occupational Health Safety.* 1995;11:461-5.

13. Blix, A. Integrating occupational health protection and health promotion: Theory and program application. *American Association of Occupational Health Nurses Journal.* 1999;47:168-71.

14. Boyle, R.G., O'Connor, P., Pronk, N., and Tan, A. Health behaviors of smokers, ex-smokers, and never smokers in an HMO. *Preventive Medicine.* 2000;31:177-82.

15. Bradbury, J.A. The policy implications of differing concepts of risk. *Science, Technology and Human Values.* 1989;14:381-96.

16. Brigham, J., Gross, J., and Stitzer, M.L. Effects of a restricted worksite smoking policy on employees who smoke. *American Journal of Public Health.* 1994;84:773-8.

17. Campbell, M., Tessaro, I., DeVellis, B., et al. Effects of a tailored health promotion program for female blue-collar workers: Health works for women. *Preventive Medicine.* 2002;34:313-23.

18. Centers for Disease Control and Prevention. *National health interview survey.* Atlanta: Centers for Disease Control and Prevention, National Center for Health Statistics; 1994.

19. Chu, C., Driscoll, T., and Dwyer, S. The health-promoting workplace: An integrative perspective. *Australian and New Zealand Journal of Public Health.* 1997;21:377-85.

20. Colditz, G. Disseminating research findings into public health practice (editorial). *Cancer Causes and Control.* 2002;13:503-4.

21. Curry, S.J., McBride, C.M., Grothaus, L.C., Louie, D., and Wagner, E.H. A randomized trial of self-help materials personalized feedback and telephone counseling with nonvolunteer smokers. *Journal of Consulting and Clinical Psychology.* 1995;63:1005-14.

22. De Bourdeaudhuij, I., Stevens, V., Vandelanotte, C., and Brug, J. Evaluation of an interactive computer-tailored nutrition intervention in a real-life setting. *Annals of Behavioral Medicine.* 2007;33:39-48.

23. DeJoy, D., and Southern, D. An integrative perspective on worksite health promotion. *Journal of Medicine.* 1993;35:1221-30.

24. Delichatsios, H.K., Friedman, R.H., Glanz, K., et al. Randomized trial of a "talking computer" to improve adults' eating habits. *American Journal of Health Promotion.* 2001;15:215-24.

25. Deloitte Development LLC. *Wellness survey.* Washington, DC: Deloitte Center for Health Solutions; 2005.

26. Dishman, R.K., Oldenburg, B., O'Neal, H., and Shephard, R.J. Worksite physical activity interventions. *American Journal of Preventive Medicine.* 1998;15:344-61.

27. Eakin, J.M., Cava, M., and Smith, T.F. From theory to practice: A determinants approach to workplace health promotion in small businesses. *Health Promotion Practice.* 2001;2:172-81.

28. Edington, M., Karjalainen, T., Hirschland, D., and Edington, D.W. The UAW-GM Health Promotion Program: Successful outcomes. *American Association of Occupational Health Nurses Journal.* 2002;50:26-31.

29. Engbers, L.H., van Poppel, M.N., Chin, A.P.M.J., and van Mechelen, W. Worksite health promotion programs with environmental changes: a systematic review. *American Journal of Preventive Medicine.* 2005;29:61-70.

30. Eriksen, M.P., and Gottlieb, N.H. A review of the health impact of smoking control at the workplace. *American Journal of Health Promotion.* 1998;13:83-104.

31. European Network for Workplace Health Promotion. *The Luxembourg declaration on workplace health promotion in the European Union.* Luxembourg: European Network for Workplace Health Promotion; 1997.

32. Evans, C.J. Health and work productivity assessment: State of the art or state of flux. *Journal of Occupational and Environmental Medicine.* 2004;46:S3-11.

33. Everson, S.A., Siobhan, C.M., Lynch, J.W., and Kaplan, G.A. Epidemiologic evidence for the relation between socioeconomic status and depression, obesity, and diabetes. *Journal of Psychosomatic Research.* 2002;53:891-5.

34. Fielding, J.E. Smoking control at the workplace. *Annual Review of Public Health.* 1991;12:209-34.

35. Fischoff, B., Bostrom, A., and Quadrel, M.J. Risk perception and communication. *Annual Review of Health.* 1993;14:183-200.

36. Galobardes, B., Morabia, A., and Bernstein, M.S. The differential effect of education and occupation on body mass and overweight

in a sample of working people of the general population. *Annals of Epidemiology.* 2000;10:532-7.

37. Geller, E.S. Chapter 29: Psychology and occupational health. In: DiNardi, R., ed. *The occupational environment: Its evaluation and control.* Fairfax, VA: American Industrial Hygiene Association Press; 1998.

38. Giovino, G., Pederson, L., and Trosclair, A. *The prevalence of selected cigarette smoking behaviors by occupation in the United States. Work, smoking and health: A NIOSH scientific workshop.* Washington, DC; NIOSH, 2000.

39. Glanz, K., Lewis, F.M., and Rimer, B. *Health behavior health education: Theory, research, and practice.* San Francisco: Jossey-Bass; 1990.

40. Glanz, K., Sorensen, G., and Farmer, A. The health impact of worksite nutrition and cholesterol intervention programs. *American Journal of Health Promotion.* 1996;10:453-70.

41. Glasgow, R.E., McKay, H., Piette, J., and Reynolds, K.D. The RE-AIM framework for evaluating interventions: What can it tell us about approaches to chronic illness management? *Patient Education and Counseling.* 2001;44:119-27.

42. Goetzel, R.Z. *Examining the value of integrating occupational health and safety and health promotion programs in the workplace. Steps to a healthier US workforce.* Washington, DC: NIOSH; 2004.

43. Goetzel, R.Z., Long, S.R., Ozminkowski, R.J., Hawkins, K., Wang, S., and Lynch, W. Health, absence, disability and presenteeism cost estimates of certain physical and mental health conditions affecting US employers. *Journal of Occupational and Environmental Medicine.* 2004;46:398-412.

44. Golaszewski, T. Shining lights: Studies that have most influenced the understanding of health promotion's financial impact. *American Journal of Health Promotion.* 2001;15:332-40.

45. Gottlieb, N., Weinstein, R., Baun, W., and Bernacki, E. A profile of health risk among blue-collar workers. *Journal of Medicine.* 1992;34:61-8.

46. Green, K.L. Issues of control and responsibility in worker's health. *Health Education Quarterly.* 1988;15:473-86.

47. Green, K.L., and Johnson, J.V. The effect of psychological work organization on patterns of cigarette smoking among male chemical plant employees. *American Journal of Public Health.* 1990;80:1368-71.

48. Hammond, S.K., Sorensen, G., Youngstrom, R., and Ockene, J.K. Occupational exposure to environmental tobacco smoke. *Journal of the American Medical Association.* 1995;37:453-60.

49. Harris, J.R., Holman, P.B., and Carande-Kulis, V.G. Financial impact of health promotion: We need to know much more, but we know enough to act. *American Journal of Health Promotion.* 2001;15:378-82.

50. Heaney, C.A., and Goetzel, R.Z. A review of health-related outcomes of multi-component worksite health promotion programs. *American Journal of Health Promotion.* 1997;11:290-308.

51. Heaney, C.A., and Israel, B.A.. Social networks and social support. In: Glanz, K., Rimer, B.K., and Lewis, F.M., ed. *Health behavior and health education: Theory, research, and practice.* 3rd ed. San Francisco: Jossey-Bass; 2002:185-209.

52. Hennrikus, D.J., and Jeffery, R.W. Worksite intervention for weight control: A review of the literature. *American Journal of Health Promotion.* 1996;10:471-98.

53. Hunt, M.K., Lederman, R., Stoddard, A.M., et al. Process evaluation of an integrated health promotion/occupational health model in WellWorks-2. *Health Education and Behavior.* 2005;32:10-26.

54. Institute of Medicine. *Safe work in the 21st century: Education and training needs for the next decade's occupational safety and health personnel.* Washington, DC: National Academy Press; 2000.

55. Institute of Medicine, Committee to Assess Worksite Preventive Health Program Needs for NASA Employees, Food and Nutrition Board. *Integrating employee health: A model program for NASA.* Washington, DC: Institute of Medicine, National Academies Press; 2005.

56. Isaac, F., and Flynn, P. Johnson & Johnson Live For Life Program: Now and then. *American Journal of Health Promotion.* 2001;15:365-7.

57. Janer, G., Sala, M., and Kogevinas, M. Health promotion trials at worksites and risk factors for cancer. *Scandinavian Journal of Work Environment and Health.* 2002;28:141-57.

58. Jeffery, R.W., French, S.A., Raether, C., and Baxter, J.E. An environmental intervention to increase fruit and salad purchases in a cafeteria. *Preventive Medicine.* 1994;23:788-92.

59. Kant, A.K., Schatzkin, A., Block, G., Ziegler, R.G., and Nestle, M. Food group intake patterns and associated nutrient profiles of the US population. *Journal of the American Dietetic Association.* 1991;91:1532-7.

60. King, D.K., Estabrooks, P.A., Strycker, L.A., Toobert, D.J., Bull, S.S., and Glasgow, R.E. Outcomes of a multifaceted physical activity regimen as part of a diabetes self-management intervention. *Annals of Behavioral Medicine.* 2006;31:128-37.

61. King, E., Rimer, B., Seay, J., Balshem, A., and Enstrom, P. Promoting mammography use through progressive interventions: Is it effective? *American Journal of Public Health.* 1994;84:104-6.

62. Kinne, S., Kristal, A.R., and White, E. Worksite smoking policies: Their population impact in Washington State. *American Journal of Public Health.* 1993;83:1031-3.

63. Kreuter, M.W., Strecher, V.J., and Glassman, B. One size does not fit all: The case for tailoring print materials. *Annals of Behavioral Medicine.* 1999;21:276-83.

64. Kroeze, W., Werkman, A., and Brug, J. A systematic review of randomized trials on the effectiveness of computer-tailored education of physical activity and dietary behaviors. *Annals of Behavioral Medicine.* 2006;31:205-23.

65. Kruger, J., Yore, M.M., Bauer, D.R., and Kohl, H.W. Selected barriers and incentives for worksite health promotion services and policies. *American Journal of Health Promotion.* 2007;21:439-47.

66. Lahiri, S., Gold, J., and Levenstein, C. Estimation of net-costs for prevention of occupational low back pain: Three case studies from the US. *American Journal of Industrial Medicine.* 2005;48:530-41.

67. Lahiri, S., Markkanen, P., and Levenstein, C. *Cost effectiveness of interventions to reduce occupational back pain. The world health report 2002: Reducing risks, promoting healthy life.* Geneva, Switzerland: World Health Organization; 2002.

68. LaMontagne, A.D., Youngstrom, R.A., Lewiton, M., et al. Assessing and intervening on OSH programs: Effectiveness evaluation of the WellWorks-2 intervention in fifteen manufacturing worksites. *Occupational and Environmental Medicine.* 2004;61:651-60.

69. Levy, B.S., and Wegman, D.H. Occupational health: Recognizing and preventing work-related disease and injury. Philadelphia: Lippincott, Williams & Wilkins; 2000.

70. Lewis, M.A., DeVellis, B.M., and Sleath, B. Social influence and interpersonal communication in health behavior. In: Glanz, K., Rimer, B.K., and Lewis, F.M., ed. *Health behavior and health education: Theory, research, and practice.* 3rd ed. San Francisco: Jossey-Bass; 2002:240-64.

71. Linnan, L., Bowling, M., Childress, J., et al. Results of the 2004 National Worksite Health Promotion Survey. *American Journal of Public Health.* In press.

72. Linnan, L.A., Sorensen, G., Colditz, G., Klar, N., and Emmons, K. Using theory to understand the multiple determinants of low participation in worksite health promotion programs. *Health Education and Behavior.* 2001;28:591-607.

73. Lutz, S.F., Ammerman, A.S., Atwood, J.R., Campbell, M.K., DeVellis, R.F., and Rosamond, W.D. Innovative newsletter interventions improve fruit and vegetable consumption in healthy adults. *Journal of the American Dietetic Association.* 1999;99:705-9.

74. Maes, S., Verhoeven, C., Kittel, F., and Scholten, H. Effects of a Dutch worksite wellness-health program: The Brabantia project. *American Journal of Public Health.* 1998;88:1037-41.

75. Marcus, A.C., Baker, D.B., and Froines, J. The ICWU cancer control and evaluation program: Research design and needs assessment. *Journal of Occupational Medicine.* 1986;28:226-36.

76. Marcus, B.H., Emmons, K.M., Abrams, D.B., et al. Restrictive workplace smoking policies: Impact on nonsmoker's tobacco exposure. *Journal of Public Health Policy.* 1992;13:42-51.

77. Martinson, B.C., Crain, A.L., Pronk, N.P., O'Connor, P.J., and Maciosek, M.V. Changes in physical activity and short-term changes in health care charges: A prospective cohort study of older adults. *Preventive Medecine.* 2003;37:319-26.

78. Matson-Koffman, D.M., Brownstein, J.N., Neiner, J.A., and Greaney, M.L. A site-specific literature review of policy and environmental interventions that promote physical activity and nutrition for cardiovascular health: What works? *American Journal of Health Promotion.* 2005;19:167-93.

79. McLeroy, K., Bibeau, D., Steckler, A., and Glanz, K. An ecological perspective on health promotion programs. *Health Education Quarterly.* 1988;15:351-77.

80. Minkler, M., and Wallerstein, N.B. Improving health through community organization and community building. In: Glanz, K., Rimer, B.K., and Lewis, F.M., ed. *Health behavior and health education: Theory, research, and practice*. 3rd ed. San Francisco: Jossey-Bass; 2002:279-311.

81. Moher M, Hey K, Lancaster T. Workplace interventions for smoking cessation. *Cochrane Database of Systematic Reviews* 2005, Issue 1. Art. No.: CD003440. DOI: 10.1002/14651858.CD003440.pub2 (First versionm published in 2003).

82. Mokdad, A.H., Ford, E.S., Bowman, B.A., et al. Prevalence of obesity, diabetes, and obesity-related health risk factors, 2001. *Journal of the American Medical Association*. 2003;289:76-9.

83. Mokdad, A.H., Marks, J.S., Stroup, D.F., and Gerberding, J.L. Actual causes of death in the United States, 2000. *Journal of the American Medical Association*. 2004;291:1238-45.

84. Morris, W., Conrad, K., Marcantonio, R., Marks, B., and Ribisl, K. Do blue-collar workers perceive the worksite health climate differently than white-collar workers? *Journal of Health Promotion*. 1999;13:319-24.

85. National Center for Health Statistics. Table 150. Persons enrolled in health maintenance organizations (HMOs) by geographic region and state: United States, selected years 1980-2002. In: National Center for Health Statistics, ed. *Health, United States 2003, with chartbook on trends in the health of Americans*. Hyattsville, MD: National Center for Health Statistics; 2003.

86. National Institute for Occupational Safety and Health. *Worker health chartbook 2000*. Washington, DC: U.S. Department of Health and Human Services; 2000.

87. O'Donnell, M.P. Health impact of workplace health promotion programs and methodological quality of the research literature. *Art of Health Promotion*. 1997;1:1-7.

88. Oenema, A., Brug, J., and Lechner, I. Web-based tailored nutrition education: Results of a randomized controlled trial. *Health Education Research*. 2001;16:647-60.

89. Office for National Statistics. *Introduction. The national statistics socio-economic classification (NS-SEC)*. London: Office for National Statistics; 2004.

90. Office of Technology Assessment. *Preventing illness and injury in the workplace*. Washington, DC: Office of Technology Assessment, Congressional Board of the 99th Congress, US Government Printing Office; 1985.

91. Ozminkowski, R.J., Dunn, R.L., Goetzel, R.Z., Cantor, R.I., Murnane, J., M. H. A return on investment evaluation of the Citibank, N.A., health management program. *American Journal of Health Promotion*. 1999;14:31-43.

92. Ozminkowski, R.J., Goetzel, R.Z., Chang, S., and Long, S. The application of two health and productivity instruments at a large employer. *Journal of Occupational and Environmental Medicine*. 2004;43:635-48.

93. Ozminkowski, R.J., Goetzel, R.Z., Smith, M.W., Cantor, R.I., Shaughnessy, A., and Harrison, M. The impact of the Citibank, NA, health management program on changes in employee health risks over time. *Journal of Occupational and Environmental Medicine*. 2000;42:502-11.

94. Ozminkowski, R.J., Ling, D., Goetzel, R.Z., et al. Long-term impact of Johnson & Johnson's Health & Wellness Program on health care utilization and expenditures. *Journal of Occupational and Environmental Medicine*. 2002;44:21-9.

95. Patterson, B., and Block, G. Food choices and the cancer guidelines. *American Journal of Public Health*. 1988;78:282-6.

96. Paulozzi, L.J., Spengler, R.F., and Gower, G.A. An evaluation of the Vermont Worksite Smoking Law. *Public Health Reports*. 1992;107:724-6.

97. Pelletier, K.R. A review and analysis of the clinical and cost-effectiveness studies of comprehensive health promotion and disease management programs at the worksite: 1993-1995 update. *American Journal of Health Promotion*. 1996;10:380-8.

98. Pelletier, K.R. A review and analysis of the clinical and cost-effectiveness studies of comprehensive health promotion and disease management programs at the worksite: 1995-1998 update (IV). *American Journal of Health Promotion*. 1999;13:333-45.

99. Pelletier, K.R. A review and analysis of the clinical and cost-effectiveness studies of comprehensive health promotion and disease management programs at the worksite: 1998-2000 update. *American Journal of Health Promotion*. 2001;16:107-16.

100. Pelletier, K.R. A review and analysis of the clinical and cost-effectiveness studies of comprehensive health promotion and disease management programs at the worksite: Update VI 2000-2004. *Journal of Occupational and Environmental Medicine*. 2005;47:1051-8.

101. Petty, R., and Cacioppo, J.T. The elaboration likelihood model of persuasion. *Advances in Experimental Social Psychology*. 1986;19:123-205.

102. Pierce, J.P., Shanks, T.G., and Pertschuk, M. Do smoking ordinances protect non-smokers from environmental tobacco smoke at work? *Tobacco Control*. 1994;3:15-20.

103. Porru, S., Donato, F., Apostoli, P., Coniglio, L., Duca, P., and Alessio, L. The utility of health education among lead workers: The experience of one program. *American Journal of Industrial Medicine*. 1993;22:473-81.

104. Powell, D.R. Characteristics of successful wellness programs. *Employee Benefits Journal*. 1999;24:15-21.

105. Proper, K., Staal, B.J., Hildebrandt, V.H., van der Beek, A.J., and van Mechelen, W. Effectiveness of physical activity programs at worksites with respect to work-related outcomes. *Scandinavian Journal of Work Environment and Health*. 2002;28:75-84.

106. Quintiliani, LM, Sattelmair, J., and Sorensen, G. *The workplace as a setting for intervention to improve diet and promote physical activity*. Geneva, Switzerland: WHO. In press.

107. Raven, B., and Rubin, J. *Social psychology: People in groups*. New York: Wiley; 1976.

108. Rimer, B.K., Orleans, C.T., Fleisher, L., et al. Does tailoring matter? The impact of a tailored guide on ratings and short-term smoking-related outcomes for older smokers. *Health Education Research*. 1994;9:69-84.

109. Robins, T., and Klitzman, S. Hazard communication in a large U.S. manufacturing firm: The ecology of health education in the workplace. *Health Education Quarterly*. 1988;15:451-72.

110. Roman, P.M., and Blum, T.C. Alcohol: A review of the impact of worksite interventions on health and behavioral outcomes. *The Science of Health Promotion*. 1996;11:136-49.

111. Rose, G. Sick individuals and sick populations. *International Journal of Epidemiology*. 1985;14:32-8.

112. Rose, G. *The strategy of preventive medicine*. New York: Oxford University Press; 1992.

113. Sarlio-Lahteenkorva, S., Silventoinen, K., and Lahelma, E. Relative weight and income at different levels of socioeconomic status. *American Journal of Public Health*. 2004;94:468-72.

114. Serxner, S., Anderson, D.R., and Gold, D. Building program participation: Strategies for recruitment and retention in worksite health promotion programs. *American Journal of Health Promotion*. 2004;18:1-6, iii.

115. Sexner, S., Gold, D., Anderson, D., and Williams, D. The impact of a worksite health promotion program on short-term disability usage. *Journal of Occupational and Environmental Medicine*. 2001;43:25-9.

116. Shepard, R.J. Worksite fitness and exercise programs: A review of methodology and health impact. *American Journal of Health Promotion*. 1996;10:436-52.

117. Skinner, C.S., Campbell, M.K., Rimer, B.K., Curry, S., and Prochaska, J.O. How effective is tailored print communication? *Annals of Behavioral Medicine*. 1999;21:290-8.

118. Sorensen, G. Smoking cessation at the worksite: What works and what is the role of occupational health? In: National Institute for Occupational Safety and Health, ed. *Work, smoking, and health, a NIOSH scientific workshop;* 2000 June 15-16. Cincinnati: U.S. Department of Health and Human Services, Public Health Service, Centers for Disease Control and Prevention, National Institute for Occupational Safety and Health; 2002. DHHS (NIOSH) Publication No. 2002-148.

119. Sorensen, G., and Barbeau, E. *Steps to a healthier US workforce: Integrating occupational health and safety and worksite health promotion: State of the science*. Washington, DC: National Institute for Occupational Safety and Health; 2004.

120. Sorensen, G., Barbeau, E., Hunt, M.K., and Emmons, K. Reducing social disparities in tobacco use: A social contextual model for reducing tobacco use among blue-collar workers. *American Journal of Public Health*. 2004;94:230-9.

121. Sorensen, G., Barbeau, E., Stoddard, A., Hunt, M.K., Kaphingst, K., and Wallace, L. Promoting behavior change among working-class, multi-ethnic workers: Results of the Healthy Directions Small Business Study. *American Journal of Public Health*. 2005;95:1389-95.

122. Sorensen, G., Barbeau, E., Stoddard, A.M., et al. Tools for Health: The efficacy of a tailored intervention targeted for construction laborers. *Cancer Causes and Control*. 2007;18:51-9.

123. Sorensen, G., Himmelstein, J.S., Hunt, M.K., et al. A model for worksite cancer prevention: Integration of health protection and health promotion in the WellWorks project. *American Journal of Health Promotion.* 1995;10:55-62.

124. Sorensen, G., Linnan, L., and Hunt, M.K. Worksite-based research and initiatives to increase fruit and vegetable consumption. *Preventive Medicine.* 2004;39:S94-100.

125. Sorensen, G., Rigotti, N., Rosen, A., Pinney, J., and Prible, R. Employee knowledge of and attitudes about a worksite nonsmoking policy: Rationale for further smoking restrictions. *Journal of Occupational Medicine.* 1991;33:1125-30.

126. Sorensen, G., Stoddard, A., Hammond, S.K., Hebert, J.R., and Ocklene, J.K. Double jeopardy: Job and personal risks for craftspersons and laborers. *American Journal of Health Promotion.* 1996;10:355-63.

127. Sorensen, G., Stoddard, A., Hunt, M.K., et al. The effects of a health promotion-health protection intervention on behavior change: The WellWorks study. *American Journal of Public Health.* 1998;88: 1685-90.

128. Sorensen, G., Stoddard, A., LaMontagne, A., et al. A comprehensive worksite cancer prevention intervention: Behavior change results from a randomized controlled trial in manufacturing worksites (United States). *Cancer Causes and Control.* 2002;13:493-502.

129. Sorensen, G., Stoddard, A., Ockene, J.K., Hunt, M.K., and Youngstrom, R. Worker participation in an integrated health promotion/ health protection program: Results from the WellWorks project. *Health Education Quarterly.* 1996;23:191-203.

130. Sorensen, G., Stoddard, A., Youngstrom, R., et al. Local labor unions' positions on worksite tobacco control. *American Journal of Public Health.* 2000;90:618-20.

131. Stave, G.M. The Glaxo Wellcome health promotion program: The contract for health and wellness. *American Journal of Health Promotion.* 2001;15:358-60.

132. Stillman, F.A., Becker, D.M., and Swank, R.T. Ending smoking at the Johns Hopkins Medical Institutions. *Journal of the American Medical Association.* 1990;246:1565-92.

133. Stokols, D., Pelletier, K., and Fielding, J. The ecology of work and health: Research and policy directions for the promotion of employee health. *Health Education Quarterly.* 1996;23:137-58.

134. Taylor, C.A. *The corporate response to rising health care costs.* Ottawa, ON: The Conference Board of Canada; 1996.

135. The Health Project. *1995 C. Everett Koop National Health Award winners: Marriott International, Inc., "Wellness & You!"* Stanford, CA: Stanford University; 1997.

136. Thompson, B., Hannon, P.A., Bishop, S.K., West, B.E., Peterson, A.K., and Beresford, S.A. Factors related to participatory employee advisory boards in small, blue-collar worksites. *American Journal of Health Promotion.* 2005;19:430-7.

137. Tosteson, A.N.A., Weinstein, M.C., Hunink, M.G.M., et al. Cost-effectiveness of population-wide educational approaches to reduce serum cholesterol levels. In press.

138. U.S. Department of Health and Human Services. *Healthy people 2010: Understanding and improving health and objectives for health.* 2nd ed. Washington, DC: U.S. Government Printing Office; 2000.

139. U.S. Department of Labor. *Emerging benefits: Access to health promotion benefits in the United States, private industry, 1999 and 2005.* Washington, DC: USDL; 2006.

140. U.S. Preventive Services Task Force. *Guide to clinical preventive services: An assessment of the effectiveness of 169 interventions.* Alexandria, VA: International Medical Publishing; 1996.

141. Velicer, W.F., Prochaska, J.O., Bellis, J.M., et al. An expert system intervention for smoking cessation. *Addictive Behaviors.* 1993;18: 269-90.

142. Walsh, D.C., Sorensen, G., and Leonard, L. Gender, health, and cigarette smoking. In: Amick, B.C.I., Levine, S., Tarlov, A.R., and Walsh, D.C., ed. *Society and health.* New York: Oxford University Press; 1995:131-71.

143. Walsh, D.W., Jennings, S.E., Mangione, T., and Merrigan, D.M. Health promotion versus health protection? Employees' perceptions and concerns. *Journal of Public Health Policy.* 1991;12:148-64.

144. Warshaw, L.J., and Messite, J. Health protection and promotion in the workplace: An overview. In: Stellman, J.M., ed. *Encyclopaedia of occupational health and safety.* Geneva Switzerland: International Labour Office; 1998:79-89.

145. Whitehead, D.A. A corporate perspective on health promotion: Reflections and advice from Chevron. *American Journal of Health Promotion.* 2001;15:367-9.

146. Woodruff, T.J., Rosbrook, B., Pierce, B., and Glantz, S.T. Lower levels of cigarette consumption found in smoke-free workplaces in California. *Archives of Internal Medicine.* 1993;153:1485-93.

147. World Health Organization. *Anexo 6: Estrategia de promocion de la salud en los lugares de trabajo de America Latina y el Caribe.* Geneva, Switzerland: World Health Organization; 2000:23.

148. World Health Organization. *Jakarta statement on healthy workplaces.* Jakarta, Indonesia: World Health Organization; 1997.

149. World Health Organization. *Ottawa charter for health promotion.* World Health Organization; 1986. (See www.who.int/hpr/NPH/docs/ ottawa_charter_hp.pdf. Accessed September 28, 2008).

150. World Health Organization. *Regional guidelines for the development of healthy workplaces.* Shanghai, China: World Health Organization, Western Pacific Regional Office; 1999:66.

Chapter 31

1. Aarts, H., Paulussen, T., and Schaalma, H. Physical exercise habit: On the conceptualization and formation of habitual health behaviours. *Health Education Research.* 1997;12(3):363-74.

2. Ainsworth, B.E., Haskell, W.L., Whitt, M.C., et al. Compendium of physical activities: An update of activity codes and MET intensities. *Medicine and Science in Sports and Exercise.* 2000;32 Suppl. 9: S498-516.

3. Asfaw, A. The effects of obesity on doctor-diagnosed chronic diseases in Africa: Empirical results from Senegal and South Africa. *Journal of Public Health Policy.* 2006;27(3):250-64.

4. Bandura, A. Social foundation of thought and action. A social cognitive theory. Englewood Cliffs, NJ: Prentice Hall; 1986.

5. Bandura, A. Social learning theory. Englewood Cliffs, NJ: Prentice Hall; 1977.

6. Blue, C.L., and Conrad, K.M. Adherence to worksite exercise programs: An integrative review of recent research. *American Association of Occupational Health Nurses Journal.* 1995;43(2):76-86.

7. Booth, S.L., Mayer, J., Sallis, J.F., et al. Environmental and societal factors affect food choice and physical activity: Rationale, influences, and leverage points. *Nutrition Reviews.* 2001;59(3): S21-39.

8. Bracht, N. *Health promotion at the community level: New advances.* Thousand Oakes, CA: Sage; 1999.

9. Central Bureau of Statistics. Lifestyle and health status of the Dutch population in 2004. 2008. Available at: http://statline.cbs.nl/StatWeb/ table.asp?PA=03799&D1=267.

10. Dishman, R.K., Oldenburg, B., O'Neal, H., et al. Worksite physical activity interventions. *American Journal of Preventive Medicine.* 1998;15:344-61.

11. Emmons, K.M., Linnan, J.M., Shadel, W.G., Marcus, B., and Abrams, D.B. The Working Healthy Project: A worksite health-promotion trial targeting physical activity, diet and smoking. *Journal of Occupational and Environmental Medicine* 1999;41(7):545-55.

12. Engbers, L.H. FoodSteps. The effects of a worksite environmental intervention on cardiovascular risk indicators [dissertation]. Amsterdam: Vrije Universiteit; 2007.

13. Engbers, L.H., van Poppel, M.N., and van Mechelen, W. Measuring stair use in two office buildings: A comparison between an objective and a self-reported method. *Scandinavian Journal of Medicine and Science in Sports.* 2007;17(2):165-71.

14. Engbers, L.H., van Poppel, M.N.M., Chin A Paw, M.J.M., and van Mechelen, W. The effectiveness of worksite health promotion programs with environmental modifications: A systematic review. *American Journal of Preventive Medicine.* 2005;29:61-70.

15. Eves, F.F., and Webb, O.J. Worksite interventions to increase stair climbing; reasons for caution. *Preventive Medicine.* 2006;43:4-7.

16. Gates, D., Brehm, B., Hutton, S., Singler, M., and Poeppelman, A. Changing the work environment to promote wellness. A focus group study. *American Association of Occupational Health Nurses Journal.* 2006;54(12):515-20.

17. Glanz, K., and Mullis, R.M. Environmental intervention to promote healthy eating: A review of models, programs and evidence. *Health Education Quarterly.* 1988;15(4):395-415.

18. Glanz, K., and Seewald-Klein, T. Nutrition at the worksite: An overview. *Journal of Nutrition Education.* 1986;15:395-415.

19. Green, L.W., and Kreuter, M.W. Health promotion planning: An educational and environmental approach. Mountain View, CA: Mayfield;1991.

20. Haslam, D.W., and James, W.P. Obesity. *Lancet.* 2005;366:1197-209.

21. Heirich, M.A., Foote, A., Erfurt, J.C., and Konopka, B. Work-site physical fitness programs. Comparing the impact of different program designs on cardiovascular risks. *Journal of Occupational Medicine.* 1993;35:510-7.

22. Kahn, E.B., Ramsey, L.T., Brownson, R.C., et al. The effectiveness of interventions to increase physical activity. A systematic review. *American Journal of Preventive Medicine.* 2002;22 Suppl. 4:73-107.

23. Kerr, J., Eves, F., and Carroll, D. Can posters prompt stair use in a worksite environment? *Journal of Occupational Health.* 2001;43:205-7.

24. Lechner, L., and De Vries, H. Participation in an employee fitness program: Determinants of high adherence, low adherence, and dropout. *Journal of Occupational and Environmental Medicine.* 1995;37(4):429-36.

25. Marshall, A., Bauman, A., Patch, C., et al. Can motivational signs prompt increases in incidental physical activity in an Australian health care facility? *Health Education Research.* 2002;17(2):743-9.

26. Matson-Koffman, D.M., Brownstein, J.N., Neiner, J.A., and Greaney, M.L. A site-specific literature review of policy and environmental interventions that promote physical activity and nutrition for cardiovascular health: What works? *American Journal of Health Promotion.* 2005;19(3):167-93.

27. Nicoll, G. Spatial measures associated with stair use. *American Journal of Health Promotion.* 2007;21 Suppl. 4;346-52.

28. Pegus, C., Bazzarre, T., Brown, J.S., and Menzin, J. Effect of the Heart at Work program on awareness of risk factors, self-efficacy, and health behaviours. *Journal of Occupational and Environmental Medicine.* 2002;44:228-36.

29. Popkin, B.M. Global nutrition dynamics: The world is shifting rapidly toward a diet linked with noncommunicable diseases. *American Journal of Clinical Nutrition.* 2008;84:289-98.

30. Popkin, B.M., Duffey, K., and Gordon-Larsen, P. Environmental influences on food choice, physical activity and energy balance. *Physiology and Behavior.* 2005;86(5):603-13.

31. Popkin, B.M., Kim, S., Rusev, E.R., Du, S., and Zizza, C. Measuring the full economic costs of diet, physical activity and obesity-related chronic diseases. *International Association for the Study of Obesity.* 2006;7:271-93.

32. Proper, K.I., Koning, M., van der Beek, A.J., Hildebrandt, V.H., Bosscher, R.J., and van Mechelen, W. The effectiveness of worksite physical activity programs on physical activity, physical fitness and health. *Clinical Journal of Sport Medicine.* 2003;13:106-17.

33. Sallis, J.F., and Owen, N. Ecological models. In: Glanz, K., Lewis, F.M., and Rimer, K., ed. *Health behavior and health education.* 2nd ed. San Francisco: Jossy-Bass; 1997:403-24.

34. Sallis, J.F., Bauman, A., and Pratt, M. Environmental and policy interventions to promote physical activity. *American Journal of Preventive Medicine.* 1998;15(4):379-97.

35. Seymour, J.D., Yaroch, A.L., Serdula, M., Blanck, H.M., and Khan, L.K. Impact of nutrition environmental interventions on point-of-purchase behavior in adults: A review. *Preventive Medicine.* 2004;39 Suppl. 2:S108-36.

36. Shephard, R.J. Worksite fitness and exercise programs: A review of methodology and health impact. *American Journal of Health Promotion.* 1996;10(6):436-52.

37. Sparling, P.B., Owen, N., Lambert, E.V., and Haskell, W.L. Promoting physical activity: The new imperative for public health. *Health Education Research.* 2000;15(3):367-76.

38. Swinburn, B., and Egger, G. The runaway weight gain train: Too many accelerators, not enough brakes. *British Medical Journal.* 2004;329:736-9.

39. Titze, S. *Promotion of health-enhancing physical activity. An individual, social and environmental approach.* Aachen, Germany: Shaker Verlag GMBH; 2003.

40. Verplanken, B., Aarts, H., van Knippenberg, A., and Moonen, A. Habit versus planned behaviour: a field experiment. *British Journal of Social Psychology.* 1998;37 Part 1:111-28.

41. Vuori, I., Oja, P., and Paronen, O. Physically active commuting to work - testing its potential for exercise promotion. *Medicine and Science in Sports and Exercise.* 1994;26:844-50.

42. Wetter, A.C., Goldberg, J.P., King, A., et al. How and why do individuals make food and physical activity choices. *Nutrition Reviews.* 2001;59(3):S11-20.

43. Wicker, A.W. An introduction to ecological psychology. Pacific Groove, CA: Brooks/Cole; 1979.

44. World Health Organization (WHO) and World Economic Forum (WEF). Preventing noncommunicable diseases in the workplace through diet and physical activity. WHO/World Economic Forum report of a joint event. 2008. Available at: www.who.int/dietphysicalactivity/workplace/en.

45. Zimring, C., Joseph, A., Nicoll, G.L., and Tsepas, S. Influences of building design and site design on physical activity: Research and intervention opportunities. *American Journal of Preventive Medicine.* 2005;28 Suppl. 2:186-93.

Chapter 32

1. Business Roundtable. Doing well through wellness: 2006-07 Survey of wellness programs at Business Roundtable member companies. 2007. Available at: www.businessroundtable.org/pdf/Health_retirement/BR_Doing_Well_through_Wellness_09192007.pdf.

2. Centers for Studying Health System Change. Health care cost and access challenges persist across country. 2007. Available at: www.businessroundtable.org/pdf/Health_Retirement/BR_Doing_Well_through_Wellness_09192007.pdf. (Accessed September 28, 2008).

3. Committee on Injury, Violence, and Poison Prevention. Poison treatment in the home. *Pediatrics.* 2003;112(5):1182-5.

4. Consumer Healthcare Products Association. Consumer survey on self-medication. 2006. Available at: www.chpa-info.org/ChpaPortal/PressRoom/Statistics/ ConsumerSurveyonSelfMedication.htm.

5. Dunnel, K., and Cartwright, C. Medicine takers, prescribers, and hoarders. Boston: Routledge & Kegan Paul; 1972:121.

6. Dzenis Haralds, J. Effectiveness of health promotion interventions upon high risk lifestyle behaviours of adult clients of health benefits organisations. Queensland University of Technology. 2007. Available at: http://adt.library.qut.edu.au./adt-qut/public/adt-QUT20051014.162500.

7. Joint Commission. Facts about patient-centered communications. 2007. Available at: www.jointcommission.org/PublicPolicy/facts_health_literacy.htm.

8. Internet World Stats. United States of America internet usage and broadband usage report. 2007. Available at: www.internetworldstats.com/am/us.htm.

9. Lewis, S. Large self-care study demonstrates significant positive results. *Employee Health and Fitness.* 1998;20(3):25-8.

10. Machlin, S.R., and Zodet, M.W. Family health care expenses, by income level, 2002. Medical Expenditure Panel Survey statistical brief #64. 2005. Available at: www.meps.ahrq.gov/mepsweb/data_files/publications/st64/stat64.pdf.

11. Mechanic, D., McAlpine, D.D., and Rosenthal, M. Are patient's office visits with physicians getting shorter? *New England Journal of Medicine.* 2001;344(3):198-204.

12. Mercer. National survey of employer-sponsored health plans. 2007. Available at: www.mercer.com/referencecontent.jhtml?indContent=1287790.

13. Oregon Health and Science University. Nurse-advice lines are the right call, study shows. 2005. Available at: www.ohsu.edu/son/news/discovery03_20_23.pdf.

14. Pew Internet & American Life Project. 2006. Available at: www.pewinternet.org.

15. Powell, D.R. How to achieve an ROI on your health care dollars. *Employee Benefits Journal.* 2002;27(1):2-5.

16. Powell, D.R. Implementing a self-care program. *Employee Benefits Journal.* 2003;28(3):40-3.

17. Powell, D.R., and Breedlove-Williams, C. The evaluation of an employee self-care program. *Health Values.* 1995;19:17-22.

18. Powell, D.R., Sharp, S.L., Farnell, S.D., and Smith, P.T. Implementing a self-care program. The effect on employee health care utilization. *American Association of Occupational Health Nurses Journal.* 1997;45(5):247-53.

19. Towers Perrin. 2008 health care cost survey 2007 press release. 2007. Available at: www.towersperrin.com.

20. U.S. Department of Army, Center for Health Promotion and Preventive Medicine, and Directors of Health Promotion and Wellness. *Soldiers self-care summary report.* Washington, DC: Author; 2006.

21. U.S. Department of Health and Human Services and Agency for Healthcare Research and Quality. *Expenses for a hospital emergency room visit, 2003. Statistical brief #111.* Rockville, MD: Agency for Healthcare Research and Quality; 2006.

22. U.S. Department of Health and Human Services, Centers for Disease Control and Prevention, and National Center for Health Statistics. *National ambulatory medical care survey: 2005 summary. Advance data from vital and health statistics; number 387.* Hyattsville, MD: National Center for Health Statistics; 2006.

23. U.S. Department of Health and Human Services, Centers for Disease Control and Prevention, and National Center for Health Statistics. *National hospital ambulatory medical care survey: 2004 emergency department summary. Advance data from vital and health statistics; number 372.* Hyattsville, MD: National Center for Health Statistics; 2006.

24. Wellness Councils of America. Self-care simplified, clearing the air on the benefits of medical self-care, a Wellness Councils of America interview, 2004 with Larry Chapman, MPH, chairman and senior consultant, Summex Corporation. 2004. (See www.welcoa.org for access to this resource).

Chapter 33

1. Agency for Healthcare Research and Quality. Health care costs: Why do they increase? What can we do? Available at: www.ahrq.gov/news/ulp/costs/ulpcosts5.htm. (Accessed September 28, 2008.)

2. American College of Physicians. *The advanced medical home: A patient-centered, physician-guided model of health care.* 2006. Available at: www.hhs.gov/healthit/ahic/materials/meeting03/cc/ACP_Initiative.pdf.

3. Blumenthal, D. Employer-sponsored insurance—riding the health care tiger. *New England Journal of Medicine.* 2006;355:195-202.

4. Committee on Quality of Health Care in America, Institute of Medicine. *Crossing the quality chasm: A new health system for the 21st century.* Washington, DC: National Academies Press; 2001.

5. Enthoven, A.C. The history and principles of managed competition. *Health Affairs.* 1993;12:24-48.

6. Farquhar, J.W., Maccoby, N., Wood, P.D., et al. Community education for cardiovascular health. *Lancet.* 1977;1:1192-5.

7. Greenfield, S., Kaplan, S., and Ware, J.E., Jr. Expanding patient involvement in care. Effects on patient outcomes. *Annals of Internal Medicine.* 1985;102:520-8.

8. Havranek, E.P. Improving the outcomes of heart failure care. *Journal of the American College of Cardiology.* 2005;45:1665-6.

9. Improving Chronic Illness Care (ICIC). The chronic care model. 2008. Available at: www.improvingchroniccare.org/index.php?p=Model_Elements&s=18.

10. Kenny, S.J., Smith, P.J., Goldschmid, M.G., Newman, J.M., and Herman, W.H. Survey of physician practice behaviors related to diabetes mellitus in the U.S.: Physician adherence to consensus recommendations. *Diabetes Care.* 1993;16:1507-10.

11. Law, M. *Evidence based rehabilitation: A guide to practice.* 2nd ed. Thorofare, NJ: Slack, Inc.; 2002:8.

12. Loeppke, R., Taitel, M., Richling, D., Parry, T., Kessler, R.C., Hymel, P., and Konicki, D. Health and productivity as a business strategy. *Occupational and Environmental Medicine.* 2007;49:712-21.

13. Mattke, S., Seid, M., and Ma, S. Evidence for the effect of disease management: Is $1 billion a year a good investment? *American Journal of Managed Care.* 2007;13:670-6.

14. McGlynn, E.A., Asch, S.M., Adams, J., Keesey, J., Hicks, J., DeCristofaro, A., and Kerr, E.A. The quality of health care delivered to adults in the U.S. *New England Journal of Medicine.* 2003;349:1866-8.

15. Midwest Business Group on Health. *Reducing the cost of poor quality health care through responsible purchasing leadership.* 2003. Available at: www.mbgh.org/ for more information

16. National Coalition on Health Care. Health insurance cost. Available at: www.nchc.org/facts/cost.shtml (Accessed September 28, 2008).

17. Perrin, J.M., Homer, C.J., Berwick, D.M., Woolf, A.D., Freeman, J.L., and Wennberg, J.E. Variations in rates of hospitalization of children in three urban communities. *New England Journal of Medicine.* 1989;320:1183-7.

18. Pinnock, H., Bawden, R., Proctor, S., et al. Accessibility, acceptability, and effectiveness in primary care of routine telephone review of asthma: Pragmatic, randomised controlled trial. *British Medical Journal.* 2003;326(7387):477-9.

19. Sackett, D.L., Rosenburg, W.M., Muir Gray, J.A., Haynes, R.B., and Richardson, W.S. Evidence based medicine: What it is and what it isn't. *British Medical Journal.* 1996;312:71-2.

20. Stockwell, D.H., Madhavan, S., Cohen, H., Gibson, G., and Alderman, M.H. The determinants of hypertension awareness, treatment, and control in an insured population. *American Journal of Public Health.* 1994;84:1768-74.

21. The Health Project. Available at: http://healthproject.stanford.edu/koop/index.html. (Accessed September 28, 2008.).

22. Wagner, E.H., Austin, B.T., and Von Korff, M. Organizing care for patients with chronic illness. *Milbank Quarterly.* 1996;74:511-44.

Chapter 34

1. Baun, W.B., and Pronk, N.P. Good program don't just happen—They're planned! *ACSM's Health & Fitness Journal.* 2006;10(3):40-3.

2. Chapman, L. Meta evaluation of worksite health promotion economic return studies: 2005. *The Art of Health Promotion.* 2005;7:1-15.

3. Pelletier, K.R. A review and analysis of the health and cost-effective outcome studies of comprehensive health promotion and disease prevention programs at the worksite: Update IV 2000-2004. *Journal of Occupational and Environmental Medicine.* 2005;47(10):1051-8.

4. U.S. Department of Health and Human Services. *Healthy people 2010. Understanding and improving health* and *Objectives for improving health.* 2 vols. Washington, DC: U.S. Government Printing Office; 2000:76.

Chapter 35

1. Ashford, R.F., Nagelburg, S., and Adkins, R. Sensitivity of the Jamar dynamometer in detecting submaximal grip effort. *Journal of Hand Surgery.* 1996;21:402-5.

2. Australian Sports Commission (ASC). *CD-ROM recording of the 20m shuttle run test.* Belconnen, Australia: Sport Education Department of Physiology and Applied Nutrition, Australian Institute of Sport; 1998.

3. Bannisterm E., Robinson, D., and Trites, D. *Ergonomics of tree planting.* FRDA report 127. Victoria, BC: Government of Canada; 1990:1-18.

4. Biffl, W.L., Moore, E.E., Moore, F.A., and Peterson, V.M. Interleukin-6 in the injured patient: Marker of injury or mediator of inflammation? *Annals of Surgery.* 1996; 224:647-64.

5. Bruunsgaard, H., Galbo, H., Halkjaer-Kristensen, J., Johansen, T.L., MacLean, D.A., and Pedersen, B.K. Exercise-induced increase in serum interleukin-6 in humans is related to muscle damage. *Journal of Physiology.* 1997;499:833-41.

6. Cady, L.D., Thomas, P.C., and Karwasky, R.J. Program for increasing health and physical fitness of firefighters. *Journal of Occupational Medicine.* 1985;27:111-4.

7. Canadian Council of Forest Ministers. National forestry database program. 2007. Available at: http://nfdp.ccfm.org.

8. Craig, B.N., Congleton, J.J., Kerk, C.J., Lawler, J.M., and McSweeney, K.P. Correlation of injury occurrence data with estimated maximal aerobic capacity and body composition in a high-frequency manual materials handling task. *AIHA Journal.* 1998;59:25-33.

9. Hodgsonn, M., Docherty, D., and Robbins, D. Post-activation potentiation: Underlying physiology and implications for motor performance. *Sports Medicine.* 2005;35:585-95.

10. Keller, C., Steensberg, A., Pilegaard, H., Osada, T., Saltin, B., Pedersen, B.K., and Neufer, P. Transcriptional activation of the IL-6 gene in human contracting muscle: Influence of muscle glycogen content. *FASEB Journal.* 2001;15(14):2748-50.

11. Knapik, J., Ang, P., Reynolds, K., and Jones, B. Physical fitness, age, and injury incidence in infantry soldiers. *Journal of Occupational Medicine.* 1993;35:598-603.

12. Musich, S., Napier, D., and Edington, D.W. The association of health risks with worker's compensation costs. *Journal of Occupational and Environmental Medicine.* 2001;43:534-41.

13. Newham, D.J., McPhail, G., Miles, K.R., and Edwards, R.H. Ultrastructural changes after concentric and eccentric contractions of human muscle. *Journal of the Neurological Sciences.* 1983;61:109-22.

14. Roberts, D. In-season physiological and biochemical status of reforestation workers. *Journal of Occupational and Environmental Medicine.* 2002;44:559-67.

15. Roberts, D. Treeplanting—Fit to plant. 2007. Available at: www.selkirk.ca/treeplanting.

16. Rohde, T., MacLean, D.A., Richter, E.A., Kiens, B., and Pedersen, B.K. Prolonged submaximal eccentric exercise is associated with increased levels of plasma IL-6. *American Journal of Physiology—Endocrinology and Metabolism.* 1997;273:E85-91.

17. Saunders, M.J., Kane, M.D., and Todd, M.K. Effects of a carbohydrate-protein beverage on cycling endurance and muscle damage. *Medicine and Science in Sports and Exercise.* 2004;36(7):1233-8.

18. Soule, R.G., and Goldman, R.F. Terrain coefficients for energy cost prediction. *Journal of Applied Physiology.* 1972;35(5):706-8.

19. Smith, D.J., and Roberts, D. Effects of high volume and/or intense exercise on selected blood chemistry parameters. *Clinical Biochemistry.* 1994;27:435-40.

20. Umphred, D.A. *Neurological rehabilitation.* 2nd ed. Toronto, ON: Mosby; 1990:606-11.

21. Wenger, H.A., and Bell, G.J. The interactions of intensity, frequency and duration of exercise training in altering cardiorespiratory fitness. *Sports Medicine.* 1986;3(5):346-56.

22. Yuhasz, M.S. Physical fitness and sports appraisal laboratory manual. London: University of Western Ontario; 1977:145-94.

Chapter 36

1. Boucher, J.L., Schaumann, J.D., Pronk, N.P., Priest, B., Ett, T., and Gray, C.M. The effectiveness of telephone-based counseling for weight management. *Diabetes Spectrum.* 1999;12(2):121-3.

2. Boyle, R.G., Pronk, N.P., and Enstad, C.J. A randomized trial of telephone counseling with adult moist snuff users. *American Journal of Health Behavior.* 2004;28(4):347-51.

3. Bravata, D.M., Smith-Spangler, C., Sundaram, V., et al. Using pedometers to increase physical activity and improve health: A systematic review. *Journal of the American Medical Association.* 2007;298(19):2296-304.

4. Goetzel, R.Z., Anderson, D.R., Whitmer, R.W., Ozminkowski, R.J., Dunn, R.L., and Wasserman, J. The relationship between modifiable health risks and health care expenditures. *Journal of Occupational and Environmental Medicine.* 1998;40(10):843-54.

5. Goetzel, R.Z., Guindon, A.M., Turshen, J., and Ozminkowski, R.J. Health and productivity management: Establishing key performance measures, benchmarks, and best practice. *Journal of Occupational and Environmental Medicine.* 2001;43:10-7.

6. Goetzel, R.Z., Hawkins, K., Ozminkowski, R.J., and Wang, S. The health and productivity cost burden of the "top 10" physical and mental health conditions affecting six large U.S. employers in 1999. *Journal of Occupational and Environmental Medicine.* 2003;45:5-14.

7. Goetzel, R.Z., Long, S., Ozminkowski, R.J., Hawkins, K., Wang, S., and Lynch, W. Health, absence, disability and presenteeism cost estimates of certain physical and mental health conditions affecting U.S. employers. *Journal of Occupational and Environmental Medicine.* 2004;46:398-412.

8. Pronk, N.P., Goodman, M.J., O'Connor, P.J., and Martinson, B.C. Relationship between modifiable health risks and short-term health care charges. *Journal of the American Medical Association.* 1999;282(23):2235-9.

9. Reilly Associates. Work productivity and activity impairment (WPAI) questionnaire. 2007. Available at: http://reillyassociates.net/WPAI_GH.html.

10. Serxner, S.A., Gold, D.B., Grossmeier, J.J., and Anderson, D.R. The relationship between health promotion program participation and medical costs: A dose response. *Journal of Occupational and Environmental Medicine.* 2003;45:1196-200.

11. VanWormer, J., Pronk, N.P., and Boucher, J.L. Experience analysis of a practice-based, online pedometer program. *Diabetes Spectrum.* 2006;19(4);197-200.

Chapter 37

1. Burton, W.N., Conti, D.J., Chen, C.Y., Schultz, A.B., and Edington, D.W. The role of health risk factors and disease on worker productivity. *Journal of Occupational and Environmental Medicine.* 1999;41:863-77.

2. Hemp, P. Presenteeism: At work—but out of it. *Harvard Business Review.* 2004;82:49-58, 155.

3. Joffe, M.M., and Rosenbaum, P.R. Invited commentary: propensity scores. *American Journal of Epidemiology.* 1999;150:327-33.

4. Kessler, R.C., Barber, C., Beck, A., et al. The World Health Organization health and work performance questionnaire (HPQ). *Journal of Occupational and Environmental Medicine.* 2003;45:156-74.

5. Loeppke, R., Taitel, M., Richling, D., et al. Health and productivity as a business strategy. *Journal of Occupational and Environmental Medicine.* 2007;49:712-21.

6. Mills, P.R. The development of a new corporate specific health risk measurement instrument, and its use in investigating the relationship between health and well-being and employee productivity. *Environmental Health.* 2005;4:1.

7. Mills, P.R., Kessler, R.C., Cooper, J., and Sullivan, S. Impact of a health promotion program on employee health risks and work productivity. *American Journal of Health Promotion.* 2007;22:45-53.

8. Pelletier, B., Boles, M., and Lynch, W. Change in health risks and work productivity over time. *Journal of Occupational and Environmental Medicine.* 2004;46:746-54.

Chapter 38

1. Andersen, R.E., Franckowiak, S.C., Snyder, J., Bartlett, S.J., and Fontaine, K.R. Can inexpensive signs encourage the use of stairs? Results of a community intervention. *Annals of Internal Medicine.* 1998;129(5):363-9.

2. Biener, L., Glanz, K., McLerran, D., et al. Impact of the Working Well Trial on the worksite smoking and nutrition environment. *Health Education and Behavior.* 1999;26(4):478-94.

3. Blamey, A., Mutrie, N., and Aitchison, T. Health promotion encouraged by stairs. *British Medical Journal.* 1995;311(7000):289-90.

4. Brownell, K.D., Stunkard, A.J., and Albaum, J.M. Evaluation and modification of exercise patterns in the natural environment. *American Journal of Psychiatry.* 1980;137(12):1540-5.

5. DeJoy, D.M., and Wilson, M.G. Organizational health promotion: Broadening the horizon of workplace health promotion. *American Journal of Health Promotion.* 2003;17(5):337-41.

6. DeJoy, D.M., Wilson, M.G., Goetzel, R.Z., et al. The development of the Environmental Assessment Tool (EAT) to measure organizational physical and social support for worksite obesity prevention programs. *Journal of Occupational and Environmental Medicine.* 2008;50(2):126-37.

7. Della, L., DeJoy, D.M., Goetzel, R.Z., Ozminkowski, R.J., and Wilson, M. Assessing management support for worksite health promotion: Psychometric analysis of the Leading by Example instrument. *American Journal of Health Promotion.* 2008;22(5):359-67.

8. French, S.A., Story, M., and Jeffery, R.W. Environmental influences on eating and physical activity. *Annual Review of Public Health.* 2001;22:309-35.

9. French, S.A., Story, M., Jeffery, R.W., Snyder, P., and Eisenberg, M. Pricing strategy to promote vegetable purchase in high school cafeterias. *Journal of the American Dietetic Association.* 1997;97(9):1008-10.

10. Goetzel, R.Z., Ozminkowski, R.J., Baase, C.M., and Billotti, G.M. Estimating return-on-investment from changes in the employee health risks on the Dow Chemical Company's health care costs. *Journal of Occupational and Environmental Medicine.* 2005;47(8):759-68.

11. Holdsworth, M., and Haslam, C. A review of point-of-choice nutrition labeling schemes in the workplace, public eating places and universities. *Journal of Human Nutrition and Dietetics.*1998;11:423-45.

12. Jeffery, R.W., French, S.A., Raether, C., and Baxter, J.E. An environmental intervention to increase fruit and salad purchases in a cafeteria. *Preventive Medicine.* 1994;23(6):788-92.

13. National Business Group on Health. *Improving health, improving business: The employer's guide to health improvement and preventive services.* Washington, DC: National Business Group on Health; 2004.

14. National Business Group on Health. Institute on the Costs and Health Effects of Obesity. 2008. Available at: www.wbgh.org/about/obesity.cfm.

15. Oldenburg, B., Sallis, J., Harris, D., and Owen, N. Checklist of health promotion environments at worksites (CHEW): Development and measurement characteristics. *American Journal of Health Promotion.* 2002;16(5):288-99.

16. Partnership for Prevention. *Leading by example: Improving the bottom line through a high performance, less costly workforce.* Washington, DC: Partnership for Prevention; 2005.

17. Russell, W.D., Dzewaltowski, D.A., and Ryan, G.J. The effectiveness of a point-of-decision prompt in deterring sedentary behavior. *American Journal of Health Promotion.* 1999;13(5):257-9,ii.

18. Sorensen, G., Morris, D.M., Hunt, M.K., et al. Worksite nutrition intervention and employees' dietary habits: The Treatwell program. *American Journal of Public Health.* 1992;82(6):877-80.

19. Wilson, M.G., Goetzel, R.Z., Ozminkowski, R.J., et al. Using formative research to develop environmental and ecological interventions to address overweight and obesity. *Obesity (Silver Spring).* 2007;15 Suppl. 1:37S-47S.

20. Zifferblatt, S.M., Wilbur, C.S., and Pinsky, J.L. A new direction for public health care: Changing cafeteria eating habits. *Journal of the American Dietetic Association.* 1980;76(1):15-20.

Index

Note: Page references followed by *f* or *t* refer to figures or tables, respectively.

About the Editor

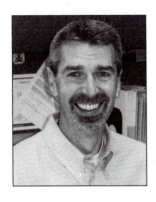

Nicolaas P. Pronk, PhD, is the vice president of health management at HealthPartners in Bloomington, Minnesota, the largest consumer-governed, nonprofit health care organization in the nation. He is also senior research investigator at HealthPartners Research Foundation and health science officer of JourneyWell, a Minneapolis-based nationwide provider of health and wellness programs.

Pronk has 20 years of experience in the health promotion field as a researcher, developer, and administrator of health promotion programs and services. Since 1993 he has directed health improvement initiatives that involve a systems approach to generating health across multiple sectors, including business and industry. He is a member of the distinguished Task Force on Community Preventive Services, an independent panel supported by the Centers for Disease Control and Prevention, which presents evidence-based recommendations to the health field.

A member of the American College of Sports Medicine (ACSM) since 1984, Pronk served as section editor and contributor for the first edition of *ACSM's Worksite Health Promotion Manual.* He currently serves as associate editor for the *ACSM's Health & Fitness Journal.* He served as the chair for the ACSM Interest Group on Worksite Health Promotion until 2008, when it morphed into the International Association for Worksite Health Promotion (IAWHP), an ACSM affiliate society. Pronk is a founding member and inaugural president of the international board of directors for the IAWHP. Previously, he was a board member of the former Association for Worksite Health Promotion (AWHP).

Pronk and his wife, Stephanie, reside in Eagan, Minnesota. He enjoys spending time with his family and dogs, watching English Football Association soccer after a Saturday-morning run, and riding his Harley on country roads in the Minnesota northland.

About the American College of Sports Medicine

ACSM advances and integrates scientific research to provide educational and practical applications of exercise science and sports medicine.

The American College of Sports Medicine, founded in 1954, is a professional membership society with more than 20,000 national, regional, and international members in more than 70 countries dedicated to improving health through science, education, and medicine. ACSM members work in a wide range of medical specialties, allied health professions, and scientific disciplines. Our members are committed to the diagnosis, treatment, and prevention of sport-related injuries and the advancement of the science of exercise.

Our members' diversity and expertise make ACSM the largest, most respected sports medicine and exercise science organization in the world. From astronauts and athletes to people with chronic diseases or physical challenges, ACSM continues to look for and find better methods to allow people to live longer and more productive lives. ACSM is leading the way in exercise science and sports medicine.

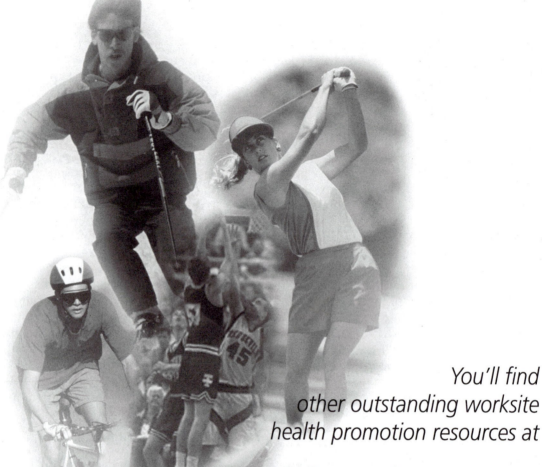

*You'll find
other outstanding worksite
health promotion resources at*

www.HumanKinetics.com

In the U.S. call

1-800-747-4457

Australia..08 8372 0999
Canada 1-800-465-7301
Europe..+44 (0) 113 255 5665
New Zealand......................................0064 9 448 1207

 HUMAN KINETICS
The Information Leader in Physical Activity
P.O. Box 5076 • Champaign, IL 61825-5076 USA